Drug
Actions and
Interactions

Notice

Medicine is an ever-changing science. As new research and clinical experience broaden our knowledge, changes in treatment and drug therapy are required. The author and the publisher of this work have checked with sources believed to be reliable in their efforts to provide information that is complete and generally in accord with the standards accepted at the time of publication. However, in view of the possibility of human error or changes in medical sciences, neither the author nor the publisher nor any other party who has been involved in the preparation or publication of this work warrants that the information contained herein is in every respect accurate or complete, and they disclaim all responsibility for any errors or omissions or for the results obtained from use of the information contained in this work. Readers are encouraged to confirm the information contained herein with other sources. For example and in particular, readers are advised to check the product information sheet included in the package of each drug they plan to administer to be certain that the information contained in this work is accurate and that changes have not been made in the recommended dose or in the contraindications for administration. This recommendation is of particular importance in connection with new or infrequently used drugs.

Drug
Actions and
Interactions

Jae Y. Choe, PhD
Professor of Pharmacology
American University of the Caribbean
School of Medicine
St. Maarten, West Indies

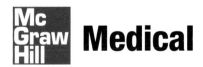

New York   Chicago   San Francisco   Lisbon   London   Madrid   Mexico City
Milan   New Delhi   San Juan   Seoul   Singapore   Sydney   Toronto

The McGraw·Hill Companies

Drug Actions and Interactions

Copyright © 2011 by the McGraw-Hill Companies, Inc. All rights reserved. Printed in China. Except as permitted under the United States Copyright Act of 1976, no part of this publication may be reproduced or distributed in any form or by any means, or stored in a database or retrieval system, without the prior written permission of the publisher.

1 2 3 4 5 6 7 8 9 0   CTP/CTP   14 13 12 11 10

ISBN 978-0-07-163475-5
MHID 0-07-163475-4

This book was set in Minion Pro by Thomson Digital.
The editors were Michael Weitz and Peter J. Boyle.
The production supervisor was Phil Galea.
Project management was provided by Shivi Sharma, Thomson Digital.
Original design by Elise Lansdon was adapted; the cover designer was Malvina D'Alterio; photo © Bodell Communications, Inc./Phototake.
China Translation & Printing Services, Ltd., was printer and binder.

This book is printed on acid-free paper.

Library of Congress Cataloging-in-Publication Data

Choe, Jae Y., 1939-
  Drug actions and interactions / by Jae Y. Choe.
      p. ; cm.
  Includes index.
  ISBN-13: 978-0-07-163475-5 (pbk.)
  ISBN-10: 0-07-163475-4 (pbk.)
1. Drug interactions. 2. Drugs—Physiological effect. 3. Drugs—Side effects. I. Title.
  [DNLM: 1. Pharmacological Phenomena—Handbooks. 2. Drug Interactions—Handbooks.
3. Pharmaceutical Preparations—adverse effects—Handbooks. QV 39]
  RM302.C46 2011
  615'.7045—dc22

                                  2010026613

McGraw-Hill books are available at special quantity discounts to use as premiums and sales promotions, or for use in corporate training programs. To contact a representative please e-mail us at bulksales@mcgraw-hill.com.

To the tempest-tossed souls of my late parents,
who went through war-torn poverty, crushing tribulations,
and frustrations but never abandoned hope, pinned on me,
by buttressing my life with an education they could not afford
for themselves.

Contents

About the Author **xii**

Preface **xiii**

Acknowledgements **xv**

Abbreviations Used in This Book **xvii**

Introduction: Drug Interactions **xxi**

PART **I**

DRUGS ACTING ON THE CARDIOVASCULAR SYSTEM 1

1. Hypertension **1**
2. Edema **13**
3. Congestive Heart Failure **21**
4. Cardiac Arrhythmia **32**
5. Angina Pectoris **45**
6. Thrombosis/Myocardial Infarction **48**
7. Hemorrhage **61**
8. Anemia **65**
9. Varicose Veins **76**
10. Hyperlipidemia **78**

PART **II**

DRUGS ACTING ON THE RESPIRATORY SYSTEM 89

11. Rhinitis /Sinusitis **89**
12. Laryngitis/Bronchitis **95**
13. Hiccups **104**
14. Tussis (Common Cough) **110**
15. Asthma **116**

PART **III**

DRUGS ACTING ON THE GASTROINTESTINAL SYSTEM 123

16. Xerostomia (Dry Mouth) **123**
17. Aphthous Ulcer (Canker Sore) **127**
18. Odontalgia (Toothache) **131**
19. Gingivitis (Gum Infection) **136**
20. Nausea/Vomiting **139**
21. Flatulence **143**
22. Peptic Ulcer **146**
23. Gastroesophageal Reflux Disease **154**
24. Dyspepsia **157**
25. Irritable Bowel Syndrome **159**
26. Intestinal Cramps **166**
27. Constipation **168**
28. Diarrhea **173**
29. Hemorrhoids **176**

PART **IV**

DRUGS ACTING ON THE GENITOURINARY SYSTEM 179

30. Erectile Dysfunction (Impotence) **179**
31. Condylomata (Genital Warts) **185**
32. Benign Prostate Hypertrophy **188**
33. Urinary Incontinence **191**
34. Nephrolithiasis (Kidney Stone) **195**
35. Cystitis /Urethritis **199**
36. Urinary Retention **206**

PART **V**

DRUGS ACTING ON THE BONES, MUSCLES, AND SKIN 209

37. Osteoporosis **209**
38. Osteoarthritis/Osteoarthrosis **217**
39. Gout **221**

40. Myasthenia Gravis **228**

41. Muscle Spasticity **234**

42. Carpal Tunnel Syndrome **239**

43. Rosacea **243**

44. Eczema **246**

45. Psoriasis **251**

PART **VI**

DRUGS ACTING ON THE NEURONAL SYSTEM 257

46. Stress and Anxiety **257**

47. Seasonal Affective Disorder **263**

48. Attention Deficit Hyperactivity Disorder **269**

49. Chronic Fatigue Syndrome **274**

50. Mental Depression **278**

51. Mania **289**

52. Psychosis **298**

53. Alzheimer Disease **301**

54. Memory Impairment **306**

55. Epilepsy **313**

56. Parkinson Disease **324**

57. Vertigo **334**

58. Motion Sickness **338**

59. Multiple Sclerosis **340**

PART **VII**

DRUGS ACTING ON THE ENDOCRINE SYSTEM 349

60. Diabetes Mellitus **349**

61. Diabetes Insipidus **360**

62. Addison Disease **362**

63. Cushing Disease **366**

64. Hyperthyroidism **369**

65. Hypothyroidism **372**

66. Hypogonadism/Infertility **376**

67. Menstrual Dysfunction **380**

68. Menopausal Symptoms **384**

69. Breast Engorgement **388**

70. Hyperemesis Gravidarum **391**

P A R T **VIII**

DRUGS ACTING ON GENERAL HEALTH **395**

71. Algesia (Physical Pain) **395**

72. Pyrexia (Fever) **408**

73. Insomnia **413**

74. Pregnancy **417**

75. Allergic Reactions **425**

76. Obesity **435**

77. Cancer **440**

78. Systemic Infections by Viruses **502**

79. Systemic Infections by Bacteria **525**

80. Systemic Infections by Fungi **537**

81. Malaria **544**

82. Dysentery **555**

83. Helminthiasis **560**

84. Chemical Poisoning **569**

APPENDIXES **589**

Appendix A: Major Drugs in Therapeutic Classifications **589**

Appendix B-1: Interactions of Beta Blockers **596**

Appendix B-2: Interactions of Alpha Blockers **600**

Appendix B-3: Interactions of ACE Inhibitors **602**

Appendix B-4: Interactions of Thiazide Diuretics **604**

Appendix B-5: Interactions of Loop Diuretics **606**

Appendix B-6: Interactions of Angiotensin-Receptor Blockers **609**

Appendix B-7: Interactions of Calcium-Channel Blockers **611**

Appendix B-8: Interactions of Alpha Agonists **614**

Appendix B-9: Interactions of Protease Inhibitors **615**

Appendix B-10: Interactions of Antihistamines, First-Generation **618**

Appendix B-11: Interactions of Antihistamines, Second-Generation **620**

Appendix B-12: Interactions of Atypical Antipsychotic Drugs **621**

Appendix B-13: Interactions of Macrolide Antibiotics **623**

Appendix B-14: Interactions of Antifungal Drugs **625**

Appendix B-15: Interactions of Belladonna Alkaloids **627**

Appendix B-16: Interactions of Benzodiazepines **629**

Appendix B-17: Interactions of Cephalosporins **631**

Appendix B-18: Interactions of Gastric Antacids **633**

Appendix B-19: Interactions of Magnesium Salts **635**

Appendix B-20: Interactions of Glucocorticoids **637**

Appendix B-21: Interactions of H2 Blockers **639**

Appendix B-22: Interactions of NSAIDs **641**

Appendix B-23: Interactions of Dopamine Agonists **646**

Appendix B-24: Interactions of Penicillins **648**

Appendix B-25: Interactions of Phenothiazine Antipsychotic Drugs **649**

Appendix B-26: Interactions of Progesterone or Progestogens **653**

Appendix B-27: Interactions of Proton-Pump Inhibitors **655**

Appendix B-28: Interactions of Quinolone Antibiotics **657**

Appendix B-29: Interactions of SSRIs (Selective Serotonin Reuptake Inhibitors) **660**

Appendix B-30: Interactions of Tetracyclines **664**

Appendix B-31: Interactions of Tricyclic Antidepressants **667**

Appendix B-32: Interactions of Opioid Analgesics **670**

Index **675**

About the Author

Jae Y. Choe received his PhD degree in pharmacology from the University of North Carolina at Chapel Hill. He did his postdoctoral work at the Northwestern University School of Medicine in Chicago, Illinois, then apprenticed for three years under Dr. Karl Folkers, an Ashbel Smith Professor and a Nobel Prize nominee, at the University of Texas at Austin.

Currently, he serves as a professor of pharmacology at the Department of Pharmacology, the AUC School of Medicine, St. Maarten, West Indies.

He published two editions of *Choe Notes: A Handbook of Pharmacology; Choe's Medical Pharmacology,* 3rd edition; and *Choe's Choices of Pharmacology: Quick Cuts to the USMLE Step #1.*

Preface

The *Chicago Tribune* of December 24, 2008 reported, quoting researchers at the University of Chicago Medical Center, that more than half of adults 65 and older in the United States were taking five or more medications, and 68 percent of those who took prescription drugs also used over-the-counter medications or dietary supplements such as vitamins and herbal remedies. In fact, physicians and other healthcare professionals frequently encounter patients asking for an alternative remedy, either prescription or nonprescription, alone or in combination.

Taking two or more incompatible drugs together may either nullify therapeutic value or stir up side effects of life-threatening consequence. Therefore, to reach the promised land of therapeutics the boons and banes of prescription drugs and alternative remedies should be carefully weighed and their possible interactions must be promptly addressed. However, in reality, no knotty problem in pharmacology can rival that of drug-drug interactions, for not only are they vast in number (thousands upon thousands) but the mechanisms of each drug interaction often defy clarification. As if that is not enough, responses to the same drug at the same dose often differ from person to person owing to differences in genetic makeup. For these reasons, many drug interactions still remain shrouded in obscurity. Although many new drug interactions are being reported continuously, the overwhelming majority of healthcare professionals are too time-constrained to digest all the information, which is where this book comes to the rescue.

Drug Actions and Interactions aims for the following objectives: (1) to review what major drugs are available for what kinds of diseases; (2) to understand how the selected drugs produce therapeutic benefits; (3) to predict side effects (or adverse effects) that might crop up while taking those drugs; and (4) to warn which drugs should be avoided in combination to steer clear of serious consequences.

At first mention and in interaction pairings, the generic name is typeset in boldface, followed in parenthesis by capitalized representative brand names. On the other hand, if one brand name medication is comprised of two or more generic drugs in mixture, the capitalized brand name is shown first and then listed in parenthesis appear the generic drugs boldfaced and joined with the "+" sign. For interactions between a prescription drug and an herbal remedy, the herbs are listed in parentheses, unlike the brand name drugs.

Molecular structures are presented to help explain mechanism of action and metabolic fate of drugs; or to inspire scientists to undertake research on those parameters in the future.

Given that it is virtually impossible to discuss interactions of each and every of several thousand drugs currently available (amounting to millions of drug interaction pairs), it was imperative to be selective. Priority was given to the top 300 most prescribed drugs in the United States. These are divided among 84 common disorders, and each drug is presented with its mechanism of action, side effects, and drug interactions, in that order.

The listings of side effects are not meant to imply that all the listed side effects would affect every patient nor that additional side effects could not crop up. In fact, a rare allergic reaction, though not listed, may precipitate an alarming situation without warning. Therefore, readers are advised to be alert to such possibilities; and, if such an emergency occurred, to notify their doctors, pharmacists, or other health-care professionals as soon as possible.

As to the descriptions of interactions in this book, a three-letter code name was assigned to each principal drug or to each principal group of drugs, and those drug interactions whose incidences recur with great clinical significance and whose mechanisms of interaction are relatively well known are put into a box labeled "Basic Concepts of Interactions," and others standing alone or whose mechanisms of interaction are poorly understood yet are of clinical significance are pooled under the heading "Miscellaneous Interactions."

In the event that one or more cytochrome (CYP) isozymes are involved in a drug's pharmacokinetic interactions, the relationship of the precipitant drug with cytochrome isozymes is provided in a separate table attached.

Appendix A at the back of the book shows major drugs currently in use in each therapeutic classification, and each of the Appendixes B-1 though B-32 are reserved for interactions between a therapeutic group of drugs and an individual drug or a group of drugs.

Given the constant influx of new drug research, the information in this book, albeit carefully collated and monitored for accuracy at the time of publication, may turn at odds with new discoveries in the future, especially in the field of CYP research. Readers therefore are asked to exercise their discretion in interpretation of the contents, and I will be indebted to those who find and bring up any such discrepancies to be rectified in the future.

Acknowledgments

I am indebted to the following educators for my graduate studies in the United States. Dr. Philip F. Hirsch and the late Dr. Paul L. Munson for their gracious invitations to scholarship at the great institution of the University of North Carolina School of Medicine at Chapel Hill. Dr. Munson, who published the book entitled *Principles of Pharmacology: Basic Concepts & Clinical Applications,* was also instrumental in my landing a postdoctoral position at the reputable institution of the Northwestern University School of Medicine in Chicago.

My gratitude is extended to the late Dr. Karl Folkers, a nominee for the Nobel Prize in Medicine, for his scientific inspirations, guidance, and personal warmth during my apprenticeship with him at the University of Texas at Austin.

I am also grateful to Byong Kak Kim, PhD, professor emeritus at the Seoul National University, for his encouragement and advice for my studies abroad; and to Mr. Joon-Seok Suh, the president of the Won-Jin Pharmaceutics Company in Seoul, South Korea, and Edward Chang, MSOM, OTRL, LAc, in Los Angeles, California, for kindly providing me with several color photos of herbal remedies; and to Yong-Zun Kwon, PhD, my former college chum, for his consistent friendship during our difficult times of studies and beyond.

The following individuals reviewed my manuscript and offered their insight and constructive suggestions: Asrar B. Malik, PhD, Distinguished Professor and the Department Head of Pharmacology, and the Director of the Center for Lung and Vascular Biology at the University of Illinois College of Medicine at Chicago; and William Thurman, MD, a former Vice President of Medical Affairs at the University of Oklahoma and the current Provost at the University of Medicine and Health Sciences, Saint Kitts, West Indies.

My book would not have come to light without supportive editorial staff at McGraw-Hill, especially Michael Weitz as my senior acquisitions editor, and Peter Boyle as my developmental editor, both of whom have been extremely helpful throughout, providing me with constructive ideas and guidance. I regret I cannot thank enough the other workers at McGraw-Hill who have toiled anonymously behind the scenes.

Finally, my thanks go to my two young daughters Carol Choe, MD, and Christina Choe, MD, at the University of Michigan at Ann Arbor and the University of Pennsylvania in Philadelphia, respectively, for reviewing and revising my manuscript; and also to my wife Midaeja K. Choe, MSN, for bringing me coffee and criticism, and for sorting pages after pages, without whose help my manuscript could not have been brought to fruition in time; and to Paul S. Tien, PhD, the founder and chancellor of the American University of the Caribbean School of Medicine at St. Maarten, West Indies, for his incessant support of my teaching career by hiring and keeping me at his proud institution for 30 consecutive years.

Abbreviations Used in This Book

ACE	angiotensin converting enzyme
ACTH	adrenocorticotropic hormone
ADH	antidiuretic hormone
ADHD	attention deficit hyperactivity disorder
ADP	adenosine diphosphate
AIDS	acquired immune deficiency syndrome
ALT	alanine aminotransferase
AQP2	aquaporin-2
AR	angiotensin receptor
AST	aspartate aminotransferase
AT_1	angiotensin 1
ATP	adenosine triphosphate
AUC	area under the plasma concentration-versus-time curve
A-V NODE	atrioventricular node
BDNF	brain-derived neurotrophic factor
BPH	benign prostatic hyperplasia
BZD	benzodiazepine
cAMP	cyclic-adenosine monophosphate
cGMP	cyclic-guanosine monophosphate
CGRP	calcitonin gene-related peptide
CNS	central nervous system
CoA	coenzyme A
COMT	catechol-o-methyltransferase
CoQ10	coenzyme Q-10
COX	cyclooxygenase
CTZ	chemoreceptor trigger zone
CYP	cytochrome P
DDC	dideoxycytidine

DDP	cis-diamminedichloroplatinum
DNA	deoxyribonucleic acid
5-dUMP	5-deoxyuridine monophosphate
EC	emergency contraception
ECF	extracellular fluid
E. coli	*Escherichia coli*
ED	erectile dysfunction
EDRF	endothelium-derived relaxing factor
EKG	electrocardiogram
FDA	food and drug administration
5-F-dUMP	5-fluoro-deoxyuridine monophosphate
FSH	follicle-stimulating hormone.
GABA	gamma-aminobutyric acid
G-CSF	granulocyte colony-stimulating factor
GERD	gastroesophageal reflux disease
GFR	glomerular filtration rate
GI	gastrointestinal
GLP-1	glucagon-like peptide-1
GM-CSF	granulocyte-macrophage colony-stimulating factor
GnRH	gonadotropin-releasing hormone
GP	glycoprotein
Hb	hemoglobin
HCG	human chorionic gonadotropin
HDL	high-density lipoproteins
HER2	human epidermal growth factor receptor 2
HIV	human immunodeficiency virus
HMG-CoA	reductase 3-hydroxy-3-methylglutaryl CoA reductase
hOAT	human organic anion transporter
5-HPETE	5-hydroperoxyeicosatetraenoic acid
H. pylori	*Helicobacter pylori*
HPV	human papilloma virus
HSV	*Herpes simplex* virus
5-HT	5-hydroxytryptamine
IBS	irritable bowel syndrome
IgE	immunoglobulin-E
IL	interleukin
IFN	interferon
IM	intramuscular
Inh	inhibitors
INR	international normalized ratio
IM	intramuscular
IOP	intraocular pressure
IV	intravenous

IVF	in vitro fertilization
LDL	low-density lipoproteins
L-DOPA	levo-3,4-dihydroxyphenylalanine (levodopa)
LH	luteinizing hormone
LMWH	low-molecular-weight heparin
LTD4	leukotriene D4
MAOIs	monoamine oxidase inhibitors
MDR	multidrug-resistance
mEH	microsomal epoxide hydrolase
mEq	milliequivalent
mg/ml	milligram per milliliter
mmol/L	millimole per liter
m-RNA	messenger-ribonucleic acid
M-1	muscarinic-1
M-3	muscarinic-3
MRSA	methicillin-resistant *Staphylococcus aureus*
MS	multiple sclerosis
mTOR	mammalian target of rapamycin
NAPQI	N-acetyl-p-benzoquinoneimine
NMDA	*N*-methyl-*D*-aspartic acid
N. meningitidis	*Neisseria meningitidis*
NNRT	nonnucleoside reverse transcriptase
NSAIDs	nonsteroidal antiinflammatory drugs
OHSS	ovarian hyperstimulation syndrome
PABA	para-aminobenzoic acid
PBP	penicillin-binding protein
P. falciparum	*Plasmodium falciparum*
PGE	prostaglandin-E
P gp	glycoprotein transporter protein
P. malariae	*Plasmodium malariae*
PNP	purine nucleoside phosphorylase
P. ovale	*Plasmodium ovale*
PPAR	peroxisome proliferator-activated receptors
PSVT	paroxysmal supraventricular tachycardia
PUD	peptic ulcer disease
P. vivax	*Plasmodium vivax*
RBC	red blood cells
REM	rapid eye movement sleep
RNA	ribonucleic acid
RT	reverse transcriptase
RTK	receptor tyrosine kinase
S-A	sinoatrial
SAD	seasonal affective disorder

SC	subcutaneous
SERM	selective estrogen receptor modulators
SIADH	syndrome of inappropriate antidiuretic hormone
SJS	Stevens-Johnson syndrome
SRSA	slow-reacting substance of anaphylaxis
SPRM	selective progesterone- receptor modulator
SSRIs	selective serotonin reuptake inhibitors
STD	sexually transmitted disease
Sub	substrate
T3	triiodothyronine
T4	tetraiodothyronine
TCA	tricarboxylic acid
TEN	toxic epidermal necrolysis
TH-1	helper-T cell-1
TPA	tissue plasminogen activator
TNF	tumor necrosis factor
TPMT	thiopurine methyltransferase
t-RNA	transfer-ribonucleic acid
TSH	thyroid stimulating hormone.
UDP	uridine diphosphate
UTIs	urinary tract infections
V_2-receptors	vasopressin-2 receptors;
VLDL	very low-density lipoprotein
WBC	white blood cells
WHO	World Health Organization

Introduction: Drug Interactions

Sir William Osler, the renowned nineteenth century physician, declared in 1894 that, "Man has an inborn craving for medicine." Indeed, humans, unlike other creatures, possess a unique fascination with medications: What drugs can treat what kinds of disease? What are the advantages and disadvantages of taking a particular medication? and What are the possible consequences of taking one drug in combination with other drugs? In keeping with these concerns, this book presents drugs or therapeutic classes of drugs with their mechanisms of action, side effects (or adverse effects), and interactions with other drugs.

It is quite common for most patients to take more than one drug in combination. The higher the number, the greater the chance of drug interactions. These introductory pages are provided to present general principles of drug interactions. The importance of drug interactions cannot be overemphasized because, while some may have a salutary effect, others are destined to have a detrimental effect on physical well-being.

Virtually all in vivo drug interactions fall into two major categories: (1) pharmacokinetic interactions, and (2) pharmacodynamic interactions. In the former, a causative drug (precipitant drug) alters the absorption, distribution, metabolism, or excretion of another drug (object drug); whereas in the latter, a causative drug alters the dose-response relationship of the object drug by influencing the biochemical or physiologic effects of the object drug, to result in an antagonistic, synergistic, or simple additive effect with the affected drug.

PHARMACOKINETIC INTERACTIONS

Drug Absorption: One drug may oppose gastrointestinal absorption of another drug, lowering its blood concentration and therapeutic effect. Mechanisms include:
1. Changes in gastric pH. For example, absorption of ketoconazole, an antifungal drug, is impaired in patients having gastric pH of 5.0 or higher.

2. Abnormal GI motility. For example, anticholinergic drugs such as scopolamine slow gastric emptying of other drugs such as procainamide.

3. Adsorption of drug. For instance, activated charcoal adsorbs tolbutamide, phenobarbital, and phenytoin; while such bile acid sequestrants as cholestyramine adsorb digoxin and warfarin, interfering with intestinal absorption.

DRUG DISTRIBUTION

1. Some drugs are bound extensively to plasma proteins, but with low affinity (e.g., coumarin anticoagulants such as dicumarol and warfarin; and sulfonylurea hypoglycemic agents such as tolbutamide). While bound they are therapeutically inactive and not subject to metabolism nor to glomerular filtration, but they are susceptible to displacement by other drugs with higher affinity for binding such as aspirin, gemfibrozil, and phenylbutazone. Once displaced, the freed drugs are apt to generate not only therapeutic effects but also undesirable side effects.

2. The P-glycoproteins (Pgps) in the small intestine, kidneys, and the brain efflux many drugs to lead to their low bioavailability. Inducers of the (Pgps) (or transporters), such as thyroxine, rifampin, and the herb St. John's Wort, can help the transporter to efflux substrate drugs, including many anticancer drugs, antiarrhythmic agents, antifungal drugs, anti-HIV protease inhibitors, antimalarial agents, some calcium-channel blockers, and many steroid hormones.

Drug Metabolism: Pharmacokinetic interactions have much to do with drug metabolism. Water-soluble drugs cannot easily be absorbed through the gastrointestinal (GI) tract to enter the circulation, which is why such drugs are administered by injection. But once in the circulatory system such drugs are readily eliminated through the kidneys. On the other hand, lipid-soluble drugs are favored for GI absorption, and elimination is suppressed because the drugs cannot readily be filtered through the glomeruli. Even those secreted through the renal tubules into the tubular fluid are destined to be reabsorbed by back diffusion because the drug concentration in the tubular fluid is usually higher than that in the blood. Hence, the lipid-soluble drugs are readily accumulated potentially to create havoc with the host system. But by drug metabolism, lipid-soluble drugs can be converted to water-soluble metabolites that are readily removed from the body.

The liver is the most important organ for this metabolism, or biotransformation. The first phase of this metabolic process includes oxidation, reduction, and hydrolysis, introducing to the parent-drug molecules a polar functional group, such as $-NH_2$, or -OH, to make them somewhat water-soluble. If these resultant metabolites are sufficiently water soluble, no more biotransformation is required. But many drugs undergo an additional, second-phase biotransformation that involves conjugation of the polar groups generated by the first phase with an endogenous molecule such as glucuronic acid, glycine, a sulfate group, or a methyl

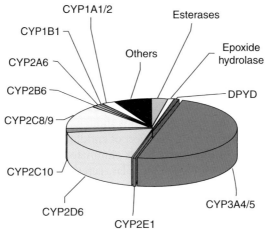

FIGURE 0-1 **CYP distributions.** Reproduced, with permission, from Brunton LL, Lazo JS, and Parker KL. *Goodman & Gilman's The Pharmacological Basis of Therapeutics.* 11th ed. New York, NY: McGraw-Hill; 2006, p 78.

or acetyl group, to generate highly ionized and water-soluble metabolites that in general are not readily bound to plasma proteins and are easily excreted in the urine.

Cytochrome P450 enzymes are responsible for metabolism of many commonly used medications. They consist of a group of isoenzymes, or isozymes, located at the microsome, that interacts with molecular oxygen (O_2) to generate monooxygen (O), which can be inserted into drug molecules to make oxidized metabolites. There are many isoenzymes, but nearly half of all drugs clinically in use are processed through the CYP3A4 (Fig. 0-1). Different drugs may be oxidized by different isozymes, and some drugs can inhibit particular isozymes, while others may induce them. The table below lists major human CYP isozymes and shows what kind of drugs serve as substrates, inhibitors, or inducers of those isozymes. Strong inhibitors are marked in red; moderate inhibitors in peach; and strong substrates in blue.

Renal Excretion of Drugs: Some drugs can interfere with renal excretions of other drugs. For example:

1. The Pgp (P-glycoprotein) transporter, which is expressed in the proximal renal tubule, utilizes energy derived from hydrolysis of ATP to efflux various natural and synthetic drugs across the luminal membranes into the tubular lumen to get rid of them. One such Pgp substrate is digoxin. Therefore, taking digoxin in conjunction with other drugs that inhibit this transporter can result in digoxin secretions being blocked with consequent rise of its blood concentration and toxicity. Such Pgp inhibitors include quinidine (an antimalarial drug) and such calcium-channel blockers as nifedipine and verapamil.

2. The urinary excretion of lithium is diminished by thiazide diuretics such as hydrochlorothiazide or by loop diuretics such as furosemide, because they mobilize sodium in the urine, and the sodium and lithium compete each with other for renal clearance.

3. Some nonsteroidal antiinflammatory drugs (NSAIDs) such as indomethacin and phenylbutazone, reduce the renal excretions of both sodium and lithium. This is probably because the NSAIDs inhibit the synthesis of prostaglandin E (PGE) which in the distal nephron is thought to inhibit sodium and water reabsorption by antagonizing the effect of antidiuretic hormone (ADH).

4. Probenecid, a uricosuric agent that is eliminated through tubular secretion, can interfere by competition with tubular secretions of weak acidic drugs such as cephalosporins, penicillins, and thiazide diuretics.

5. A carbonic anhydrase inhibitor such as acetazolamide or methazolamide makes the urine alkaline to promote nonionization of such basic drugs as procainamide and quinidine. The more nonionized the form, the greater the diffusion back to circulation, raising their serum concentrations and toxicities.

6. Low doses of aspirin (less than 2 grams a day) may oppose the uricosuric effect of probenecid or sulfinpyrazone, probably by competing with uric acid for secretions through the renal proximal tubules.

PHARMACODYNAMIC INTERACTIONS

Pharmacodynamic interaction is due either to competition at the same receptor site or to different pharmacologic activities of concurrently administered drugs, with no change in plasma concentrations of the interacting drugs. For instance:

1. Epinephrine, by activation of beta-receptors of the heart, increases heart rate, contractility, and cardiac output whereas propranolol, a beta-blocker, can oppose or reverse those effects.

2. Alcohol can enhance the sedative effect of benzodiazepines (antianxiety drugs), probably by altering the milieu or responsiveness of the brain tissues.

3. Thyroxine and other thyroid hormones accelerate inactivation of blood clotting factors and thereby enhance the anticoagulant effects of Coumarin derivatives such as dicumarol and warfarin.

4. Salicylates such as aspirin and salsalate inhibit synthesis of thromboxane, opposing platelet aggregation and generating a hypoprothrombinemic effect; hence, they can enhance the hemorrhagic tendency of other drugs taken in combination. Such affected drugs include anticoagulants such as dicumarol and warfarin, antiplatelet agents such as clopidogrel, ticlopidine, and dipyridamole, and thrombolytic agents such as streptokinase, urokinase, and tissue plasminogen activator (TPA).

5. Indomethacin and phenylbutazone each cause sodium retention as explained above and thus can oppose the blood pressure lowering effect of many antihypertensive agents.

DANGER OF DRUG INTERACTIONS

In many cases, drug interactions do not create life-threatening consequences, especially when dealing with drugs that have a great margin of safety. This is why incidences of life-threatening drug interactions are not high, but special caution should be exercised with any drugs that can affect the cardiovascular or the respiratory systems. The following are a few examples where life-threatening drug interactions could occur.

1. Ventricular arrhythmia may be produced by a digitalis glycoside if it is administered in combination with a potassium depleting diuretic agent such as chlorothiazide or furosemide, since the toxicity of the digitalis can be increased by hypokalemia.

2. Hypertensive emergency can arise when a drug that inhibits monoamine oxidase (MAO) such as procarbazine or tranylcypromine is taken together with a food containing tyramine. As the oxidative destruction of food tyramine by the MAO is blocked, the tyramine causes an excessive release of norepinephrine, raising the blood pressure to an alarming degree.

3. Internal bleeding may occur when an anticoagulant such as dicumarol or warfarin is administered with a drug that has a higher affinity for binding to proteins such as phenylbutazone or a salicylate because the latter drugs can displace the former from their protein binding sites as stated above.

4. Respiratory muscles can be paralyzed when two drugs, both of which have a neuromuscular blocking effect, are used in combination (e.g., when succinylcholine is used with an aminoglycoside antibiotic such as neomycin or tobramycin).

5. Excessive hypoglycemia can result when an oral hypoglycemic agent such as chlorpropamide or tolbutamide is used in combination with a drug that has a higher affinity for binding to proteins, or with a drug that also can induce hypoglycemia.

The data in Table 0 were compiled from the "Drug Development and Drug Interactions: Table of Substrates, Inhibitors, and Inducers" (http://www.fda.gov/cder/drug/drugInteractions/tableSubstrates.htm, accessed September 2006), published by the U.S. Food and Drug Administration, and have been updated by incorporating new discoveries or new interpretations of previous discoveries. This table shows whether an individual drug is an inhibitor, a substrate, or an inducer of certain cytochrome isozymes. Strong inhibitors are shown in red; moderate inhibitors, in gold; and strong substrates, in blue.

TABLE 0 Major Drugs in Relationship with Cytochrome (CYP) P-450 Isozymes

CYP	Enzyme Inhibitors	Enzyme Substrates	Enzyme Inducers
1A1	Isoniazid, Nitrous oxide, Propofol, Retinol *(CYP1A1 is not normally expressed in human liver and is unlikely to play a role)*	Dacarbazine, Docetaxel, Ellipticine, Erlotinib, Tamoxifen	
1A2	Acyclovir, Alosetron, Amiodarone, Amitriptyline, Amlodipine, Anastrozole, Aprindine, Atazanavir, Bepridil, Bortezomib, Bromocriptine Buprenorphine, Caffeine, Cimetidine, Ciprofloxacin, Citalopram, Clarithromycin, Clotrimazole, Clozapine, Delavirdine Dexmedetomidine, Diclofenac, Diltiazem, Disulfiram, Drospirenone, Duloxetine, *Echinacea*, Enoxacin, Entacapone, Erythromycin, Estradiol, Estrogens conjugated, Famotidine, Flecainide, Fluconazole, Fluoroquinolones, Fluoxetine, Fluphenazine, Flutamide, Fluvastatin, Fluvoxamine, Furafylline, Gemfibrozil, Ginseng, Grapefruit, Grepafloxacin, Imipramine, Interferon, Isoniazid, Josamycin, Ketoconazole, Levofloxacin, Lidocaine, Lomefloxacin, Losartan, Mestranol, Methimazole, Methoxsalen, Mexiletine, Mibefradil, Miconazole, Mirtazapine, Moclobemide, Nalidixic acid, Nefazodone, Nelfinavir, Nevirapine,	Acenocoumarol, Acetaminophen, Alosetron, Aminophylline, Amitriptyline, Betaxolol, Caffeine, Chlorpromazine, Cinacalcet, Clomipramine, Clozapine, Cyclobenzaprine, Dacarbazine, Docetaxel, Doxepin, Duloxetine, Ellipticine, Erlotinib, Erythromycin, Estradiol, Estrogens, conjugated (synthetic & equine), Estrone, Estropipate, Etoposide, Fluphenazine, Flutamide, Fluvoxamine, Frovatriptan, Guanabenz, Haloperidol, Imatinib, Imipramine, Lidocaine, Melatonin, Metoclopramide, Mexiletine, Mirtazapine, Naproxen, Nicardipine, Olanzapine, Ondansetron, Perphenazine, Phenacetin, Pimozide, Propafenone, Propranolol, Ramelteon, Rasagiline, Retinal, Retinol, Riluzole, Ropinirole, Ropivacaine, Tacrine, Terbinafine, Theophylline, Thioridazine, Thiothixene, Tizanidine, Toremifene, Trifluoperazine, Verapamil, R-Warfarin, Zileuton, Ziprasidone, Zolmitriptan, Zotepine	Amino-glutethimide, *Broccoli* Beta-naphthoflavone Brussels sprout, Carbamazepine, Charbroiled foods, Esomeprazole, Griseofulvin, Insulin, Lansoprazole, Methyl-cholanthrene, Marijuana, Modafinil, Moricizine, Nafcillin, Nicotine, Omeprazole, Phenobarbital, Phenytoin, Primidone, Rifampin, Ritonavir Tobacco smoking

CYP	Enzyme Inhibitors	Enzyme Substrates	Enzyme Inducers
	Nifedipine, Nisoldipine, Norfloxacin, Ofloxacin, Olanzapine, Omeprazole, Ondansetron, Orphenadrine, Paroxetine, Peginterferon, Pentoxifylline, Perfloxacin, Perphenazine, Phenacetin, Primaquine, Propafenone, Propofol, Propranolol, Ritonavir, Quercetin, Ranitidine, Rofecoxib, Ropinirole, Selegiline, Sertraline, Sildenafil, Sulconazole, Tacrine, Tenofovir, Theophylline, Thiabendazole, Thioridazine, Ticlopidine, Tioconazole, Tipranavir, Tocainide, Tranylcypromine, Verapamil, Zafirlukast, Zileuton		
1B1		Docetaxel, Ellipticine, Mitoxantrone, Tamoxifen.	
2A6	Letrozole, Methoxsalen, Pilocarpine, Ritonavir, Tranylcypromine	Coumarin, Cyclophosphamide, Docetaxel, Ifosfamide, Letrozole, Nicotine.	Dexamethasone, phenobarbital, rifampin
2B6	Clopidogrel, Efavirenz, Fluoxetine, Fluvoxamine, Itraconazole, Memantine, Nelfinavir, Norfluoxetine, Orphenadrine, Paroxetine Phencyclidine, Ritonavir, Sertraline, Thiotepa, Ticlopidine.	Altretamine, Artemisinin, Benzphetamine, Bupropion, Cyclophosphamide, Docetaxel, Diazepam, Efavirenz, Ifosfamide, Ketamine, Meperidine, Mephenytoin, Mephobarbital, Propofol, Methadone, Nevirapine, Nicotine, Procarbazine, Selegiline, Sertraline, Tamoxifen, Testosterone Thiotepa	Artemisinin, Cyclophosph-amide, Lopinavir/ritona-vir, Nevirapine, Phenobarbital, Phenytoin, Primidone, Rifampin,

CYP	Enzyme Inhibitors	Enzyme Substrates	Enzyme Inducers
2C8	Anastrozole, Bezafibrate, Cimetidine, Etoposide, Gemfibrozil, Irbesartan, Montelukast, Nicardipine, Omeprazole, Quercetin, Retinol, Rosiglitazone, Tamoxifen, Trimethoprim, Verapamil	Amiodarone, Amodiaquine, Carbamazepine, Cerivastatin, Chloroquine, Cyclophosphamide, Diazepam, Docetaxel, Ifosfamide, Nicardipine, Paclitaxel, Phenytoin, Pioglitazone, Repaglinide, Retinoic acid, Retinol, Rosiglitazone, Taxol, Tolbutamine, Torsemide, Tretinoin, Verapamil, Warfarin, Zopiclone	Cyclophosphamide, Dexamethasone, Phenobarbital, Primidone, Rifampin
2C9	Amiodarone, Anastrozole, Capecitabine, Chloramphenicol, Cimetidine, Clopidogrel, Co-trimoxazole (Sulfamethoxazole-trimethoprim), Delavirdine, Diclofenac, Disulfiram, Doxifluridine, Efavirenz, Fenofibrate, Flecainide, Fluconazole, Fluorouracil, Fluoxetine, Flurbiprofen, Fluvastatin, Fluvoxamine, Gemfibrozil, Irbesartan, Imatinib, Isoniazid, Itraconazole, Ketoconazole, Ketoprofen, Leflunomide, Lovastatin, Metronidazole, Miconazole, Modafinil, Nicardipine, Omeprazole, Orphenadrine, Oxandrolone, Paroxetine, Phenylbutazone, Probenecid, Ritonavir, Sertraline, Sorafenib, Sulfamethoxazole, Sulfaphenazole, Sulfinpyrazone, Sulfonamides, Tamoxifen, Teniposide, Ticlopidine, Tipranavir, Tranylcypromine, Trimethoprim, Troglitazone, Valproic Acid, Voriconazole, Zafirlukast	Aceclofenac, Alosetron, Amitriptyline, Bexarotene, Bosentan, Candesartan, Celecoxib, Cerivastatin, Chloramphenicol, Chlorpromazine, Chlorpropamide, Cyclophosphamide, Dextromethorphan, Diazepam, Diclofenac, Docetaxel, Doxorubicin, Dronabinol, Ellipticine, Estradiol, Etodolac, Etravirine, Fluoxetine, Flurbiprofen, Fluvastatin, Fosphenytoin, Glibenclamide, Glimepiride, Glipizide, Glyburide, Ibuprofen, Idarubicin, Ifosfamide, Imatinib, Indomethacin, Irbesartan, Ketoprofen, Lornoxicam, Losartan, Mefenamic acid, Meloxicam, Mephenytoin, Mestranol, Methadone, Metronidazole, Montelukast, Naproxen, Nateglinide, Nicardipine, Omeprazole, Ondansetron, Phenobarbital, Phenytoin, Piroxicam, Progesterone, Ramelteon, Rosiglitazone, Rosuvasartan, Sertraline, Sulfamethoxazole, Suprofen, Tamoxifen, Tenoxicam, Terbinafine, Tetrahydrocannabinol,	Amino-glutethimide, Aprepitant (long term), Bosentan, Carbamazepine, Cyclophosphamide, Ethanol, Griseofulvin, Phenobarbital, Primidone, Rifabutin, Rifampin, Secobarbital, St. John's Wort

CYP	Enzyme Inhibitors	Enzyme Substrates	Enzyme Inducers
		Tolbutamide, Torsemide, Tretinoin, Valsartan, Valdecoxib, Valproic acid, Verapamil, S-Warfarin, Zafirlukast	
2C18	Cimetidine	Mephenytoin, Propranolol, Warfarin.	
2C19	Amitriptyline, Artemisinin, Chloramphenicol, Cimetidine, Citalopram, Clopidogrel, Delavirdine, Disulfiram, Efavirenz, Esomeprazole, Felbamate, Fluconazole, Fluoxetine, Fluvoxamine, Imipramine, Indomethacin, Isoniazid, Ketoconazole, Lansoprazole, Letrozole, Loratadine, Modafinil, Nicardipine, Norfluoxetine, Omeprazole, Oxcarbazepine, Pantoprazole, Paroxetine, Probenecid, Rabeprazole, Retinol, Ritonavir, Sorafenib, Teniposide, Ticlopidine, Tipranavir, Tolbutamide, Topiramate, Tranylcypromine, Troglitazone, Valproic acid, Voriconazole	Ambrisentan, Amitriptyline, Aripiprazole, Carisoprodol, Chloramphenicol, Chloroguanide , Chlorpropamide, Cilostazol, Citalopram, Clomipramine, Clopidogrel, Clozapine, Cyclophosphamide, Desipramine, Dextromethorphan, Diazepam, Diphenhydramine, Diphenylhydantoin, Doxepin, Escitalopram, Esomeprazole, Esoprazole, Flunitrazepam, Fluoxetine, Hexobarbital, Ifosfamide, Imatinib, Imipramine, Indomethacin, Lansoprazole, Malarone, Mephenytoin, Mephobarbital, Meprobamate, Methadone, Moclobemide, Nelfinavir, Nilutamide, Olanzapine, Omeprazole, Pantoprazole, Pentamidine, Phenobarbital, Phenobarbitone , Phenytoin, Prazepam, Primidone, Progesterone, Proguanil, Propranolol, Rabeprazole, Sertraline, Tamoxifen, Teniposide, Thalidomide, Tolbutamide, Topiramate, Trimipramine, Valproic acid, Venlafaxine, Voriconazole, R-Warfarin	Amino-glutethimide, Artemisinin, Carbamazepine, Gingko biloba, Norethindrone, Pentobarbital, Phenobarbital, Phenytoin, Prednisone, Primidone, Rifampin, Ritonavir, Rifapentine, St. John's Wort Topiramate, Valproic acid.

CYP	Enzyme Inhibitors	Enzyme Substrates	Enzyme Inducers
2D6	Amiodarone, Amitriptyline, Aprindine, Brompheniramine, Bupropion, Celecoxib, Chloroquine, Chlorpheniramine, Chlorpromazine, Cimetidine, Cinacalcet, Citalopram, Clemastine, Clomipramine, Clozapine, Cocaine, Cyclosporine, Delavirdine, Desipramine, Dextropropoxyphene, Diphenhydramine, Doxepin, Doxorubicin, Duloxetine, Escitalopram, Imatinib, Felbamate, Flecainide, Fluoxetine Fluphenazine, Fluvoxamine, Goldenseal, Halofantrine, Haloperidol, Hydroxychloroquine, Hydroxyzine, Imatinib, Imipramine, Labetalol, Lansoprazole, Levomepromazine, Lomustine, Mepyramine, Methadone, Metoclopramide, Mibefradil, Meclobemide, Miconazole, Midodrine, Nefazodone , Nicardipine, Norfloxacin, Norfluoxetine, Orphenadrine, Paroxetine, Pergolide, Perphenazine, Pimozide, Probenecid, Propafenone, Propoxyphene. Quercetin, Quinidine, Quinine, Ranitidine, Risperidone, Ritonavir, Ropinirole, Sertindole, Sertraline, Terbinafine, Thioridazine, Thiothixene, Ticlopidine, Tipranavir, Tripelennamine, Triprolidine, Valproic acid, Venlafaxine, Vinblastine, Vinorelbine	Alprazolam, Alprenolol, Amitriptyline, Amphetamine, Aprindine, Aripiprazole, Atomoxetine, Azelastine, Benztropine, Betaxolol, Bisoprolol, Bufuralol, Captopril, Carteolol, Carvedilol, Cevimeline, Chlorpheniramine, Chlorpromazine, Citalopram, Clomipramine, Clozapine, Codeine, Cyclobenzaprine, Darifenacin, Debrisoquine, Desipramine, Dexfenfluramine, Dextromethorphan, Dihydrocodeine , Diphenhydramine, Docetaxel, Dolasetron, Donepezil, Doxepin, Doxorubicin, Duloxetine, Efavirenz, Encainide, Escitalopram, Fenfluramine, Fentanyl, Flecainide, Fluoxetine, Fluphenazine, Fluvoxamine, Galantamine, Haloperidol, Hydrocodone, Hydroxyzine, Idarubicin, Imatinib, Imipramine. Labetalol, Lidocaine, Loratadine, Maprotiline, Meclobemide, Meperidine, Mequitazine, Methadone, MDMA (ecstasy), Methamphetamine, Methoxyamphetamine, Methylphenidate, Metoclopramide, Metoprolol, Mexiletine, Mianserin, Minaprine, Mirtazapine, Modafinil, Morphine, Nebivolol, Nefazodone, Nelfinavir, Nicardipine, Nortriptyline, Olanzapine, Ondansetron, Orphenadrine, Oxycodone, Palonosetron, Paroxetine,	

CYP	Enzyme Inhibitors	Enzyme Substrates	Enzyme Inducers
		Perhexiline, Perphenazine, Phenacetin, Phenformin, Pindolol, Procainamide, Prochlorperazine, Promethazine, Propafenone, Propranolol, Protriptyline, Quetiapine, Risperidone, Ritonavir, Sertindole, Sertraline, Sparteine Tamoxifen, Thioridazine, Timolol, Tiotropium, Tolterodine, Tramadol, Tranylcypromine, Trazodone, Tropisetron, Venlafaxine, Zuclopenthixol.	
2E1	Cimetidine, Diethyldithiocarbamate, Disulfiram, Dithiocarbamate, Econazole, Garlic, Miconazole, Ritonavir, Tranylcypromine	Acetaminophen, Alcohols, Caffeine, Chlorzoxazone, Cisplatin, Dacarbazine, Dapsone, Dextromethorphan, Docetaxel, Enflurane, Ethanol, Etoposide, Felbamate, Halothane, Isoflurane, Methoxyflurane, Ondansetron, Propranolol, Rifampin, Sevoflurane, Theophylline, Tolbutamide, Tretinoin, Venlafaxine, Vesnarinone	Carbamazepine, Ethanol, Isoniazid, Nicotine
3A3-7	Amiodarone, Amprenavir, Anastrozole, Aprepitant, Atazanavir, Azithromycin, Bromocriptine, Cannabinoids, Chloramphenicol, Cimetidine, Ciprofloxacin, Clarithromycin, Clomipramine, Clotrimazole, Conivaptan, Cyclosporine, Danazol, Darunavir, Dasatinib, Delavirdine, Dexamethasone Diethyldithiocarbamate, Diltiazem, Disulfiram, Doxycycline, Echinacea,	Albendazole, Alclometasone, Alfentanil, Alfuzosin, Almotriptan, Alprazolam, Amcinonide, Amiodarone, Amitriptyline, Amlodipine, Amprenavir, Aprepitant, Aripiprazole, Artemisinin, Astemizole, Atazanavir, Atorvastatin, Azelastine, Barnidipine, Beclomethasone, Bepridil, Betamethasone, Bexarotene, Bezafibrate, Bortezomib, Bosentan, Bromocriptine, Budesonide, Buprenorphine, Bupropion, Buspirone, Busulfan, Cafergot,	Amino-glutethimide, Aprepitant (long-term), Barbiturates, Bexarotene, Bosentan, Carbamazepine, Efavirenz, Felbamate, Fosphenytoin, Glucocorticoids, Griseofulvin, Growth Hormone, Modafinil, Nafcillin, Oxcarbazepine, Phenobarbital, Phenylbutazone,

CYP	Enzyme Inhibitors	Enzyme Substrates	Enzyme Inducers
	Enoxacin, Ergotamine, Erythromycin, Ethinylestradiol, Fluconazole, Fluoxetine, Fluvoxamine, Fosamprenavir, Gestodene, Goldenseal, Grapefruit juice, Haloperidol, Imatinib, Indinavir, Isoniazid, Isotretinoin, Itraconazole, Josamycin, Ketoconazole, Lapatinib, Metronidazole, Mibefradil, Miconazole, Mifepristone, Milk Thistle, Nefazodone, Nelfinavir, Norfloxacin, Norfluoxetine, Omeprazole, Oxiconazole, Paroxetine, Pimozide, Posaconazole, Progesterone, Propofol, Propoxyphene, Quercetin, Quinidine, Quinupristin, Ranitidine, Ritonavir, Sage, Saquinavir, Sertindole, Sertraline, Tacrolimus, Tamoxifen, Telithromycin, Troleandomycin, Valspodar, Venlafaxine, Verapamil, Vinblastine, Vincristine, Voriconazole, Zafirlukast, Zileuton	Caffeine, Cannabinoids, Carbamazepine, Cerivastatin, Cevimeline, Chloroquine, Chlorpheniramine, Chlorpromazine, Cilostazol, Cinacalcet, Cisapride, Cisplatin, Citalopram, Clarithromycin, Clindamycin, Clobetasol, Clocortolone, Clomipramine, Clonazepam, Clopidogrel, Clozapine, Cocaine, Codeine, Colchicine, Conivaptan, Cortisol, Cortisone, Cyclobenzaprine, Cyclophosphamide, Cyclosporine, Cytarabine, Dapsone, Darifenacin, Darunavir, Dasatinib, Delavirdine, Desipramine, Desloratadine, Desogestrel, Desonide, Dexamethasone, Dextromethorphan, DHEA, Diazepam, Diclofenac, Diergotamine, Diflorasone, Dihydroergotamine, Diltiazem, Disopyramide, Disulfiram, Docetaxel, Dofetilide, Domperidone, Donepezil, Doxazosin, Doxepin, Doxorubicin, Doxycycline, Droperidol, Dutasteride, Ebastine, Efavirenz, Eletriptan, Ellipticine, Enalapril, Eplerenone, Ergonovine, Ergotamine, Erlotinib, Erythromycin, Escitalopram, Esomeprazole, Estazolam, Estradiol, Estramustine, Estrogens, Estropipate, Eszopiclone, Ethinylestradiol, Ethosuximide, Etoposide, Etravirine, Everolimus, Exemestane, Felbamate, Felodipine, Fentanyl, Fexofenadine, Finasteride, Flecainide, Fludrocortisone, Flunisolide, Fluocinolone, Fluocinonide,	Phenytoin, Pioglitazone, Prednisone, Primidone, Rifabutin, Rifampin, Rifapentine, John's Wort, Sulfinpyrazone, Taxol, Topiramate,

CYP	Enzyme Inhibitors	Enzyme Substrates	Enzyme Inducers
		Fluorometholone, Fluoxetine, Flurandrenolide, Flurazepam, Flutamide, Fluticasone, Fluvastatin, Fosamprenavir, Fulvestrant, Galantamine, Gefitinib, Gemfibrozil, Gleevec, Glyburide, Granisetron, Halcinonide, Halobetasol, Halofantrine, Haloperidol, Hydrocodone, Hydrocortisone, Ifosfamide, Imatinib, Imipramine, Indinavir, Irinotecan, Isradipine, Itraconazole, Ketamine, Ketoconazole, Lansoprazole, Lapatinib, Lercanidipine, Letrozole, Levomethadyl, Lidocaine, Lignocaine, Loperamide, Lopinavir, Loratadine, Losartan, Loteprednol, Lovastatin, Medroxyprogesterone, Medrysone, Mefloquine, Meperidine, Methadone, Methylprednisolone, Midazolam, Mifepristone, Mirtazapine, Mitoxantrone, Modafinil, Mometasone, Montelukast, Nateglinide, Nefazodone, Nelfinavir, Nevirapine, Nicardipine, Nifedipine, Nimodipine, Nisoldipine, Nitrendipine, Norethindrone, Nortriptyline, Omeprazole, Ondansetron, Orphenadrine, Oxybutynin, Oxycodone, Paclitaxel, Paricalcitol, Paroxetine, Phencyclidine, Pimecrolimus, Pimozide, Pioglitazone, Prazepam, Praziquantel, Prednicarbate, Prednisolone, Prednisone, Progesterone, Propafenone, Propoxyphene, Propranolol, Protriptyline, Quazepam, Quetiapine, Quinacrine,	

CYP	Enzyme Inhibitors	Enzyme Substrates	Enzyme Inducers
		Quinidine, Quinine, Ramelteon, Ranolazine, Repaglinide, Retinal, Retinol, Rifabutin, Rifampin, Rimexolone, Risperidone, Ritonavir, Ropivacaine, Salmeterol, Saquinavir, Sertindole, Sertraline, Sibutramine, Sildenafil, Simvastatin, Sirolimus, Solifenacin, Sorafenib tosylate, Sufentanil, Sunitinib, Tacrolimus, Tadalafil, Tamoxifen, Tamsulosin, Taxol, Telithromycin, Temazepam, Teniposide, Terfenadine, Terbinafine, Testosterone, Theophylline, Thiotepa, Tiagabine, Tinidazole, Tiotropium, Tipranavir, Tirilazad, Tolterodine, Topiramate, Topotecan, Toremifene, Tramadol, Trazodone, Tretinoin, Triamcinolone, Triazolam, Trimipramine, Trofosfamide, Valdecoxib, Valproic acid, Vardenafil, Venlafaxine, Verapamil, Vesnarinone, Vinblastine, Vincristine, Vindesine, Vinorelbine, Voriconazole, R-Warfarin, Zaleplon, Zileuton, Ziprasidone, Zolpidem, Zonisamide, Zopiclone, Zotepine.	

CHAPTER

1

Hypertension

The American Heart Association defines hypertension (high blood pressure) as systolic pressure consistently at or greater than 140 mmHg, or diastolic pressure at or greater than 90 mmHg. If left untreated, hypertension can lead to kidney failure, heart attack, arteriosclerosis, and stroke. Medications shown effective in the treatment of hypertension include: (1) such beta blockers as **acebutolol, atenolol, bisoprolol, carvedilol, labetalol** (Normodyne, Trandate), **metoprolol** (Toprol-XL), **nadolol, pindolol, propranolol** (Inderal), and **timolol;** (2) such alpha-1 blockers as **doxazosin,** and **terazosin;** (3) such alpha-2 activators as **clonidine, guanfacine,** and **methyldopa;** (4) such angiotensin-converting enzyme (ACE) inhibitors as **benazepril, captopril, enalapril, fosinopril, lisinopril, moexipril, quinapril** (Accupril), and **ramipril;** (5) such angiotensin-receptor blockers as **candesartan** (Atacand), Avalide (**irbesartan + hydrochlorothiazide**), **eprosartan** (Teveten), **irbesartan** (Avapro), **losartan** (Cozaar, Hyzaar), **olmesartan** (Benicar), **telmisartan** (Micardis), and **valsartan** (Diovan); (6) such calcium-channel blockers as **amlodipine** (Caduet, Lotrel, Norvasc), **diltiazem** (Cartia XT), **isradipine** (Dynacirc), **nifedipine, nitrendipine** (Bayotensin), and **verapamil;** and (7) such diuretics as **bumetanide** (Bumex), **chlorthalidone, ethacrynic acid** (Edecrin), and **furosemide** (Lasix).

BETA BLOCKERS

Acebutolol, atenolol, bisoprolol, carvedilol, labetalol, metoprolol, nadolol, pindolol, propranolol, and **timolol**

Atenolol is often used in combination with chlorthalidone, a diuretic; and bisoprolol is often used in combination with hydrochlorothiazide, another diuretic.

MECHANISM OF ACTION

The beta blockers block the adrenergic beta-receptors at the myocardium to weaken cardiac contractility with consequent reduction of cardiac output and blood pressure. Chlorthalidone (Fig. 1-1) is a diuretic that promotes urine output to shrink blood volume to further lowering of the pressure by atenolol. Hydrochlorothiazide (HCTZ) (Fig. 1-2) is another diuretic that is often used in combination with bisoprolol to further lowering of blood pressure. Carvedilol (Fig. 1-3) and labetalol (Fig. 1-4) are unusual in that they have not only a beta-blocking effect but also an alpha-blocking effect that relaxes blood vessels to ease lowering of the pressure by their beta-blocking effect.

SIDE EFFECTS

Some patients may experience one or more of the following adverse effects. If the symptoms get worse or a side effect not listed here emerges, a warning to take emergency action is warranted. The frequent side effects of these drugs may include low

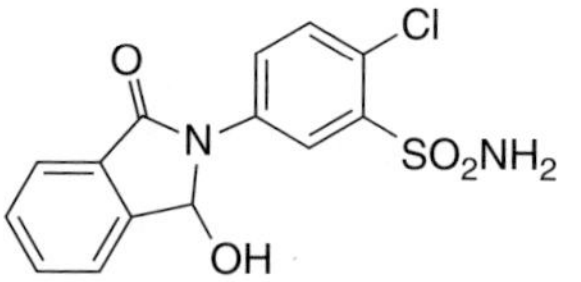

FIGURE 1-1 Molecular structure of chlorthalidone.

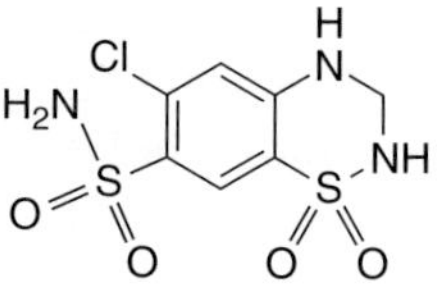

FIGURE 1-2 Molecular structure of hydrochlorothiazide.

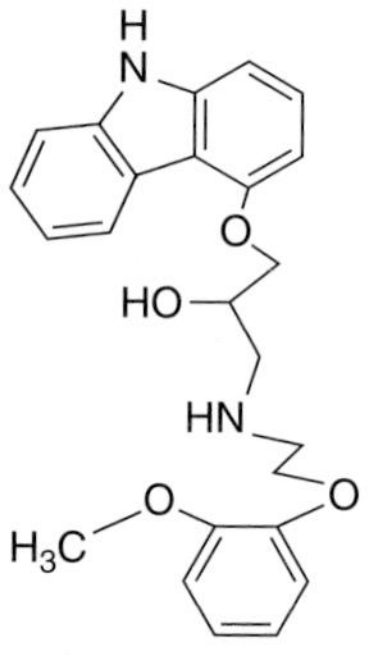

FIGURE 1-3 Molecular structure of carvedilol.

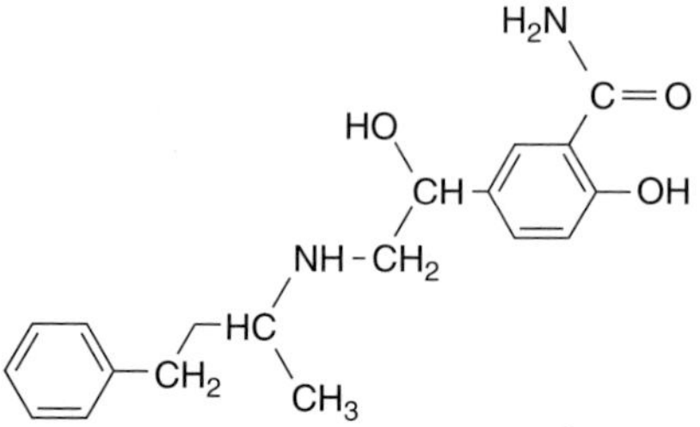

FIGURE 1-4 Molecular structure of labetalol.

blood pressure; shortness of breath or wheezing; abdominal cramps, nausea, diarrhea, and constipation; fatigue; memory loss; lightheadedness; and insomnia. They also tend to raise blood triglyceride levels and reduce so-called "good-cholesterol" (HDL) levels, and tend to lower blood glucose levels, but atenolol and metoprolol are less likely to cause this problem of hypoglycemia.

DRUG INTERACTIONS

See Appendix B-1: Interactions of Beta Blockers.

ALPHA-1 BLOCKERS

Doxazosin (Fig. 1-5) and **terazosin** (Fig. 1-6)

MECHANISM OF ACTION

They block the adrenergic neuronal alpha-1 receptors located at the blood vessels. Since blood vessels are constricted by activation of the alpha-1 receptors, the blockade allows the blood vessels to dilate toward lowering the pressure.

SIDE EFFECTS

Some patients may experience one or more of the following adverse effects. If the symptoms get worse or a side effect not listed here emerges, a warning to take emergency action is warranted. The possible side effects of these drugs include

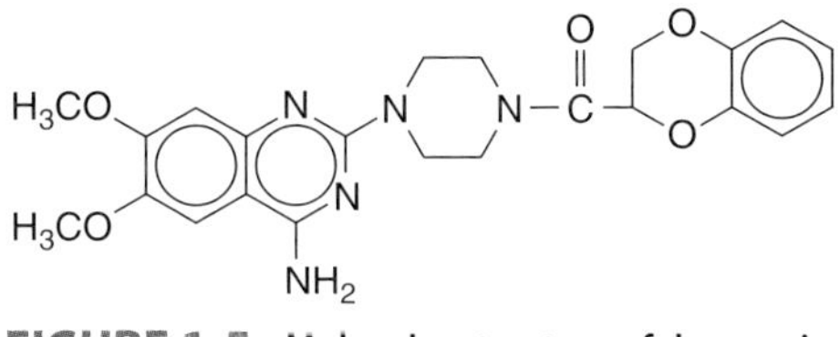

FIGURE 1-5 Molecular structure of doxazosin.

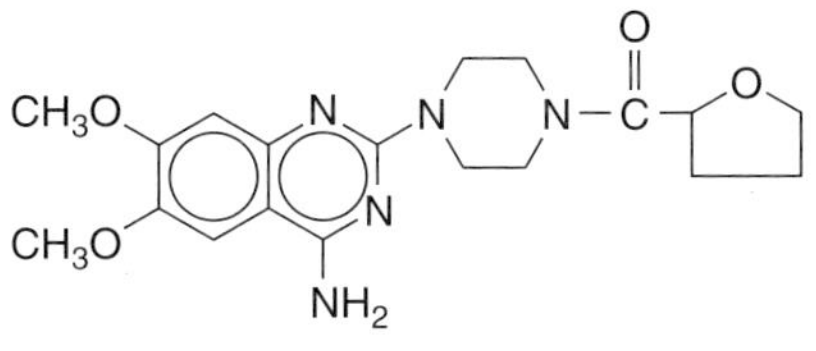

FIGURE 1-6 Molecular structure of terazosin.

excessive fall of blood pressure; runny nose or stuffy nose; priapism (painful sustained penile erection lasting four or more hours); decreased sex drive; and severe dizziness, drowsiness, fainting, fatigue, and insomnia.

DRUG INTERACTIONS

See Appendix B-2: Interactions of Alpha Blockers

ALPHA-2 ACTIVATORS

Clonidine (Fig. 1-7), **guanfacine** (Fig. 1-8), and **methyldopa** (Fig. 1-9)

MECHANISM OF ACTION

They activate the neuronal alpha-2 receptors located at the presynaptic adrenergic nerves to stop the release of norepinephrine. As no vasoconstrictive neurotransmitter is released to act, the high pressure cannot be sustained.

SIDE EFFECTS

Some patients may experience one or more of the following adverse effects. If the symptoms get worse or a side effect not listed here emerges, a warning to take emergency action is warranted. The frequent side effects of these drugs include bradycardia (fewer than 60 beats per minute); dry mouth, nausea, and vomiting; and dizziness, drowsiness, and tiredness.

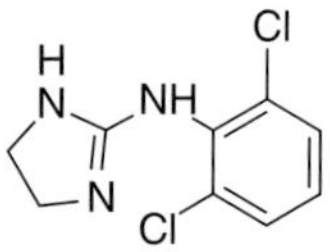

FIGURE 1-7   Molecular structure of clonidine.

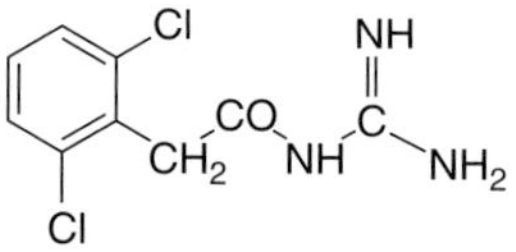

FIGURE 1-8   Molecular structure of guanfacine.

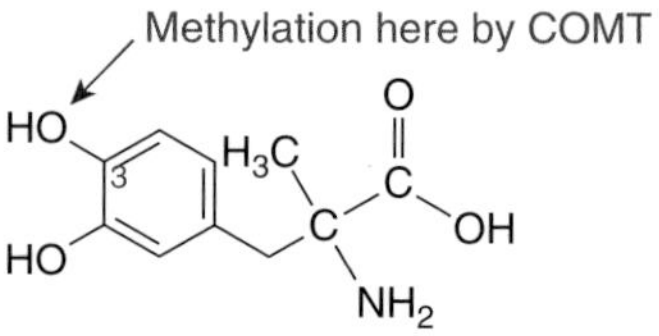

FIGURE 1-9   Molecular structure of methyldopa.

BOX 1-1

Basic Concepts of Alpha-2 Activators Interactions

1. Alpha-2 activators have CNS side effects of sedation and drowsiness. If both interacting parties have a sedative effect they may cause extreme drowsiness or dizziness, as a result of pharmacodynamic interaction. Examples include: **alcohol** and **antihistamines** (*See* Ω-19 in Appendix A).

2. If both interacting parties have a tendency to lower blood pressure, they may create additive or supra-additive effect to result in a severe fall of blood pressure. Examples include: **beta blockers; nitroprusside sodium** (used for the immediate control of very high blood pressure); **verapamil; chlorpromazine; olanzapine** (a medication useful for schizophrenia and manic episodes associated with bipolar disorder); and **prazosin**.

3. Interleukin (IL-2) or aldesleukin taken in combination can potentiate the therapeutic effects of above-mentioned antihypertensive medications. To stem excessive fall of pressure, all antihypertensive agents should be stopped at least 24 hours before treatment with IL-2.

DRUG INTERACTIONS

See Box 1-1.

Miscellaneous Interactions of Alpha-2 Activators (ATA)

ATA ⟷ Beta Blockers (non-cardioselective beta blockers, such as nadolol and propranolol): When the vasodilating beta-receptors at arterial vessels are blocked, peripheral vasoconstriction will prevail to amplify the rebound hypertension caused by waning doses of the above alpha-2 activators.

ATA ⟷ Insulin: Hypoglycemia induced by insulin triggers sympathetic activation to elevate blood levels of both epinephrine and norepinephrine to cause such hypoglycemic symptoms as tachycardia and diaphoresis, whereas the above alpha-2 activators suppress the blood levels of epinephrine and norepinephrine to mask the hypoglycemic signs and symptoms.

ATA ⟷ Prazosin: Prazosin is an alpha-1 blocker, but at high doses it can block the alpha-2 receptors as well to undercut therapeutic effectiveness of the above alpha-2 activators in lowering blood pressure.

ATA ⟷ Tricyclic Antidepressants: (*See* Ω-76 in Appendix A.) Tricyclic antidepressants tend to inhibit central alpha-2 receptors to undermine therapeutic effectiveness of the above alpha-2 activators in lowering blood pressure.

ATA ⟷ Verapamil: All the above alpha-2 activators tend to depress the atrioventricular (AV) nodal conduction at the heart, as does verapamil, to culminate in the atrioventricular (A-V) nodal blockade.

Clonidine (CLD); Guanfacine (GFC); Methyldopa (MTD)

CLD ⟷ Cyclosporine: This combination is apt to increase blood levels and adverse effects of cyclosporine. The mechanisms behind this observation remain unknown.

GFC ⟷ Bupropion: This combination is apt to cause grand mal seizures. The mechanisms behind this observation remain unclear.

MTD ⟷ Entacapone: Methyldopa (*See* Figure 1-9) is degraded to 3-O-methylated product by the enzyme COMT (catechol-O-methyltransferase), whereas entacapone inhibits this very enzyme to raise blood levels and adverse effects of methyldopa such as excessive cardiac arrhythmias and fall of blood pressure.

MTD ⟷ Lithium: Methyldopa used in combination is thought to reduce the rate of renal excretions of lithium to raise its blood levels and toxicity.

ACE INHIBITORS

Benazepril, captopril, enalapril, fosinopril, lisinopril, moexipril, quinapril, and **ramipril**

Except for captopril and lisinopril, each of which is active by itself, all others above are a prodrug (Fig.1-10), which have to be deesterified (cleavage of their ester linkage) by esterases in the liver to form an active metabolite. Each of the active metabolites carries the suffix (-at). For instance, enalaprilat is the active form of enalapril; and ramiprilat is the active form of ramipril.

MECHANISM OF ACTION

Unlike angiotensin-1, a peptide having ten amino acids (NH_2-Asp-Arg-Val-Tyr-Ile-His-Pro-Phe-His-Leu-COOH), angiotensin-2, a peptide having eight amino acids (NH_2-Asp-Arg-Val-Tyr-Ile-His-Pro-Phe-COOH), is a very powerful vasoconstrictive substance to raise blood pressure, and it also causes release of aldosterone from the adrenal cortex to retain sodium and water to further raise pressure. The

BENAZEPRIL

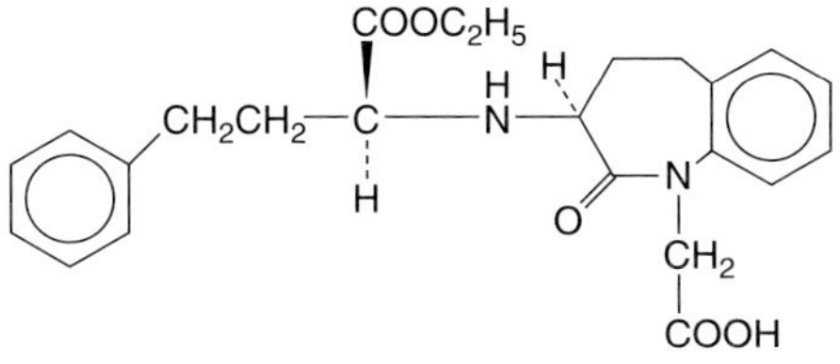

COOC$_2$H$_5$

CH$_2$CH$_2$—C—N
H

H

N

O

N

CH$_2$

COOH

H

CAPTOPRIL

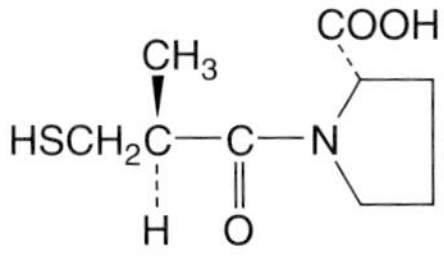

CH$_3$

COOH

HSCH$_2$C—C—N

H

O

ENALAPRIL

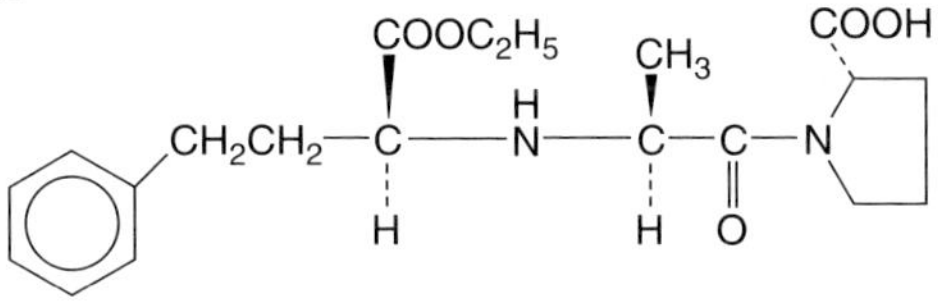

COOC$_2$H$_5$ CH$_3$ COOH

CH$_2$CH$_2$—C—N—C—C—N
H H O

H

ENALAPRILAT

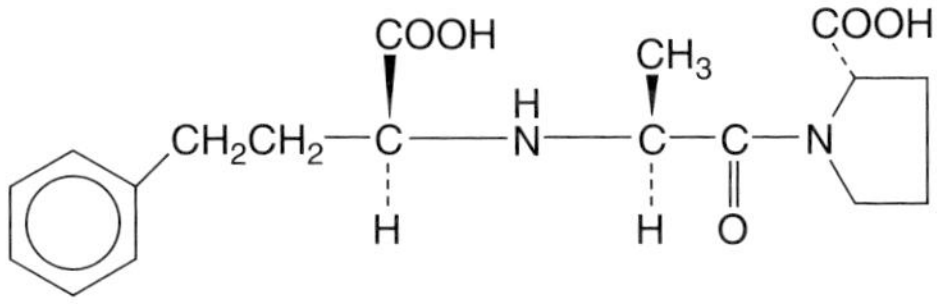

COOH CH$_3$ COOH

CH$_2$CH$_2$—C—N—C—C—N
H H O

H

FOSINOPRIL

O COOH

CH$_2$CH$_2$CH$_2$CH$_2$—P—CH$_2$—C—N

O O

CH$_3$CH$_2$COOCHCH(CH$_3$)$_2$

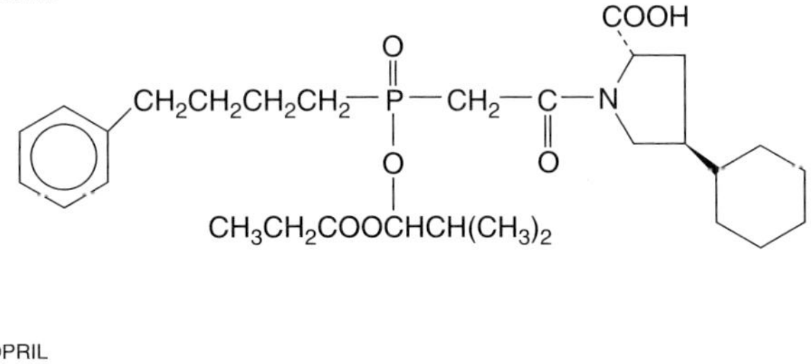

LISINOPRIL

NH$_2$

COOH (CH$_2$)$_4$ COOH

CH$_2$CH$_2$C—N—C—C—N
H H O

H

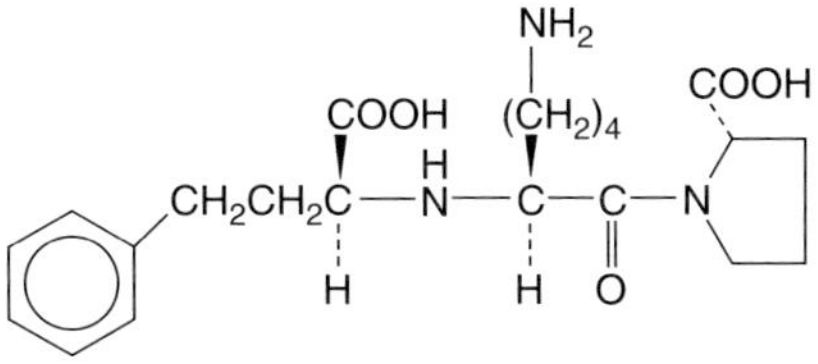

MOEXIPRIL

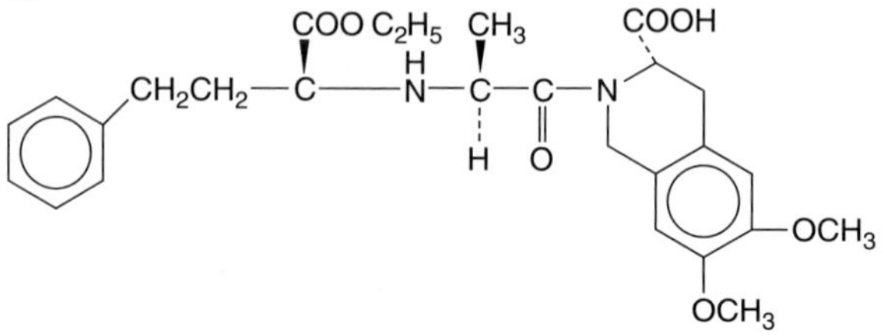

PERINDOPRIL

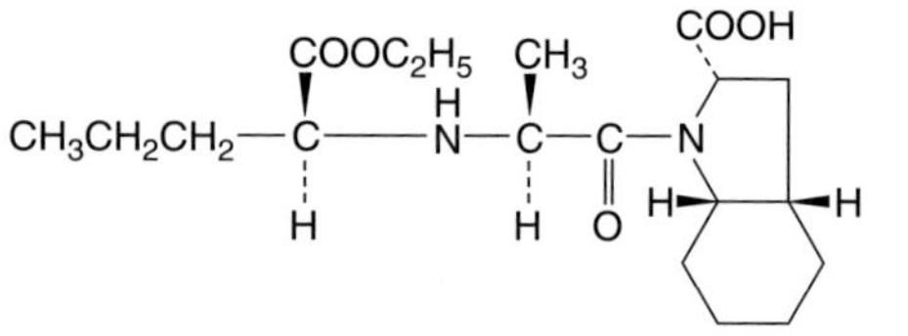

QUINAPRIL

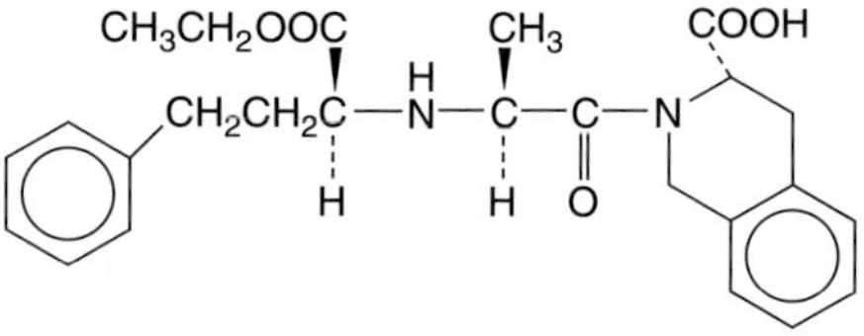

RAMIPRIL

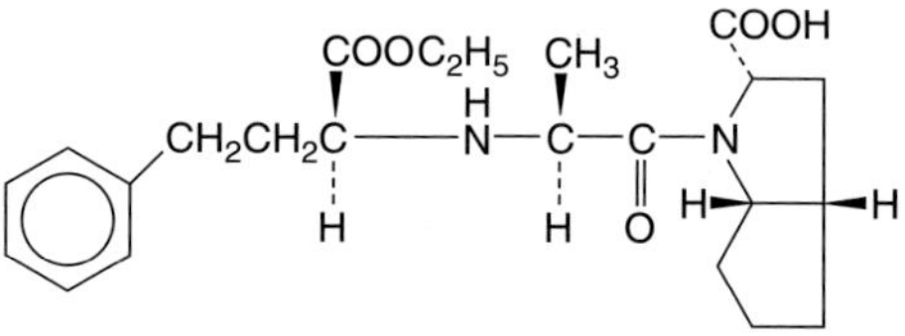

TRANDOLAPRIL

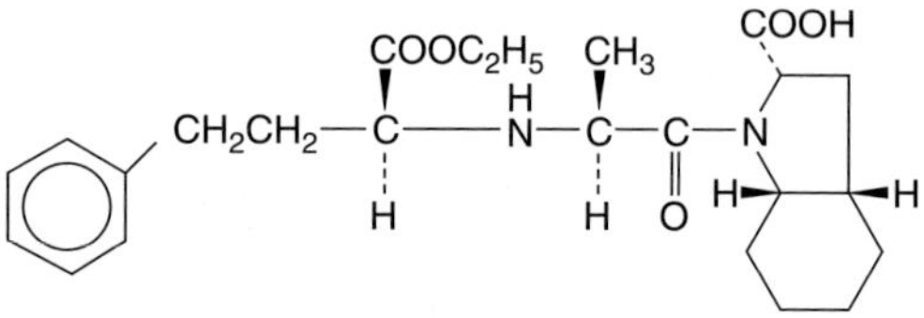

FIGURE 1-10   Molecular structures of ACE inhibitors.

angiotensin-converting enzyme (ACE) inhibitors inhibit the activity of ACE, the enzyme that is involved in the production of angiotensin-2 from angiotensin-1 by removal of two amino acids (His-Leu) at the -COOH terminal. They thereby oppose generation of angiotensin-2 to help lower blood pressure. Lisinopril is often used in combination with such a diuretic as hydrochlorothiazide (HCTZ) that promotes urine output to reduce blood volume, thereby enhancing the antihypertensive effect of the former.

SIDE EFFECTS

Possible side effects of these drugs include irregular heartbeat; nausea and vomiting; rarely, renal insufficiency such as ischemic renal tubular necrosis and glomerulonephritis; sexual impotence; fever and chills (flu-like symptoms); and dizziness, drowsiness, fainting, and insomnia.

DRUG INTERACTIONS

See Appendix B-3: Interactions of ACE Inhibitors.

ANGIOTENSIN-RECEPTOR BLOCKERS

Candesartan, eprosartan, irbesartan, losartan, olmesartan, telmisartan, and **valsartan**

Hyzaar contains both losartan and hydrochlorothiazide, a diuretic, whereas Avalide contains both irbesartan and hydrochlorothiazide.

MECHANISM OF ACTION

The above angiotensin-receptor blockers (ARBs) block the receptors with which vasoconstrictive angiotensin interacts. Angiotensin is a dreaded substance in hypertensive patients, for it not only strongly constricts blood vessel but also causes sodium retention to elevate the blood volume and pressure. Hence, ARBs can thwart these undesirable influences to help lower blood pressure. However, ARBs are usually reserved for patients who are intolerant of the ACE blockers mentioned above.

SIDE EFFECTS

The frequent side effects of the above ARBs include irregular heartbeat; hyperkalemia; diarrhea; and mild fatigue, dizziness, and lightheadedness. Rarely they may also cause failures of the liver and kidney. ARBs should not be taken after the third month of pregnancy, for it may cause renal injury, oligohydramnios (too little amniotic fluid), or even birth defects such as additional fingers and/or toes. Fetal morphology scan and monitoring the volume of amniotic fluid should be performed if the above drugs were prescribed accidentally. ARBS are not recommended for use in children who have severely decreased kidney function, as their safety and effectiveness in this population has not been ascertained.

DRUG INTERACTIONS:

See Appendix B-6: Interactions of Angiotensin-Receptor Blockers

CALCIUM-CHANNEL BLOCKERS

Amlodipine, diltiazem, isradipine, nifedipine, nitrendipine, and **verapamil**

Amlodipine is often used in combination with benazepril, an ACE inhibitor.

MECHANISM OF ACTION

All of these drugs work by blocking the so-called L-type calcium-channels located at the blood vessels and at the heart muscle. Calcium is normally required for constriction of blood vessels and for strengthening of the heart contractility to raise blood pressure. Hence, a calcium-channel blocker (CCB) helps to lower the pressure.

SIDE EFFECTS

Some patients may experience one or more of the following adverse effects. If the symptoms get worse or a side effect not listed here emerges, a warning to take emergency action is warranted. The frequent side effects of these drugs include irregular heartbeats; stuffy nose; appetite loss and stomach pain; jaundice (yellowing of the skin or eyes); tiredness; and headache, fainting, and dizziness.

DRUG INTERACTIONS

See Appendix B-7: Interactions of Calcium-Channel Blockers.

DIURETIC DRUGS

Chlorthalidone; and **loop diuretics (bumetanide** [Fig. 1-11], **ethacrynic acid** [Fig. 1-12], and **furosemide** [Fig. 1-13])

MECHANISM OF ACTION

Diuretic drugs increase urinary excretions of sodium and water to shrink extracellular fluid (ECF) volume and thereby to help reduce the blood pressure.

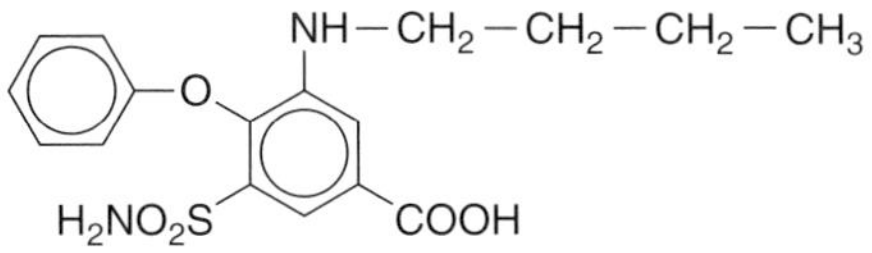

FIGURE 1-11 Molecular structure of bumetanide.

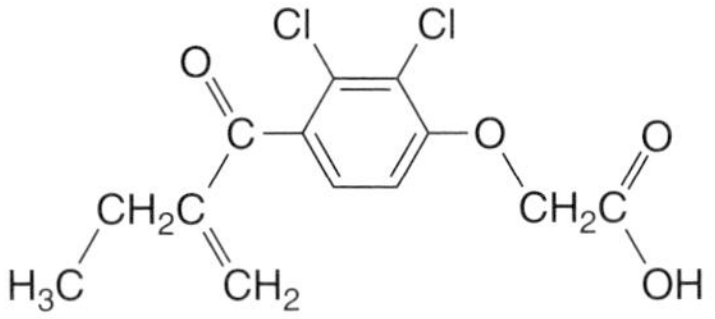

FIGURE 1-12 Molecular structure of ethacrynic acid.

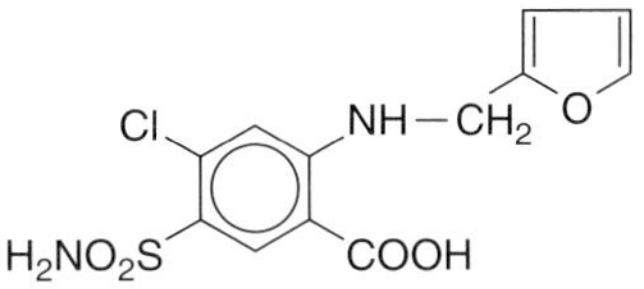

FIGURE 1-13 Molecular structure of furosemide.

SIDE EFFECTS

Chlorthalidone: This drug may cause orthostatic hypotension; thrombocytopenia, leucopenia; nausea, vomiting, diarrhea, and constipation; jaundice; pancreatitis; photosensitivity (vasculitis); and dizziness and headache.

Loop Diuretics: These diuretics may cause hypotension; electrolyte disturbances, hyperuricemia; dehydration; nausea, diarrhea, and abdominal pain; jaundice; pancreatitis; increased sensitivity to light; tinnitus; skin rash; dizziness; and, very rarely, ototoxicity, such as hearing loss, especially by ethacrynic acid, which is seldom used because of this side effect.

DRUG INTERACTIONS

Chlorthalidone: *See* Box 1-2.

Loop Diuretics: *See* Appendix B-5: Interactions of Loop Diuretics

Miscellaneous Interactions of Chlorthalidone (CTD)

CTD ◆▶ Digoxin: Chlorthalidone induces hypokalemia, a condition that can stir up the cardiac arrhythmic tendency of digoxin.

CTD ◆▶ Lithium: Chlorthalidone used in combination reduces the kidney's ability to eliminate lithium with a consequence of elevated blood levels and toxicities of lithium.

BOX 1-2

Basic Concepts of Chlorthalidone Interactions

1. Chlorthalidone is prone to produce hypokalemia, which prolongs the Q-T interval. Hence, when chlorthalidone is taken concurrently with drugs that elongate the interval, it may worsen the elongation to possibly lead to fatal torsade de pointes. Drugs that may elongate the Q-T include: **bepridil** (a calcium-channel blocker useful to treat angina pectoris); **chloroquine; amiodarone** (paradoxical cardiac arrhythmia may ensue by this anti-arrhythmic drug in the presence of hypokalemia); and less frequently, **chlorpromazine** (an antipsychotic drug).

2. If both interacting parties have a tendency to lower blood levels of potassium, they may create an additive or supra-additive effect to cause excessive hypokalemia that portends cardiac arrhythmia. Examples of such drugs include: **loop diuretics** (*See* Ω-49 in Appendix A) and sennosides (hydroxyanthracene glycosides derived from senna leaves, useful as laxatives).

CTD ↔ NSAIDs: (*See* Ω-54 in Appendix A.) Virtually all NSAIDs are apt to cause sodium retention by inhibiting the synthesis of prostaglandins and thereby can counteract diuretic effectiveness of chlorthalidone and of other diuretics.

CTD ↔ Toremifene: Side effects of toremifene include hypercalcemia, and chlorthalidone also tends to raise blood levels of calcium by reducing its renal excretion. Hence, their use in combination may create an additive or supra-additive effect toward excessive hypercalcemia.

2

Edema

Edema refers to an excessive accumulation of fluid in interstitial spaces or in a body cavity. Edema may not only cause swelling of such tissues as the legs and eyelids but even may contribute to elevation of blood pressure. Pulmonary edema is the most critical form of edema requiring urgent treatment.

The following classes of drugs may be administered to treat edema: (1) diuretics such as **hydrochlorothiazide, bumetanide, ethacrynic acid,** and **furosemide;** (2) vasodilators such as **nitroglycerin** (Nitro-Bid, Nitrolingual, Nitroquick, Nitro-Dur, Nitrostat, Transderm-Nitro, Minitran, Deponit, Nitrol), and **sodium nitroprusside** (Nitropress); and (3) inhibitors of angiotensin-converting enzyme (ACE) such as **captopril** (Capoten), **benazepril, enalapril** (Vasotec), **lisinopril,** and **ramipril** (Tritace, Ramace, Altace).

DIURETIC AGENTS

Hydrochlorothiazide and loop diuretics

The loop diuretics include **bumetanide, ethacrynic acid,** and **furosemide.** These diuretics are often used to treat edema associated with congestive heart failure, hepatic cirrhosis, or with renal insufficiency; or to treat edema caused by steroids or estrogen. Since continuous administration of **hydrochlorothiazide** or of a loop diuretic is apt to cause serious hypokalemia that could lead to muscle pain and weakness, it is wise to take these medications with **potassium chloride** (Klor-Con) to prevent hypokalemia. There are some milder diuretics that can save rather than deplete potassium. They include **spironolactone** (Aldactone) and **triamterene.** In fact, triamterene is often used in combination with hydrochlorothiazide as is exemplified by Dyazide. In treatment of life-threatening pulmonary edema, powerful and rapid-acting loop diuretics, such as bumetanide and furosemide, are preferred. However, all oral drug products containing potassium chloride at doses 100 mg or above per dosage unit were withdrawn from the United States market as they were decided unsafe.

MECHANISM OF ACTION

Hydrochlorothiazide, a thiazide diuretic, inhibits electroneutral Na^+-Cl^- reabsorption pump located at the distal convoluted tubules, causing increased excretions of sodium, water, and potassium, whereas the loop diuretics mentioned above work by blocking the Na^+,K^+-Cl_2 cotransport system available at the medullary portion of the thick ascending limb of loop of Henle (Fig. 2-1). They are the most prompt and most powerful diuretic agents currently available. Thus, the above diuretics both increase output of urine to reduce blood volume, and dilate blood vessels to reduce the pulmonary fluid pressure that contributes to pulmonary edema. In fact, the power of furosemide is so great and its onset of action so rapid that it can quickly reverse edema.

SIDE EFFECTS

Hydrochlorothiazide: Side effects of hydrochlorothiazide may include hypotension; electrolyte disturbances; hyperglycemia; nausea and abdominal discomfort;

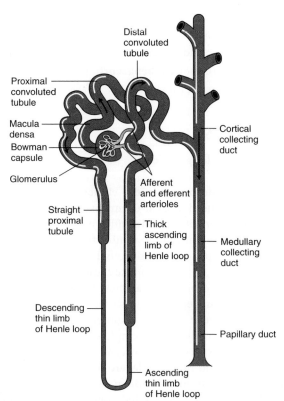

FIGURE 2-1   **Loop of Henle of the kidney.** Reproduced, with permission, from DiPiro JT, Talbert RL, Yee GC, Matzke GR, Wells BG, and Posey LM, eds. *Pharmacotherapy: A Pathologic Approach.* 7th ed. New York, NY: McGraw-Hill; 2008, p 706.

jaundice; pancreatitis; muscle weakness; impotence; skin rash caused by sunlight; and allergic reaction especially in patients who are allergic to sulfonamide chemo-therapeutic agents.

Dyazide **(hydrochlorothiazide + triamterene):** Similar to the side effects of hydrochlorothiazide but with lower incidences of hypokalemia. Triamterene may give urine a blue-green tint, but this does not lead to medical emergency.

Loop Diuretics: Their common side effects include hypotension; electrolyte disturbances and hyperuricemia; dehydration; nausea, diarrhea, and abdominal pain; jaundice; pancreatitis; increased sensitivity to light; tinnitus; skin rash; and dizziness; and very rarely, ototoxicity (such as hearing loss) especially by ethacrynic acid, which is seldom used because of this side effect.

Potassium Chloride: Its side effects may include irregular heartbeats; nausea, vomiting, bloody diarrhea, and hyperkalemia (excessive blood potassium may cause unusual tiredness and weakness). Its use is contraindicated in patients with renal insufficiency.

DRUG INTERACTIONS

Hydrochlorothiazide: *See* Appendix B-4: Interactions of Thiazide Diuretics.

Loop Diuretics: *See* Appendix B-5: Interactions of Loop Diuretics.

Potassium Chloride: *See* Box 2-1.

BOX 2-1

Basic Concepts of Potassium Chloride Interactions

1. Potassium chloride elevates blood levels of potassium. If both interacting parties have a tendency to elevate blood levels of potassium they may create an additive or supra-additive effect resulting in excessive hyperkalemia, a condition that slows down the heartbeat, weakens skeletal muscles, and blurs mental judgments. Examples include: **ACE inhibitors** (*See* Ω-1 in Appendix A), where the ACE inhibitors cause loss of sodium and retention of potassium; **aldosterone antagonists** (*See* Ω-3 in Appendix A) which retain potassium in exchange for sodium excreted; **amiloride** (a potassium-sparing diuretic); and **triamterene** (another potassium-sparing diuretic); and to a lesser extent, **(dandelion).** Roots of dandelion (Fig. 2-2), an herb that has a diuretic effect mobilizing sodium for its excretion, are a rich source of potassium and hence the combination may increase the risk of hyperkalemia.

continued

BOX 2-1 *(continued)*

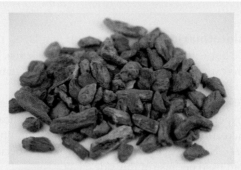

FIGURE 2-2   **Cut and dried root of dandelion.**

2. If both interacting parties have a tendency to slow down impulse conduction speed at the A-V node of the heart (Fig. 2-3), they may create an additive or supra-additive effect to cause A-V conduction blockade. Examples include: **digoxin** and **quinidine**.

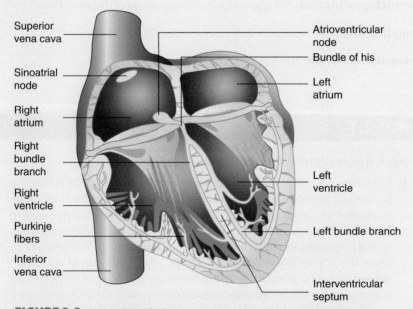

FIGURE 2-3   **A-V node at the heart.**   Reproduced, with permission, from Goldman MJ. *Principles of Clinical Electrocardiography*, 12th ed. Originally published by Appleton & Lange, copyright 1986 by McGraw-Hill, p 493.

VASODILATORS

Nitroglycerin (Fig. 2-4) and **sodium nitroprusside** (Fig. 2-5). They mimic actions of endogenous nitric oxide (NO). Nitroglycerin may be taken sublingually or by applying its transdermal patches (such as Deponit and Nitrol). Sodium nitroprusside is commonly injected by IV.

MECHANISM OF ACTIONS

Nitroglycerin: Nitroglycerin is chemically glyceryl trinitrate (*See* Figure 2-4), which is converted by mitochondrial aldehyde dehydrogenase to 1,2-glycerol dinitrate and nitrite, and the nitrate group interacts with enzymes and intracellular sulfhydryl (-SH) groups that reduce the nitrate group to nitric oxide (NO), or to S-nitrosothiol (Fig. 2-6) which then is converted to nitric oxide (NO). Nitric oxide activates soluble guanylyl cyclase in smooth muscles to form c-GMP, which causes vasodilation by several mechanisms including: (1) inhibition of calcium entry into the cell, thereby decreasing intracellular calcium concentrations and (2) activation of a calcium-sensitive potassium channel through the cyclic GMP-dependent protein kinase.

Sodium Nitroprusside: Nitric oxide (NO) is released from the molecule of this drug [$Na_2Fe(CN)_5NO.2H_2O$], and the NO activates guanylate cyclase to raise intracellular levels of cyclic-GMP that can induce quick vasodilation as stated above.

SIDE EFFECTS

Nitroglycerin: Its possible side effects include drop in blood pressure and increased heart rate; flushing of the head and neck; nausea, vomiting, and dry

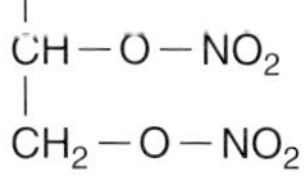

$$CH_2-O-NO_2$$
$$|$$
$$CH-O-NO_2$$
$$|$$
$$CH_2-O-NO_2$$

FIGURE 2-4 Molecular structure of nitroglycerin.

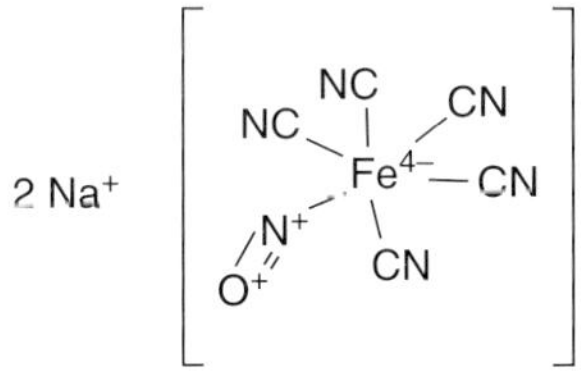

FIGURE 2-5 Molecular structure of sodium nitroprusside.

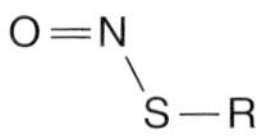

$$O=N$$
$$\backslash$$
$$S-R$$

FIGURE 2-6 Molecular structure of S-nitrosothiol.

mouth; weakness; headache and dizziness; and, rarely, may cause allergic reactions such as skin hives.

Sodium Nitroprusside: Its frequent side effects include irregular pulse; trouble in breathing; nausea and stomach pain; muscle spasms or muscle weakness; and dizziness and headache.

DRUG INTERACTIONS
Nitroglycerin

Isosorbide has similar interactions as nitroglycerin. *See* Box 2-2.

Miscellaneous Interactions of Nitroglycerin (NGR)

NGR ◆▶ N-Acetylcysteine: Continuous administration of nitroglycerin usually leads to development of drug tolerance (lost effectiveness). N-acetylcysteine taken intravenously helped to reverse nitroglycerin tolerance in patients with unstable angina, and transdermal nitroglycerin plus N-acetyl cysteine taken orally at 600 mg three times per day was also associated with fewer failures of nitroglycerin effectiveness than nitroglycerin alone. However, N-acetyl

BOX 2-2

Basic Concepts of Nitroglycerin Interactions

Nitroglycerin induces rapid fall of blood pressure. If both interacting parties have a hypotensive effect they may create an additive or supra-additive effect to cause a precipitous fall of blood pressure. Examples include: **ACE inhibitors** (*See* Ω-1 in Appendix A); **alpha blockers** (*See* Ω-6 in Appendix A); **beta blockers** (*See* Ω-27 in Appendix A (*note:* **labetalol** causes excessive fall of blood pressure more so than by other pure beta blockers because labetalol is unusual in that it has not only a beta-blocking effect but also has a selective alpha-1 blocking effect as well); **calcium-channel blockers** (*See* Ω-31 in Appendix A); **ganglionic blockers** (*See* Ω-41 in Appendix A); **anesthetic agents** (*See* Ω-9 in Appendix A); and **erectile dysfunction (ED) drugs** (*See* Ω-38 in Appendix A). Sildenafil (Viagra), tadalafil (Cialis), and vardenafil (Levitra) each have their own vasodilating effect to contribute to unsafe fall of blood pressure, leading to syncope and myocardial infarction. Hence, their combination with nitroglycerin should be contraindicated.

cysteine taken in combination with nitroglycerin was associated with intolerable headaches.

NGR ⟷ Alcohol: Alcohol, when consumed during nitroglycerin therapy, may cause additive effect resulting in unsafe fall of blood pressure and may cause circulatory collapse in extreme cases.

NGR ⟷ Alteplase: Nitroglycerin may reduce the serum levels and pharmacological effectiveness of alteplase. Hence, it is best to avoid this combination.

NGR ⟷ Aspirin: The vasodilatory effects of nitroglycerin may be enhanced by concomitant administration of aspirin because the latter reportedly increases maximum concentrations of nitroglycerin by almost 70%, to cause severe headache and even syncope by nitroglycerin. The underlying mechanism behind this interaction is poorly understood.

NGR ⟷ L-Carnitine: L-carnitine can cause severe headache and hypotension if taken with nitroglycerin or with isosorbide dinitrate.

NGR ⟷ L-Cysteine: Concurrent use of nitroglycerin and L-cysteine (100 micro mole) enhanced nitroglycerin-induced vasodilation of coronary vessels.

NGR ⟷ Diuretics: (*See* Ω-49 and Ω-73 in Appendix A.) Concurrent use of nitroglycerin and diuretics (water pills) may cause precipitous fall of blood pressure.

NGR ⟷ Heparin: Nitroglycerin may reduce the pharmacologic effects of heparin sodium. Nitroglycerin appears to decrease the serum concentration of heparin. Hence, monitoring of partial thromboplastin time to adjust heparin dosage is recommended during intravenous nitroglycerin.

NGR ⟷ Neuromuscular Blockers: (*See* Ω-53 in Appendix A): Nitroglycerin may increase the pharmacological effects of neuromuscular blockers to cause prolonged respiratory depression.

NGR ⟷ Vitamin C: Vitamin C, when taken at 500 mg or more three times a day in combination, may help to keep the vasodilation sustained, caused by nitroglycerin, with little therapeutic tolerance developed to nitroglycerin.

Sodium Nitroprusside

See Box 2-3.

BOX 2-3

Basic Concepts of Sodium Nitroprusside Interactions

If both interacting parties each have a tendency to lower blood pressure they may create an additive or supra-additive effect to cause excessive fall of pressure. Such examples include **erectile dysfunction (ED) drugs** (*See* Ω-38 in Appendix A). While sodium nitroprusside releases nitric oxide which mediates increased levels of c-GMP to cause vasodilation, the ED drugs, on the other hand, inhibit phosphodiesterase-5, the enzyme that destroys c-GMP and hence, the combination of the two can cause the additive effect of severe hypotension.

ACE INHIBITORS

Captopril, benazepril, enalapril, lisinopril, and **ramipril**

Rapid improvement of acute pulmonary edema can be obtained by sublingual administration of captopril. Lisinopril is often used in combination with hydrochlorothiazide, a diuretic; benazepril is often used in combination with amlodipine, a calcium-channel blocker, as is exemplified by Lotrel. Except for captopril and lisinopril, each of which is active by itself, all the currently available ACE inhibitors are prodrugs that must be activated by esterases in the liver, the enzymes that detach ester groups from prodrug molecules. For instance, enalapril, quinapril, and ramipril are each metabolized *in vivo* to the active form enalaprilat, quinaprilat, and ramiprilat, respectively.

MECHANISM OF ACTION

Drugs in this group inhibit the activity of ACE, the enzyme that is involved in production of angiotensin-2, an autacoid that stimulates synthesis and secretion of the hormone aldosterone from the adrenal cortex, which in turn decreases renal excretions of sodium to incite edema formation.

SIDE EFFECTS

Their frequent side effects may include persistent cough; nausea, vomiting, loss of appetite, abdominal pain, and diarrhea; and dizziness, fatigue, and headache.

DRUG INTERACTIONS

See Appendix B-3: Interactions of ACE Inhibitors.

CHAPTER

Congestive Heart Failure 3

Congestive heart failure is a condition in which the heart muscle is too weak to pump enough blood to sustain normal body functions. This condition may result in shortness of breath due to an insufficient blood supply to the lungs.

Medications shown effective to treat congestive heart failure include: (1) inhibitors of angiotensin-converting enzyme (ACE) such as **captopril** (Capoten), **enalapril** (Vasotec), and **lisinopril** (Prinivil, Zestril); (2) angiotensin-receptor blockers such as **losartan,** and **valsartan**; (3) beta-adrenergic blockers such as **bisoprolol** (Zebeta), **carvedilol** (Coreg), and **metoprolol** (Lopressor); (4) diuretic agents such as **bumetanide** (Bumex), **ethacrynic acid** (Edecrin*)*, and **furosemide** (Lasix); (5) aldosterone-receptor blockers such as **eplerenone** (Inspra) and **spironolactone** (Aldactone); and (6) a digitalis glycoside such as **digoxin** (Digitek, Lanoxin).

ACE INHIBITORS

Captopril, enalapril, and **lisinopril**

MECHANISM OF ACTION

By blocking the ACE, they oppose formation of the vasoconstricting substance angiotensin. The resultant arterial vasodilation improves outflow of blood from the heart, lessening the undue workload of the heart. Captopril and lisinopril are active by themselves, whereas enalapril is a prodrug that must be de-esterified *in vivo* to the active form enalaprilat by enzyme esterases. Lisinopril is the lysine-analog of the active agent enalaprilat.

SIDE EFFECTS

Their frequent side effects include uneven or fast heartbeat; fainting spells; irritating cough (their major side effect) and difficulty in breathing; loss of taste; and fatigue, tiredness, dizziness, and lightheadedness. For patients who cannot tolerate the side effect of cough, an angiotensin-receptor blocker is an alternative to be recommended.

DRUG INTERACTIONS

See Appendix B-3: Interactions of ACE Inhibitors.

ANGIOTENSIN-RECEPTOR BLOCKERS

Losartan and **valsartan**

They share many of the beneficial effects and side effects of ACE inhibitors, but without much persistent cough.

MECHANISM OF ACTION

They block the angiotensin receptors so that angiotensin-II cannot activate these receptors. The consequence of the blockade is vasodilation and opposed secretions of both aldosterone and vasopressin.

SIDE EFFECTS

Their frequent side effects include slow and weak heartbeats; chest pain; muscle weakness; painful or difficult urination; and muscle numbness or tingling.

DRUG INTERACTIONS

See Appendix B-6: Interactions of Angiotensin-Receptor Blockers.

BETA-ADRENERGIC BLOCKERS

Bisoprolol, carvedilol, and **metoprolol**

MECHANISM OF ACTION

Beta blockers inhibit the release of renal enzyme renin to lower the ECF volume and thereby reduce workload of the heart.

SIDE EFFECTS

Possible side effects of these drugs include low blood pressure; shortness of breath or wheezing; abdominal cramps, nausea, diarrhea, and constipation; fatigue; memory loss; lightheadedness; and insomnia. They also tend to raise blood triglyceride levels and reduce levels of so-called "good-cholesterol" (HDL), and reduce blood glucose levels (hypoglycemia), but metoprolol is less likely to cause hypoglycemia.

DRUG INTERACTIONS

See Appendix B-1: Interactions of Beta Blockers.

DIURETIC DRUGS

Bumetanide, ethacrynic acid, and **furosemide**

MECHANISM OF ACTION

They promote urine output and thereby decrease the body fluid retained, lessening the workload for the heart to pump. The decrease of fluid retained in the lungs allows easier breathing.

SIDE EFFECTS

The frequent side effects of these diuretics include loss of potassium and magnesium to cause fast or uneven heartbeat; nausea, stomach pain, diarrhea, and constipation; jaundice (yellowing of the skin or eyes); muscle pain or weakness; and lightheadedness. Further, ethacrynic acid, among the above, is most likely to cause ototoxicity.

DRUG INTERACTIONS

See Appendix B-5: Interactions of Loop Diuretics.

ALDOSTERONE ANTAGONISTS

Eplerenone (Fig. 3-1) and **spironolactone** (Fig. 3-2)

MECHANISM OF ACTION

They block the receptors with which aldosterone, a mineralocorticoid, interacts, and by so doing inhibit sodium reabsorption coupled to potassium excretion at the collecting ducts of the kidney. This blockade culminates in retention of potassium and increased urinary excretion of sodium. Their beneficial effect in the treatment of congestive heart failure derives from their diuretic effect that reduces ECF volume, relieving edema and reducing the workload of the heart.

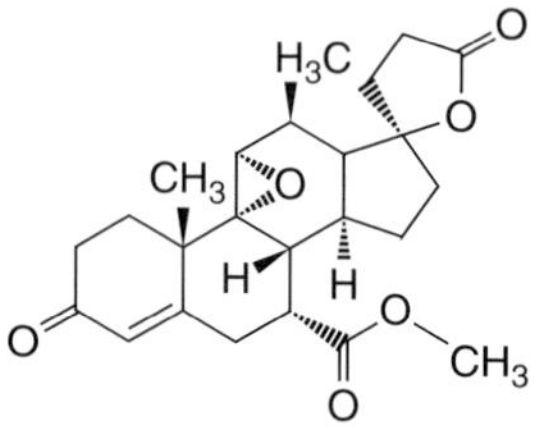

FIGURE 3-1   Molecular structure of eplerenone.

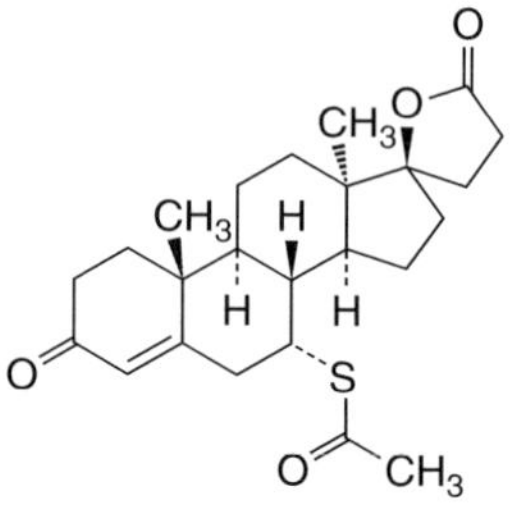

FIGURE 3-2   Molecular structure of spironolactone.

SIDE EFFECTS

Their frequent side effects include renal impairment with excessive retention of potassium to weaken muscle tone, especially with spironolactone.

DRUG INTERACTIONS

See Box 3-1

Miscellaneous Interactions of Aldosterone Antagonists (ADA)

Parentheses below indicate an herb.

ADA ⟷ CYP Isozymes: *See* Table 3-1.

ADA ⟷ Digoxin: Spironolactone and, to a lesser extent, eplerenone reduce renal clearance of digoxin used in combination, leading to an increased half-life and toxicity of digoxin.

BOX 3-1

Basic Concepts of Aldosterone Antagonist Interactions

Aldosterone antagonists retain potassium in exchange for excreted sodium. If both interacting parties have a tendency to retain potassium they may create an additive or supra-additive effect of severe hyperkalemia that may cause heart failure, especially when renal impairment is present as is the case with an aldosterone antagonist. Examples include: **ACE inhibitors** (*See* Ω-1 in Appendix A); **angiotensin-receptor blockers** (*See* Ω-10 in Appendix A); and **potassium chloride**.

TABLE 3-1 Eplerenone vs. CYP Enzymes

Drug Name	1A2	2A6	2B6	2C8	2C9	2C18	2C19	2D6	2E1	3A4
Eplerenone										Sub

Abbreviations: Sub, substrate of the enzyme; Inh, inhibits the enzyme; Ezi, induces the enzyme

1. Spironolactone , unlike eplerenone, either does not interact with cytochrome P450 isozymes or its nature of interaction with CYP is not clearly elucidated.
2. Metabolic clearance of eplerenone requires the presence of microsomal CYP3A4, and hence inhibition of this enzyme by any other drug taken together may raise blood levels of eplerenone to possibly perk up its adverse effects. (*See* the left-hand column of Table-0 at the 'Introduction' for possible inhibitors of this enzyme).

ADA ⟷ (Licorice): Glycyrrhetinic acid, an ingredient in licorice, inhibits breakdown of aldosterone to raise its blood levels and to possibly aggravate its adverse effects.

ADA ⟷ NSAIDs: (*See* Ω-54 in Appendix A.) Since non-steroidal anti-inflammatory drugs (NSAIDs), such as ibuprofen, indomethacin, and naproxen, can oppose renal excretions of sodium to retain water, they may undercut diuretic effects of aldosterone antagonists when used in combination.

DIGITALIS GLYCOSIDE

Digoxin is the most frequently prescribed digitalis glycoside (Digitek, Lanoxin). Formation of digoxin involves hydroxylation at position 12 of digitoxin (Fig. 3-3).

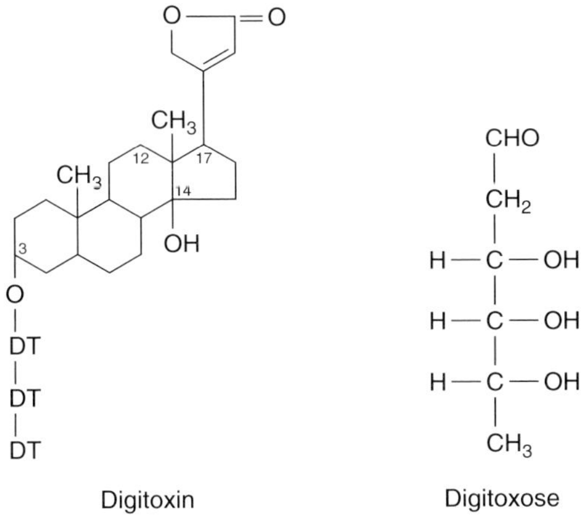

FIGURE 3-3 Molecular structure of digitoxin and digitoxose.

MECHANISM OF ACTION

Digoxin binds to and inhibits the Na^+/K^+-ATPase pump of the cardiac cell membranes to cause accumulation of sodium inside the cardiac cells, which slows extrusion of calcium ions by sodium-calcium exchange, resulting in retention of calcium ions that strengthen contractility of cardiac muscle, improving cardiac output.

SIDE EFFECTS

Digoxin may cause changes in heart rate; nausea, vomiting, loss of appetite, diarrhea, and stomach pain; gynecomastia (breast development in males); blurred vision and changed perception of color such as yellow vision; and dizziness, headache, and confusion.

DRUG INTERACTIONS

See Box 3-2.

BOX 3-2

Basic Concepts of Digoxin Interactions

1. Digoxin slows atrioventricular conduction speed, and if both interacting parties have a tendency to slow conduction they may create an additive or supra-additive slowing of the cardiac conduction speed. Examples include: **adenosine; beta blockers** (*See* to Ω-27 in Appendix A); and **potassium chloride**.

2. Hypokalemia generated by other drugs can enhance arrhythmogenic tendency of digoxin. Examples include: **amphotericin-B** (antifungal drug); **chlorthalidone** (a diuretic drug); **fludrocortisone; potassium-depleting diuretics** (*See* Ω-49 and Ω-73 in Appendix A); **sodium polystyrene sulfonate** (high doses of sodium polystyrene sulfonate can cause hypokalemia, a condition that can stir up arrhythmogenicity of digoxin).

3. The cardiac arrhythmic tendency of digoxin is enhanced in the presence of sympathomimetic drugs. Examples include: **amphetamine** (Fig. 3-4), **epinephrine** (Fig. 3-5), **pseudoephedrine** (Fig. 3-6), and other **sympathomimetic drugs** (*See* Ω-71 in Appendix A).

4. Digoxin is a substrate of the efflux P-gp transporter proteins in the intestines, and therefore if digoxin is co-administered with an inhibitor of this transporter, the blood levels of digoxin rise to possibly whip up its adverse effects such

BOX 3-2 *(continued)*

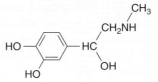

FIGURE 3-4 Molecular structure of amphetamine.

FIGURE 3-5 Molecular structure of epinephrine.

FIGURE 3-6 Molecular structure of pseudoephedrine.

as cardiac arrhythmia. Examples include: **statin drugs** (*See* Ω-69 in Appendix A) and other **P-gp transporter inhibitors** (*See* Ω-57 in Appendix A).

5. Digoxin is a substrate for efflux P-gp transporter proteins in the renal tubules as well, and when taken together with another drug that inhibits this efflux transporter it will impair renal clearance of digoxin to elevate its serum concentration and may cause adverse effects such as cardiac arrhythmia. Examples include: **itraconazole; ketoconazole; calcium-channel blockers** (*See* Ω-31 in Appendix A); **quinine** or **quinidine,** and possibly **chloroquine** and **hydroxychloroquine**.

6. Digoxin is slowly hydrolyzed by gastric acid to digoxigenin and hence, intestinal absorption of digoxin is enhanced by an elevated gastric pH. Examples of drugs that tend to raise the pH include proton-pump inhibitors (*See* Ω-61 in Appendix A). Proton-pump inhibitors block secretions of gastric acid and the elevated gastric pH can increase the absorption of digoxin (peak plasma concentrations increased by about 30%). However, gastric antacids, though they elevate gastric pH, lower intestinal absorption of digoxin (*See* 7. below).

7. Some drugs can adsorb digoxin to hinder its intestinal absorption. Examples include: **gastric antacids** and some **bile acid sequestrants** (*See* Ω-28 in Appendix A). Intestinal absorption of digoxin can be impaired by cholestyramine but little affected by colestipol.

continued

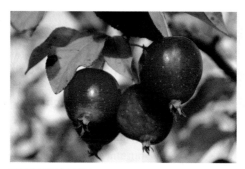

FIGURE 3-10   A. Hawthorn berries. (courtesy of William Vann/www.edupic.net)

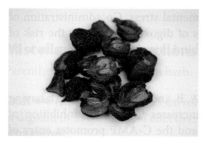

FIGURE 3-10   B. Hawthorn berries (cut & dried).

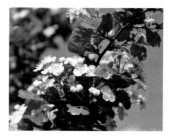

FIGURE 3-10   C. Hawthorn flowers. (courtesy of Bo Jensen in Copenhagen, Denmark)

DGX ⟷ Penicillamine: Penicillamine may decrease the blood levels of digoxin to undercut its therapeutic effectiveness. The mechanism of action behind this observation still remains to be elucidated.

DGX ⟷ Phenytoin: Phenytoin, when taken together, may undercut therapeutic efficacy of digoxin, by an unknown mechanism.

DGX ⟷ Procarbazine: Procarbazine was shown to impair intestinal absorption of digoxin, and thereby may it lower the blood levels and therapeutic efficacies of digoxin.

DGX ⟷ Propafenone: It is postulated that Propafenone decreases the volume of distribution and non-renal elimination of digoxin, leading to increased blood levels and toxicities of digoxin.

DGX ⟷ Quininolone Antibiotics: (*See* Ω-62 in Appendix A.) When taken in combination, the quinolone antibiotics may raise serum levels of digoxin.

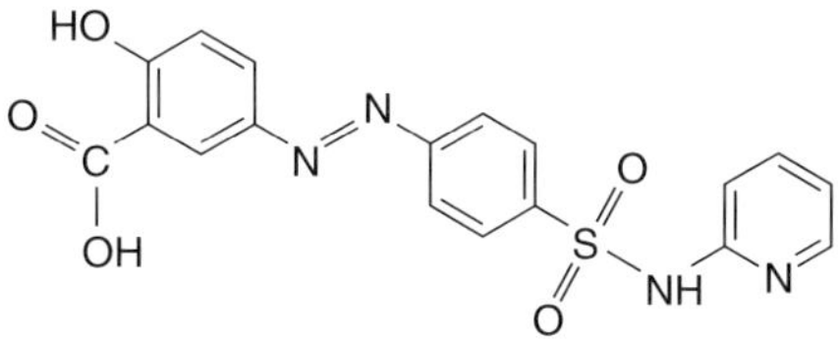

FIGURE 3-11   Molecular structure of sulfasalazine.

DGX ⟷ SSRIs: (*See* Ω-68 in Appendix A.) All of the SSRI members can displace digoxin from its protein-binding sites, raising its free drug concentrations and adverse effects.

DGX ⟷ Spironolactone: Spironolactone (Aldactone), probably by inhibiting the distal tubular secretions, decreases the renal clearance of digoxin to raise its blood levels and adverse effects.

DGX ⟷ Sulfamethoxazole/Trimethoprim: Co-administration of digitalis with antibiotic sulfamethoxazole-trimethoprim (Bactrim) may increase blood levels of digoxin by unknown mechanism, and may increase the risk of its adverse effects.

DGX ⟷ Sulfasalazine: When used in combination, intestinal absorption of digoxin can be impaired by such antibiotics as sulfasalazine (Azulfidine) (Fig. 3-11) by an unknown mechanism. Sulfasalazine may turn urine dark yellow to orange-red, but this does not usually amount to medical emergency.

DGX ⟷ Telmisartan: Telmisartan, unlike losartan, appears to quicken and enhance absorption of digoxin to increased blood levels and toxicities of digoxin.

DGX ⟷ Thyroid Preparations: (*See* Ω-75 in Appendix A.) Thyroid drugs or hyperthyroidism tend to cause heart palpitations and their co-administration with digoxin may further the cardiac arrhythmia.

DGX ⟷ Trazodone: When digoxin is used together with trazodone, serum levels of digoxin may be elevated by unknown mechanism.

CHAPTER

4

Cardiac Arrhythmia

Cardiac arrhythmia refers to irregular heartbeats caused by a defect in the cardiac muscle or electrical conduction system of the heart. Arrhythmias include tachycardia (abnormally fast heart rate) and bradycardia (abnormally slow heart rate as compared to normal). Some arrhythmias can be life-threatening, as they can result in cardiac arrest and death.

Medications shown effective in the treatment of cardiac arrhythmia include: (1) **amiodarone** (Cordarone, Pacerone); (2) sodium-channel blockers such as **lidocaine** (Xylocaine), **procainamide** (Procan, Procanbid, Pronestyl), **quinidine** (Quinaglute, Quinidex, Quinora), and **tocainide** (Tonocard); (3) calcium-channel blockers such as **diltiazem** (Cardizem, Cartia, Dilacor, Diltia, Tiazac) and **verapamil** (Calan, Covera, Isoptin, Verelan); (4) adrenergic beta blockers such as **esmolol** (Brevibloc), **propranolol** (Inderal), and **sotalol** (Betapace); and (5) miscellaneous antiarrhythmic drugs such as **adenosine** (Adenocard), and **cibenzoline** (Cipralan). Drugs containing adenosine-5-monophosphate were removed from the United States market in 1973 because they were determined to be unsafe.

AMIODARONE

MECHANISM OF ACTION

Amiodarone works by blocking the K^+-channel at the myocardial cells and by blocking, to a lesser degree, the Na^+ and Ca^{++} channels as well.

SIDE EFFECTS

Amiodarone may cause elongation of the Q-T interval with tendency to proarrhythmia (a new arrhythmia or worsening of existing arrhythmia), and rarely congestive heart failure and bradycardia; interstitial pneumonitis or alveolitis; vomiting, diarrhea, stomach upset; hepatotoxicity with yellowing of the skin or eyes; bluish-gray skin discoloration; blurred vision and dizziness; and allergic reactions such as interstitial pneumonitis with difficulty in breathing and swelling of the lips, tongue, or face; and skin hives.

DRUG INTERACTIONS

See Box 4-1.

Miscellaneous Interactions of Amiodarone (AMD)

Parentheses below indicate an herb.

AMD ↔ Cholestyramine: Co-administration of oral amiodarone with cholestyramine impairs absorption of amiodarone to its reduced serum levels with therapeutic insufficiency.

BOX 4-1

Basic Concepts of Amiodarone Interactions

1. Amiodarone is prone to elongate the Q-T interval (Fig. 4-1), and concurrent administration of amiodarone with other drugs that also tend to elongate the Q-T interval may result in the life-threatening torsade de pointes (Fig. 4-2).

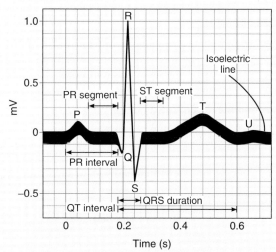

FIGURE 4-1 Q-T interval. Reproduced, with permission, from Barrett KE, Barman SM, Boitano S, and Brooks HL. *Ganong's Review of Medical Physiology*. 23rd ed. New York, NY: McGraw-Hill; 2010, p 494.

continued

BOX 4-1 *(continued)*

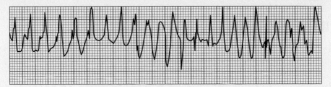

FIGURE 4-2   Torsade de pointes.

Examples include: **chlorpromazine** (an antipsychotic drug); **moxifloxacin** (an antibiotic drug); and **disopyramide** (an antiarrhythmic drug).

2. Hypokalemia generated by other drugs tends to arouse the arrhythmogenic tendency of amiodarone when taken together, as hypokalemia worsens the elongated Q-T interval of amiodarone, possibly leading to torsade de pointes. Examples include: **loop diuretics** (*See* Ω-49 in Appendix A); **thiazide diuretics** such as chlorthalidone (*See* Ω-73 in Appendix A); and **sennosides.** Sennosides may cause hypokalemia and hypomagnesemia.

3. Amiodarone rarely causes congestive heart failure and bradycardia. When amiodarone is taken concurrently with other drugs that cause negative inotropic and chronotropic effects, it may cause a drastic fall in cardiac output and sinus arrest. Examples include: **calcium-channel blockers** (*See* Ω-31 in Appendix A) and **fentanyl** (Fig. 4-3) (a narcotic analgesic drug that can rarely cause myocardial depression).

4. Side effects of amiodarone include interstitial pneumonitis or alveolitis, and concurrent intake of this drug with other drugs that also cause similar side effects may lead to severe (sometimes fatal) pulmonary complications. Examples include: **methotrexate** (an anticancer drug) and **cyclophosphamide** (an anticancer drug).

FIGURE 4-3   Molecular structure of fentanyl.

TABLE 4-1 Amiodarone vs CYP Enzymes

Drug Name	1A2	2A6	2B6	2C8	2C9	2C18	2C19	2D6	2E1	3A4
Amiodarone				Sub						Sub+
	Inh				Inh			Inh		Inh

Abbreviations: Sub, substrate of the enzyme; Inh, inhibits the enzyme; Ezi, induces the enzyme

1. The N-deethylation of amiodarone to desethylamiodarone is catalyzed by CYP2C8.

2. Amiodarone is processed by both CYP2C8 and CYP3A4 and both enzymes are inhibited by cimetidine to elevate blood levels and adverse effects of amiodarone. (*See* the left-hand column of Table-0 at the 'Introduction' for other possible inhibitors of these enzymes).

3. Rifampin is a potent inducer of both CYP3A4 and CYP2C8. Administration of rifampin in combination with oral amiodarone has resulted in a decrease in serum concentrations of amiodarone to undercut its therapeutic effectiveness. (*See* the right-hand column of Table-0 at the 'Introduction' for other possible inducers of the enzyme.)

4. Amiodarone inhibits CYP1A2, 2C9, 2D6, and CYP3A4; and dextromethorphan is cleared through CYP2C9, 2C19, 2D6, and CYP3A4. When amiodarone is used in combination with dextromethorphan the former inhibits clearance of the latter to raise its blood levels and adverse effects. (*See* the middle column of Table-0 at the 'Introduction' for other possible substrates of the enzyme.)

   Theophylline and amiodarone used in combination can increase the serum levels and the risk of toxicity of theophylline, a strong substrate of CYP1A2.

5. Amiodarone may interfere with clearances of cyclosporine and simvastatin (both substrates of CYP3A4) to increase their blood levels and the risks of nephrotoxicity and rhabdomyolysis, respectively.

6. Amiodarone can oppose metabolic clearance of metoprolol (a substrate of CYP2D6) to increase its blood levels and adverse effects. (*See* the middle column of Table-0 at the 'Introduction' for other possible substrates of the enzyme.).

7. Amiodarone can increase the blood levels and anticoagulant effects of S-warfarin which is mostly processed through CYP 2C9, the enzyme amiodarone inhibits.

AMD ⬌ CYP Isozymes: (*See* Table 4-1.) Amiodarone (Fig. 4-4) is metabolized to desethylamiodarone (Fig. 4-5) by the cytochrome P450 enzyme group, specifically cytochrome P450-3A4 (CYP3A4) and CYP2C8.

AMD ⬌ Digoxin: Co-administration of amiodarone with digoxin can increase blood levels and toxicities of digoxin. Therefore doses of digoxin should be reduced

FIGURE 4-4 Molecular structure of amiodarone.

FIGURE 4-5 Molecular structure of N-desethylamiodarone.

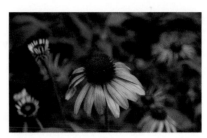

FIGURE 4-6   Echinacea flowers. (attribution: Wikipedia)

or discontinued. The cause of this interaction has not been known, but it does not appear due to a change in the renal clearance of digoxin.

AMD ⟷ (Echinacea): Some of the alkaloids found in echinacea (Fig. 4-6), an herb believed to be an immunomodulator that can shorten the duration of the common cold and flu, may be harmful to the liver. Thus it should not be taken together with any other drugs that are also known to be toxic to the liver, such as amiodarone (Cordarone).

SODIUM-CHANNEL BLOCKERS

Lidocaine (Fig. 4-7), **procainamide** (Fig. 4-8), **quinidine** (Fig. 4-9), and **tocainide** (Fig. 4-10)

MECHANISM OF ACTION

Lidocaine, procainamide, quinidine, and tocainide all block sodium channels to generate some local anesthetic effect, especially lidocaine, to depress the phase-0 slope generated by the influx of sodium ions thereby elevating the threshold of myocardial excitation. Procainamide and quinidine are classified as class-1a drugs as they also increase the duration of action potential with slowed repolarization (Q-T elongation). On the other hand, lidocaine and tocainide are classified as class-1b drugs as they shorten the duration of action potential by quickening repolarization of the myocardium.

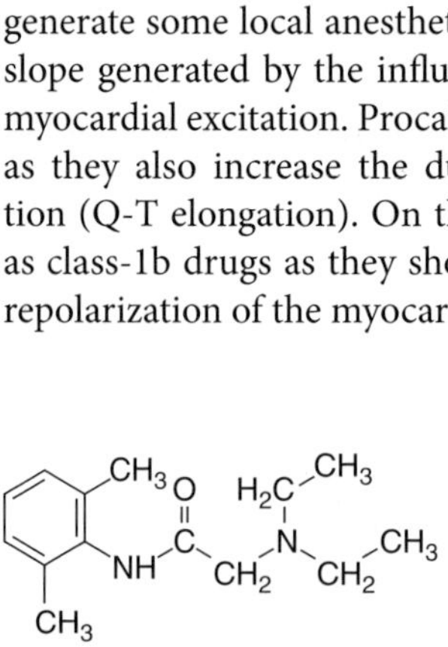

FIGURE 4-7   Molecular structure of lidocaine.

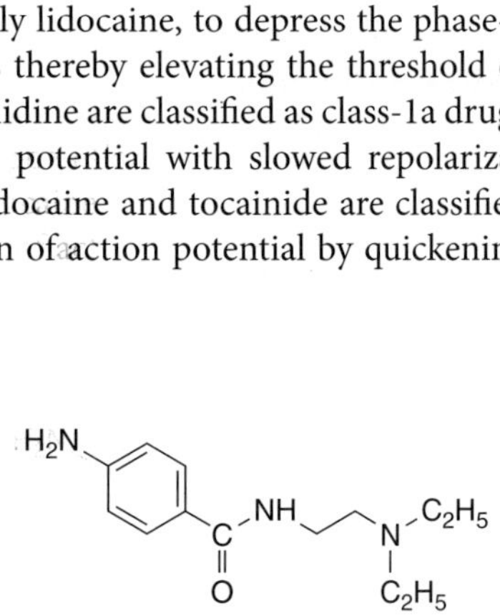

FIGURE 4-8   Molecular structure of procainamide.

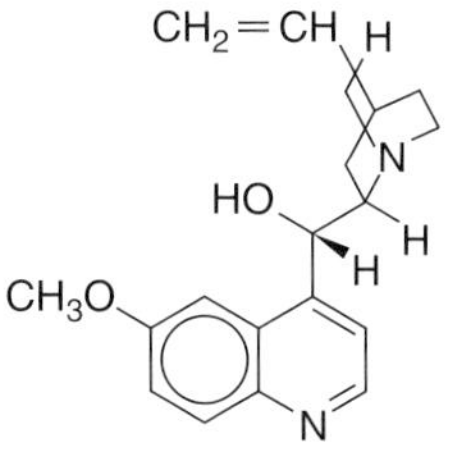

FIGURE 4-9   Molecular structure of quinidine.

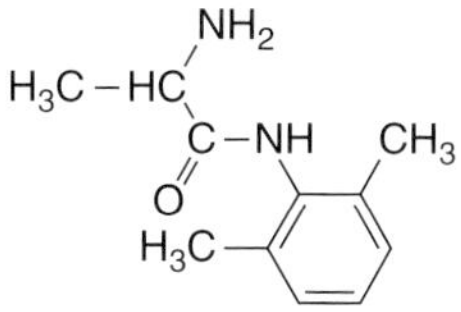

FIGURE 4-10   Molecular structure of tocainide.

SIDE EFFECTS

Some patients may experience one or more of the following adverse effects. If the symptoms get worse or a side effect not listed here emerges, a warning to take emergency action is warranted. The side effects of these drugs may include Q-T elongation (especially by procainamide and quinidine); proarrhythmia (a new type of arrhythmia or aggravation of existing arrhythmia); shortness of breath or wheezing; loss of appetite, bitter taste (especially quinidine), nausea, vomiting, stomach pain, constipation; ringing in the ears (especially by quinidine); numbness, dizziness and drowsiness (especially by lidocaine).

DRUG INTERACTIONS

Lidocaine or tocainide (LPT)

LPT ⟷ Acetazolamide: Acetazolamide being a carbonic anhydrase inhibitor can make the urine alkaline, promoting nonionization of such basic drugs as lidocaine (*See* Fig. 4-7) and tocainide (*See* Figure 4-10), and thereby increasing their reabsorption through the renal tubules, consequently increasing their blood levels and adverse effects.

LPT ⟷ Antiarrhythmic Drugs: (*See* Ω-12 in Appendix A.) Toxic effects of these antiarrhythmic drugs may become synergistic if lidocaine or tocainide is used together with any member of the antiarrhythmic drugs in combination.

LPT ⟷ CYP Isozymes: *See* Table 4-2.

DRUG INTERACTIONS

Procainamide
See Box 4-2.

TABLE 4-2   Lidocaine and Tocainide vs CYP Enzymes

Drug Name	1A2	2A6	2B6	2C8	2C9	2C18	2C19	2D6	2E1	3A4
Lidocaine	Sub + Inh							Sub		Sub
Tocainide	Inh									

Abbreviations: Sub, substrate of the enzyme; Inh, inhibits the enzyme; Ezi, induces the enzyme

1. Cimetidine is an inhibitor of many microsomal cytochrome P450 isozymes, including CYP 1A2, CYP 2D6, and CYP 3A4. Therefore, elimination of lidocaine that utilizes these enzymes for its clearance will be impaired by combined use with cimetidine, resulting in elevated blood levels and adverse effects of lidocaine.

2. Both lidocaine and tocainide inhibit CYP1A2 and hence, administration of either drug in combination with drugs that require this enzyme for hepatic clearance may raise their blood levels, potentially exacerbating their adverse effects. Those drugs include alosetron, duloxetine, theophylline, and tizanidine. (*See* the middle column of Table-0 at the 'Introduction' for other possible substrates of the enzyme.)

Miscellaneous Interactions of Procainamide (PCM)

PCM ⟷ Antiarrhythmic Drugs: (*See* Ω-12 in Appendix A.) Toxic effects of procainamide may become synergistic if it is used together with one or more of the other antiarrhythmic drugs.

PCM ⟷ CYP Isozymes: *See* Table 4-3.

BOX 4-2

Basic Concepts of Procainamide Interactions

1. Hypokalemia generated by other drugs concurrently taken tends to further the Q-T elongation of procainamide possibly leading to torsade de pointes. Examples include: **thiazide diuretics** (*See* Ω-73 in Appendix A) and **loop diuretics** (*See* Ω-49 in Appendix A).

2. Alkaline pH of urine generated by other drugs can promote nonionization of procainamide to increase its reabsorption through the renal tubules with consequent rise in its blood levels and adverse effects. **Acetazolamide** (a carbonic anhydrase inhibitor that can make the urine alkaline) is an example of such a drug.

3. Procainamide is prone to elongate the Q-T interval, and concurrent administration with other drugs that also tend to elongate it may create an additive or supra-additive effect on the interval. Examples include: **indapamide**, a nonthiazide diuretic that tends to prolong the Q-T interval.

TABLE 4-3 **Procainamide & Quinidine vs CYP Enzymes**

Drug Name	1A2	2A6	2B6	2C8	2C9	2C18	2C19	2D6	2E1	3A4
Procainamide								Sub		
Quinidine								Inh		Sub+ Inh

Abbreviations: Sub, substrate of the enzyme; Inh, inhibits the enzyme; Ezi: induces the enzyme

1. Procainamide requires CYP2D6 for its metabolic clearance and hence inhibition of this enzyme by other drugs taken together can impair its metabolic clearance to elevate its blood levels and adverse effects. (*See* the left-hand column of Table-0 at the 'Introduction' for possible inhibitors of this enzyme.)

2. Quinidine: (1) has a strong inhibitory effect of CYP2D6, the enzyme required for activation of the prodrug codeine, and hence combined use may lead to lessened analgesic effects of codeine; and (2) has inhibitory effect on CYP3A4 and hence administration of it in combination with other drugs that require this enzyme for their metabolic clearance may result in elevated blood levels, possibly inciting their adverse effects to surface. (*See* the middle column of Table-0 at the 'Introduction' for possible substrates of the enzyme) .

3. Metabolic clearance of Quinidine requires the presence of microsomal CYP3A4, and hence inhibition of this enzyme by any other drug taken together may raise blood levels of Quinidine to perk up its adverse effects.

PCM ↔ Trimethoprim: Trimethoprim is an inhibitor of renal cationic secretions, and when used in combination can decrease the renal tubular secretions of procainamide to raise its blood levels and adverse effects.

DRUG INTERACTIONS

Quinidine
See Box 4-3.

Miscellaneous Interactions of Quinidine (QND)

QND ↔ Chlorpromazine: When these two drugs, both tending to cause elongation of the Q-T interval, are taken in combination, they may result in the life-threatening arrhythmia of torsade de pointes.

QND ↔ CYP Isozymes: *See* Table 4-3.

QND ↔ Digoxin: Quinidine is thought to inhibit the renal excretions of digoxin without affecting the glomerular filtration rate. Quinidine thus used in combination can increase serum levels of digoxin to foment its adverse effects of cardiac arrhythmia.

QND ↔ Loperamide: Quinidine is an inhibitor of the transporter for loperamide, and when used in combination opposes efflux of loperamide to raise blood concentrations and adverse effects of loperamide.

BOX 4-3

Basic Concepts of Quinidine Interactions

1. Hypokalemia is a most significant Q-T prolonging factor. If quinidine, which itself prolongs the Q-T interval, is taken together with other drugs that cause hypokalemia, it may generate further elongation. Examples include **diuretics** (See Ω-49 and Ω-73 in Appendix A).

2. Alkaline urine promotes nonionization of such basic drugs as quinidine to increase its reabsorption through the renal tubules to raise its blood levels and adverse effects. An example of drugs that can cause alkaline urine pH is **acetazolamide** (Fig. 4-11), a carbonic anhydrase inhibitor.

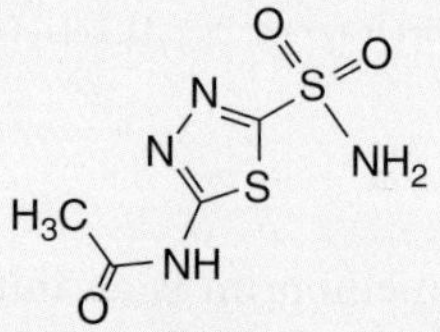

FIGURE 4-11   Molecular structure of acetazolamide.

3. Quinidine markedly slows the A-V conduction speed, and hyperkalemia also tends to slow the A-V conduction speed. Hence when quinidine is taken concurrently with other drugs that generate hyperkalemia it may possibly lead to complete heart block. Examples include: **potassium chloride** and **amiloride**, a potassium-sparing diuretic agent (Fig. 4-12).

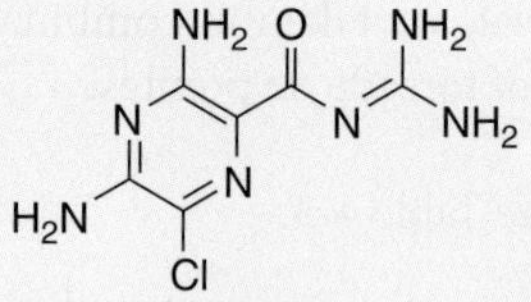

FIGURE 4-12   Molecular structure of amiloride.

4. Quinidine markedly slows the A-V conduction speed and when taken concurrently with other drugs that also slow the conduction, it may further prolong the P-R interval. Examples include **calcium-channel blockers** (See Ω-31 in Appendix A).

BOX 4-3 (continued)

5. Quinidine possesses anticholinergic activities to decrease vagal tone, and hence when used in conjunction with other drugs that work either by accumulation of acetylcholine, such as those used in the treatment of myasthenia gravis, or by directly activating the muscarinic receptors, it may diminish the therapeutic effects of those other drugs, which include: **neostigmine** and **pyridostigmine**, both anticholinesterase agents to accumulate acetylcholine; and **bethanechol** (a muscarinic agonist). Therefore, it is prudent to hold off combinations of quinidine with these drugs.

CALCIUM-CHANNEL BLOCKERS

The most frequently prescribed calcium-channel blockers to treat cardiac arrhythmia include **diltiazem** (Fig. 4-13) (Cardizem, Cartia, Dilacor, Diltia, Tiazac) and **verapamil** (Fig. 4-14) (Calan, Covera, Isoptin, Verelan).

MECHANISM OF ACTION

The calcium-channel blockers inhibit flux of calcium ions from ECF into the S-A node, the A-V node, and the cardiac muscle. They, by doing so, depress the rate of discharge of the S-A node, and slow the conduction speed at the A-V node to prolong the refractory period at the node. They are effective by intravenous administration in the treatment of supraventricular tachycardia and to reduce the ventricular rate in patients having atrial fibrillation, but they are not indicated to treat Wolf-Parkinson-White syndrome in which the QRS complex is widened.

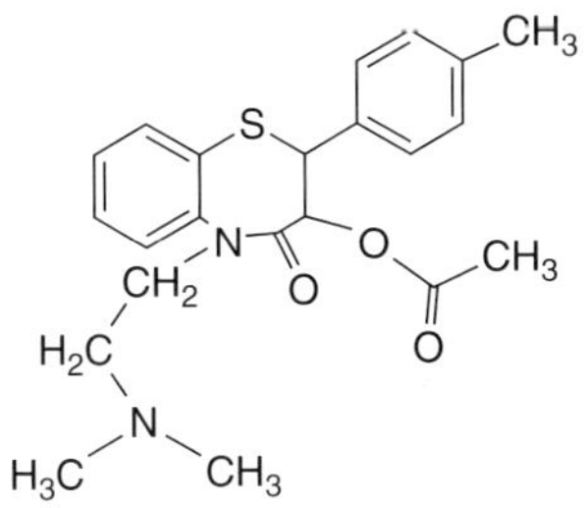

FIGURE 4-13 Molecular structure of diltiazem.

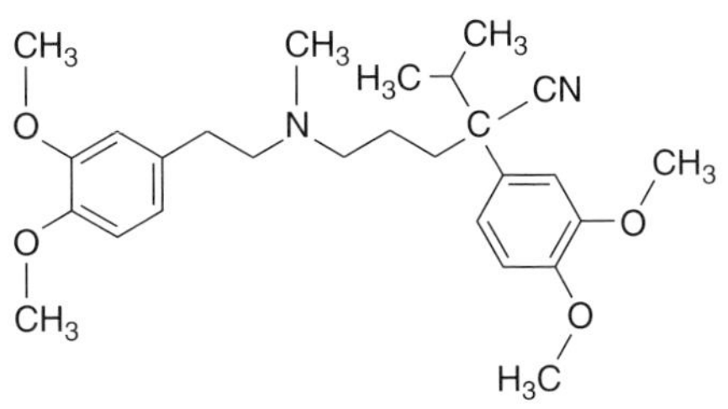

FIGURE 4-14 Molecular structure of verapamil.

SIDE EFFECTS

Their frequent side effects may include slowed heart rates, postural hypotension; wheezing or difficulty in breathing; constipation; swelling of the lower extremities; skin rash; headache, and dizziness.

DRUG INTERACTIONS

See Appendix B-7: Interactions of Calcium-Channel Blockers .

BETA BLOCKERS

Esmolol (Fig. 4-15), **propranolol** (Fig. 4-16), and **sotalol** (Fig. 4-17)

MECHANISM OF ACTION

These adrenergic beta blockers can depress the phase-4 slope elevated by catecholamines. Esmolol is a cardioselective beta blocker that is used by intravenous infusion to obtain rapid (in a few minutes) control of ventricular arrhythmia in patients with atrial flutter or fibrillation. These adrenergic beta blockers prolong the P-R interval by slowing the impulse conduction speed at the A-V node, but have little effect on the QRS width or the Q-T interval.

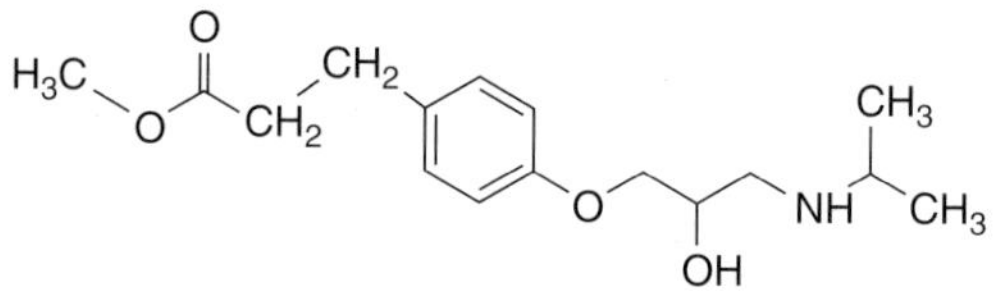

FIGURE 4-15   Molecular structure of esmolol.

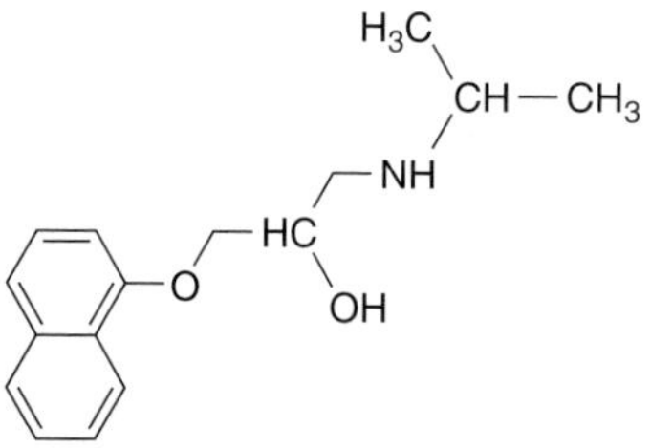

FIGURE 4-16   Molecular structure of propranolol.

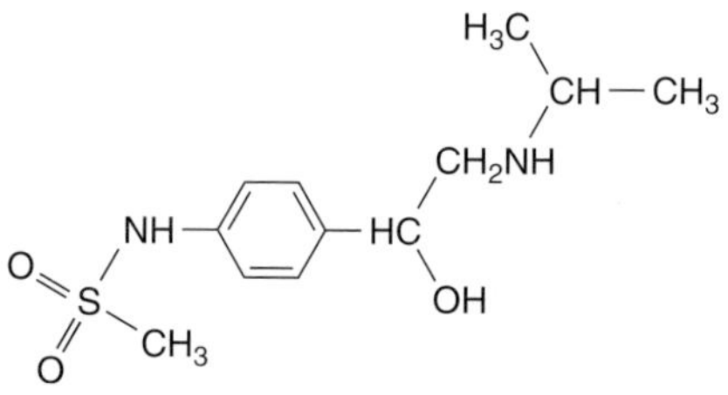

FIGURE 4-17   Molecular structure of sotalol.

SIDE EFFECTS

Frequent side effects of the beta blockers may include bradycardia (slow heart-beats); bronchial spasms, cough; nausea, stomach pain, loss of appetite; hypoglycemia (but esmolol is less likely to cause this problem); decreased sexual desire; jaundice (yellowing of the skin or eyes); muscle weakness and pain; blurred vision; dizziness, drowsiness, lightheadedness, mental confusion; and impotence especially by propranolol; and rarely may they cause allergic reactions such as difficulty in breathing; and skin hives.

DRUG INTERACTIONS

See Appendix B-1: Interactions of Beta Blockers.

MISCELLANEOUS ANTIARRHYTHMIC DRUGS

Adenosine and **cibenzoline**. Adenosine (Adenocard) may be administered by IV to suppress ventricular arrhythmias associated with acute myocardial infarction.

MECHANISM OF ACTION

Adenosine: Adenosine has a selective depressant effect on the abnormal accessory A-V node, where it, probably by increasing efflux of potassium ions, hyperpolarizes the node to slow the abnormal impulse conduction speed and to interrupt reentry of retrograde impulses through the node. However, adenosine is not effective in converting rhythms other than PSVT, and is not effective in treating atrial flutter or atrial fibrillation.

Cibenzoline: Cibenzoline is a new class antiarrhythmic drug that can thwart shortening of action potential in hypoxic condition. Cibenzoline has little anticholinergic activity and hence has less tendency toward proarrhythmia. Though regarded as one of the class-1a antiarrhythmic drugs, cibenzoline blocks the ATP-sensitive K^+ channels, rather than the sodium channel, in the heart to increase duration of action potential with a slowed repolarization.

SIDE EFFECTS

Adenosine: Possible side effects by adenosine include fast or irregular heartbeats, pressure in the chest, and flushing of the face; bronchoconstriction; nausea; dizziness and lightheadedness; and such allergic reactions as skin rash, hives, and itching.

Cibenzoline: Possible side effects by cibenzoline include proarrhythmia, though rarer than by others; hypoglycemia; liver and renal dysfunctions; and diaphragmatic neuromuscular blockade.

BOX 4-4

Basic Concepts of Adenosine Interactions

Adenosine slows the A-V conduction speed, and when it is taken together with other drugs that also slow that speed it may possibly lead to bradycardia and even complete heart block. Examples include: **digoxin; dipyridamole** (a coronary vasodilator and a known inhibitor of adenosine reuptake, which can slow A-V conduction; and **verapamil** (a calcium-channel blocker).

DRUG INTERACTIONS

Adenosine

See Box 4-4.

Miscellaneous Interactions of Adenosine (ADS)

ADS ⟷ Caffeine: Caffeine administered together with adenosine can competitively antagonize pharmacologic effects of adenosine and may require an increased dose of the latter. Caffeine appears to be a nonselective antagonist of a certain adenosine receptor, but the exact mechanism behind this cardiac effect remains obscure.

ADS ⟷ Theophylline: Theophylline when taken together can competitively antagonize pharmacologic effects of adenosine. Theophylline appears to be a nonselective antagonist of a certain adenosine receptor, but the exact mechanism behind this cardiac effect remains to be elucidated.

Cibenzoline

Hepatic inactivation of cibenzoline appears to require the presence of microsomal CYP3A4, and hence inhibition of this enzyme by any other drug such as cimetidine taken together may raise its blood levels and adverse effects.

Angina Pectoris

Angina pectoris literally means "pain of the chest." This pain or discomfort is due to an inadequate supply of oxygen and nutrition to the heart muscle. A crushing chest pain may be felt just behind the sternum (breastbone) and usually spreads to the left arm. Often, the pain is accompanied by a sensation of faintness and difficulty in breathing. This pain may last about 15 minutes.

Medications shown effective to prevent or relieve a sudden attack of angina include: (1) vasodilators such as **isosorbide mononitrate** (Imdur, Ismo) and **nitroglycerin sublingual** (Nitroquick, Nitrostat); (2) beta blockers such as **acebutolol** (Sectral), **bisoprolol** (Zebeta), **metoprolol** (Lopressor, Toprol XL), **nadolol** (Corgard), **pindolol** (Visken), and **propranolol;** and (3) calcium-channel blockers such as **diltiazem** and **verapamil.**

VASODILATORS

Isosorbide mononitrate and **nitroglycerin sublingual**

MECHANISM OF ACTION

Both isosorbide mononitrate and nitroglycerin are converted to nitric oxide in the body by mitochondrial aldehyde dehydrogenase. Nitric oxide (NO) in turn activates guanylate cyclase to raise intracellular levels of cyclic-GMP that can induce quick vasodilation.

SIDE EFFECTS

Their possible side effects include cardiac arrhythmia; dry mouth, nausea, and vomiting; warmth, redness, or tingling under the skin; headache and dizziness; and may rarely cause allergic reactions such as skin hives and itching

DRUG INTERACTIONS

See Box 5-1.

BOX 5-1

Basic Concepts of Isosorbide & Nitroglycerin Interactions

Both isosorbide mononitrate and nitroglycerin cause rapid fall of blood pressure. When either drug is taken concurrently with other drugs that cause hypotension, a precipitous fall of pressure may result. Examples include: **ACE Inhibitors** (*See* Ω-1 in Appendix A); **alpha blockers** (*See* Ω-6 in Appendix A); **calcium-channel blockers** (*See* Ω-31 in Appendix A); and **beta blockers** (*See* Ω-27 in Appendix A) (labetalol is unusual in that it has not only a beta blocking effect but also a selective alpha-1 blocking effect—hence this combination will cause a greater fall of blood pressure than by combination with other pure beta blockers); **ganglionic blockers** (*See* Ω-41 in Appendix A); **anesthetic agents** (See Ω-9 in Appendix A) (most general anesthetic agents have a slight hypotensive effect of their own); and **erectile dysfunction drugs** (See Ω-38 in Appendix A) (sildenafil (Viagra), tadalafil (Cialis), and vardenafil (Levitra) each have their own vasodilating effect).

Miscellaneous Interactions of Nitroglycerin (NGR)

NGR ⟷ Alteplase: Nitroglycerin when used in combination may reduce the serum levels and thrombolytic effect of alteplase. Nitroglycerin appears to increase blood flow and help increase metabolism of alteplase in the liver.

NGR ⟷ L-Carnitine: L-Carnitine is thought to help the heart to produce energy more efficiently and may enable it to get by with less oxygen. However, L-carnitine reduces tolerance to nitroglycerin in patients with angina, permitting severe headache and hypotension when it is taken together with nitroglycerin or with isosorbide mononitrate.

NGR ⟷ Heparin: Nitroglycerin used in combination may reduce the anticoagulant effects of heparin sodium even at low doses. The exact mechanism involved remains unclear but it appears to result from acceleration of heparin elimination by nitroglycerin.

NGR ⟷ Neuromuscular Blockers: (*See* Ω -53 in Appendix A) Nitroglycerin used in combination may increase the pharmacological effects of neuromuscular blockers, such as pancuronium, tubocurarine, and vecuronium, to prolong respiratory depressions. Though the mechanism behind this observation is unclear, concurrent administration of nitroglycerin and pancuronium, therefore, is not recommended.

BETA BLOCKERS

Acebutolol, bisoprolol, metoprolol, nadolol, pindolol, and **propranolol**

MECHANISM OF ACTION

They lessen cardiac contractility and heart rates by blocking myocardial beta receptors, and thereby prevent exercise-induced increase in oxygen demands by the heart. Thus, they are only for the prevention of angina and not for treatment of acute angina attack or variant angina.

SIDE EFFECTS

The frequent side effects of these beta blockers include hypotension; shortness of breath or wheezing; abdominal cramps, nausea, diarrhea, and constipation; fatigue; memory loss; and lightheadedness and insomnia. They also raise blood triglyceride levels while reducing blood levels of both "good-cholesterol" (HDL) and glucose. Metoprolol is less likely to cause hypoglycemia.

DRUG INTERACTIONS

See Appendix B-1: Interactions of Beta Blockers.

CALCIUM-CHANNEL BLOCKERS

Diltiazem and **verapamil**

MECHANISM OF ACTION

They, by blocking membrane calcium-channels, depress contractility of myocardium and induce coronary vasodilation to lessen oxygen demand by the heart and to improve oxygen supply to the myocardium, respectively.

SIDE EFFECTS

Possible side effects of calcium-channel blockers include cardiac arrhythmia; nausea, diarrhea, and jaundice (yellowing of the skin); headache, fatigue, and tiredness; and may they rarely cause allergic reactions too.

DRUG INTERACTIONS

See Appendix B-7: Interactions of Calcium-Channel Blockers.

CHAPTER 6

Thrombosis/Myocardial Infarction

Thrombosis refers to obstruction of a blood vessel by a thrombus (blood clot). If a blood clot forms in a deep vein, most commonly in the femoral vein of the leg, the clot may break off and be carried by the blood into the pulmonary artery. This clot, now called an embolus, may block the artery and cause a life-threatening event. Platelet aggregation is often involved in blood clotting and consequent obstruction of coronary blood flow that leads to myocardial infarction.

The term myocardial infarction refers to destruction of the heart tissue due to obstruction of one or more of the coronary arteries that supply blood to the heart. Myocardial infarction can precipitate cardiac arrhythmia, heart failure, and cardiogenic shock.

Medications shown effective in the prevention of thrombosis include: (1) **heparin** or **low-molecular-weight heparin** (LMWH) such as **enoxaparin** (Lovenox, Clexane); (2) **lepirudin** (Refludan); and (3) oral anticoagulants such as **warfarin** (Coumadin).

Medications shown effective to lessen the chance of myocardial infarction include (4) **clopidogrel** (Plavix); (5) glycoprotein llb/llla receptor antagonists such as **abciximab** and **eptifibatide;** and (6) thrombolytic agents (drugs that dissolve blood clots already formed) such as **alteplase, anistreplase, reteplase, streptokinase,** and **urokinase.** Anistreplase is a complex molecule, where the p-anisoyl group (Fig. 6-1) is conjugated to the complex of a bacteria-derived streptokinase and human plasma-derived Lys-plasminogen proteins.

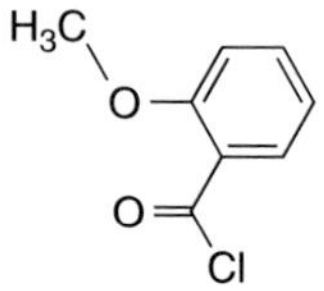

FIGURE 6-1 Molecular structure of anisoyl group.

HEPARIN OR LOW-MOLECULAR-WEIGHT HEPARIN

Injection of heparin or a low-molecular-weight heparin (LMWH), such as **enoxaparin,** opposes formation of a new blood clot. The LMWH is usually injected subcutaneously to obtain a longer duration of action than regular heparin. Heparin is the only drug that can produce rapid anticoagulation. The onset of its action is immediate following intravenous injection, and about 30 minutes after its subcutaneous injection.

MECHANISM OF ACTION

Heparin works by binding to antithrombin-lll, an alpha-2 globulin in the blood; and the heparin-antithrombin-lll complex then enhances inactivation of thrombin (Fig. 6-2) by binding to it. The anticoagulant effect of enoxaparin derives mainly from its inhibition of the coagulation factor Xa, which catalyzes the conversion of prothrombin to thrombin. As formation of thrombin is decreased, it helps prevent fibrin clot formation. However, these anticoagulants mentioned above do not dissolve blood clots already formed.

SIDE EFFECTS

Their possible side effects include nausea and vomiting; sweating, thrombocytopenia (a low platelet count in the blood) with bleeding episodes even for several weeks after termination of heparin; osteoporosis (loss of bone minerals leading to brittle bones); and some allergic reactions such as hives, itching, trouble breathing, and swelling of face, lips, tongue, or throat.

DRUG INTERACTIONS

See Box 6-1.

Miscellaneous Interactions of Heparin or LMWH (HPN)

Parentheses below indicate an herb.

HPN ⟷ Cefamandole: Cephalosporins (Fig. 6-3) containing an N-methylthiotetrazole or a similar side chain, such as cefamandole (Fig. 6-4), have caused hypoprothrombinemia and bleeding even when used alone. Concurrent use of them with heparin or LMWH may further the risk of excessive hemorrhage.

HPN ⟷ Dextran: Dextran interferes with fibrin polymerization and enhances fibrinolysis mediated by plasmin; and hence co-administration of it with either heparin or a LMWH may further the tendency toward excessive hemorrhage.

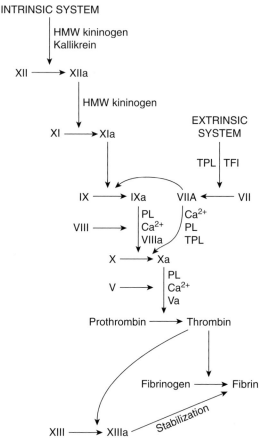

FIGURE 6-2   Thrombin site of action. Reproduced, with permission, from Barrett KE, Barman SM, Boitano S, and Brooks HL. *Ganong's Review of Medical Physiology*. 23rd ed. New York, NY: McGraw-Hill; 2010, p 533.

BOX 6-1

Basic Concepts of Heparin or LMWH Interactions

1. Heparin or LMWH is prone to produce hemorrhage, and concurrent administration of either of them with drugs that have a similar tendency may result in excessive bleeding. Examples include: **human antithrombin-III; argatroban,** a synthetic anticoagulant that inhibits thrombin-catalyzed reactions such as fibrin formation and activation of coagulation factors VIII and XIII; **antiplatelet drugs** (*See* Ω-22 in Appendix A); and **thrombolytic agents** (*See* Ω-74 in Appendix A).

BOX 6-1 *(continued)*

2. Co-administration of either Heparin or LMWH with any drug that inhibits synthesis of thromboxane by blocking the COX-1 enzyme can increase the tendency toward excessive bleeding. Those drugs include: **non-steroidal anti-inflammatory drugs** (*See* Ω -54 in Appendix A) including **salicylates** (*See* Ω-64 in Appendix A).

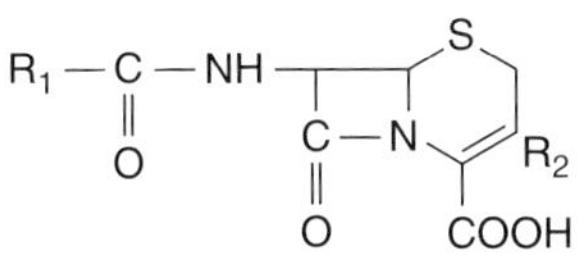

FIGURE 6-3 Basic Molecular structures of cephalosporins.

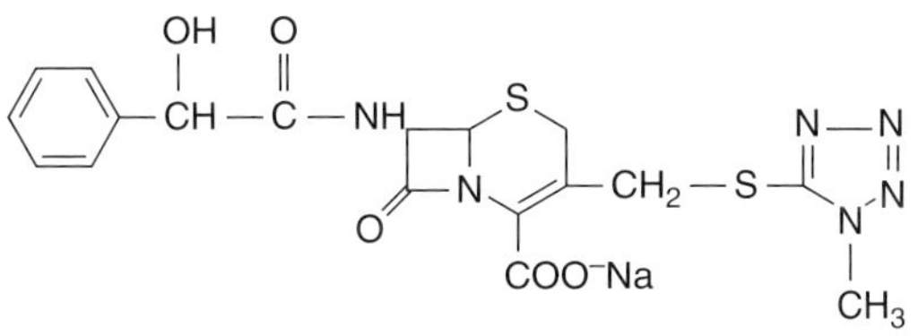

FIGURE 6-4 Molecular structure of cefamandole.

HPN ⟷ Fludrocortisone: Side effects of fludrocortisone include thrombophlebitis and hypercoagulability, and its use in combination may oppose the anticoagulants effects of heparin. It is recommended to have their blood clotting time (INR) regularly monitored.

HPN ⟷ (Chamomile): Some coumarins, such as 7-methoxycoumarin, are detected in chamomile and hence, co-administration with either heparin or a LMWH may result in excessive bleeding.

HPN ⟷ Valproic Acid: Valproic acid can reduce the number of platelets or inhibit the ability of platelets to aggregate, and hence valproic acid used in combination with heparin or with such a low-molecular-weight heparin as enoxaparin (Lovenox) can cause excessive hemorrhage.

LEPIRUDIN

In case thrombocytopenia has developed as a result of an antibody-mediated reaction to heparin, lepirudin (Refludan) is another option to prevent blood clotting.

MECHANISM OF ACTION

Lepirudin is a protein derived from the saliva of a medicinal leech. The protein is a highly specific, direct inhibitor of thrombin, insomuch as one molecule of

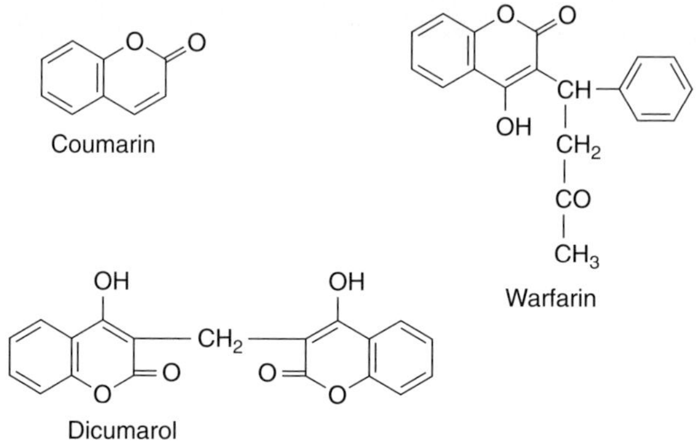

FIGURE 6-5   Molecular structures of coumarin derivatives.

lepirudin, even in the absence of antithrombin-lll, binds one molecule of thrombin to make it dysfunctional, opposing formation of blood clot.

SIDE EFFECTS

Lepirudin may cause easy bruising or bleeding; nausea, vomiting, and bloody stools; allergic reactions such as skin rash; difficulty in breathing; tightness in the chest; and swelling of the mouth, face, lips, or tongue.

DRUG INTERACTIONS

If co-administered with the following drugs, the bleeding tendency of lepirudin will be increased: such anticoagulants as dicumarol and warfarin (Fig. 6-5); and such thrombolytic agents as alteplase, streptokinase, and urokinase.

ORAL ANTICOAGULANTS

Oral anticoagulants shown effective in the treatment of thrombosis include **warfarin** (*Coumadin*). Warfarin (*See* Fig. 6-5) is a racemic mixture, and the S-isomer possesses about three times the anticoagulant effect of the R-isomer.

MECHANISM OF ACTION

Warfarin works by inhibition of vitamin K epoxide reductase, the enzyme important to make the active form of vitamin K, an essential vitamin required for blood coagulation.

SIDE EFFECTS

Warfarin may cause nausea, vomiting, stomach pain, and loss of appetite; jaundice (yellowing of the skin or conjunctiva); bleeding (such as nosebleeds, bleeding gums, and blood in the urine); headache and confusion; and allergic reactions such as skin hives and itching.

DRUG INTERACTIONS

See Box 6-2.

BOX 6-2

Basic Concepts of Warfarin Interactions

1. Co-administration of warfarin with a drug that also has a bleeding tendency may result in excessive hemorrhage. Such drugs include: **cefamandole** (an antibiotic drug); **cefoperazone** (an antibiotic drug); **cefotetan** (an antibiotic drug); **dextrothyroxine** (Choloxin); and **heparin.**

2. Warfarin is weakly bound to plasma albumin and can be displaced if used in combination with drugs that have a higher affinity for binding. This displacement raises blood levels and adverse effects of free warfarin. Those high affinity drugs include: **aspirin** and other salicylates (*also see* non-steroidal anti-inflammatory drugs [NSAIDs]; many **sulfonamides** (chemotherapeutic agents); **duloxetine** (a drug used to treat major depression); **etoposide** (an anticancer drug); **mefloquine** (an antimalarial drug); **propoxyphene** (an analgesic drug); **SSRIs** (*See* Ω-68 in Appendix A) (all these SSRIs are highly protein-bound to displace warfarin from its protein-binding sites); **trastuzumab** (a drug used for breast cancer that might displace warfarin from its protein-binding sites); and **NSAIDs** (*See* Ω-54 in Appendix A): When taken together, warfarin may be displaced from its protein-binding sites by many NSAIDs, especially indomethacin, ketoprofen, naproxen, and by a metabolite of nabumetone; and furthermore, all of the NSAIDs, with possible exception of celecoxib, meloxicam, and nabumetone (Fig. 6-6), may also inhibit platelet aggregation to enhance the anticoagulant effects of warfarin.

3. Warfarin taken with an antiplatelet agent may result in excessive bleeding. (*See* Ω-22 in Appendix A for a list of the agents).

4. Warfarin works by suppression of availability of the active form of vitamin K, and when taken with other drugs that also have some anti-vitamin-K activity, it may potentiate the anticoagulant effect of warfarin. Those drugs

continued

BOX 6-2 (continued)

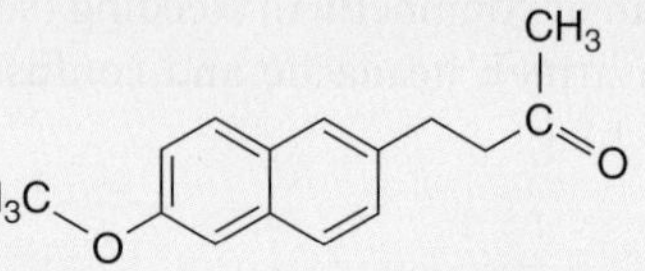

FIGURE 6-6   Molecular structure of nabumetone.

include: **propylthiouracil** (an antithyroid drug); **quinine,** which appears to depress the hepatic enzyme system that synthesizes vitamin K–dependent clotting factors; **aminoglycoside antibiotics** (*See* Ω-7 in Appendix A), which can suppress vitamin K–producing intestinal flora; **methimazole,** a drug useful to treat hyperthyroidism that has some anti-vitamin-K activity similar to warfarin; **tetracycline antibiotics** (*See* Ω-72 in Appendix A), all of which not only chelate the calcium ions required for blood clotting, but also kill vitamin K–producing intestinal flora; and **thyroid preparations** (*See* Ω-75 in Appendix A)—thyroid hormones increase catabolism of vitamin K–dependent clotting factors.

Miscellaneous Interactions of Warfarin (WFR)

Parentheses below indicate an herb.

WFR ⟷ Anabolic Steroids: (*See* Ω-8 in Appendix A.) Anabolic steroids such as testosterone and oxandrolone can enhance the effectiveness of such oral anticoagulants as warfarin when used in combination, probably by their opposing formation of blood clotting factors and by enhancing their degradations.

WFR ⟷ Bismuth Subsalicylate: Bismuth subsalicylate is a salicylate that can cause a bleeding problem when used alone in patients with ulcers. Its concurrent intake with heparin or with an oral anticoagulant such as warfarin may increase the risk of bleeding.

WFR ⟷ Cholestyramine: Co-administration of cholestyramine with warfarin can reduce gastrointestinal absorption of the latter to undercut its therapeutic effectiveness.

WFR ⟷ Clofibrate: Co-administration of warfarin with clofibrate, a lipid-lowering drug, was shown to cause excessive bleeding. Clofibrate did not displace

TABLE 6-1   Warfarin vs CYP Enzymes

Drug Name	1A2	2A6	2B6	2C8	2C9	2C18	2C19	2D6	2E1	3A4
R-Warfarin	Sub					Sub	Sub			Sub
S-Warfarin				Sub	**Sub**					

Abbreviations: Sub, substrate of the enzyme; Inh, Inhibits the enzyme; Ezi, induces the enzyme

1. CYP3A4 is extensively involved in the metabolism of many drugs, and its presence in the small intestine is responsible for poor oral bioavailability of many drugs such as R-warfarin.

2. Warfarin requires several microsomal enzymes for its metabolic clearance, as are shown in this table and hence, inhibition of these enzymes by drugs administered together can raise blood levels and the adverse effects of warfarin. Those inhibitory drugs include: chloramphenicol, cimetidine, disulfiram, erythromycin, metronidazole, and quinidine. (*See* the left-hand column of Table-0 at the 'Introduction' for other possible inhibitors of those enzymes.)

3. If tamoxifen (an inhibitor of CYP2C9) is used in combination with S-warfarin (a strong substrate of CYP2C9), it interferes with clearance of warfarin to increase its blood levels and adverse effects, such as excessive bleeding.

4. Aminoglutethimide can induce CYP1A2, CYP3A4, CYP2C9, and CYP2C19, those enzymes involved in metabolic clearance of warfarin. Hence, concurrent intake of aminoglutethimide can quicken clearance of warfarin to reduce its therapeutic effectiveness.

5. Zafirlukast, an inhibitor of CYP1A2, CYP2C9, and CYP3A4, taken together can oppose elimination of warfarin to raise its blood levels and adverse effects.

warfarin from its protein-binding sites nor delayed its elimination, and it is believed that clofibrate potentiates the activity of warfarin by interaction at its receptor site.

WFR ⟷ Cyclophosphamide: Cyclophosphamide itself can reduce production of platelets to cause bleeding in the bladder. When used in combination warfarin is likely to increase such bleeding incidences by cyclophosphamide.

WFR ⟷ CYP Isozymes: *See* Table 6-1.

WFR ⟷ Gemfibrozil: When taken together, gemfibrozil can increase the risk of bleeding caused by warfarin.

WFR ⟷ (Coumarin-Like Herbs): Some herbal remedies contain coumarin-like substances so as to promote bleeding when taken with warfarin. They include **(chamomile)** and **(licorice).**

WFR ⟷ (Herbs Opposing Platelets): Some herbal remedies contain ingredients that inhibit synthesis of thromboxane (Fig. 6-7), interfering with platelet aggregation; or interrupting directly the functions of blood platelets so as to promote bleeding when taken together with warfarin. Those herbs include **(dong quai)** (Fig. 6-8 A and B), an herb known in Chinese medicine to treat menstrual

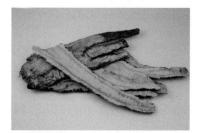

FIGURE 6-7   Molecular structure of thromboxane.

disturbance and amenorrhea; **(feverfew)** (Fig. 6-9), an herb that reduces fever and headache; **(garlic)**; **(ginger)**; **(hawthorn)**; and **(turmeric).**

WFR ⟷ (Herbs Promoting Metabolic Clearance of Warfarin): Some herbal remedies appear to contain ingredients that occasionally enhance the metabolic clearance of warfarin to lower its serum levels and anticoagulant efficacy. These herbs include **(ginseng),** which when taken at daily doses for two weeks had caused reduced serum levels of warfarin.

WFR ⟷ Glucagon: If glucagon and warfarin are taken together, the blood is much less likely to clot. The mechanism behind this interaction is yet to be elucidated.

WFR ⟷ Grape Juice: Grape juice used in combination can enhance anticoagulant effectiveness of warfarin. Grape juice is known to oppose metabolic inactivation of warfarin through CYP enzymes.

WFR ⟷ Leflunomide: Leflunomide (a drug to treat rheumatoid arthritis) when used in combination may raise blood levels and increase the anticoagulant effects of warfarin. One possible mechanism of this interaction is that S-warfarin is mainly cleared through CYP2C9 and leflunomide is inhibitory to this enzyme.

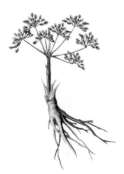

FIGURE 6-8   **A. Image of dong quai.**
(courtesy of Vita Green International, Inc.
at http://www.vitagreen.com/)

FIGURE 6-8   **B. Dong quai (sliced root).**

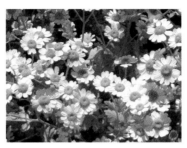

FIGURE 6-9   **Feverfew flowers.** (attribution: Wikipedia at
http://www.herbal-supplement-resource.com/feverfew-herb.html)

WFR ⟷ Omega-3 Fatty Acids: Omega-3 fatty acids (Fig. 6-10) are a family of polyunsaturated fatty acids, each of which has at least three double bonds starting at the third carbon from the methyl group (the omega end). Studies have shown that omega-3 fatty acids reduce platelet aggregability. The omega-3 fatty acids in flaxseed oil may increase the blood-thinning effects of warfarin or other anticoagulants taken in combination.

WFR ⟷ Piracetam: Piracetam (a drug used in cognitive disorders and dementia) causes an increase in prothrombin time and is currently being investigated as a complement to warfarin. Concurrent administration of piracetam with warfarin is apt to increase the tendency toward excessive bleeding.

WFR ⟷ Tramadol: If tramadol (an analgesic drug) is taken with warfarin, which is highly bound to plasma albumin but with a low affinity, it can displace warfarin, resulting in elevated plasma levels and potentially exacerbating warfarin's adverse effects.

WFR ⟷ Valproic Acid: Valproic acid (an antiepileptic drug) tends to oppose the formation of a blood clot. Hence, if used in combination with anticoagulants such as dicumarol, heparin, warfarin (Coumadin), and Lovenox, a LMWH, valproic acid can cause excessive bleeding.

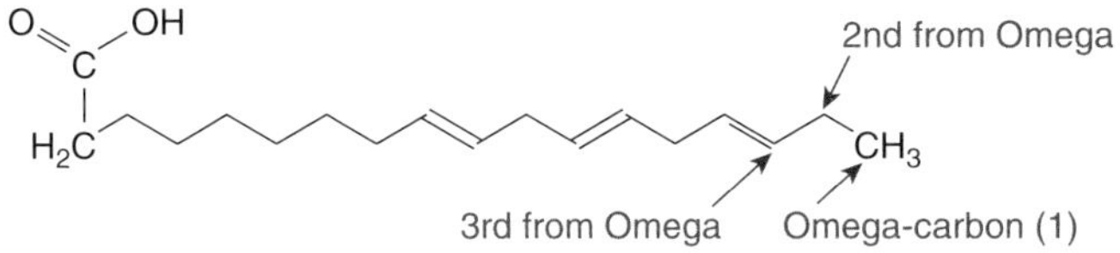

FIGURE 6-10   Molecular structure of linolenic acid (an omega-3 fatty acid).

CLOPIDOGREL

Clopidogrel (Plavix) has been shown effective to lessen the chance of stroke or heart attack.

MECHANISM OF ACTION

Clopidogrel (Fig. 6-11) is an inactive prodrug. The majority of clopidogrel is destroyed by hydrolysis by esterases in the liver to a carboxylic acid derivative, and the rest has to be activated by microsomal cytochrome P450 (CYP) to become active. Clopidogrel was first oxidized mainly by CYP 2C19 to 2-oxo-clopidogrel, a thiolactone, which in turn undergoes a second step of oxidation, mainly by CYP3A4 and to a lesser degree by CYP2C19, to a thiol acid, the active metabolite of clopidogrel. The final active metabolite contains a free thiol group that is able to block the ADP receptor on the platelets by forming a disulfide bridge with a cysteine residue of the platelet ADP receptor to prevent linking of fibrinogen to the receptor, without which platelets cannot aggregate to cause myocardial infarction or stroke.

SIDE EFFECTS

Clopidogrel may cause irregular heartbeat; bleeding (such as nosebleed, vomiting of blood, and blood in urine or stools); shortness of breath; stomach pain or sore throat; difficult urination; headache; and fever, chills; and anxiety.

DRUG INTERACTIONS

Clopidogrel (CDG)

CDG ↔ Abciximab: Both clopidogrel and abciximab are classified as antiplatelet agents and hence, when taken together may result in excessive bleeding.

CDG ↔ Aspirin: Aspirin inhibits the synthesis of thromboxane which promotes platelet aggregation. When used in combination it may increase the risk of hemorrhage caused by clopidogrel, a potent oral antiplatelet agent.

CDG ↔ CYP Isozymes: *See* Table 6-2.

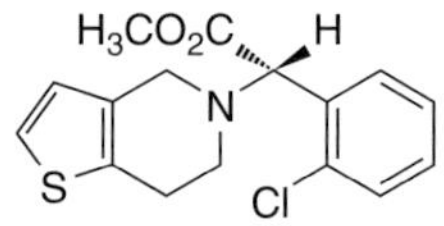

FIGURE 6-11   Molecular structure of clopidogrel.

TABLE 6-2 Clopidogrel vs CYP Enzymes

Drug Name	1A2	2A6	2B6	2C8	2C9	2C18	2C19	2D6	2E1	3A4
Clopidogrel							Sub+			Sub
			Inh		Inh		Inh			

Abbreviations: Sub, substrate of the enzyme; Inh, inhibits the enzyme; Ezi, induces the enzyme

1. The prodrug clopidogrel is activated mainly by CYP3A4 and CYP3A5 (not shown) to its active metabolite. Hence, inhibitors of the enzyme, such as erythromycin, can oppose activity of clopidogrel. (*See* the left-hand column of Table-0 at the 'Introduction' for other possible inhibitors of those enzymes.)
2. Clopidogrel functions as an inhibitor of CYP 2B6, CYP2C9, and 2C19; and hence co-administration of it with other drugs that require these enzymes for hepatic clearance may raise their blood levels to possibly whip their adverse effects into action. (*See* the middle column of Table-0 at the 'Introduction' for possible substrates of those enzymes).

CDG ⟷ NSAIDs: (*See* Ω-54 in Appendix A.) Non-steroidal anti-inflammatory drugs (NSAIDs) oppose synthesis of thromboxane. Co-administration of clopidogrel with an NSAID may increase the tendency toward gastrointestinal bleeding.

CDG ⟷ Omeprazole: Omeprazole (Prilosec), when used in combination, can undercut the effectiveness of clopidogrel, probably because omeprazole is a strong inhibitor of CYP2C19, more so than any other proton-pump inhibitors, preventing activation by oxidation of clopidogrel by this enzyme.

CDG ⟷ Valproic Acid: Valproic acid can lower the counts of platelets and inhibit their ability to form a blood clot. Hence valproic acid can cause excessive bleeding if used in combination with clopidogrel.

CDG ⟷ Warfarin: Co-administration of clopidogrel and warfarin is apt to increase the general tendency toward excessive bleeding.

GLYCOPROTEIN IIb / IIIa RECEPTOR ANTAGONISTS

Abciximab and **eptifibatide**

MECHANISM OF ACTION

Both of the above drugs bind to the glycoprotein (GP) IIb/IIIa receptors of human platelets and inhibit aggregation of platelets. They are mainly used during and after angioplasty to prevent platelets from forming a thrombus within the coronary artery.

SIDE EFFECTS

Abciximab and eptifibatide may cause bradycardia, hypotension, and bleeding due to thrombocytopenia; nausea, vomiting, and abdominal pain; chest pain; back pain; and headache.

DRUG INTERACTIONS

Both abciximab and eptifibatide can induce thrombocytopenia that can last for five days after initial administration of either drug. Hence use caution when either drug is to be used together with any drug that has a tendency to cause bleeding such as dicumarol, heparin, warfarin (Coumadin), and other thrombolytics or antiplatelet agents.

THROMBOLYTIC AGENTS

Alteplase, anistreplase, reteplase, streptokinase, and **urokinase**

These drugs can dissolve blood clots already formed, hence their classification as thrombolytic agents.

MECHANISM OF ACTION

Anistreplase, the anisoylated analog of the active form of the streptokinase-plasminogen complex, is a prodrug that has to have the anisoyl (or methoxybenzoyl) group (*See* Fig. 6-1) detached to become active. Those above drugs bind to fibrin first to activate fibrin-bound plasminogen and then the activated plasminogen dissolves clot fibrins.

SIDE EFFECTS

The most frequent adverse effect of all of the above drugs is bleeding. Other possible side effects include irregular heartbeat; stomach pain and nausea; fatigue or weakness; and headache or dizziness. Streptokinase may be prone to generate allergic reactions such as skin rash, itching, swelling; trouble breathing; and hypotension.

DRUG INTERACTIONS

It is not known whether other medications will interact with these thrombolytic agents, except that when any of them are used in combination with an oral anticoagulant, excessive bleeding may ensue.

7

Hemorrhage

Hemorrhage refers to excessive discharge of blood from a ruptured or wounded blood vessel.

Medications shown effective to stem hemorrhage include: (1) **oxymetazoline** (Afrin) or **phenylephrine** (Neosynephrine) to suppress nosebleed; (2) **vasopressin** to stem variceal hemorrhage; (3) **oxytocin** to prevent postpartum bleeding; and (4) loop diuretics such as **bumetanide** (Bumex) or **furosemide** to stop subarachnoid hemorrhage caused by increased intracranial pressure.

OXYMETAZOLINE OR PHENYLEPHRINE

MECHANISM OF ACTION

Both oxymetazoline (Fig. 7-1) and phenylephrine (Entex) (Fig. 7-2) have an adrenergic alpha-agonistic effect to constrict the small arterioles of the nasal passages to thwart blood flow.

SIDE EFFECTS

These two drugs may cause irregular or fast heartbeat; difficulty in breathing; nausea or vomiting; and sweating; and headache, insomnia, dizziness, or lightheadedness.

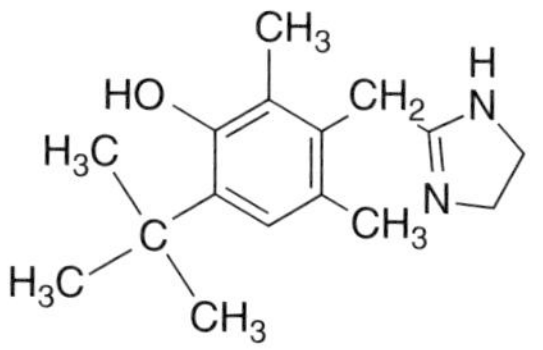

FIGURE 7-1 Molecular structure of oxymetazoline.

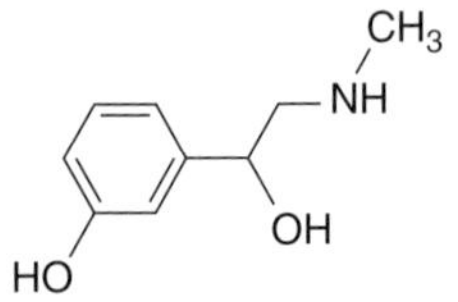

FIGURE 7-2   Molecular structure of phenylephrine.

DRUG INTERACTIONS

Chance of serious drug interactions is rather small between either drug used topically and other drugs taken orally, but *See* Appendix B-8: Interactions of Alpha Agonists for more information.

VASOPRESSIN

MECHANISM OF ACTION

Vasopressin (Fig. 7-3) is the so-called antidiuretic hormone (ADH), as it activates its receptor (V-2) at the kidney to increase water reabsorption. Vasopressin also acts on its receptor (V-1) at the smooth muscle of blood vessels to cause vasoconstriction. The Food and Drug Administration in 2010 has granted orphan drug status to intravenous use of terlipressin, an analog of vasopressin, for the treatment of Type-1 hepato-renal syndrome (HRS), where a rapid renal failure develops due to liver cirrhosis. Terlipressin activates vasopressin (V-1) receptor to cause constriction of splanchnic vessels to increase arterial volume and improve renal blood flow, thereby improving renal function in patients with HRS.

SIDE EFFECTS

Side effects of vasopressin may include high blood pressure, slowed heartbeat; pale skin due to reduction of blood flow; nausea, stomach bloating, abdominal cramps, diarrhea; blurred vision; dizziness and headache; and rarely, allergic reactions.

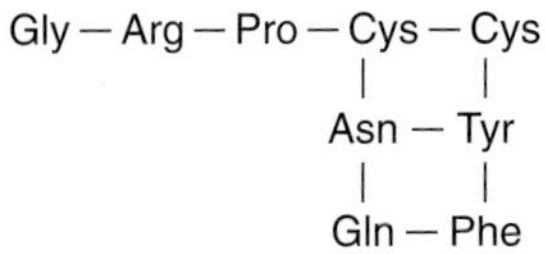

FIGURE 7-3   Molecular structure of vasopressin.

DRUG INTERACTIONS

No serious interaction reported with vasopressin or terlipressin, and it is not known whether other medications will interact with either of these two drugs.

OXYTOCIN

MECHANISM OF ACTION

Oxytocin (Fig. 7-4) activates its specific receptors at the uterine myometrium to increase concentrations of intracellular calcium ions, which in turn stimulate contractility of uterine smooth muscle, and the contraction is accompanied by reduced blood flow to the uterus.

SIDE EFFECTS

Oxytocin may cause irregular heartbeat; difficulty in breathing; nausea, vomiting; rupture of the uterus; dizziness, headache, confusion, and convulsions (seizures).

DRUG INTERACTIONS

Oxytocin (OXT)

Parentheses below indicated an herb.

OXT ⟷ (Sage): Sage, an herb, (Fig. 7-5) is known to have estrogen-like substances and can amplify oxytocin-induced uterine muscle contractility.

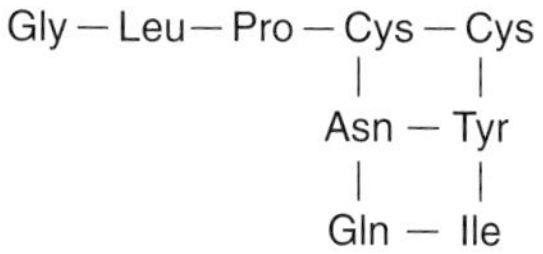

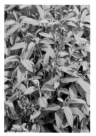

Gly — Leu — Pro — Cys — Cys
                   | |
           Asn — Tyr
            | |
           Gln — Ile

FIGURE 7-5 Sage leaves in nature.
(courtesy of Leo Michels at http://luirig.altervista.org/ schedeit/pz/salvia_officinalis.htm)

FIGURE 7-4 Molecular structure of oxytocin.

OXT ⟷ Vasopressors: (*See* Ω-79 in Appendix A.) Avoid taking oxytocin in combination with another vasoconstrictive drug, as a severe hypertension may ensue.

LOOP DIURETICS

Bumetanide and **furosemide**

These loop diuretics are useful to stop subarachnoid hemorrhage.

MECHANISM OF ACTION

Loop diuretics induce rapid lowering of the blood pressure to lessen the pressure involved in the subarachnoid hemorrhage.

SIDE EFFECTS

Possible side effects of loop diuretics include cardiac arrhythmia; hyperglycemia, hypokalemia, hyperuricemia; dry mouth, nausea, vomiting, stomach pain; ototoxicity (hearing loss); and allergic reactions such as swelling of the face, lips, tongue, or throat; and skin hives.

DRUG INTERACTIONS

See Appendix B-5: Interactions of Loop Diuretics.

CHAPTER

8

Anemia

Anemia is a condition in which the blood has insufficient numbers of red blood cells (RBCs) or insufficient quantity of hemoglobin, giving rise to such symptoms as fatigue, weakness, headache and dizziness. The hemoglobin in the RBCs is vital for transportation of oxygen to the mitochondria for generation of energy. Anemia may arise from deficiency of iron, folic acid, or vitamin B-12.

Medications shown effective in the treatment of anemia include: (1) **ferrous sulfate** or **ferrous fumarate** for microcytic hypochromic anemia; (2) **folic acid** for megaloblastic anemia; (3) **cyanocobalamin** (vitamin B-12) for pernicious anemia; (4) immunosuppressive agents such as **antithymocyte globulin** and **cyclosporine** to treat aplastic anemia; (5) **darbepoetin alfa** or **epoetin alfa** to stimulate production of RBCs originated from the stem cells within the bone marrow; (6) **granulocyte colony-stimulating factor** (GCSF) or **granulocyte-macrophage colony-stimulating factor** (GM-CSF) to help stimulate the bone marrow to produce new blood cells.

FERROUS SULFATE OR FERROUS FUMARATE

MECHANISM OF ACTION

Ferrous sulfate or ferrous fumarate provides iron, an essential component in the synthesis of heme for hemoglobin.

SIDE EFFECTS

When ingested, ferrous sulfate or ferrous fumarate may cause stomach cramping, staining of teeth, constipation, nausea, vomiting, and dark stools.

DRUG INTERACTIONS

Concurrent ingestion of either drug with an antibiotic within two hours of each other may impair intestinal absorption of the antibiotic. Those antibiotics that may be affected include: **ciprofloxacin** (Cipro), **demeclocycline** (Declomycin), **doxycycline** (Adoxa, Doryx, Oracea, Vibramycin), **levofloxacin** (Levaquin), **lomefloxacin** (Maxaquin), **minocycline** (Dynacin, Minocin, Solodyn, Vectrin), **norfloxacin** (Noroxin), **ofloxacin** (Floxin), and **tetracycline** (Brodspec, Panmycin, Sumycin, Tetracap).

FOLIC ACID

MECHANISM OF ACTION

Folic acid (chemically, pteroyl glutamic acid) (Fig. 8-1) is reduced first to dihydrofolate and then to tetrahydrofolate, which in turn is converted to $N^{5,10}$-CH_2-FH_4, a one-carbon carrier, important in the methylation of uracil at its position 5 to form thymine (5-methyl uracil) of the DNA. Hence, if no folic acid is available, no thymine is formed, and DNA cannot be synthesized. Macrocytic cells arise when mitosis of the RBC precursor cells in the bone marrow is impaired due to interrupted DNA synthesis. Therefore, folic acid helps to promote DNA synthesis so as to treat megaloblastic anemia.

SIDE EFFECTS

Folic acid may rarely cause nausea, decreased appetite, flatulence, and insomnia.

DRUG INTERACTIONS

Folic Acid (FLA)

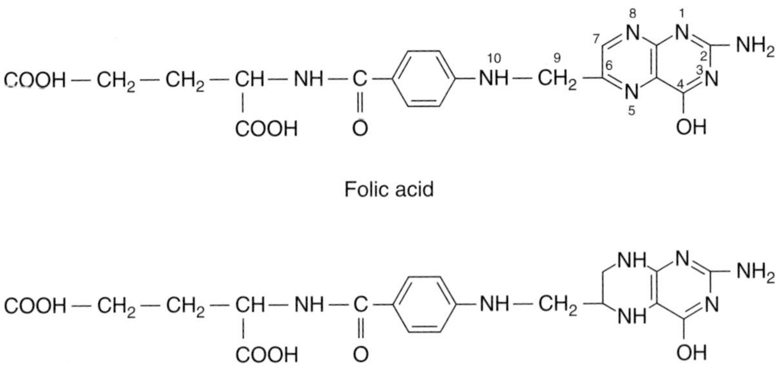

Folic acid

Tetrahydrofolic acid

FIGURE 8-1   Molecular structures of folic acid and THFA.

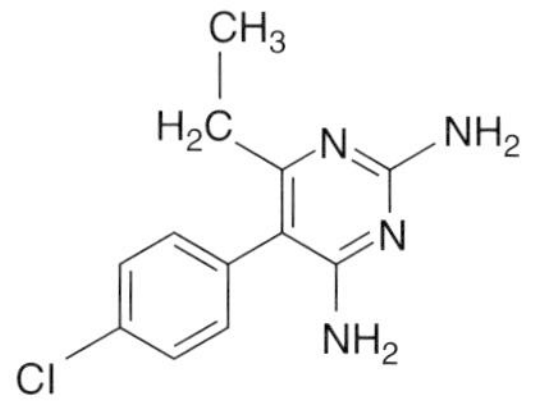

FIGURE 8-2   Molecular structure of pyrimethamine.

FLA ⟷ Cholesterol-Lowering Drugs: (*See* Ω-33 in Appendix A.) The cholesterol-lowering agents such as cholestyramine and colestipol have the ability to adsorb folic acid to impair its intestinal absorption.

FLA ⟷ Phenytoin: Concurrent use of large doses of folic acid and phenytoin (Dilantin) has resulted in decreased serum concentrations of phenytoin to undercut its therapeutic effectiveness, allowing increased seizure frequency. The mechanism behind this observation remains unclear.

FLA ⟷ Pyrimethamine: Pyrimethamine (Fig. 8-2), a drug commonly used as an antimalarial agent, works by inhibition of the enzyme dihydrofolate reductase to oppose the formation of tetrahydrofolate required for DNA synthesis in the malarial parasite. Therefore, folic acid taken together may win the above enzyme over to supply dihydrofolate and to undercut therapeutic effectiveness of pyrimethamine.

FLA ⟷ Sulfasalazine: Intestinal absorption of dietary folic acid is likely impaired by concurrent administration of sulfasalazine, a chemotherapeutic for ulcerative colitis. Sulfasalazine appears to compete with folic acid for intestinal absorption.

CYANOCOBALAMIN

MECHANISM OF ACTION

Cyanocobalamin (or vitamin B-12) (Fig. 8-3) is required for conversion of $(N^5\text{-}CH_3)\text{-}FH_4$, a storage form of folate, to FH_4, a form of folate useful for the formation of thymine from uracil. Hence, if no cyanocobalamin is present, no storage form of folate can be mobilized to synthesize DNA in the RBC precursor cells, to result in the production of macrocytic cells in megaloblastic anemia. Additionally, cyanocobalamin is required for the conversion of methylmalonyl CoA to succinyl CoA to enter the TCA cycle (or Kreb cycle). Therefore, in the absence of cyanocobalamin, methylmalonyl CoA accumulates and competes with natural malonyl CoA for the synthesis of fatty acids to be incorporated into

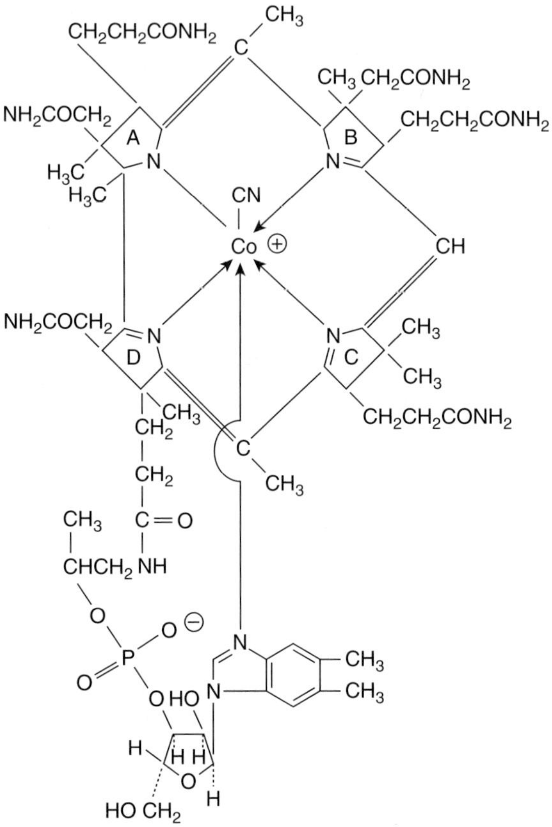

FIGURE 8-3   **Molecular structure of vitamin B-12.** Reproduced, with permission, from Barrett KE, Barman SM, Boitano S, and Brooks HL. *Ganong's Review of Medical Physiology.* 23rd ed. New York, NY: McGraw-Hill; 2010, p 434.

phospholipids of the neuronal membrane, and this can result in the production of aberrant phospholipids with consequent neurological disturbances.

SIDE EFFECTS

Cyanocobalamin may rarely cause irregular heartbeat; diarrhea; muscle weakness or cramping; fever or chills; and allergic reactions such as swelling of the mouth, face, lips, or tongue.

DRUG INTERACTIONS

See Box 8-1.

BOX 8-1

Basic Concepts of Cyanocobalamin Interactions

If gastric pH rises by taking other drugs in combination, the intestinal absorption of cyanocobalamin (vitamin B-12) is impaired. Such drugs include: (1) **gastric antacids** such as aluminum hydroxide; **H-2 blockers** (*See* Ω-45 in Appendix A); and **proton-pump inhibitors** (*See* Ω-61 in Appendix A).

Miscellaneous Interactions of Cyanocobalamin (CBM)

CBM ⟷ Alcohol: Intestinal absorption of cyanocobalamin (vitamin B-12) tends to be impaired when taken together with alcohol.

CBM ⟷ Chloramphenicol: Chloramphenicol (at serum levels of 25 mcg/ml or more) used in combination may cause depression of bone marrow, making it unresponsive to the therapeutic effects of cyanocobalamin.

CBM ⟷ Neomycin: Intestinal absorption of cyanocobalamin (vitamin B-12) tends to be decreased to lower its blood concentrations when taken together with neomycin, an antibiotic drug, but prolonged use of large doses of neomycin is needed to induce pernicious anemia. Neomycin appears to cause mucosal damage, and inhibits pancreatic enzymes to cause malabsorption.

CBM ⟷ Tetracycline: Cyanocobalamin, as well as all the vitamin B complex members taken concurrently with tetracycline, impairs its intestinal absorption to undercut the therapeutic effectiveness of tetracycline.

IMMUNOSUPPRESSIVE AGENTS

Antithymocyte globulin and **cyclosporine**

To treat aplastic anemia, these immunosuppressive agents may be used until stem cell transplantation can be performed. Antithymocyte globulin is usually used in combination with cyclosporine.

MECHANISM OF ACTION

The precise mechanisms of action of these immunosuppressants remain obscure, but it is suggested that antithymocyte globulin has an inhibitory effect on the

CD8-positive T-lymphocytes (T8-cells, CD8 T-cells, or also called suppressor T-cells, as they recognize antigens on the surface of a virus-infected cell and bind to the infected cell to destroy it, and likewise to suppress growth of virus-infected hematopoietic precursor cells to lead to aplastic anemia). Antithymocyte globulin also appears to stimulate production of hemoglobin-containing erythroid cells. Cyclosporine, on the other hand, impairs production of interleukin-2 and thereby opposes secondary proliferation of cytotoxic T-lymphocytes that suppress growth of hematopoietic precursor cells.

SIDE EFFECTS

Antithymocyte Globulin: It may cause muscle aches and joint pain; serum sickness; and allergic reactions such as difficulty in breathing, skin rash, hives, and fever. The drug may be excreted into breast milk to cause serious side effects to the baby.

Cyclosporine: This drug may cause elevated blood pressure, hyperkalemia; nausea, abdominal cramps, and diarrhea; liver toxicity (yellowing of the skin or eyes); muscle or joint pain (myopathy); tremor or tingling of the hands or feet; loss of hair; mental confusion, headache, or blurred vision; coma and seizures; and, rarely, allergic reactions.

DRUG INTERACTIONS

Antithymocyte Globulin: There are no well known interactions, but when the doses of corticosteroids administered in combination are reduced, some previously masked reactions to antithymocyte globulin may rise to the surface.

Cyclosporine: *See* Box 8-2.

Miscellaneous Interactions of Cyclosporine (CSP)

CSP ⟷ Acetazolamide: Acetazolamide, when used in combination with cyclosporine, may increase the adverse effects of the latter, such as nephrotoxicity and neurotoxicity, by an unknown mechanism.

CSP ⟷ Caspofungin: Co-administration of cyclosporine and caspofungin is not recommended, for when taken together, cyclosporine can increase the serum levels of caspofungin to perk up its adverse effects such as elevated serum levels of aspartate aminotransferase (AST) and alanine transaminase (ALT), enzymes that are leaked out into the blood stream when the liver is damaged. Given that caspofungin is acetylated and hydrolyzed in the liver and little is excreted in the urine as unchanged form, the elevated blood levels of caspofungin is not due to impaired

GRANULOCYTE COLONY-STIMULATING FACTOR OR GRANULOCYTE-MACROPHAGE COLONY-STIMULATING FACTOR

MECHANISM OF ACTION

Aplastic anemia is characterized by hypoplastic bone marrow with pancytopenia, including neutropenia. Use of GCSF or GM-CSF in aplastic anemia is justified because of their ability to stimulate production of neutrophil precursors and to enhance functions of mature neutrophils so as to protect host immunity and to reduce early mortality by various infections.

SIDE EFFECTS

Possible side effects to be generated by these drugs include bone pain, and allergic reactions such as difficulty in breathing; swelling of lips; chest tightness; or skin rash.

DRUG INTERACTIONS

No clinically important interactions reported.

9

Varicose Veins

A varicose vein refers to a superficial vein, most commonly in the legs, that is abnormally dilated, giving rise to a sensation of pain. In a normal vein, valves keep bloods flowing toward the heart, but in a varicose vein the valves are weakened and do not function properly, allowing blood to accumulate in the vein to swell it.

Medications shown effective in the treatment of varicose vein include: (1) **polidocanol;** (2) **ethanolamine oleate;** and (3) **sodium morrhuate.**

POLIDOCANOL

One-time injection of 2 ml of 3% polidocanol (Aethoxysclerol) is of help but if the varicose vein is extensive, the drug may have to be injected more than once at monthly treatment intervals.

MECHANISM OF ACTION

There must be a proper concentration of polidocanol that causes damage to the endothelium of the abnormal vein to be sclerosed, while leaving the adjacent normal veins unaffected.

SIDE EFFECTS

Polidocanol may cause necrosis at the site of injection and may damage endothelia of the nearby normal vessels to result in a thrombosis or sepsis.

DRUG INTERACTIONS

It is not known whether other medications will interact with this medication.

ETHANOLAMINE OLEATE

MECHANISM OF ACTION

Intravenous injection of ethanolamine oleate generates an inflammatory reaction to lead to fibrosis and occlusion of the varicose vein.

SIDE EFFECTS

This medication can cause high incidences of ulceration and anaphylactic reactions. Thus, it is rarely used.

DRUG INTERACTIONS

It is not known whether other medications will interact with this drug.

SODIUM MORRHUATE

MECHANISM OF ACTION

Sodium morrhuate generates inflammation in the intima of varicose veins, causing the formation of a thrombus. The consequent occlusion can result in obliteration of the malfunctioning vein. Injection of hypertonic (20% or 23.4%) solution of sodium chloride into the varicose vein also may be of help.

SIDE EFFECTS

Sodium morrhuate can cause a very high incidence of ulceration and anaphylactic reactions. As such, this drug is rarely used.

DRUG INTERACTIONS

It is not known whether other medications will interact with this drug.

10

Hyperlipidemia

Hyperlipidemia refers to presence in the blood of an excess amount of fats or lipids such as cholesterol and triglycerides. Cholesterol is a vital substance for human survival as it serves as an essential precursor for the formation of many sex hormones, adrenal corticosteroids, bile acids, and vitamin D in the body. However, an excess of it can be oxidized to form plaque that clogs blood vessels to cause atherosclerosis. Likewise, though triglycerides are an important source of energy for daily activities, their excess can bring about acute pancreatitis and even coronary occlusion. Ideally, total cholesterol in the blood should be less than 200 mg/dL; the low-density lipoprotein (LDL)-cholesterol ("bad" cholesterol), less than 100 mg/dL; the high-density lipoprotein (HDL)-cholesterol ("good" cholesterol), at least 40 mg/dL; and the triglycerides, less than 150 mg/dL.

Medications shown effective mainly to lower cholesterol include: (1) statins, such as **atorvastatin, fluvastatin, lovastatin, pravastatin, rosuvastatin** (Crestor), and **simvastatin;** and (2) **ezetimibe** (Vytorin, Zetia); whereas medications shown effective mainly to lower triglycerides include: (3) such fibrates as **fenofibrate** (Tricor) and **gemfibrozil;** and medications effective to lower both cholesterol and triglycerides include: (4) **niacin** (Niaspan).

STATINS

Atorvastatin, fluvastatin, lovastatin, pravastatin, rosuvastatin, and **simvastatin**

These statins (Fig. 10-1) are useful to lower blood levels of cholesterol.

MECHANISM OF ACTION

They inhibit biosynthesis of cholesterol in the liver. They inhibit the enzyme HMG-CoA reductase (3-hydroxy-3-methylglutaryl CoA reductase), the enzyme required for formation of mevalonic acid from 3-hydroxy-3-methylglutaryl CoA, the rate-limiting step in the biosynthesis of cholesterol (Fig. 10-2). As the synthesis

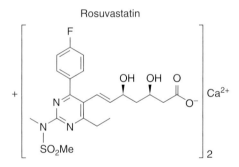

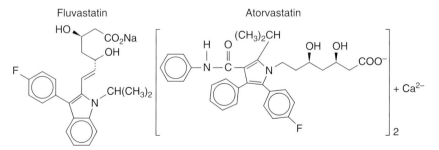

FIGURE 10-1   Molecular structures of statins. Reproduced, with permission, from Brunton LL, Lazo JS, and Parker KL. *Goodman and Gilman's The Pharmacological Basis of Therapeutics*. 11th ed. New York, NY: McGraw-Hill; 2006, p 949.

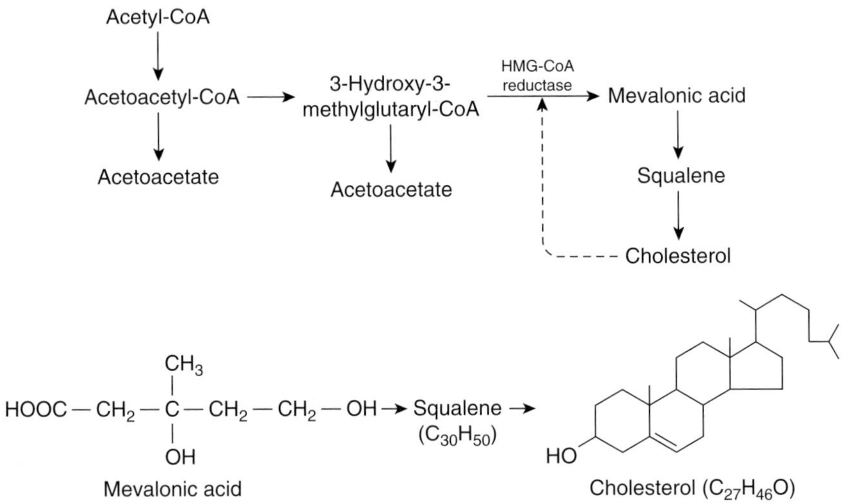

FIGURE 10-2   **HMG CoA reductase site of action.** Reproduced, with permission, from Barrett KE, Barman SM, Boitano S, and Brooks HL. *Ganong's Review of Medical Physiology*. 23rd ed. New York, NY: McGraw-Hill; 2010, p 27.

of cholesterol is inhibited, there are an increased number of LDL-cholesterol receptors developed in the liver to promote uptake of cholesterol from the blood.

SIDE EFFECTS

Frequent side effects of these drugs include bloating, stomach upset, and heartburn; hepatitis; muscle pain and tenderness (rhabdomyolysis); and rarely, allergic reactions.

DRUG INTERACTIONS

See Box 10-1.

Miscellaneous Interactions of Statins (STN)

Parentheses below indicate an herb.

STN ⟷ Cholestyramine: Co-administration of cholestyramine, which is known to adsorb many drugs, and such HMG-CoA reductase inhibitors as fluvastatin can result in reduced gastrointestinal absorption of the latter to undercut their therapeutic values.

BOX 10-1

Basic Concepts of Statins Interactions

Statins are prone to cause muscle pain and tenderness, and concurrent administration with other drugs that tend to generate similar side effects may cause rhabdomyolysis and other myopathies. Examples include: **cyclosporine** (an immunosuppressant); **clofibrate** (used to treat hyperlipidemia); **fenofibrate** (used to treat hypertriglyceridemia); and **gemfibrozil** (used to treat hypertriglyceridemia).

STN ⟷ CYP Isozymes: *See* Table 10-1.

STN ⟷ Digoxin: Concurrent administration of atorvastatin with digoxin can elevate plasma levels of digoxin. However, fluvastatin and simvastatin may raise digoxin levels to a clinically insignificant degree, whereas lovastatin and pravastatin have little such reported effect on the digoxin levels.

STN ⟷ (Gotu Kola): This herb (Fig. 10-3), which is used in Chinese medicine to treat bacterial, viral, or parasitic infections, may raise blood levels of cholesterol to undermine effectiveness of above statin drugs taken in combination.

[Lovastatin (LVS) and Simvastatin (SVS)]

LVS ⟷ Exenatide: Exenatide slows gastric emptying of lovastatin, a drug that is mainly absorbed from the small intestine. Exenatide therefore decreases the absorption of lovastatin to lower its blood levels, undercutting its effectiveness as a cholesterol-lowering drug. Exenatide may exert a similar effect on other statin drugs.

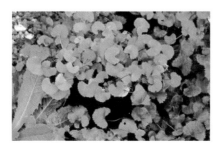

FIGURE 10-3   Gotu Kola leaves. (courtesy of Mim Beim at http://www.beamingwithhealth.com.au/tisanes/herbs/gotu-kola)

TABLE 10-1 Statins vs CYP Enzymes

Drug Name	1A2	2A6	2B6	2C8	2C9	2C18	2C19	2D6	2E1	3A4
Atorvastatin										Sub
Fluvastatin	Inh				Sub+ Inh					Sub
Lovastatin					Inh					Sub
Simvastatin										Sub

Abbreviations: Sub, substrate of the enzyme; Inh, inhibits the enzyme; Ezi, induces the enzyme

1. Pravastatin unlike others above is not a substrate of any CYP isozyme and the CYP system does not extensively metabolize it.

2. Cytochrome p450 metabolism of rosuvastatin (not shown) appears to be minimally mediated by the 2C9 enzyme, with little involvement of CYP 3A4.

3. Atorvastatin, fluvastatin, lovastatin, and simvastatin require CYP3A4, and hence concurrent administration of any of them with an inhibitor of this enzyme can cause elevated blood levels of unmetabolized drugs with increased potential for their adverse effects. Proven inhibitors of CP3A4 include cyclosporine , nefazodone, telithromycin, and verapamil. (*See* the left-hand column of Table-0 at the 'Introduction' for other possible inhibitors of those enzymes.)

4. Atorvastatin, fluvastatin, lovastatin, and simvastatin require CYP3A4, and hence concurrent administration of any of them with an inducer of this enzyme taken together can quicken their elimination to undercut their pharmacologic effectiveness. The inducers of CYP3A4 include carbamazepine and rifampin. (*See* the right-hand column of Table-0 at the 'Introduction' for other possible inducers of the enzyme.

5. Fluvastatin exerts inhibitory effect on CYP1A2 and hence administration of it in combination with other drugs that require this enzyme for their metabolic clearance may result in elevated blood levels, possibly inciting their adverse effects to surface. (*See* the middle column of Table-0 at the 'Introduction' for possible substrates of the enzyme.)

6. Both fluvastatin and lovastatin exert inhibitory effects on CYP2C9 and hence administration of either of them in combination with other drugs that require this enzyme for their metabolic clearance may result in elevated blood levels to instigate their adverse effects. (*See* the middle column of Table-0 at the 'Introduction' for possible substrates of the enzyme.)

SVS ⟷ Verapamil: When used in combination verapamil can raise blood levels of simvastatin to stir up its adverse effects such as rhabdomyolysis. One possible mechanism of this interaction is that simvastatin is cleared mainly through CYP3A4 and verapamil is a strong inhibitor of this enzyme. *See* Table 10-1 and the left-hand column of Table-0 at the 'Introduction' for other possible inhibitors of this enzyme.

EZETIMIBE

MECHANISM OF ACTION

Ezetimibe (Fig. 10-4) decreases absorption of cholesterol in the small intestine. It may be used alone or in combination with a statin drug when cholesterol levels are not controlled by a statin drug used alone.

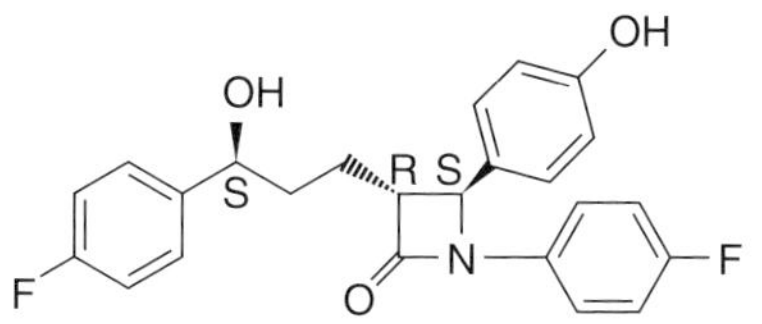

FIGURE 10-4   Molecular structure of ezetimibe.

SIDE EFFECTS

Its possible side effects include stomach pain, nausea, loss of appetite, and diarrhea; jaundice (yellowing of the skin or conjunctiva); chest pain, back pain, and joint or muscle pain; fatigue; dizziness and headache; and, rarely, may it cause allergic reaction such as difficulty in breathing; and skin rash.

DRUG INTERACTIONS

See Box 10-2.

Miscellaneous Interactions of Ezetimibe (EZT)

EZT ⟷ Cyclosporine: Ezetimibe, when taken together, may raise blood levels of cyclosporine by unknown mechanism.

BOX 10-2

Basic Concepts of Ezetimibe Interactions

1. Concurrent administration of ezetimibe with drugs that can decrease its intestinal absorption diminishes its effectiveness. This is because ezetimibe, though active by itself, is normally absorbed and quickly metabolized to its more active glucuronide form in the liver. Hence, the smaller the amount absorbed, the lesser its effectiveness. Those drugs that inhibit its absorption include: **cholestyramine,** and **antacids**. (*See* Ω-11 in Appendix A.)

2. Ezetimibe is apt to increase cholesterol excretions into the bile. Hence, taking ezetimibe concurrently with other drugs that have a similar effect may lead to increased risk of cholelithiasis (gallstone formation). Examples include: **fenofibrate** (a drug used mainly to reduce high blood triglyceride levels); **gemfibrozil** (a drug used mainly to reduce elevated blood triglyceride levels); and **clofibrate** (a drug used to reduce elevated blood triglyceride and cholesterol levels).

EZT ⟷ Saturated Fat: Avoid eating foods rich in saturated fat or cholesterol. Otherwise, ezetimibe cannot be as effective in lowering blood cholesterol levels.

FIBRATES

Fenofibrate (Fig. 10-5) and **gemfibrozil** (Fig. 10-6)

MECHANISM OF ACTION

These fibrates are classified as agonists of peroxisome proliferator-activated receptor-α (PPAR-α). Fenofibrate is a prodrug, and it has to be converted to fenofibric acid (Fig. 10-7), its active metabolite that acts as an agonist of the PPAR-α. The above fibrate drugs activate the nuclear PPAR-α receptors (1) to increase hydrolysis of plasma triglycerides by induction of lipoprotein lipase and to reduce production of apoC-III (an inhibitor of the enzyme activity); (2) to increase mitochondrial beta-oxidation in the liver; (3) to stimulate cellular uptake of fatty acid and its conversion to acetyl-CoA by increased expressions of genes for fatty acid transport protein and acetyl-CoA synthetase; and (4) to decrease synthesis of fatty acids and triglycerides, and to decrease the production of VLDL (very low-density lipoprotein) in the liver.

SIDE EFFECTS

They may cause irregular heartbeat; tendency toward bleeding; nausea, vomiting, and stomach pain; yellowing of the skin or eyes (jaundice); muscle pain; and headache, dizziness, or drowsiness. Use of gemfibrozil or fenofibrate is contraindicated

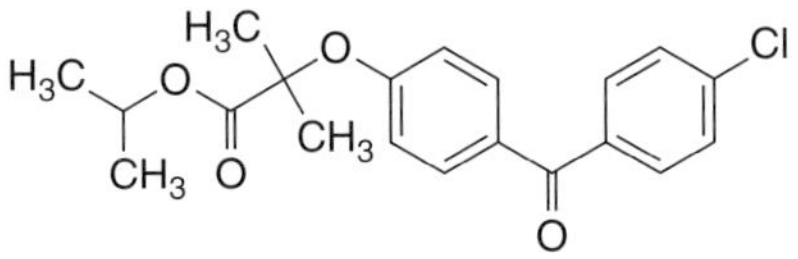

FIGURE 10-5   Molecular structure of fenofibrate.

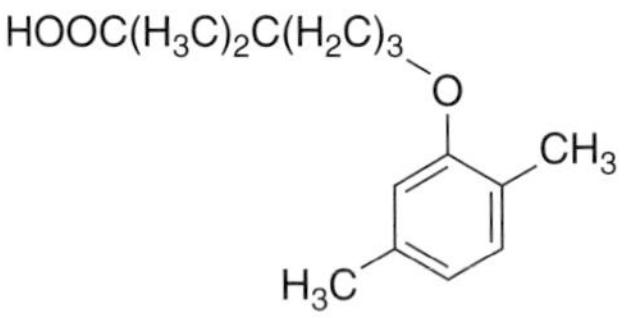

FIGURE 10-6   Molecular structure of gemfibrozil.

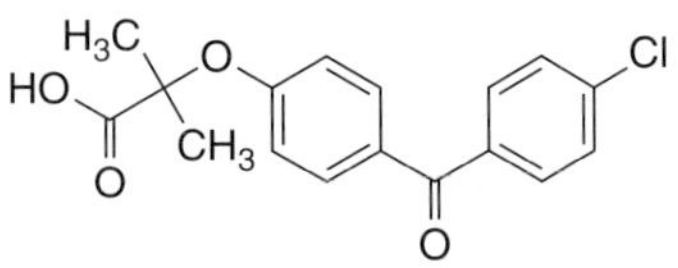

FIGURE 10-7   Molecular structure of fenofibric acid.

BOX 10-3

Basic Concepts of Fenofibrate or Gemfibrozil Interactions

1. Fibrate drugs have myopathy as a side effect, and when either of the drugs mentioned is used in combination with drugs that generate similar side effects, rhabdomyolysis and other myopathies may result. Those drugs include: **HMG-CoA reductase inhibitors** (*See* Ω-46 in Appendix A) or **statin drugs** (*See* Ω-69 in Appendix A).

2. Fibrate drugs have a tendency toward bleeding. Hence, taking either of these drugs with other drugs that cause bleeding may lead to excessive hemorrhage. Those drugs include: **anticoagulants** (*See* Ω-16 in Appendix A [the dosage of the anticoagulant should be reduced to maintain the prothrombin time at the desired level to prevent bleeding complications]).

---

in patients having biliary cirrhosis and in patients having severely impaired renal function.

DRUG INTERACTIONS

See Box 10-3.

Miscellaneous Interactions of Fenofibrate or Gemfibrozil (FGF)

Parentheses below indicate an herb.

FGF ⟷ Bile Acid Sequestrants: (*See* Ω-28 in Appendix A.) Bile acid sequestrants such as cholestyramine and colestipol can adsorb both fenofibrate and gemfibrozil, to reduce their intestinal absorptions to their insufficient therapeutic effectiveness.

FGF ⟷ (Bitter Gourd): This herb has some triglyceride-lowering and cholesterol-lowering effects, and may have additive effects with drugs used to lower blood triglyceride and cholesterol levels.

FGF ⟷ Cyclosporine: Renal excretion is the primary means of elimination for fibrate drugs, and hence co-administration of any of them with cyclosporine, a known nephrotoxic drug that decreases creatinine clearance, can raise blood levels of the above drugs to their increased therapeutic and adverse effects.

FGF ⟷ Ezetimibe: Both fibrates and ezetimibe promote excretions of cholesterol from the liver into the bile. When taken together they may pull together toward increased risk of cholelithiasis (gallstones formation).

FGF ⟷ (Gotu Kola): This herb may raise blood levels of cholesterol to undercut the cholesterol-lowering effect of both gemfibrozil and fenofibrate (Tricor).

FGF ⟷ Repaglinide: Co-administration of gemfibrozil, a strong inhibitor of CYP2C8, with repaglinide, an antidiabetic drug and a strong substrate of CYP2C8, resulted in a significant increase in blood levels of repaglinide.

NIACIN

Nicotinic acid

MECHANISM OF ACTION

Niacin (Fig. 10-8) lowers blood levels of both cholesterol and triglycerides by (1) increasing the activity of lipoprotein lipase to promote entry of triglyceride into the fat cells; (2) inhibiting the hydrolysis of stored triglycerides in the fat cells as a result of inhibition of the internal lipase. As the release of fatty acids into the blood is diminished, there is reduced entry of fatty acids into the liver to cut down synthesis of triglycerides in the liver. As the VLDL-triglyceride can be the source from which LDL-cholesterol derives, niacin can also lower the blood levels of LDL-cholesterol as well.

SIDE EFFECTS

Possible side effects of niacin include racing heartbeat; shortness of breath; nausea, vomiting, abdominal pain, and diarrhea; skin flushing and itching; and headache.

DRUG INTERACTIONS

See Box 10-4.

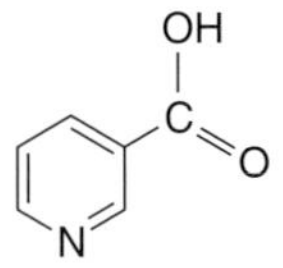

FIGURE 10-8   Molecular structure of nicotinic acid.

BOX 10-4

Basic Concepts of Niacin Interactions

Niacin is prone to cause peripheral vasodilation and thus, concurrent administration with other drugs that tend to cause vasodilation may lead to postural hypotension or excessive fall of blood pressure. Examples include: **diazoxide** (a drug used orally to treat hypoglycemia related to islet cell dysfunction, and intravenously to treat severe hypertension); other **vasodilators** (*See* Ω-78 in Appendix A); **alcohol** (concomitant intake of alcohol may increase the side effects of flushing and pruritus, and should be avoided around the time of niacin intake); and **mecamylamine** (niacin may potentiate the effects of this ganglionic blocking agent to result in postural hypotension or even serious syncope).

Miscellaneous Interactions of Niacin (NCN)

Parentheses below indicate an herb.

NCN ◆▸ Aspirin: Pretreatment of patients with aspirin can lower incidences of skin flushing and pruritus caused by niacin. The skin flushing response to niacin appears mediated by the release of vasodilatory prostaglandin-E from the skin, and aspirin inhibits the synthesis of this prostaglandin.

NCN ◆▸ Oral Hypoglycemic Agents: (*See* Ω-55 in Appendix A.) Niacin tends to produce hyperglycemia so as to reduce the effectiveness of acarbose or of other antidiabetic drugs such as repaglinide, when taken in combination.

NCN ◆▸ (Bitter Gourd): Bitter gourd (Fig. 10-9), which is used as an antidiabetic agent in Chinese medicine, has some triglyceride-lowering and cholesterol-lowering effects of its own, and when used in combination can generate additive effects with niacin in lowering blood levels of the lipids.

NCN ◆▸ Colestipol: Niacin is heavily bound to bile acid-binding resins especially to colestipol and less extensively to cholestyramine, and hence the bile sequestrants decrease intestinal absorption of niacin. At least four to six hours should elapse between the ingestion of such bile acid-binding resins and the administration of niacin.

NCN ◆▸ (Gotu Kola): The herb gotu kola raises blood levels of cholesterol to undermine effectiveness of niacin in lowering blood levels of cholesterol.

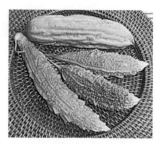

FIGURE 10-9   Bitter gourd. Cut and dried form of bitter gourd.
(courtesy of Andrew Grygus at www.clovegarden.com)

NCN ⟷ Statins: (*See* Ω-69 in Appendix A.) Niacin can rarely cause rhabdomyolysis or liver failure. Concomitant use of it with statins can potentiate such adverse effects. Hence, niacin should never be combined with statin drugs, as otherwise it may cause a potentially fatal rhabdomyolysis.

CHAPTER

11

Rhinitis/Sinusitis

Rhinitis refers to inflammation of the mucous membrane of the nasal passage-way, engendering such symptoms as rhinorrhea (runny nose), sneezing, and nasal congestion. Seasonal rhinitis (hay fever) is the most common of all allergic diseases and is due to an allergic reaction to pollen in the air. In contrast, vasomotor rhinitis (non-allergic rhinitis) is due to abnormal neuronal control of the nasal blood vessels.

Sinusitis, on the other hand, refers to inflammation of the membranes lining the sinuses (hollow areas) within the bones around the nose. Sinusitis is usually caused by an infection and less commonly by an allergic reaction. If the sinus lining is swollen and the normal sweeping action of the cilia (hair cells) is interrupted, mucus has nowhere to go but trapped in the sinuses, which facilitates growth of infectious bacteria to cause fever and create an uncomfortable pressure, resulting in headache.

Medications shown effective in the treatment of rhinitis/sinusitis include: (1) glucocorticoid nasal sprays such as **beclomethasone** (Beconase, Vancenase), **budesonide** (Rhinocort Aqua), **fluticasone** (Flonase), and **triamcinolone** (Nasacort AQ); (2) a mast-cell stabilizer such as **cromolyn sodium;** (3) an antihistaminic antiserotonin agent such as **cyproheptadine** (Periactin); (4) a sympathomimetic agent such as **pseudoephedrine** (Sudafed); and (5) first-generation antihistaminic agents such as **brompheniramine, chlorpheniramine, clemastine, diphenhydramine, doxylamine, hydroxyzine, meclizine, pyrilamine,** and

triprolidine or such second-generation antihistamines as **azelastine** (*astelin*), **cetirizine** (Zyrtec), **desloratadine** (Clarinex), and **fexofenadine** (Allegra). Among the above, azelastine, an antihistamine as well as a mast-cell stabilizer, is available as a nasal spray, whose prophylactic use may reduce the occurrence of sinusitis. Fexofenadine above is often used in combination with pseudoephedrine (for example, Allegra-D 12 Hour).

GLUCOCORTICOIDS

Beclomethasone, budesonide, fluticasone, and **triamcinolone**

The glucocorticoids are probably the most effective treatment for hay fever as well as for perennial allergic rhinitis. To prevent seasonal allergic rhinitis, it is best to start taking a corticosteroid spray one or two weeks prior to the expected rise in pollen counts.

MECHANISM OF ACTION

Glucocorticoids have their own specific receptors in cytosol and binding to those receptors invariably leads to suppression of inflammation, for the receptor-bound glucocorticoids enhance expression of anti-inflammatory proteins in the nucleus while suppressing the MAP (mitogen-activated protein) kinases (also referred to as extracellular signal-regulated protein kinases) required for proinflammatory gene activation that appears to cause joint degeneration in osteoarthritis.

SIDE EFFECTS

Possible side effects include coughs, sneezing, and dry or irritated nose or throat; unpleasant taste or smell, nausea, vomiting, and loss of appetite; white patches or sores inside the mouth or on the lips; dizziness and changes in vision; and headache.

DRUG INTERACTIONS

It is not known whether other medications will interact with any of the above glucocorticoids applied topically. *See* Appendix B-20: Interactions of Glucocorticoids for a list of interactions that may result from oral ingestion or extensive absorption from the site of application.

CROMOLYN SODIUM

MECHANISM OF ACTION

The mast cells, residents of the conjunctiva and mucosa of the mouth, nose, and lungs, are beneficially involved in wound healing and play a protective role for the host by

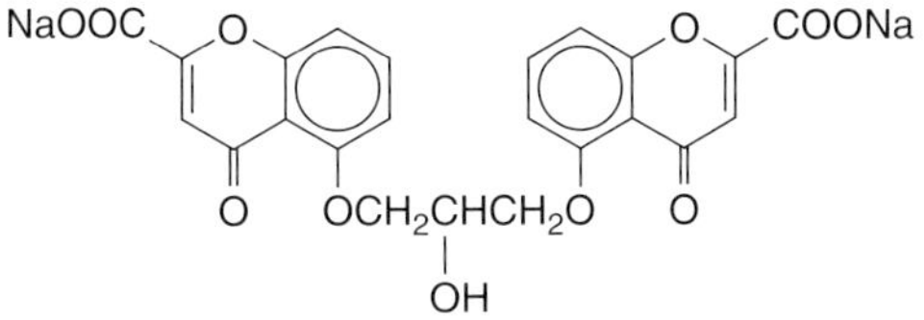

FIGURE 11-1   Molecular structure of cromolyn sodium.

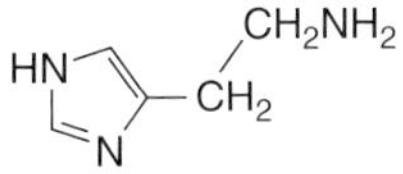

LT A4

LT B4

FIGURE 11-2   Molecular structure of histamine.

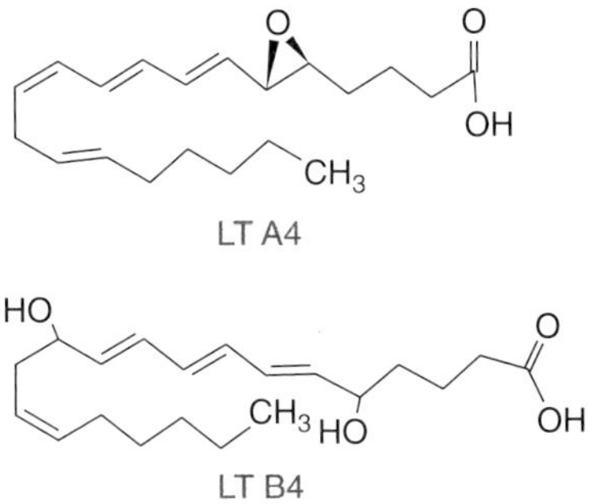

FIGURE 11-3   Molecular structures of leukotrienes.

fending off pathogens. They also play an important role in the genesis of allergy and anaphylaxis. Cromolyn sodium (Fig. 11-1), classified as a mast-cell stabilizer, inhibits degranulation of sensitized mast cells to prevent the release of inflammatory substances such as histamine (Fig. 11-2) and leukotrienes (Fig. 11-3).

SIDE EFFECTS

Side effects of cromolyn sodium may include coughing; dry mouth and nausea; increased pressure in the eyes or tearing of the eyes. It may rarely cause allergic reactions such as skin hives and swelling of the lips, tongue, throat, or face.

DRUG INTERACTIONS

There is no clinically important interaction reported.

CYPROHEPTADINE

MECHANISM OF ACTION

Cyproheptadine (Fig. 11-4) has antagonistic effects against both histamine (*See* Fig. 11-2) and serotonin (Fig. 11-5). Cyproheptadine does not prevent the release

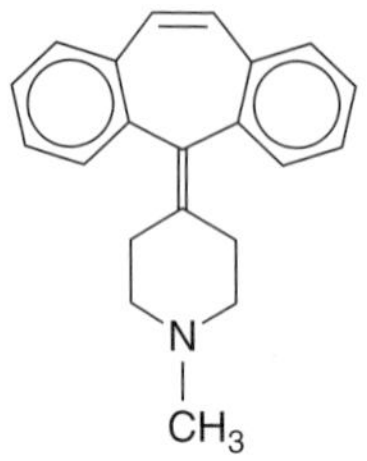

FIGURE 11-4 Molecular structure of cyproheptadine.

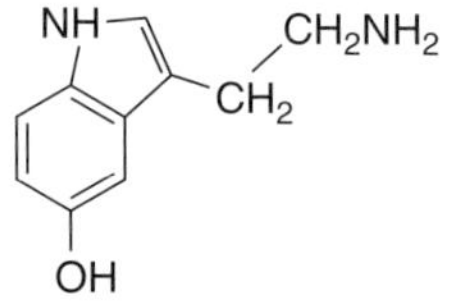

FIGURE 11-5 Molecular structure of serotonin.

of histamine but blocks its receptors located at large blood vessels and at the smooth muscles of the bronchial and respiratory tract, to fend off allergic reactions. Cyproheptadine, as it competes with serotonin at its receptor sites in the smooth muscles of blood vessels, may also be beneficial to treat vascular headache. Antagonism of serotonin in the central neurons may account for its appetite-stimulant effect useful to treat anorexia.

SIDE EFFECTS

Possible side effects of cyproheptadine include irregular heartbeat; upset stomach and increased appetite; weight gain; thickening of mucus in the nose or throat; dark urine and difficulty in urination; yellowing of the eyes and skin; blurred vision; and dizziness and drowsiness.

DRUG INTERACTIONS

At the time of publication, there has been no convincing evidence that cyproheptadine would interact with any other drugs to a serious consequence, even though there was a report that when cyproheptadine was taken together with fluoxetine (Prozac), an antidepressant, the mental depression was worsened, probably because the serotonin accumulated by fluoxetine could not work as it should in the presence of cyproheptadine, a blocker of serotonin receptors.

PSEUDOEPHEDRINE

MECHANISM OF ACTION

Pseudoephedrine is a sympathomimetic amine that activates adrenergic alpha receptors to cause vasoconstriction. Nasal vasoconstriction thus obtained shrinks the swollen mucosal tissue in the nasal cavity, often associated with colds or allergies, to open up the air pathway and thus, this drug is commonly used as a nasal decongestant.

SIDE EFFECTS

Possible side effects of pseudoephedrine include palpitations; stomach pain and vomiting; tremor; and nervousness, dizziness, and insomnia.

DRUG INTERACTIONS

See Appendix B-8: Interactions of Alpha Agonists.

ANTIHISTAMINIES

Brompheniramine, chlorpheniramine, clemastine, diphenhydramine, doxylamine, hydroxyzine, meclizine, pyrilamine, and **triprolidine** (all first-generation); and less-sedating or non-sedating antihistamines such as **azelastine, cetirizine, desloratadine,** and **fexofenadine** (all second-generation).

MECHANISM OF ACTION

Both the first- and the second-generation antihistamines are capable of blocking histamine receptors to ward off histamine-mediated allergic reactions. The major difference between these two classes is presence or absence of a sedating effect. The sedation by first-generation antihistamines appears to arise from their ability to enter the brain, probably due to lack of their efflux by P-glycoprotein located at the blood-brain barrier. Second-generation antihistamines, on the other hand, are relatively non-sedating, probably due to their P-glycoprotein-mediated efflux not allowing them to enter into the brain.

SIDE EFFECTS

First-Generation Antihistamines: Their possible side effects include low blood pressure and palpitations; drying of the laryngeal mucosa and drying and thickening of oral and other respiratory secretions; loss of appetite, nausea, stomach distress, and constipation; urinary retention; disturbed muscle coordination and tremor; blurred vision and double vision; and sedation, tiredness, dizziness, and confusion.

Second-Generation Antihistamines: Their possible side effects include dry mouth and sore throat; nausea and vomiting; weakness; weight gain; fatigue and jitteriness; and headache.

DRUG INTERACTIONS

First-Generation Antihistamines: *See* Appendix B-10: Interactions of Antihistamines, First-Generation.

Second-Generation Antihistamines: *See* Appendix B-11: Interactions of Antihistamines, Second-Generation.

Interactions of Fexofenadine + Pseudoephedrine (Allegra-D 12 Hour [ALG])

ALG ⟷ Antacids: (*See* Ω-11 in Appendix A.) If taken orally together, gastric antacids, such as aluminum hydroxide and magnesium hydroxide, can oppose intestinal absorption of fexofenadine and, to a lesser extent, pseudoephedrine.

ALG ⟷ Digitalis: Co-administration of pseudoephedrine with a digitalis glycoside can enhance cardiac arrhythmia caused by the digitalis glycoside. This is because arrhythmogenic tendency of digoxin is increased in the presence of a sympathomimetic drug.

ALG ⟷ MAO Inhibitors: (*See* Ω-51 in Appendix A.) If this preparation is used in combination with an inhibitor of monoamine oxidase, an enzyme that inactivates pseudoephedrine (*See* Fig. 3-6) contained in this preparation, it can possibly bring about hypertension.

ALG ⟷ Rifampin: Rifampin, when used in combination, significantly decreases the peak blood concentration of fexofenadine. The mechanisms of interaction assumed include: (1) rifampin induces P-glycoprotein to efflux fexofenadine and (2) rifampin induces CYP3A4 to quicken metabolic clearance of fexofenadine, which is a substrate of CYP3A4.

ALG ⟷ Sodium Bicarbonate: If urine pH is made alkaline by administration of sodium bicarbonate, the urinary excretion of pseudoephedrine, a basic drug, will be decreased in order to raise its blood level. This will result in longer-lasting therapeutic and adverse effects of this drug.

Laryngitis/Bronchitis

12

Laryngitis refers to inflammation of the lower part of the larynx, including the vocal cords. If the vocal cord is involved, the voice may become hoarse. Laryngitis may be caused by viral infections (most common), bacterial infections (often by streptococcus), allergies, and by smoking. Acid reflux from the stomach into the larynx also may cause the so-called reflux laryngitis.

Bronchitis, on the other hand, refers to acute or chronic inflammation of the mucous membranes of the trachea and bronchi. Acute bronchitis is usually caused by viral and less commonly by bacterial infections. Common symptoms of bronchitis include coughing, mild fever, and wheezing. Virus-caused laryngitis and bronchitis are self-limited and do not require treatment with an antibiotic.

Medications shown effective in the treatment of laryngitis or bronchitis caused by bacteria include: (1) penicillins such as **amoxicillin, ampicillin** (Omnipen, Polycillin, Principen), and **penicillin-V** (Veetids); (2) cephalosporin antibiotics such as **cefaclor, cefdinir, cefpodoxime** (Vantin), **cefprozil, cefuroxime**, and **cephalexin;** (3) a fluoroquinolone antibiotic such as **ciprofloxacin;** (4) macrolide antibiotics such as **azithromycin, clarithromycin, erythromycin,** and **telithromycin;** and (5) aminoglycoside antibiotics such as **gentamicin** and **tobramycin.**

PENICILLIN ANTIBIOTICS

Amoxicillin, ampicillin, and **penicillin V**

MECHANISM OF ACTION

Penicillin antibiotics kill susceptible bacteria. They bind to the penicillin-binding protein (PBP) located at the bacterial cell envelope to inhibit transpeptidase, the bacterial enzyme involved in cross-linking of two peptide chains, without which the bacteria cannot complete synthesis of their cell wall in the third stage. In addition, penicillins bind to the PBP to release autolysins, the bacterial enzymes that destroy the already formed bacterial cell wall.

SIDE EFFECTS

Their possible side effects include sore throat; nausea, vomiting, stomach pain, and bloody diarrhea; body aches; fever and chills; convulsions; and allergic reactions such as difficulty in breathing; swelling of the face, lips, tongue, or throat; and skin hives. However, incidence of penicillin allergy is difficult to predict; for example, among those patients with negative allergic reactions to a penicillin in the past, the incidence of penicillin allergy is still about 0.5% of such patients, whereas in those strongly positive patients in the past, 90% of them would not react with an allergy to penicillin.

DRUG INTERACTIONS

See Appendix B-24: Interactions of Penicillins.

CEPHALOSPORIN ANTIBIOTICS

Cefaclor, cefdinir, cefpodoxime, cefprozil, cefuroxime, and **cephalexin** (Fig. 12-1)

MECHANISM OF ACTION

Their mechanism of antibacterial action is identical to that of penicillin antibiotics, discussed earlier.

SIDE EFFECTS

Possible side effects of the above cephalosporin antibiotics include nausea, vomiting, bloody diarrhea, and stomach pain; nephrotoxicity (probably except ceftriaxone); headache, dizziness, and convulsions; and allergic reactions such as skin hives; difficulty in breathing; and swelling of the face, lips, tongue, or throat.

DRUG INTERACTIONS

See Appendix B-17: Interactions of Cephalosporins.

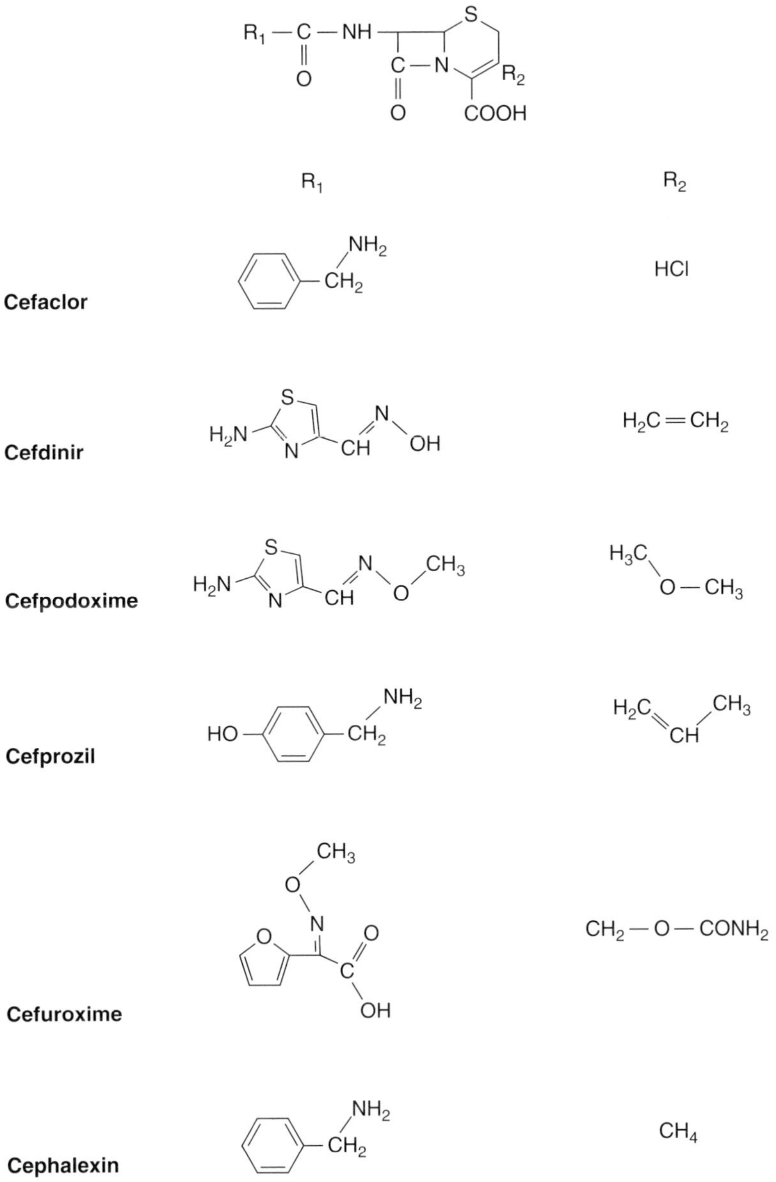

FIGURE 12-1 Molecular structures of cephalosporins (Cefaclor, Cefdinir, Cefpodoxime, Cefprozil, Cefuroxime, and Cephalexin).

CIPROFLOXACIN

MECHANISM OF ACTION

Ciprofloxacin, like other quinolone antibiotics, generates its antibacterial effect by inhibiting DNA gyrase, an essential bacterial enzyme that catalyzes the ATP-dependent introduction of negative super-coiling of double-stranded bacterial DNA, required for DNA replication.

SIDE EFFECTS

Ciprofloxacin may cause nausea, vomiting, diarrhea, and abdominal pain; nephrotoxicity; headache and restlessness; rarely, seizures; and allergic reactions such as anaphylaxis (shock), skin hives, and rash.

DRUG INTERACTIONS

See Appendix B-28: Interactions of Quinolone Antibiotics.

MACROLIDE ANTIBIOTICS

Azithromycin, clarithromycin, erythromycin, and **telithromycin** (Fig. 12-2 and Fig. 12-3)

MECHANISM OF ACTION

They bind to the 50s subunit of the bacterial 70s ribosome to inhibit bacterial protein synthesis. The binding blocks translocation of the amino acid t-RNA from the A-site to the P-site, and as the A-site remains occupied, no new amino acid carried over by another t-RNA can attach to keep feeding into the growing end of the peptide chain (Fig. 12-4).

SIDE EFFECTS

Azithromycin: Its possible side effects include uneven heartbeats; nausea, vomiting, stomach pain, bloody diarrhea; dizziness, tiredness, headache; and rarely may it cause such allergic reactions as skin hives; and difficulty in breathing.

Clarithromycin: Its possible side effects include nausea, vomiting, stomach upset, diarrhea; and rarely cardiac arrhythmia and pseudomembranous colitis due to resistant bacteria.

Erythromycin: Its possible side effects include loss of appetite, stomach cramps, vomiting, diarrhea; liver dysfunction; yellowing of the skin or eyes; transient

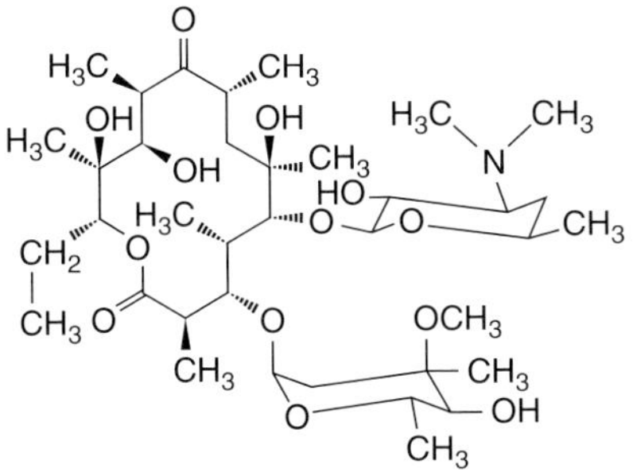

Erythromycin

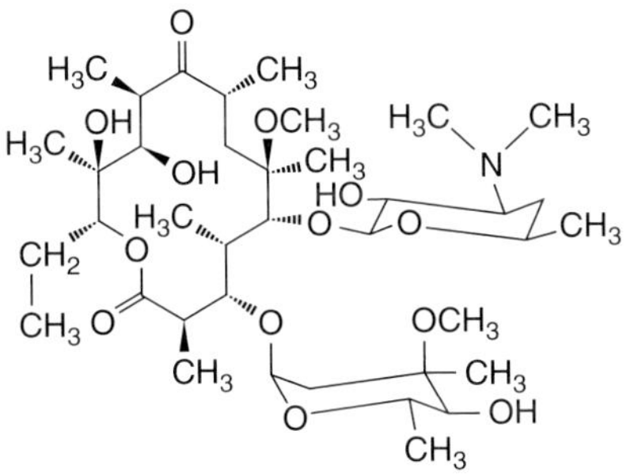

Clarithromycin

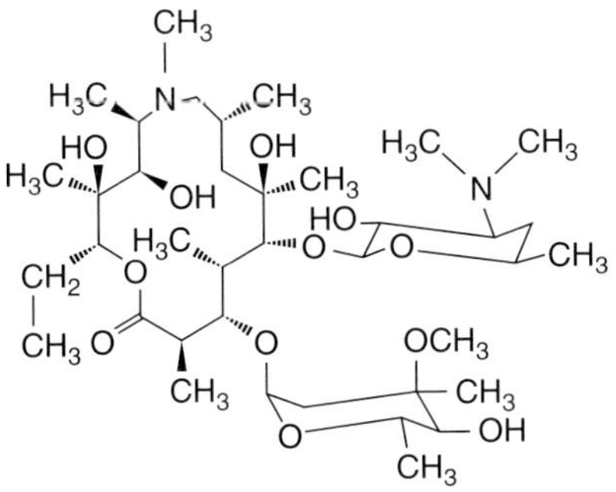

Azithromycin

FIGURE 12-2 Molecular structures of azithromycin, clarithromycin, and erythromycin.

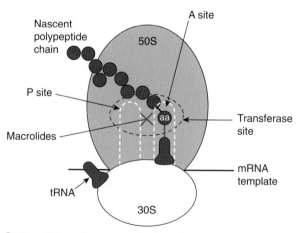

FIGURE 12-3   Molecular structure of telithromycin.

hearing disturbance; dryness, burning or itching of the skin. It may very rarely cause allergic reactions.

Telithromycin: This drug may cause a strange taste in the mouth, nausea, vomiting, mild diarrhea; dark urine; yellowing of the eyes or skin; visual disturbances (blurred vision, double vision, difficult focusing); headache, dizziness, and anxiety.

FIGURE 12-4   **Macrolide antibiotics: mechanism of action.** Reproduced, with permission, from Brunton LL, Lazo JS, and Parker KL. *Goodman and Gilman's The Pharmacological Basis of Therapeutics.* 11th ed. New York, NY: McGraw-Hill; 2006, p 1183.

Besides, this medication may rarely cause a severe pseudomembranous colitis due to resistant bacteria.

DRUG INTERACTIONS

Azithromycin: *See* Appendix B-13: Interactions of Macrolide Antibiotics.

Clarithromycin: *See* Appendix B-13: Interactions of Macrolide Antibiotics.

Erythromycin: *See* Appendix B-13: Interactions of Macrolide Antibiotics.

Telithromycin: *See* Appendix B-13: Interactions of Macrolide Antibiotics.

AMINOGLYCOSIDE ANTIBIOTICS

Gentamicin and **tobramycin**

Gentamicin and tobramycin, among aminoglycoside antibiotics, are often indicated to treat laryngitis or bronchitis. Tobramycin is preferred over gentamicin for treatment of bronchitis or bronchopneumonia caused by *Pseudomonas aeruginosa,* because of its greater bactericidal activity and better penetration into the lung and bronchial tree.

MECHANISM OF ACTION

They appear to bind to the 30s subunit of the bacterial ribosome to interfere with proper binding of incoming new aminoacyl t-RNA to the m-RNA codons, causing either failure to initiate protein synthesis or misreading of genetic codons resulting in synthesis of nonfunctional proteins or premature termination of protein synthesis.

SIDE EFFECTS

Gentamicin: It may cause loss of appetite, nausea, vomiting, stomach upset, and diarrhea; ringing in the ears; dizziness; and, rarely, allergic reaction such as trouble breathing; skin rash, and itching.

Tobramycin: Its side effects may be very similar to those of gentamicin mentioned above.

DRUG INTERACTIONS

See Box 12-1.

BOX 12-1

Basic Concepts of Aminoglycoside Antibiotics Interactions

1. All the aminoglycosides are prone to cause nephrotoxicity and concurrent administration with drugs that tend to generate similar side effects may lead to enhanced renal toxicities. Examples include: **amphotericin** (an antifungal drug); **azathioprine** (an immunosuppressant); **cisplatin** (an anticancer drug); **cyclophosphamide** (an anticancer drug); **cyclosporine** (an immunosuppressant); **ifosfamide** (an anticancer drug); and **vancomycin** (an antibiotic).

2. The above aminoglycoside antibiotics can suppress vitamin K-producing intestinal flora and thereby increase the anticoagulant effects of other drugs that work by opposing the availability of the active form of vitamin K. Those drugs include: **dicumarol** and **warfarin.**

3. The above aminoglycoside antibiotics generate neuromuscular blockage as a side effect and hence, combined use with drugs that have a similar side effect may lead to respiratory paralysis. Those drugs include: **pancuronium** and **succinylcholine.**

Miscellaneous Interactions of Aminoglycoside Antibiotics (AGA)

See extra individual interactions in brackets below.

AGA ⟷ Anticholinesterase Agents: (*See* Ω-15 in Appendix A.) An aminoglycoside antibiotic, such as amikacin, kanamycin, streptomycin or tobramycin, has a neuromuscular blocking effect to oppose therapeutic effectiveness of such anticholinesterase agents as neostigmine and pyridostigmine, when used in combination.

AGA ⟷ Cationic Drugs: Cationic drugs such as calcium and magnesium preparations can dilute the intracellular negative charge of bacteria, the driving force for the infiltration of an aminoglycoside antibiotic, diminishing access of the aminoglycosides into the germs to cause their insufficient antibacterial effect.

AGA ⟷ Clindamycin: Clindamycin itself does not cause renal toxicity, but acute renal failure is not unlikely when clindamycin is used in combination with gentamicin or another member of the aminoglycosides. The mechanism behind this observation remains unclear.

AGA ⟷ Loop Diuretics: (*See* Ω-49 in Appendix A.) Both parties have a tendency to cause ototoxicity, especially by ethacrynic acid, and when they are used in combination they may pull together toward increased risk of the toxicity.

AGA ⟷ Topotecan: Both parties are exclusively eliminated from the body by the kidney. Aminoglycosides are primarily excreted into the urine by glomerular filtration and then partly reabsorbed in the proximal renal tubule, whereas the renal elimination of topotecan involves tubular secretion in addition to glomerular filtration. If topotecan is co-administered with an aminoglycoside antibiotic, the nephrotoxicity and ototoxicity by the aminoglycoside may be enhanced, probably due to interference with its renal excretions.

[Gentamicin (GTM)]

GTM ⟷ Bacitracin: Co-administration of gentamicin and bacitracin can result in renal dysfunction and respiratory paralysis.

GTM ⟷ Polymyxin B: Co-administration of gentamicin and polymyxin B can also result in renal dysfunction and respiratory paralysis.

13

Hiccups

Hiccup, also written as hiccough, is a spasmodic, erratic inhalation due to sudden involuntary contraction of the diaphragm accompanied by closure of the glottis (vocal apparatus of the larynx). The closure interrupts the otherwise smooth inflow of air, generating the characteristic sharp, cough-like "hic" sound. Hiccups are medically treated only in persistent and severe cases.

Medications that may possibly be effective in the treatment of hiccups include: (1) phenothiazines such as **chlorpromazine** (Thorazine) and **prochlorperazine** (Compazine); (2) **baclofen;** and (3) **metoclopramide** (Reglan).

PHENOTHIAZINES

Chlorpromazine (Fig. 13-1) and **prochlorperazine** (Fig. 13-2)

MECHANISM OF ACTION

Chlorpromazine and prochlorperazine block dopamine receptors in the hypothalamus, but their exact mechanism for suppression of hiccup remains obscure.

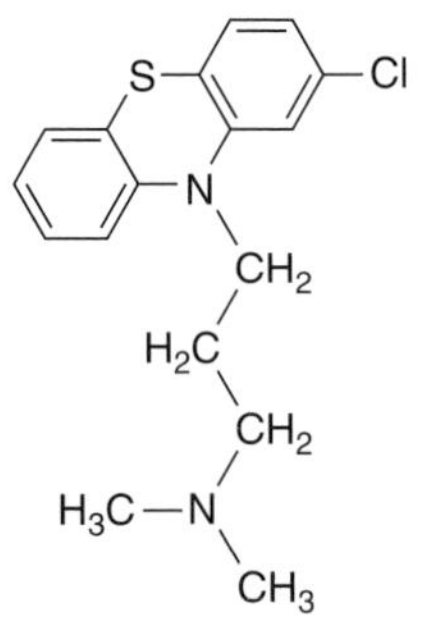

FIGURE 13-1 Molecular structure of chlorpromazine.

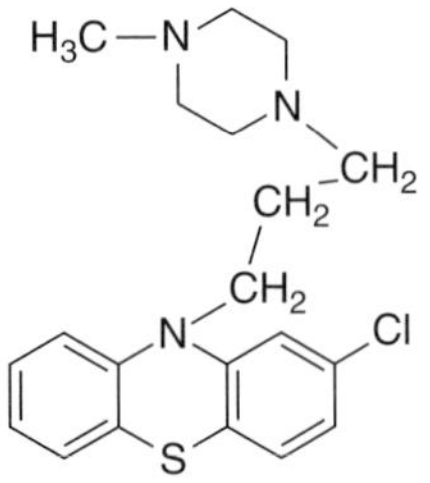

FIGURE 13-2 Molecular structure of prochlorperazine.

SIDE EFFECTS

They may cause Q-T elongation, fainting; dry mouth, constipation; jaundice (yellowing of the skin or eyes); stuffy nose; uncontrollable movements of the tongue, face, lips, arms, or legs; and drowsiness. Chlorpromazine may turn urine dark, and prochlorperazine turns urine red, but these changes do not usually lead to medical emergency.

DRUG INTERACTIONS

See Appendix B-25: Interactions of Phenothiazine Antipsychotic Drugs.

BACLOFEN

Baclofen (Fig. 13-3) is structurally related to tricyclic antidepressants.

MECHANISM OF ACTION

In severe or persistent hiccups, the anti-spasmodic effect of baclofen may help with suppression. Baclofen may reduce excitability so as to suppress reflex hiccup activity.

SIDE EFFECTS

Baclofen may generate uneven heartbeat; increased blood levels of glucose; nausea, constipation; and muscle weakness; drowsiness, dizziness, seizure (convulsions), headache, confusion, and hallucinations.

DRUG INTERACTIONS

See Box 13-1.

Miscellaneous Interactions of Baclofen (BCF)

BCF ⟷ Alcohol: Administration of baclofen in conjunction with other central nervous system depressants, such as alcohol, may lead to additional depression of brain function.

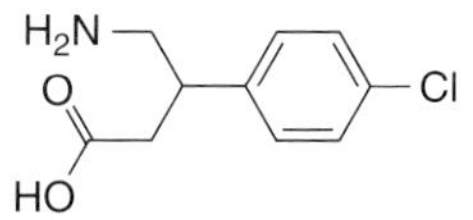

FIGURE 13-3 Molecular structure of baclofen.

BOX 13-1

Basic Concepts of Baclofen Interactions

1. Baclofen has a centrally acting muscle relaxant effect, and when taken with drugs that tend to cause muscle relaxation, it can bring about additional muscle weakness. Those other drugs include **tricyclic antidepressants** (*See* Ω-76 in Appendix A).

2. Administration of baclofen in conjunction with an inhibitor of monoamine oxidase can result in extreme depression of brain function with serious fall of blood pressure. Such MAO inhibitors include: **phenelzine** (Fig. 13-4) (Nardil, a drug to treat atypical, neurotic depression) and **tranylcypromine** (Parnate, an antidepressant) (Fig. 13-5).

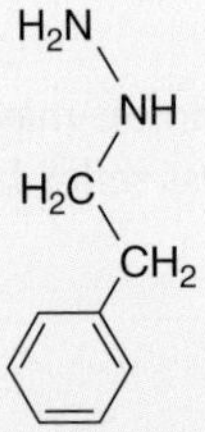

FIGURE 13-4   Molecular structure of phenelzine.

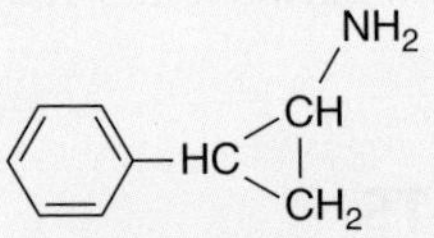

FIGURE 13-5   Molecular structure of tranylcypromine.

BCF ⟷ Ibuprofen: Ibuprofen may induce renal insufficiency to decrease excretion of baclofen used in combination, to raise its blood levels and adverse effects.

BCF ⟷ Morphine: The continuous use of baclofen (by intrathecal injection) and morphine (by epidural injection) used in combination has relieved a spasticity-related pain for months to years, but it has caused hypotension and dyspnea by unknown mechanism.

BCF ⟷ Oral Hypoglycemic Agents: (*See* Ω-55 in Appendix A.) Baclofen can increase blood glucose levels to offset the therapeutic value of antidiabetic drugs used in combination, requiring their increased doses to become effective.

BCF ⟷ Tricyclic Antidepressants: Administration of baclofen in conjunction with such tricyclic antidepressants as amitriptyline (Elavil) and doxepin (Sinequan) may cause additional loss of muscle power.

METOCLOPRAMIDE

MECHANISM OF ACTION

Metoclopramide was shown to induce dramatic relief of intractable hiccup. When administered orally or by injection the relief was observed within 30 minutes to last up to 8 hours. Metoclopramide, by its dopamine antagonist effect, appears to suppress the hiccup reflex arc at the hypothalamus, and its cholinergic activity appears to impart normal esophageal smooth muscle functions.

SIDE EFFECTS

Possible side effects of metoclopramide include tachycardia; dry mouth, nausea, diarrhea; trembling of the hands, muscle spasms; sweating, high fever; dizziness, drowsiness, confusion, restlessness, fatigue, and headache.

DRUG INTERACTIONS:

See Box 13-2.

Miscellaneous Interactions of Metoclopramide (MCP)

Parentheses below indicate an herb.

BOX 13-2

Basic Concepts of Metoclopramide Interactions

1. Since metoclopramide accelerates stomach emptying, it can increase absorption of many drugs from the small intestine and thus, their decreased doses may be required to avoid undesirable side effects. Such affected drugs include: **acetaminophen** (an analgesic); **cyclosporine** (an immunosuppressant); **diazepam** (an antianxiety drug); **levodopa; mefloquine** (an antimalarial drug); **phenothiazine antipsychotic drugs** (*See* Ω-58 in Appendix A); and **tetracycline antibiotics** (*See* Ω-72 in Appendix A).

2. Metoclopramide's effect on gastrointestinal motility is antagonized by certain drugs. Examples include: **anticholinergic agents** (*See* Ω-14 in Appendix A) and **narcotic analgesics** (*See* Ω-52 in Appendix A).

3. The pharmacologic effects of metoclopramide, a dopamine antagonist, may be counteracted by combined use with dopamine agonistic drugs. Examples include: **bromocriptine** (a drug used to treat Parkinson disease) and other authentic **dopamine agonists** (*See* Ω -37 in Appendix A).

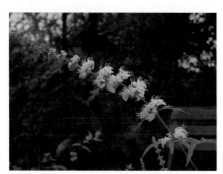

FIGURE 13-6   A, Partial feature of chasteberry in nature. (Courtesy of Wouter Hagens, the image owner)

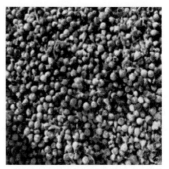

FIGURE 13-6   B, Cut and dried form of chasteberry fruit. (Attribution: Original source of image unidentified)

MCP ⟷ Alcohol: As common side effects of metoclopramide include drowsiness, restlessness, fatigue, and mental depression, it can potentiate the sedative effect of alcohol or sleeping pills when taken in combination.

MCP ⟷ Cabergoline: Metoclopramide is a dopamine antagonist, whereas cabergoline, a drug useful to treat breast engorgement by excessive secretions of prolactin, is a dopamine agonist. Hence, when they are used in combination they may counteract each other's therapeutic effectiveness.

MCP ⟷ (Chasteberry): Chasteberry (Fig. 13-6 A and B), an herb used for dysmenorrhea, and premenstrual stress in Chinese medicine, is known to contain dopaminergic compounds, and its use may offset the therapeutic effectiveness of metoclopramide.

MCP ⟷ Cyclosporine: Metoclopramide can increase the intestinal absorption of cyclosporine to raise its blood levels and toxicities.

MCP ⟷ CYP Isozymes: *See* Table 13-1 below.

MCP ⟷ Digoxin: Though metoclopramide does not affect P-glycoprotein transporter, it can decrease the intestinal absorption of digoxin as much as one-third, undercutting its therapeutic effectiveness.

MCP ⟷ MAO Inhibitors: (*See* Ω-51 in Appendix A.) Since metoclopramide can release catecholamines whose inactivation requires MAO, it should not be used with any drug that inhibits the enzyme MAO, especially in patients having essential hypertension, as otherwise a serious hypertensive crisis may ensue.

TABLE 13-1   Metoclopramide vs CYP Isozymes

Drug Name	1A2	2A6	2B6	2C8	2C9	2C18	2C19	2D6	2E1	3A4
Metoclopramide	Sub							Sub + Inh		

Abbreviations: Sub, substrate of the enzyme; Inh, inhibits the enzyme; Ezi: induces the enzyme

Metoclopramide exerts an inhibitory effect on CYP2D6 and thus, administration of this drug in combination with other drugs that require this enzyme for their metabolic clearance may result in elevated blood levels, possibly inciting their adverse effects. (*See* the middle column of Table-0 at the 'Introduction' for possible substrates of the enzyme.)

MCP ⟷ SSRIs: (*See* Ω-68 in Appendix A.) Metoclopramide is an antagonist at both the dopamine receptors and the 5HT-3 receptors. Nevertheless, when it is taken with a member of the selective serotonin reuptake inhibitors (SSRIs), it may foster incidences of serotonin syndrome, which results from overstimulation of 5-HT-1A receptors in the central gray nuclei and the medulla.

MCP ⟷ Succinylcholine: The enzyme plasma cholinesterase can be inhibited by metoclopramide and whose co-administration with a drug that requires this enzyme for inactivation can prolong and amplify effects of the latter. Those affected drugs include mivacurium and succinylcholine, leading to paralysis of respiratory muscles.

CHAPTER

14

Tussis (Common Cough)

Tussis (cough) refers to rapid expulsions of air from the lungs in an attempt to clear fluid, mucus, or other material from the air pathway.

Medications shown effective in the treatment of tussis include: (1) **hydrocodone** (Hycoclear, Lortab, Norco, Vicodin); (2) **codeine;** (3) **dextromethorphan** (Benylin-DM); (4) **tiotropium** (Spiriva); and (5) **benzonatate.** Among the above, hydrocodone is often used in combination with **chlorpheniramine,** an antihistamine (for example, Tussionex); and codeine is often used together with **promethazine.**

HYDROCODONE

MECHANISM OF ACTION

Hydrocodone is used to suppress a dry, hacking cough. This drug may directly suppress the cough center and the cough reflex. At excess doses, it may depress respiration itself. Hydrocodone (Fig.14-1) is an inactive prodrug that must be o-demethylated mainly by CYP2D6 to its active metabolite, hydromorphone (Dilaudid) (Fig.14-2), a more potent opioid analgesic than morphine, which is then metabolized by CYP3A4 to its final inactive norhydrocodone (Fig.14-3). Hydromorphone itself was once officially approved as a drug but was removed from the United States market in 2005 due to high incidence of risk when taken with alcohol.

SIDE EFFECTS

Hydrocodone: It may cause difficulty in breathing; dry mouth, stomach cramps, and pain, nausea and vomiting, constipation; difficulty in urination; decreased libido (sex drive); exaggerated sense of well-being or fear; dizziness, drowsiness, and mental clouding.

Tussionex **(Chlorpheniramine + Hydrocodone):** This combined preparation may induce cardiac arrhythmia; dry mouth, loss of appetite, upset stomach, vomiting, and constipation; difficulty in urination; and dizziness, drowsiness, anxiety, hallucinations, and seizures.

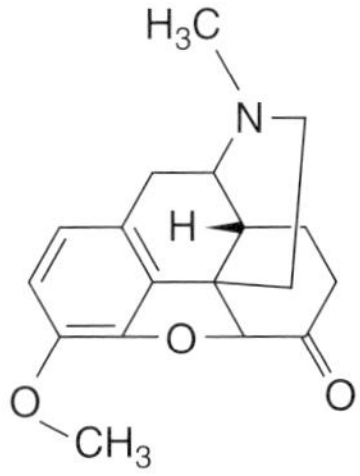

FIGURE 14-1   Molecular structure of hydrocodone.

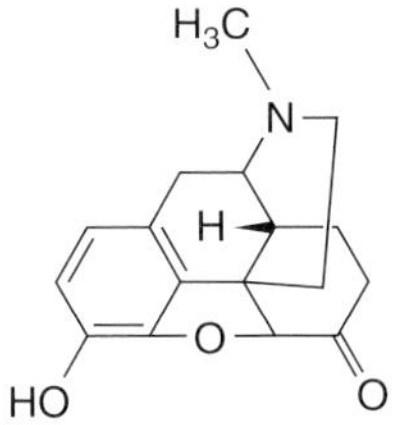

FIGURE 14-2   Molecular structure of hydromorphone.

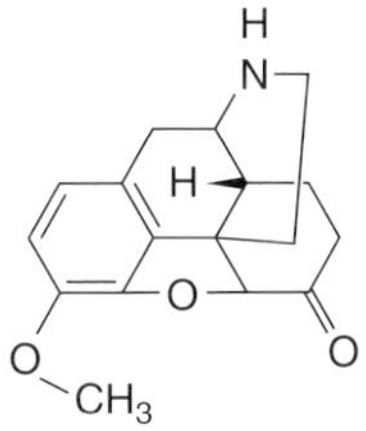

FIGURE 14-3   Molecular structure of norhydrocodone.

DRUG INTERACTIONS

Hydrocodone: *See* Appendix B-32: Interactions of Opioid Analgesics.

Tussionex (Chlorpheniramine + Hydrocodone): For chlorpheniramine, *See* Appendix B-10: Interactions of Antihistamines, First-Generation; and for hydrocodone, *See* Appendix B-32: Interactions of Opioid Analgesics.

CODEINE

Medications shown effective in the treatment of bad coughs due to colds, influenza, or hay fever include codeine or syrup containing both **codeine** and **promethazine**. Codeine activates the brain morphine receptor (μ-receptors) to suppress coughs. Codeine also produces analgesia and sedation but to a lesser degree than by morphine (Duramorph). Promethazine is an antihistamine that dries up nasal secretions and suppresses the cough reflex.

MECHANISM OF ACTION

Codeine: Codeine is used to suppress a dry, hacking cough. However, codeine is a prodrug (Fig.14-4) that has to be demethylated at its position 3 by CYP2D6

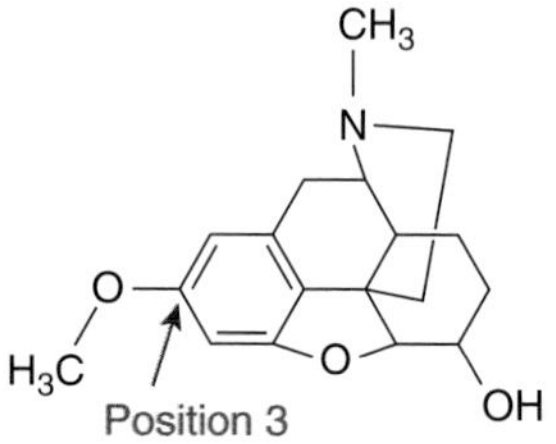

FIGURE 14-4   Molecular structure of codeine.

(*See* Table 14-1) to morphine (Fig.14-5), its active form. Codeine, after conversion to its active form, may directly suppress the cough center and cough reflex, but in excess doses, it may depress respiration itself.

Promethazine: Promethazine is an antihistamine that also has antiemetic, anticholinergic, and local anesthetic effects.

SIDE EFFECTS

Codeine: Frequent side effects of codeine include shortness of breath; nausea, vomiting, abdominal pain, constipation; lightheadedness, dizziness, drowsiness, and

TABLE 14-1   Codeine, Dextromethorphan, and Tiotropium vs CYP Enzymes

Drug Name	1A2	2A6	2B6	2C8	2C9	2C18	2C19	2D6	2E1	3A4
Codeine								Sub		Sub
Dextromethorphan					Sub		Sub	Sub	Sub	Sub
Tiotropium								Sub		Sub

Abbreviations: Sub, substrate of the enzyme; Inh, inhibits the enzyme; Ezi, induces the enzyme

1. Activation by O-demethylation of the prodrug codeine to morphine occurs in the liver and this activation is processed by the hepatic CYP2D6. Codeine is also N-demethylated by CYP3A4 to norcodeine, which has little therapeutic effectiveness. Hence, co-administration of codeine with an inhibitor of CYP2D6 can make codeine either ineffective or insufficiently active. For instance, paroxetine (Paxil), fluoxetine (Prozac), propoxyphene (Darvon), quinidine, and cimetidine are inhibitors of CYP 2D6, and if codeine is taken together with any of them, the therapeutic effectiveness of codeine may be impaired. (*See* the left-hand column of Table-0 at the 'Introduction' for other possible inhibitors of this enzyme.)

2. Dextromethorphan is cleared through CYP 2C9, 2C19, 2D6, 2E1, and CYP3A4; and fluoxetine inhibits all these enzymes except CYP2E1. Hence, co-administration with dextromethorphan may raise blood levels and adverse effects of dextromethorphan.

3. Tiotropium is metabolized to a limited extent by the cytochrome CYP2D6 and CYP3A4, and therefore, inhibitors of those enzymes may elevate its blood levels to some degree, but its clinical significance is questioned.

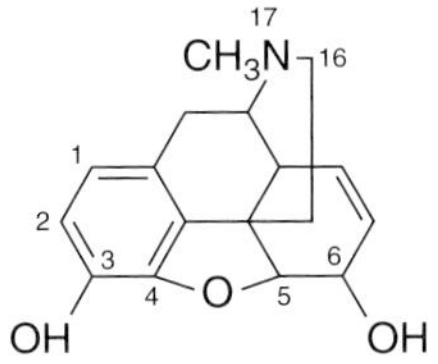

FIGURE 14-5   Molecular structure of morphine.

mental clouding with an exaggerated sense of well-being or fear. Other side effects of codeine may include allergic reactions. Codeine is also habit-forming—mental and physical dependence may occur, and when codeine is suddenly withdrawn after prolonged use, symptoms of withdrawal may develop. Hence, the dose of codeine should be reduced gradually, but dependency is unlikely when codeine is used for short-term pain relief.

Promethazine: Side effects of promethazine include dry mouth and constipation; difficulty in urination; paresthesias, fatigue, and muscle tremors; and drowsiness, dizziness, and very rarely, respiratory depression. Promethazine may turn urine blue-green, but this does not usually indicate medical emergency.

DRUG INTERACTIONS

Codeine: Morphine is the major active metabolite of codeine. Codeine-6-glucuronide has some analgesic effects, but to a much lesser extent than does morphine. For drug interactions of codeine, *See* Appendix B-32 and for its relationship with CYP enzymes, *See* Table 14-1.

Promethazine: *See* Appendix B-10: Interactions of Antihistamines, First-Generation.

DEXTROMETHORPHAN

MECHANISM OF ACTION

Dextromethorphan binds to the N-methyl-D-aspartic acid (NMDA) (Fig.14-6) receptor in the cough center of the medulla to oppose binding of L-glutamate, the major excitatory neurotransmitter in the mammalian central nervous system, with consequent reduction in discharge of the neuronal impulses down the efferent nerves to the muscles involved in coughing.

SIDE EFFECTS

Dextromethorphan may cause stomach upset; and dizziness and anxiety.

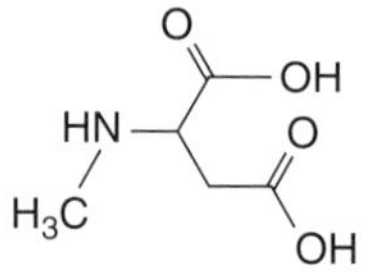

FIGURE 14-6   Molecular structure of NMDA.

BOX 14-1

Basic Concepts of Dextromethorphan Interactions

Co-administration of dextromethorphan with a central nervous system (CNS) stimulant tends to increase incidences of untoward CNS side effects such as drowsiness, restlessness, vertigo, and ataxia with muscle rigidity. Those CNS stimulant drugs include **amphetamine** and **caffeine.**

DRUG INTERACTIONS:

See Box 14-1.

Miscellaneous Interactions of Dextromethorphan (DMP)

DMP ⟷ Alcohol: If dextromethorphan is taken together with ethanol, it slows reactivity during driving and reduces clarity of thinking.

DMP ⟷ CYP Isozymes: *See* Table 14-1.

DMP ⟷ MAO Inhibitors: (*See* Ω-51 in Appendix A.) Dextromethorphan enhances serotonin activity by inhibiting its reuptake. Hence, never take dextromethorphan (Robitussin-DM) within 14 days of using an MAO inhibitor, otherwise, a serious, life-threatening hyperpyrexia and hypotension may ensue.

TIOTROPIUM

Tiotropium is administered by dry powder inhalation.

MECHANISM OF ACTION

Tiotropium (Fig.14-7) is a long-acting anticholinergic drug that induces broncho-dilation by blocking the M1 and M3 receptors. This drug minimizes the release of

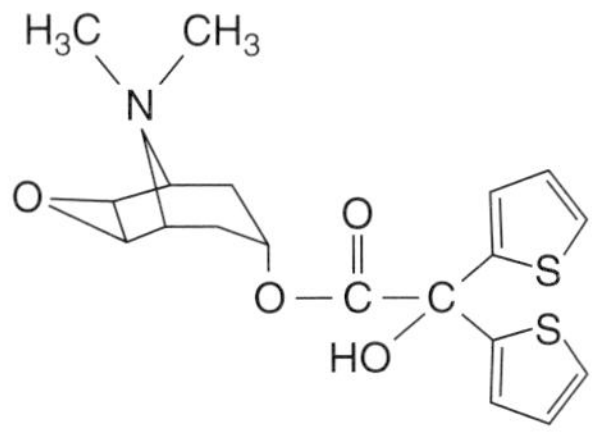

FIGURE 14-7   Molecular structure of tiotropium.

acetylcholine as well. It is therefore thought that tiotropium inhibits cough reflex sensitivities.

SIDE EFFECTS

Tiotropium may cause tachycardia (increased heart rate); difficulty in breathing; dry mouth, constipation; difficult or painful urination; narrow-angle glaucoma with eye pain or discomfort; and blurred vision.

DRUG INTERACTIONS

See Table 14-1.

BENZONATATE

Its oral preparation is used to relieve a cough due to colds or allergies for up to eight hours.

MECHANISM OF ACTION

When applied topically, benzonatate dulls the cough reflex. It binds to the voltage-gated sodium channels within the intracellular portion of the neuronal membrane to decrease the rate of depolarization, generating a local anesthetic effect on the stretch receptors of the vagal afferent fibers in the bronchi and alveoli of the lungs.

SIDE EFFECTS

Benzonatate may cause nasal congestion, bronchospasm, and difficulty in breathing; nausea, vomiting, and constipation; numbness of the chest and tremor; dizziness, drowsiness, headache, and convulsions; and, rarely, skin rash.

DRUG INTERACTIONS

There is no clinically important drug interaction reported.

CHAPTER

15

Asthma

Asthma is a chronic inflammatory disease of the lower airways. The inflammation causes the airways to constrict, generating symptoms such as coughing, wheezing, dyspnea, and paroxysmal (recurrent spasms of) chest tightness. About 60% of asthma in the United States is due to allergic reactions to such allergens as pollen, mold, dust mites, and animal dander.

The following medications have been shown effective in controlling asthma symptoms: (1) **montelukast** (Singulair): (2) adrenergic beta-2 agonists such as **albuterol aerosol, albuterol nebulizer solution,** Combivent **(albuterol + ipratropium)**, and **levalbuterol** (Xopenex); (3) xanthine derivative such as **dyphylline** (Dilor, Lufyllin); (4) glucocorticoids such as **budesonide** (Pulmicort Respules), **fluticasone** (Flonase, Flovent HFA), **methylprednisolone** (Medrol), **mometasone** (Nasonex), **prednisolone, prednisone,** and **triamcinolone**.

MONTELUKAST

MECHANISM OF ACTION

Montelukast selectively blocks the LTD4 (leukotriene D4) receptors and thereby staves off leukotriene-induced bronchoconstriction.

SIDE EFFECTS

Montelukast may cause upset stomach, nausea, and diarrhea; muscle weakness; and dizziness and headache.

DRUG INTERACTIONS

See Table 15-1.

TABLE 15-1   Montelukast vs CYP Isozymes

Drug Name	1A2	2A6	2B6	2C8	2C9	2C18	2C19	2D6	2E1	3A4
Montelukast				Inh	Sub					Sub

Abbreviations: Sub, substrate of the enzyme; Inh, inhibits the enzyme; Ezi, induces the enzyme

1. Montelukast has some inhibitory effect against CYP2C8. However, there was no evidence of adverse interactions when this drug was taken with diazepam, a CYP2C8 substrate. Nevertheless, it may be prudent to assume that its combination with a CYP2C8 substrate may result in elevated blood levels and adverse effects. (*See* the middle column of Table-0 at the 'Introduction' for other possible substrates of the enzyme.)

2. Montelukast is a substrate of both CYP2C9 & CYP3A4 and hence, inducers of these enzymes, such as phenobarbital and rifampin, may quicken metabolic clearance of montelukast to diminish its therapeutic effectiveness.

ADRENERGIC BETA-2 AGONISTS

Albuterol aerosol, **albuterol nebulizer solution**, Combivent **(albuterol + ipratropium)**, and **levalbuterol**

Levalbuterol mentioned above is a levo-isomer of traditionally used racemic albuterol. A greater effectiveness of levalbuterol over albuterol is claimed but its cost effectiveness is questioned. It is important that nebulized drugs should be used properly, so as to assure they get into the lungs.

MECHANISM OF ACTION
By activation of the adrenergic beta-2 receptors at the bronchial tree, they increase c-AMP causing dilation of the bronchial smooth muscles for easier breathing.

SIDE EFFECTS
Albuterol or **Levalbuterol:** They may cause irregular heartbeats; dry mouth; nausea, vomiting, or diarrhea; tremor; and headache, dizziness, and nervousness.

Combivent **(Albuterol + Ipratropium):** This preparation may cause cardiac arrhythmia, increased blood pressure; dry mouth, unusual taste in the mouth, nausea, vomiting, upset stomach; difficulty in urination; headache, dizziness, nervousness; and blurred vision.

DRUG INTERACTIONS
Albuterol or Levalbuterol (ALT)
It is not known whether other medications will interact with these medications applied topically, but if absorbed extensively from their site of application the following interactions may take place.

ALT ↔ Beta Blockers: (non-cardioselective) (*See* Ω-27 in Appendix A.) If a non-cardioselective beta blocker, such as propranolol or sotalol, is coadministered with a bronchodilator such as albuterol or levalbuterol, their bronchodilation through adrenergic beta receptors in the bronchial tree may be abated or nullified to allow a serious bronchoconstriction.

ALT ↔ Fludrocortisone: Both albuterol and levalbuterol induce uptake of potassium into tissue cells to lower blood levels of potassium and are effective in the treatment of hyperkalemia (excessive blood levels of potassium). If either of the drugs is used in combination with other drugs that also lower blood levels of potassium, such as fludrocortisone, which loses potassium in exchange for sodium retained, they can pull together toward excessive hypokalemia, a condition that may spawn cardiac arrhythmia.

ALT ↔ MAO Inhibitors: (*See* Ω-51 in Appendix A.) Albuterol is metabolized mainly by sulfate conjugation, which is followed by renal excretion. However, if albuterol or levalbuterol is administered in combination with an MAO inhibitor such as phenelzine, it may cause agitations, and invite dangerous cardiovascular side effects such as tachycardia.

ALT ↔ Sympathomimetic Drugs: (*See* Ω-71 in Appendix A.) If either one of the above is co-administered with a sympathomimetic drug, it may precipitate dangerous cardiovascular effects such as palpitations, flattening of the T-wave, prolongation of the Q-Tc interval, and depression of the S-T segment.

Combivent (CBV) **(Albuterol + Ipratropium)**

As an inhalation aerosol this preparation has often been used concomitantly with other sympathomimetic bronchodilators, or with theophylline, a bronchodilating xanthine, or with steroids. It is not known whether other medications will interact with this preparation applied topically, but if absorbed extensively from its site of application, the following interactions may take place.

CBV ↔ Anticholinergic Agents: (*See* Ω-14 in Appendix A.) Although ipratropium (Fig. 15-1), an anticholinergic agent, is minimally absorbed into systemic circulation, there is some potential for interaction with other anticholinergic medications used in combination to generate additive side effects.

CBV ↔ Beta Blockers: (*See* Ω-27 in Appendix A.) A beta blocker used in combination can oppose the bronchodilating effect of either of the above drugs.

CBV ↔ Digoxin: Both albuterol and levalbuterol may decrease serum levels of digoxin by about 20%, by yet unclear mechanism.

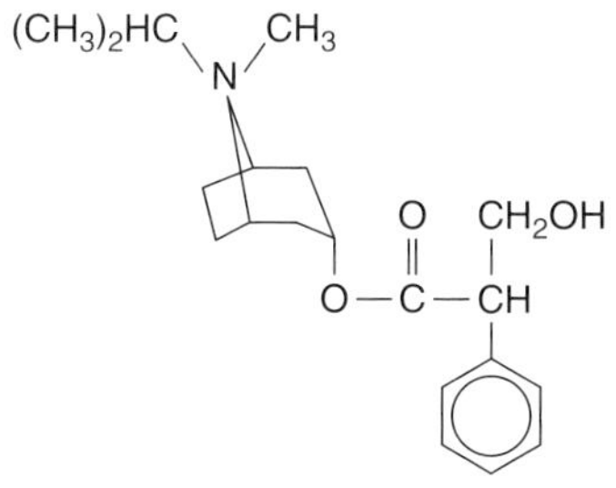

FIGURE 15-1   Molecular structure of ipratropium.

CBV ⟷ MAO Inhibitors: (*See* Ω-51 in Appendix A.) Avoid taking an inhibitor of MAO within two weeks of discontinuation of albuterol or levalbuterol, to thwart dangerous adverse cardiovascular effects.

CBV ⟷ Sympathomimetic Drugs: (*See* Ω-71 in Appendix A.) Co-administration of albuterol or levalbuterol with any other sympathomimetic drugs may lead to dangerous consequences on the cardiovascular system.

CBV ⟷ Tricyclic Antidepressants: (*See* Ω-76 in Appendix A.) Caution is advised in co-administration of albuterol or levalbuterol with a member of the tricyclic antidepressants, because the tricyclic blocks the reuptake of norepinephrine to potentiate the action of albuterol or levalbuterol on the cardiovascular system.

DYPHYLLINE

Chemically, dyphylline is (7-[2,3-dihydroxypropyl] theophylline) (Fig. 15-2) and hence, it is a xanthine derivative. This oral drug is used to relieve acute bronchial asthma and for bronchospasm associated with chronic bronchitis or emphysema.

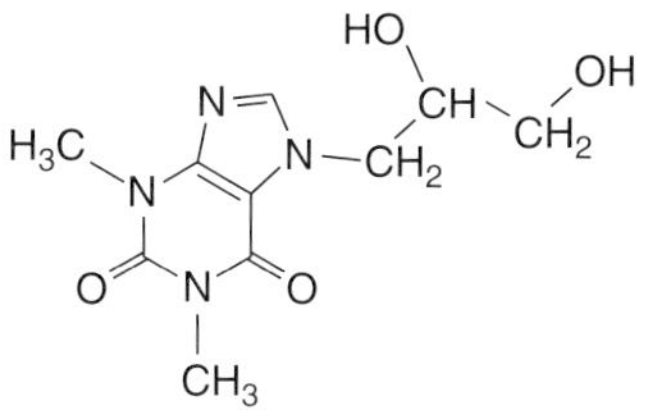

FIGURE 15-2   Molecular structure of dyphylline.

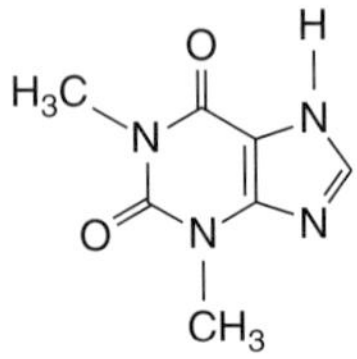

FIGURE 15-3   Molecular structure of theophylline.

MECHANISM OF ACTION

Dyphylline accumulates c-AMP by inhibition of phosphodiesterase, the enzyme that destroys c-AMP. The accumulated c-AMP in turn causes relaxation of bronchial smooth muscle to generate bronchodilation.

SIDE EFFECTS

Possible side effects of dyphylline include palpitation, flushing, and hypotension; tachypnea (rapid breathing); nausea, vomiting, epigastric pain, and diarrhea; muscle twitching; hyperglycemia; and headache, irritability, restlessness, and insomnia.

DRUG INTERACTIONS

Though dyphylline is a derivative of theophylline (Fig. 15-3), it is not converted to theophylline itself or other metabolites in the liver, but excreted unchanged in the urine. The urinary excretion of dyphylline is reduced by concomitant administration of probenecid, resulting in elevated blood levels and adverse effects of dyphylline.

GLUCOCORTICOIDS

Budesonide, fluticasone, methylprednisolone, mometasone, prednisolone, prednisone, and **triamcinolone**

Advair Diskus is a preparation containing fluticasone, a glucocorticoid, and salmeterol, an activator of the bronchial adrenergic beta-2 receptor that causes bronchodilation. The above mentioned glucocorticoids reduce itching and swelling of bronchial tissues associated with asthma. Methylprednisolone above is particularly useful to treat status asthmaticus.

MECHANISM OF ACTION

Inflammation of the airways is an integrated feature of asthma, which can cause bronchoconstriction and increased mucous secretion to generate classic asthma

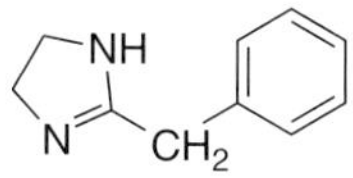

FIGURE 16-1 Molecular structure of tolazoline.

CVM ⟷ Tolazoline: Tolazoline (Fig. 16-1) is an alpha-adrenergic blocker that causes vasodilation and relieves spasms of the peripheral blood vessels. Tolazoline taken in combination may generate additive cholinomimetic signs of cevimeline.

PILOCARPINE

Pilocarpine is often indicated for the treatment of radiation-induced xerostomia and symptoms of dry mouth in patients with Sjögren syndrome.

MECHANISM OF ACTION

Pilocarpine is a cholinomimetic agent that activates M-3 receptors at the exocrine glands to increase secretions from the salivary glands.

SIDE EFFECTS

Pilocarpine may cause irregular heartbeats; nausea; runny nose; tearing; sweating; increased urge to urinate; changes in vision; and dizziness and headache.

DRUG INTERACTIONS

Pilocarpine (PLP)

PLP ⟷ Anticholinergic Agents: (*See* Ω-14 in Appendix A.) Pilocarpine, a cholinergic muscarinic agonist, may offset the effectiveness of such antimuscarinic drugs as atropine and ipratropium, when taken together.

PLP ⟷ Beta Blockers: (*See* Ω-27 in Appendix A.) Pilocarpine tends to slow the A-V nodal conduction of the heart. If it is taken together with a beta blocker, the A-V conduction may further be slowed to a detrimental consequence.

PLP ⟷ Cholinomimetic Drugs: (*See* Ω-34 in Appendix A.) Adverse effects of cholinomimetic drugs may become aggravated when administered concurrently with pilocarpine.

PLP ⟷ CYP Isozymes: *See* Table 16-1.

SORBITOL

Chewing on a piece of sugarless gum containing sorbitol for five to ten minutes every two hours may help to increase secretions of saliva. Numoisyn lozenges that contain both sorbitol and malic acid are claimed to stimulate salivation at least temporarily in patients with normal perceptions of taste and with some secretory functions of the salivary glands.

MECHANISM OF ACTION

Its mechanism of action remains unclear, but Numoisyn lozenges are claimed to increase the salivary secretions by chemical binding of their ingredients to taste bud receptors, thereby sending impulses to the salivary nuclei in the brain stem and then through the efferent gustatory axons to the parasympathetic secretomotor innervating the salivary glands.

SIDE EFFECTS

Sorbitol may induce nausea, gas, diarrhea, stomach cramps, or anal irritation. Caution is advised when using this drug in the elderly or in children because they may be more sensitive to its effects; and sorbitol is not recommended during pregnancy or breast-feeding. Sorbitol may turn urine brown or brownish black, but this does not amount to a medical emergency.

DRUG INTERACTIONS

No specific interactions with Sorbitol are known at the time of publication. It is a good practice to drink a lot of water to relieve xerostomia, but avoid drinking soda or orange juice, which is rich in citric acid that can erode the tooth enamel. Also avoid smoking or drinking alcohol, as they dry out the mouth. Avoid drinking coffee or tea, as their caffeine can also dry out the mouth. Avoid taking spicy or salty foods, as they may generate pain in a dry mouth.

17

Aphthous Ulcer (Canker Sore)

Aphthous ulcer (canker sore) is a small ulcer in the lining of the oral cavity, giving rise to pain and increased sensitivity to acids.

Medications that may possibly be effective in the treatment of canker sore include: (1) **amlexanox** (Aphthasol); (2) **sulfonated phenol topical solution** (Debacterol); (3) **tetracycline;** and (4) **dexamethasone** or **triamcinolone**.

AMLEXANOX

Amlexanox has been developed as a five percent topical oral paste, and was the first FDA-approved drug specifically for the treatment of aphthous ulcer (canker sore). Amlexanox works best if it is taken as soon as such ulcers are diagnosed.

MECHANISM OF ACTION

The mechanism of action by which amlexanox helps to heal a canker sore is poorly understood. A postulation is that amlexanox inhibits the formation and release of histamine and inflammatory substances such as leukotrienes from the mast cells, basophils, and neutrophils.

SIDE EFFECTS

Amlexanox may cause stinging or burning at the application site, and it may generate allergic reactions such as skin rash and itching; difficulty in breathing; and swelling of the face, lips, tongue, or throat. Discontinue this drug if skin rash or contact mucositis develops, and seek medical help. Amlexanox may pass into breast milk and caution is advised during periods of nursing. (It is recommended to wash hands immediately after applying amlexanox and to flush eyes with water promptly if they come in contact with the paste.)

DRUG INTERACTIONS

Its interactions with other medications are not well documented, but patients allergic to any drugs, or patients with weak immune systems caused by disease or by taking certain anticancer drugs, may best avoid taking amlexanox.

SULFONATED PHENOL TOPICAL SOLUTION

Debacterol: This topical solution contains 280 mg of sulfonated phenol and 500 mg of sulfuric acid per each milliliter of preparation. This medication is for external use only. For canker sores, cotton-tipped swab may be used to apply the product for one to three minutes. The treatment is followed by a rinse with a neutralizing solution of sodium bicarbonate (baking soda), one-half teaspoonful dissolved in 4 ounces (or 120 ml) of water.

MECHANISM OF ACTION

This preparation appears to burn and damage the exposed sensory nerves in the open sore area to promote scabbing over. This scab wards off the sensation of pain associated with the ulceration.

SIDE EFFECTS

This preparation may cause irritation at the applied area or generate a temporary stinging sensation immediately after application. If excess irritation occurs, it is recommended to rinse with a baking soda solution to chemically neutralize the acidic medication.

DRUG INTERACTIONS

It is not known whether other medications will interact with this medication applied topically.

TETRACYCLINE

Rinsing with tetracycline mouth wash several times a day was shown to reduce the pain and quicken healing of canker sores. However, it is important not to use tetracycline in pregnant patients or in children under the age of eight because of permanent discoloration of the teeth. For safety concerns, all liquid oral products containing tetracycline in a concentration greater than 25 mg/ml were withdrawn from the market in the United States.

MECHANISM OF ACTION

Tetracycline works by inhibition of bacterial protein synthesis. It binds competitively to the 30S subunit of the bacterial ribosome to block the proper attachment of amino acyl t-RNA, thus preventing incorporation of a new amino acid onto the growing end of a peptide chain.

SIDE EFFECTS

The most frequent side effects of tetracycline include nausea, abdominal pain, vomiting, and diarrhea. Tetracycline may cause permanent discoloration of teeth if used in patients below eight years of age; jaundice and liver damage, especially in patients with renal impairment; and its continuous use may cause superinfections by such tetracycline-resistant microbes as pseudomonas, staphylococcus, and candida. Rarely, tetracycline may cause allergic reactions too. Doxycycline and minocycline, both members of tetracycline family, increase sensitivity to sunlight.

DRUG INTERACTIONS

It is not known whether other medications will interact with this medication applied topically. *See* Appendix B-30: Interactions of Tetracyclines for a list of interactions that may take place if it is absorbed extensively from the site of application.

DEXAMETHASONE OR TRIAMCINOLONE

Use of mouthwash containing glucocorticoids such as dexamethasone (Fig. 17-1) and triamcinolone (Fig. 17-2) may help heal the canker sore.

MECHANISM OF ACTION

These glucocorticoids are powerful anti-inflammatory agents in the treatment of canker sore. They bind to glucocorticoid receptors in cytosol and the bound steroid-receptor complex migrates to the nucleus to inhibit the

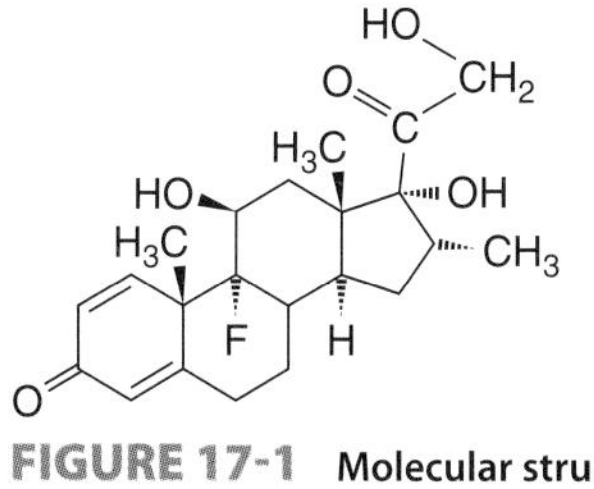

FIGURE 17-1 Molecular structure of dexamethasone.

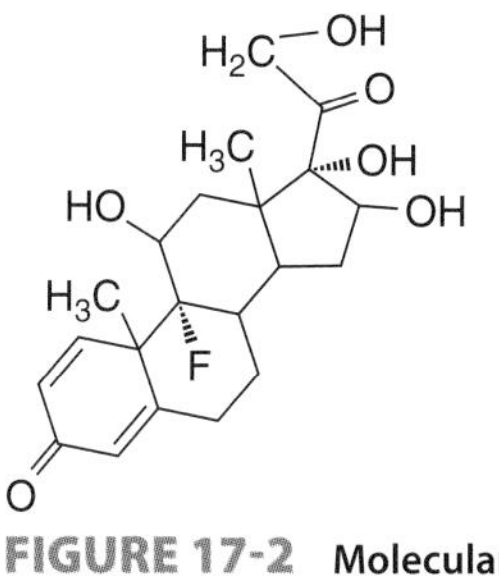

FIGURE 17-2 Molecular structure of triamcinolone.

transcriptions of most cytokines and chemokines, both of which cause inflammations.

SIDE EFFECTS

They may cause skin rash; upset stomach; swelling of the face, lower legs, or ankles; muscle weakness; headache; and dizziness and insomnia.

DRUG INTERACTIONS

See Appendix B-20: Interactions of Glucocorticoids.

Odontalgia (Toothache)

18

Odontalgia (toothache) refers to pain in or near a tooth, possibly due to infections or inflammations of the gingiva (tooth gum). The most common cause is a dental cavity that exposes nerve endings to external stimuli.

Medications that may possibly be effective in the treatment of toothache include: (1) lozenges or dental creams, containing anesthetics such as **benzocaine** (Anbesol, Benzodent, Numzident), Chloraseptic **(benzocaine + menthol)**, **dyclonine** (Sucrets), or **lidocaine** (Xylocaine); (2) **a 3% hydrogen peroxide solution;** and (3) oral analgesic drugs such as **aspirin** and **acetaminophen** (Tylenol).

LOCAL ANESTEHTICS

Benzocaine (Fig. 18-1), **dyclonine** (Fig. 18-2), and **lidocaine** (*See* Fig. 4-7)

MECHANISM OF ACTION

A charged molecule of a local anesthetic agent apparently competes with calcium ions for binding to a receptor, which in a neuronal membrane is located on the

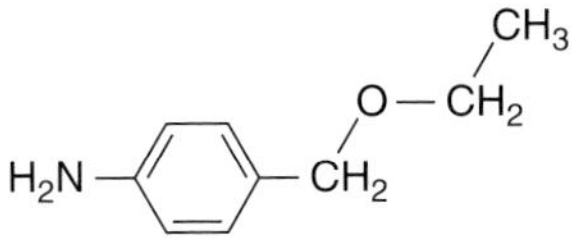

FIGURE 18-1 Molecular structure of benzocaine.

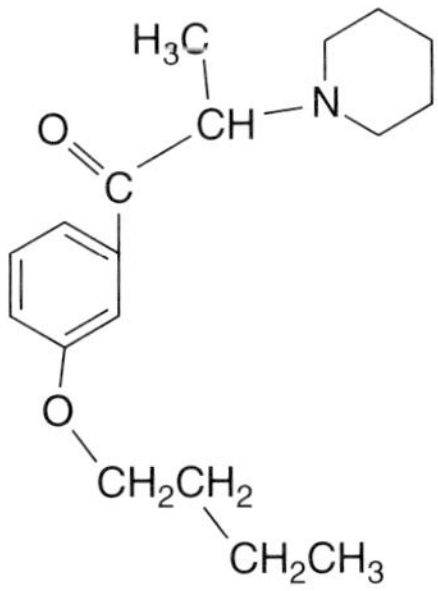

FIGURE 18-2 Molecular structure of dyclonine.

131

inner side of the sodium channel. Once bound, the local anesthetic agent may block the channel, opposing sodium influx and thereby impeding depolarization of the neuron. Nerve impulse conduction for pain sensation is similarly affected.

SIDE EFFECTS

Their frequent side effects include numbness of the mouth; rectal bleeding; and rarely, allergic reactions such as skin rash and itching.

DRUG INTERACTIONS

Their interactions are not yet well documented.

HYDROGEN PEROXIDE

Rinsing for 30 seconds with a mouthful of 3% hydrogen peroxide solution can kill bacteria in the mouth cavity. Spit it out before rinsing with clean water a few times.

MECHANISM OF ACTION

Catalase, which is ubiquitously available, catalyzes decomposition of hydrogen peroxide to water and nascent oxygen. This oxygen can generate antibacterial and antiviral activities, but this germicidal effect is diminished in the presence of organic matter.

SIDE EFFECTS

Hydrogen peroxide may cause a burning or stinging sensation, unpleasant taste, and very rarely, allergic reactions such as skin itching. However, hydrogen peroxide is such an unstable compound that when it is applied over a wound or cut, it is disintegrated into oxygen and water without being absorbed into system. Hence, it poses little harm to other parts of the body.

DRUG INTERACTIONS

Interactions of hydrogen peroxide with other drugs are not well documented.

ACETAMINOPHEN OR ASPIRIN

Acetaminophen is often used in combination with butalbital and caffeine to obtain analgesia. Endocet is a preparation containing both acetaminophen and oxycodone.

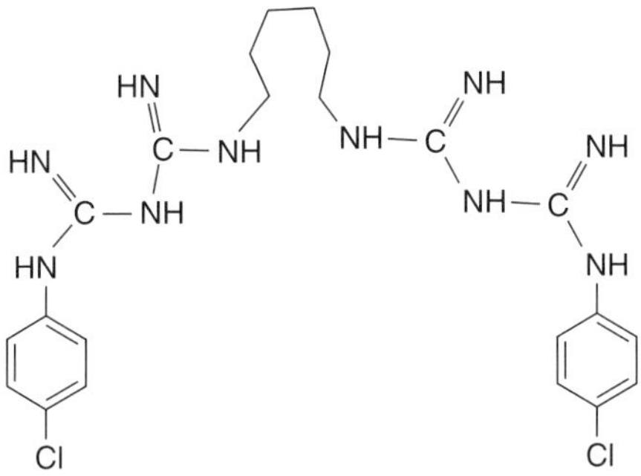

FIGURE 19-1 Molecular structure of chlorhexidine.

DRUG INTERACTIONS

There is no clinically important interaction reported.

DOXYCYCLINE OR MINOCYCLINE

Doxycycline or minocycline gel put in the tooth pockets might suppress bacteria and reduce the size of periodontal pockets.

MECHANISM OF ACTION

These tetracyclines (Fig. 19-2) work by inhibiting bacterial protein synthesis. They bind competitively to the 30S subunit of bacterial ribosomes to block the proper attachment of amino acyl t-RNA, thus preventing incorporation of a new amino acid onto the growing end of a peptide chain.

SIDE EFFECTS

The most frequent side effects of theirs include nausea, abdominal pain, vomiting, and diarrhea. They may cause permanent discoloration of teeth if used in patients below eight years of age; jaundice and liver damage especially in patients with renal impairment; increased sensitivity to sunlight; and their continuous use may cause superinfections by such tetracycline-resistant microbes as pseudomonas, staphylococcus, and candida. Rarely, they may cause allergic reactions too.

DRUG INTERACTIONS

See Appendix B-30: Interactions of Tetracyclines.

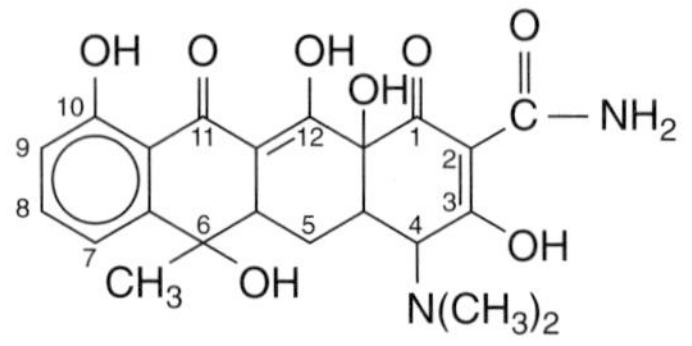

TETRACYCLINE

CONGENER	SUBSTITUENT(S)	POSITION(S)
Chlortetracycline	$-Cl$	7
Oxytetracycline	$-OH,-H$	5
Demeclocycline	$-OH,-H; -Cl$	6; 7
Methacycline	$-OH,-H; -CH_2$	5; 6
Doxycycline	$-OH,-H; -CH_3, -H$	5; 6
Minocycline	$-H,-H; -N(CH_3)_2$	6; 7

FIGURE 19-2   Molecular structures of tetracyclines. Reproduced, with permission, from Brunton LL, Lazo JS, and Parker KL. *Goodman and Gilman's The Pharmacological Basis of Therapeutics*. 11th ed. New York, NY: McGraw-Hill; 2006, p 1174.

HYDROGEN PEROXIDE

Mix half of one tablespoonful of 3% hydrogen peroxide solution with half of one tablespoonful of warm water to use as mouth gargle. Swishing this mixture inside the mouth for 30 seconds, three times a week, may inhibit growth of oral bacteria.

MECHANISM OF ACTION

See Chapter 18.

SIDE EFFECTS

See Chapter 18.

DRUG INTERACTIONS

While hydrogen peroxide is good for cleaning scabs, it is not the best choice for sterilizing wounds closed with absorbable sutures, because hydrogen peroxide could harm the stitches' integrity.

Nausea/Vomiting

Nausea refers to a sensation of queasiness with an urge to vomit. Vomiting refers to the expulsion of stomach contents through the mouth, usually as a result of reflexive spasmodic movements.

Medications that may possibly be effective in the treatment of nausea/vomiting include: (1) **ondansetron;** (2) **metoclopramide;** (3) antihistamines such as **dimenhydrinate** (Dramamine, Gravol) **meclizine** (Bonine), and **promethazine** (Phenergan). Note that dimenhydrinate is diphenhydramine (Fig. 20-1) complexed with 8-chlorotheophylline (Fig. 20-2).

ONDANSETRON

Ondansetron is used mainly to treat nausea and vomiting following chemotherapy.

MECHANISM OF ACTION

Ondansetron is a selective blocker of 5-HT3 receptors, which are located peripherally at the vagal nerve terminals and centrally at the chemoreceptor

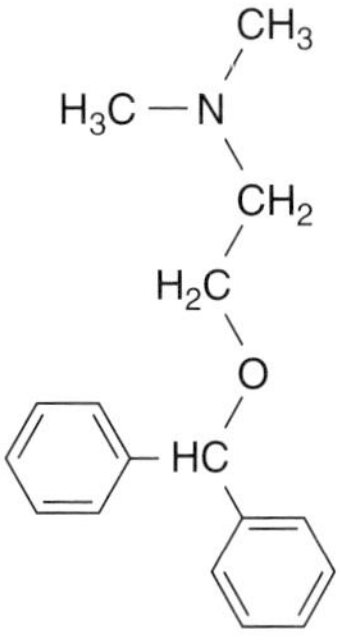

FIGURE 20-1 Molecular structure of diphenhydramine.

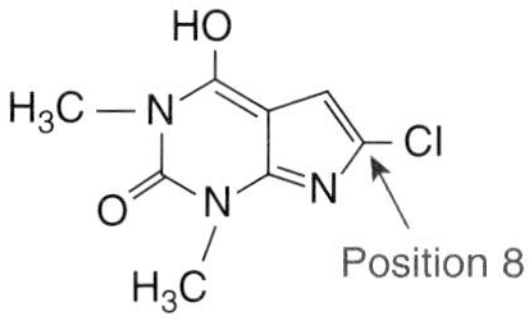

FIGURE 20-2 Molecular structure of 8-chlorotheophylline.

TABLE 20-1   Ondansetron vs CYP Isozymes

Drug Name	1A2	2A6	2B6	2C8	2C9	2C18	2C19	2D6	2E1	3A4
Ondansetron	Sub + Inh				Sub			Sub	Sub	Sub

Abbreviations: Sub, Substrate of the enzyme; Inh, Inhibits the enzyme; Ezi, Induces the enzyme

1. Ondansetron is mainly metabolized through CYP3A4 and thus, its intake with rifampin, an antibiotic and an inducer of this enzyme, can result in quickened elimination of ondansetron with diminished antiemetic effects. (*See* the right-hand column of Table-0 at the 'Introduction' for other possible inducers of the enzyme.)

2. Ondansetron is an inhibitor of hepatic microsomal enzyme CYP1A2 and thus, administration of this drug in combination with drugs that require this enzyme for hepatic clearance may raise their blood levels and potentially exacerbate their adverse effects. (*See* the middle column of Table-0 at the 'Introduction' for possible substrates of this enzyme.)

trigger zone of the area postrema in the medulla oblongata. Ondansetron may be used by intravenous infusion to prevent nausea and vomiting caused by an emetogenic cancer chemotherapeutic agent such as cisplatin, which appears to release serotonin that induces nausea and vomiting apparently by activation of the 5-HT3 receptors.

SIDE EFFECTS

Side effects of ondansetron may include diarrhea or constipation; chest pain; blurred vision; headache, lightheadedness, and drowsiness; and very rarely, it may cause allergic reaction such as skin rash and itching, and difficulty in breathing.

DRUG INTERACTIONS

See Table 20-1.

METOCLOPRAMIDE

Metoclopramide is also used in the prevention and treatment of chemotherapy-induced nausea or vomiting.

MECHANISM OF ACTION

Dopamine agonists are known to cause nausea and vomiting by stimulating the dopamine receptors. Metoclopramide blocks dopamine receptors in the chemoreceptor trigger zone (CTZ) situated in the area postrema of the medulla.

SIDE EFFECTS

Metoclopramide may cause dry mouth and diarrhea; muscle stiffness; trembling of the hands; high fever and sweating; and severe dizziness, drowsiness, and restlessness.

DRUG INTERACTIONS

See Chapter 13.

DIMENHYDRINATE, MECLIZINE & PROMETHAZINE

Dimenhydrinate (Fig. 20-3) is an 8-chlorotheophylline salt of a diphenhydramine, and is regarded as a prodrug of diphenhydramine (See Fig. 20-1). These antihistamines are useful for the prevention and treatment of nausea, vomiting, or dizziness associated with motion sickness. They are not effective in the treatment of nausea and vomiting associated with cancer chemotherapy.

MECHANISM OF ACTION

The vomiting center is responsible for the feeling of nausea and for generation of the vomiting reflex. However, the antiemetic and antivertigo effects of the above drugs are not fully understood, although it is postulated that they exert anticholinergic effects that suppress activation of the CTZ in the medulla and suppress excitability of the middle ear labyrinth. They also block histamine (H1-) receptors in the vomiting center located in the dorsolateral portion of the reticular formation of the medulla oblongata, which are activated upon receiving nerve messages from the vestibular apparatus in the middle ear.

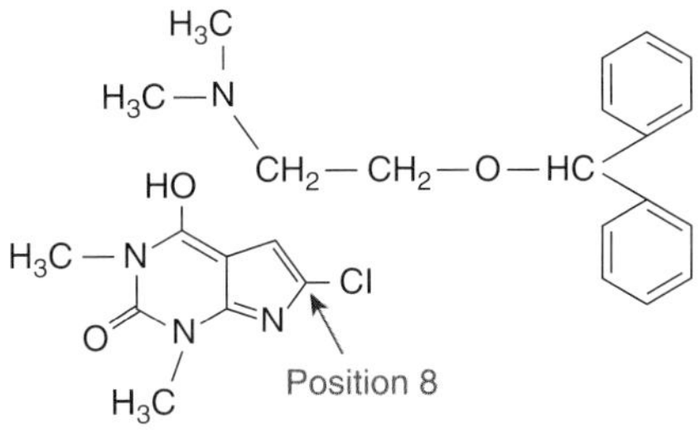

FIGURE 20-3 Molecular structure of dimenhydrinate.

SIDE EFFECTS

These antihistamines may cause irregular or fast heartbeat; depressed respiration; dry mouth, nose, or throat; constipation; urinary retention; impotence; mydriasis (dilated pupils), blurred vision; dizziness; restlessness; and sedation or insomnia.

DRUG INTERACTIONS

See Appendix B-10: Interactions of Antihistamines, First-Generation. *See* below for additional interactions of promethazine.

DRUG INTERACTIONS
Promethazine (PMZ)

PMZ ⟷ CYP Isozymes: *See* Table 20-2.

PMZ ⟷ MAO Inhibitors: (*See* Ω-51 in Appendix A.) Concurrent use of promethazine with an inhibitor of MAO may result in additive sedation and anticholinergic effects.

TABLE 20-2 **Promethazine vs CYP Enzymes**

Drug Name	1A2	2A6	2B6	2C8	2C9	2C18	2C19	2D6	2E1	3A4
Promethazine								Sub		

Abbreviations: Sub, substrate of the enzyme; Inh, inhibits the enzyme; Ezi, induces the enzyme

1. Metabolic clearance of promethazine requires the presence of microsomal CYP2D6 and thus, inhibition of this enzyme by any drug taken concomitantly may raise blood levels of promethazine and possibly exacerbate its adverse effects. (*See* the left-hand column of Table-0 at the 'Introduction' for other possible inhibitors of this enzyme.)

2. As promethazine requires CYP2D6 for its metabolic clearance, as do many tricyclic antidepressants such as amitriptyline, desipramine, and doxepin, concurrent administration of promethazine with such tricyclics may cause competition for their clearance, possibly resulting in elevated blood levels of the unmetabolized tricyclic and exacerbating their adverse effects. (*See* the middle column of Table-0 at the 'Introduction' for other possible substrates of the enzyme.)

C H A P T E R

21

Flatulence

Flatulence results from excessive gas formation in the gastrointestinal tract, giving rise to symptoms such as bloating, belching, and discomfort or pain in the abdomen.

Medications shown effective in the treatment of flatulence include: (1) **simethicone** (Mylicon); (2) **rifaximin** (Xifaxan); and (3) **activated charcoal**.

SIMETHICONE

Simethicone (Fig. 21-1) chemically represents polydimethylsiloxane to which silica, or silicon dioxide (SiO_2), is added. It can break up small gas bubbles in flatulence.

MECHANISM OF ACTION

Simethicone is thought to decrease the surface tension of the foam film of gas bubbles to rupture the liquid films, allowing escape of air in the digestive tract.

SIDE EFFECTS

There have been no reported serious side effects with simethicone.

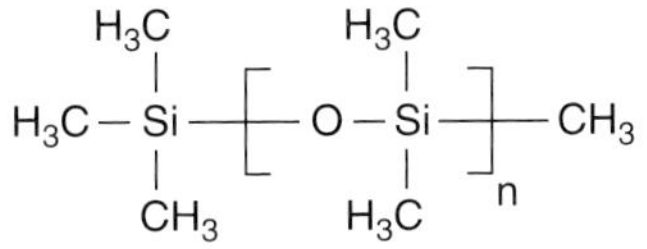

Dimethylsiloxane in the
parenthesis; n = 200–350

FIGURE 21-1 Molecular structure of simethicone.

143

DRUG INTERACTIONS

There are no known drug interactions with simethicone, but avoid taking any carbonated beverages or gas-forming foods together with simethicone, lest it undermines the drug's effectiveness.

RIFAXIMIN

Rifaximin is a derivative of the antibiotic rifampin (Fig. 21-2) used to treat diarrhea caused by *Escherichia coli* (*E. coli*). This drug was shown to reduce the production and frequency of intestinal gas, and may be beneficial for chronic abdominal bloating and flatulence.

MECHANISM OF ACTION

Rifaximin is a gastrointestinal-specific antibiotic to which no clinically relevant bacterial resistance develops. Rifaximin is mainly used to treat *E. coli*-induced diarrhea, and is not recommended to treat diarrhea due to pathogens other than *E. coli*. Rifaximin inhibits bacterial RNA synthesis in *E. coli* by binding to bacterial DNA-dependent RNA polymerase. Since *E. coli* creates gas while tackling human foods, rifaximin may help prevent formation of such gas.

SIDE EFFECTS

Side effect of rifaximin may include stomach pain, nausea, vomiting, constipation; vaginal itching or discharge; fever and headache. Rarely may it also cause allergic reactions such as skin rash and hives.

DRUG INTERACTIONS

No clinically important interactions between this drug and CYP enzymes have been reported.

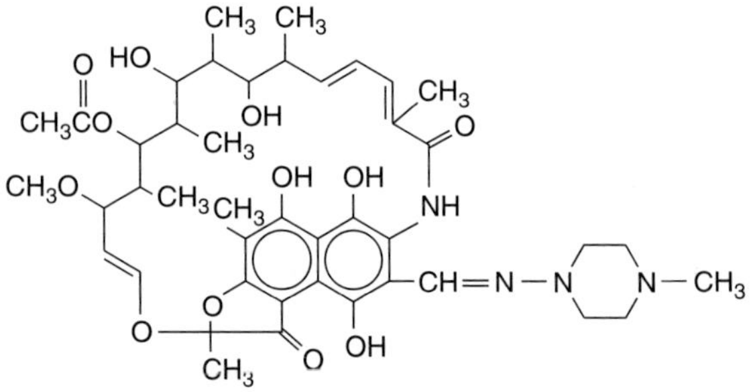

FIGURE 21-2   Molecular structure of rifampin.

ACTIVATED CHARCOAL

Activated charcoal was shown effective in reducing formation of flatulence when taken immediately before food prone to cause flatulence.

MECHANISM OF ACTION

Activated charcoal is believed to adsorb chemical substances important in sustaining the structure of gas foam.

SIDE EFFECTS

Activated charcoal may blacken the stool, cause constipation, tend to stain the oral mucosa, and rarely, may induce allergic reactions such as skin rash.

DRUG INTERACTIONS

Activated Charcoal (ATC)

ATC ⟷ Ipecac: For treatment of poisoning by many drugs, both activated charcoal and ipecac syrup are recommended but they should not be taken simultaneously because activated charcoal adsorbs ipecac to oppose its intestinal absorption. Hence, activated charcoal should not be taken within 30 minutes after intake of ipecac.

ATC ⟷ Minerals: Activated charcoal when used in combination may interfere with absorption of many minerals and vitamins.

ATC ⟷ Oral Medications: Activated charcoal when used in combination may interfere with absorption of many oral medications. Hence, activated charcoal should be taken two hours after other oral medications.

CHAPTER

22

Peptic Ulcer

Peptic (or gastric) ulcers result from erosions of the lining of the stomach by gastric acid, which is secreted from the parietal cells in the stomach. The lining of the stomach may also be eroded by the germ *Helicobacter pylori (H. pylori)*. Complications of peptic ulcer disease (PUD) include gastrointestinal bleeding and perforation.

Medications shown effective in the treatment of peptic ulcers include: (1) gastric antacids such as **aluminum hydroxide, calcium carbonate**, and **magnesium hydroxide;** (2) H2 blockers such as **cimetidine, famotidine, nizatidine,** and **ranitidine;** (3) proton-pump inhibitors such as **esomeprazole** (Nexium), **lansoprazole** (Prevacid), **omeprazole** (Prilosec), and **pantoprazole** (Protonix); (4) **bismuth subsalicylate** (Pepto-Bismol); (5) **sucralfate** (Carafate); (6) **misoprostol** (Cytotec); (7) anticholinergic medications such as **glycopyrrolate** (Robinul); and (8) antibiotics to eradicate *H. pylori* such as **amoxicillin** (Amoxil), **clarithromycin** (Biaxin), and **metronidazole** (Flagyl). Note that amoxicillin is often combined with **potassium clavulanate,** which inhibits the enzyme penicillinase that destroys amoxicillin. Augmentin XR is a commercial preparation that represents such a combined preparation.

GASTRIC ANTACIDS

Aluminum hydroxide, calcium carbonate, and **magnesium hydroxide**

MECHANISM OF ACTION

The antacids mentioned above chemically neutralize gastric acids including gastric hydrochloride to raise gastric pH. Removal of the acids lessens their etching effect, and the raised pH lessens digestion of stomach tissue by pepsin, a proteolytic enzyme.

SIDE EFFECTS

Aluminum Hydroxide or **Calcium Carbonate:** They may cause loss of appetite, constipation, stomach cramps, vomiting, dark stools, and eructation (especially with calcium carbonate).

Magnesium Hydroxide: This drug, unlike aluminum hydroxide or calcium carbonate, may cause diarrhea and its use must be dissuaded in the presence of rectal bleeding with black stools.

DRUG INTERACTIONS

Aluminum Hydroxide or **Calcium Carbonate:** *See* Appendix B-18: Interactions of Gastric Antacids.

Magnesium Hydroxide: *See* Appendix B-19: Interactions of Magnesium Salts.

H2 BLOCKERS

Cimetidine, famotidine, nizatidine, and **ranitidine**

MECHANISM OF ACTION

H2 blockers oppose action of histamine at the H2 subtype of histamine receptors to block secretions of acid from the gastric parietal cells.

SIDE EFFECTS

They may cause cardiac arrhythmia; diarrhea, nausea, and constipation; yellowing of the skin or conjunctiva; and headache and dizziness.

DRUG INTERACTIONS

See Appendix B-21: Interactions of H2 Blockers.

PROTON-PUMP INHIBITORS

Esomeprazole, lansoprazole, omeprazole, and **pantoprazole**

MECHANISM OF ACTION

Proton-pump inhibitors (Fig. 22-1) block the H^+/K^+-ATPase proton pump located at the parietal cell membrane, which is responsible for secreting H^+ ions into the gastric lumen.

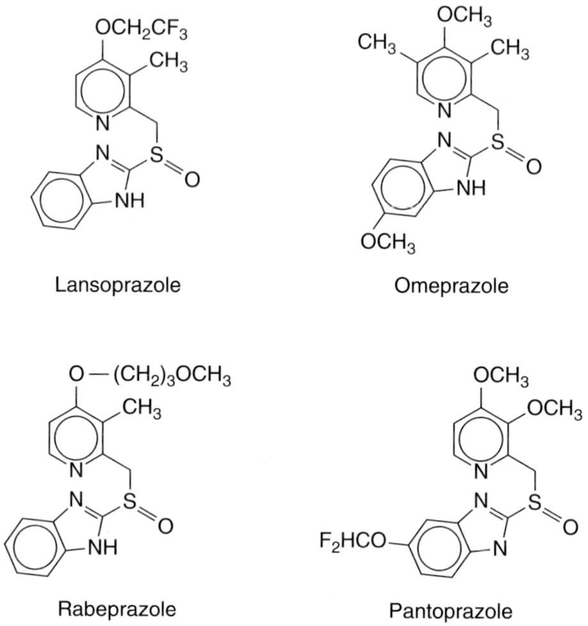

FIGURE 22-1   Molecular structures of proton- pump inhibitors.

SIDE EFFECTS

They may cause nausea, vomiting, diarrhea, stomach pain, and gas; headache; and rarely, they may cause allergic reactions such as skin hives.

DRUG INTERACTIONS

See Appendix B-27: Interactions of Proton-Pump Inhibitors.

BISMUTH SUBSALICYLATE

Bismuth subsalicylate should be avoided by persons who are allergic to aspirin.

MECHANISM OF ACTION

Bismuth subsalicylate protects the lining of the stomach and was shown to have an antibacterial activity against most susceptible strains of *H. pylori* isolated from patients with duodenal ulcers. This drug also binds bacterial toxins produced by *Escherichia coli*; and when hydrolyzed to salicylic acid, it inhibits the synthesis of prostaglandin-E, which is responsible for intestinal inflammations.

SIDE EFFECTS

Bismuth subsalicylate may cause severe constipation; ringing in the ears; allergic reactions such as skin rash and hives; difficulty in breathing; and swelling of the face, lips, tongue, or throat. Bismuth subsalicylate also causes gray to black stool that can last for several days, but it is harmless and presents no reason to be alarmed.

DRUG INTERACTIONS

See Box 22-1.

Miscellaneous Interactions of Bismuth Subsalicylate (BSS)

BSS ⟷ Aspirin: Patients allergic to aspirin should avoid taking bismuth subsalicylate alone or in combination.

BSS ⟷ Oral Hypoglycemic Agents: (*See* Ω-55 in Appendix A.) Salicylates are known to increase glycolysis by activation of glucose oxidase, and impair gluconeogenesis from amino acids or other non-carbohydrate precursors; and hence, concurrent intake of bismuth subsalicylate with an oral antidiabetic drug or with insulin may result in excessive fall of blood glucose.

BSS ⟷ Tetracycline Antibiotics: (*See* Ω-72 in Appendix A.) Bismuth subsalicylate may reduce gastrointestinal absorption of tetracyclines to diminish their antibiotic effects.

BOX 22-1

Basic Concepts of Bismuth Subsalicylate Interactions

1. Bismuth Subsalicylate competes with uric acid for tubular secretions to hinder the uricosuric effect of other drugs taken in combination. Those uricosuric agents so affected include: **sulfinpyrazone** and **probenecid.**

2. Concurrent intake of bismuth subsalicylate with other drugs may increase the risk of bleeding. Those drugs include **anticoagulants** (*See* Ω-16 in Appendix A) and **thrombolytic agents** (*See* Ω-74 in Appendix A).

SUCRALFATE

Sucralfate is sucrose (glucose-fructose disaccharide) complexed with sulfated aluminum hydroxide. It is not an antacid. This oral medication is primarily indicated for the treatment of active duodenal ulcers.

MECHANISM OF ACTION

Sucralfate, in the normally acidic condition of the stomach, becomes a viscous gel that can form a complex with proteins on the surface of ulcers, such as albumin and fibrinogen. This complex can protect peptic erosion from damage by acids and pepsin for up to eight hours after a single dose.

SIDE EFFECTS

Sucralfate may cause nausea, upset stomach, and constipation; dizziness and sleepiness; and rarely, allergic reactions such as skin rash and itching.

DRUG INTERACTIONS

Sucralfate may decrease gastrointestinal absorption of aluminum hydroxide, ciprofloxacin, digoxin, ketoconazole, levothyroxine, norfloxacin, penicillamine, phenytoin, quinidine, tetracycline, theophylline, and warfarin. Therefore, take these medications two hours before taking sucralfate.

MISOPROSTOL

Misoprostol (Fig. 22-2) is a methylated analog of prostaglandin E1, (Fig. 22-3) and is used to inhibit gastric acid secretions and to promote secretions of protective gastric mucus.

MECHANISM OF ACTION

Misoprostol competes with PGE1 for binding to its receptor site at the gastric parietal cells, and by so doing inhibits gastric acid secretions. Misoprostol also provides cytoprotection by several mechanisms, including increased secretions

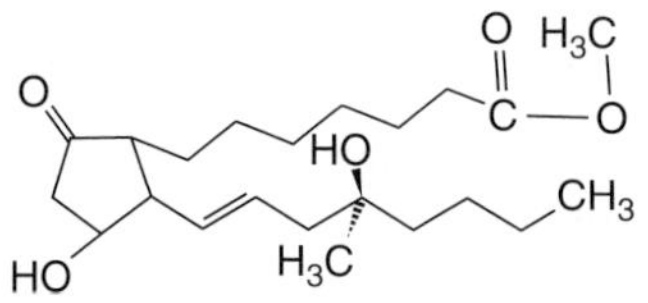

FIGURE 22-2   Molecular structure of misoprostol.

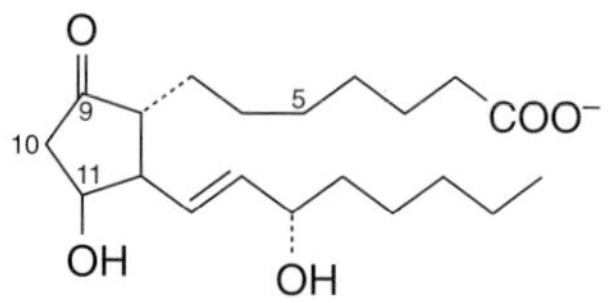

FIGURE 22-3   Molecular structure of prostaglandin E-1.

of bicarbonate ions, and increased thickness of the protective mucous layer by improved regeneration of the gastric mucosal layer.

SIDE EFFECTS

Misoprostol may cause pounding heartbeat; lowered blood pressure; troubled breathing; nausea, vomiting, abdominal pain, heartburn, indigestion, and diarrhea; vaginal bleeding; and headache.

DRUG INTERACTIONS

Misoprostol can increase the adverse effects of oxytocin on the uterus. Hence, don't administer oxytocin until 6 to 12 hours after misoprostol.

GLYCOPYRROLATE

This drug is used to treat ulcers in the stomach and small intestine. When taken orally it does not enter the brain to generate unwanted central nervous system side effects.

MECHANISM OF ACTION

Glycopyrrolate binds to the muscarinic receptors for acetylcholine to block its action at the parasympathetic secretory glands, including the parietal cells of the stomach, to inhibit gastric acid secretions.

SIDE EFFECTS

Its possible side effects include irregular heartbeat; flushing of the face; dry mouth; constipation; difficulty in urination; sexual impotence; blurred vision and increased sensitivity to light; and dizziness, drowsiness, confusion, nervousness, and headache.

DRUG INTERACTIONS

There has been no convincing evidence that this drug would interact with any other drugs to cause a serious consequence.

ANTIBIOTICS

Amoxicillin, clarithromycin, and **metronidazole**

These antibiotics are used to eradicate *H. pylori*, a type of anaerobic bacteria that may be causative of peptic ulcer.

MECHANISM OF ACTION

Amoxicillin: Amoxicillin is a penicillin antibiotic. It binds to the penicillin-binding protein (PBP) located at the bacterial cell envelope to inhibit transpeptidase, the bacterial enzyme involved in the cross-linking of two peptide chains, without which the bacteria cannot complete synthesis of the bacterial cell wall in the third stage; and it also releases autolysins, the bacterial enzymes that destroy the already-formed bacterial cell wall.

Clarithromycin: Clarithromycin (*See* Fig. 12-2) is a semisynthetic macrolide antibiotic related to erythromycin (*See* Fig. 12-2). Clarithromycin binds to the 50s subunit of the bacterial 70s ribosome to inhibit bacterial protein synthesis. The binding blocks translocation of amino acid-t-RNA from the A-site to the P-site; and as the A-site remains occupied, no new amino acid carried by another t-RNA can attach to keep feeding into the growing end of a peptide chain.

Metronidazole: Metronidazole is amebicidal, bactericidal, and trichomonacidal. Its non-ionized drug molecule (Fig. 22-4) is readily taken up by anaerobic organisms. The drug's selectivity for anaerobic bacteria is a result of the ability of these organisms to reduce the NO_2 group of the drug to NH_2 by nitrogen reductase, an enzyme which works in conjunction with ferredoxin, an iron-sulfur protein that functions as an electron carrier in the anaerobic parasites. During this reduction process, it generates a superoxide radical which in turn reacts with DNA to destroy the phosphodiesterase bondage of the DNA. Therefore, metronidazole inhibits synthesis of DNA in those affected organisms to eventually result in their cell death. Metronidazole is equally effective against dividing and non-dividing cells.

SIDE EFFECTS

Amoxicillin: It may cause nausea, vomiting, abdominal pain, diarrhea, and heartburn; vaginal yeast infection; dizziness and insomnia; and allergic reactions such as itching and swelling of tissues.

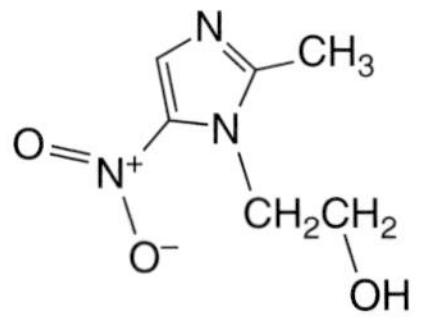

FIGURE 22-4   Molecular structure of metronidazole.

Clarithromycin: It is generally well tolerated as its side effects are usually mild and transient. However, commonly reported side effects include nausea, diarrhea, abnormal taste, dyspepsia, and abdominal pain; and headache.

Metronidazole: Its common side effects include nausea, loss of appetite, and metallic taste; and headaches. Serious side effects of metronidazole are rare but may include seizures and damage of nerves to result in numbness and tingling of extremities (peripheral neuropathy). Metronidazole should be stopped if these rare symptoms appear. Metronidazole may turn the urine brown-black, but this does not amount to medical emergency.

DRUG INTERACTIONS

Amoxicillin: *See* Appendix B-24: Interactions of Penicillins.

Clarithromycin: *See* Appendix B-13: Interactions of Macrolide Antibiotics.

Metronidazole: *See* Chapter 18.

CHAPTER

23

Gastroesophageal Reflux Disease

Heartburn refers to a painful, burning sensation in the chest. It is caused by hydrochloric acid refluxed from the stomach into the esophagus, and hence, heartburn is medically called gastroesophageal reflux disease (GERD). The burning sensation can extend to the neck and throat, and prolonged exposure of the lower part of the esophagus to the acid may result in abnormal changes by the damage (Barrett esophagus).

Medications that may possibly be effective in the treatment of GERD include: (1) **metoclopramide** (Reglan); (2) **bethanechol** (Urecholine); and (3) **drugs for peptic ulcers.** Drugs that inhibit secretions of gastric acid also help to prevent GERD. For those antacids, *See* Chapter 22.

METOCLOPRAMIDE

Metoclopramide is a commonly used drug to treat GERD in infants.

MECHANISM OF ACTION

Metoclopramide promotes intestinal peristaltic activities and strengthens the lower esophageal sphincter to prevent backflow of stomach acid into the esophagus.

SIDE EFFECTS

Metoclopramide may cause dry mouth and diarrhea; muscle stiffness; trembling of the hands; high fever and sweating; and severe dizziness, drowsiness, and restlessness.

DRUG INTERACTIONS

See Chapter 13.

BETHANECHOL

Bethanechol (Fig. 23-1) is sometimes given orally or subcutaneously to treat urinary retention resulting from general anesthesia or from diabetic neuropathy of the bladder (it is a cholinergic drug of choice to treat urinary retention) or to treat gastrointestinal atony (lack of muscular tone). Bethanechol, to treat GERD, may be used in conjunction with acid-suppressing drugs.

MECHANISM OF ACTION

Bethanechol has little or no effect on nicotinic receptors, but has a more selective agonistic effect on the muscarinic receptors at the gastrointestinal tract and urinary bladder than do most other cholinergic drugs. In patients with postoperative abdominal distention or with GERD, bethanechol activates M-2 muscarinic receptors on the gastrointestinal tracts to increase their amplitude of peristaltic contractions, resulting in improved esophageal transit to help prevent the reflux of acids.

SIDE EFFECTS

Bethanechol may cause stomach ache; excessive sweating; dizziness and lightheadedness; flushing; and increased salivation during the first few days of the body's adjustment to the medication.

DRUG INTERACTIONS

Miscellaneous Interactions of Bethanechol (BTC)

BTC ⟷ Ganglionic Blockers: (*See* Ω-41 in Appendix A.) Bethanechol may cause a rapid fall in blood pressure, and when is used in combination with a ganglionic blocker such as mecamylamine, it may entail a severe hypotension.

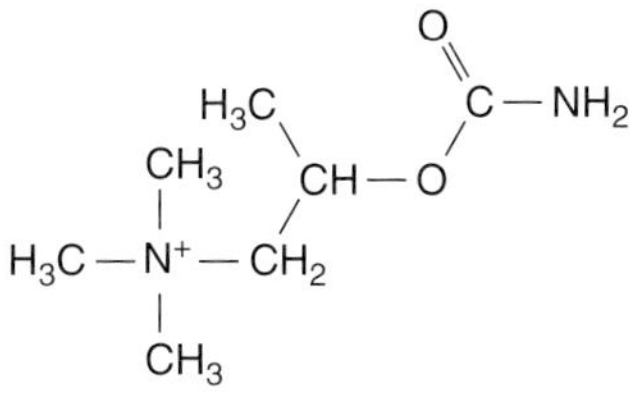

FIGURE 23-1   Molecular structure of bethanechol.

BOX 23-1

Basic Concepts of Bethanechol Interactions

1. Bethanechol has a cholinergic effect and thus, concurrent use with another drug that also has a cholinergic effect may result in a cholinergic crisis. Those drugs include: **cevimeline** and **tacrine.**

2. Bethanechol is a cholinergic drug and thus, concurrent use with other drugs that have an anticholinergic effect may result in the therapeutic actions of bethanechol being counteracted. Those drugs include: **procainamide, quinidine,** and **scopolamine.**

DRUGS FOR PEPTIC ULCERS

Many drugs that inhibit secretions of gastric acid also help to prevent GERD. For those gastric antacids, H2 blockers, and proton-pump inhibitors, *See* Chapter 22.

Dyspepsia

24

Dyspepsia (indigestion) refers to an inability to digest foods, giving rise to symptoms such as fullness, bloating, and abdominal discomfort. The underlying causes of dyspepsia are still in dispute, but too much acid secretions or sluggish stomach emptying are suspected as causes. If dyspepsia is associated with heartburn, the medications useful to treat GERD, such as H2 receptor antagonists, or antibiotics that suppress *Helicobacter pylori* may be tried first (*See* Chapter 23). However, if dyspepsia is free of such reflux heartburn (GERD), the following two drugs may be of help: (1) **domperidone** and (2) **metoclopramide** (Reglan).

DOMPERIDONE

MECHANISM OF ACTION

Activation of dopamine-2 receptors in the gut is known to decrease gastric emptying and intestinal motility. Domperidone has a dopamine-receptor blocking activity and thus, can speed up the emptying of the stomach and increase intestinal motility to decrease small bowel transit time.

SIDE EFFECTS

Domperidone may cause irregular heartbeat; dry mouth and stomach cramps; difficulty in urination; leg cramps; flushing and hot flashes; and nervousness, irritability, dizziness, headache, and insomnia.

DRUG INTERACTIONS

See Box 24-1.

Miscellaneous Interactions of Domperidone (DMP)

DMP ⟷ CYP Isozymes: *See* Table 24-1.

BOX 24-1

Basic Concepts of Domperidone Interactions

1. Domperidone is prone to cause elongation of the Q-T interval, and concurrent administration with other drugs that tend to generate Q-T elongation may result in the life-threatening ventricular arrhythmia of torsade de pointes. Examples include: **amiodarone** (an antiarrhythmic drug); **bepridil** (a calcium-channel blocker useful for angina pectoris); **chloroquine** (an antimalarial drug); **disopyramide** (an antiarrhythmic drug); **ibutilide** (an antiarrhythmic drug); and **quinidine** (an antiarrhythmic drug).

2. Some drugs are apt to cause hypokalemia, a condition that favors cardiac arrhythmia. When domperidone, which causes Q-T elongation, is taken concurrently with such drugs, it may generate the life-threatening ventricular arrhythmia of torsade de pointes. Examples include: **chlorthalidone** and other thiazide diuretics (*See* Ω-73 in Appendix A) and **furosemide** and other loop diuretics (*See* Ω-49 in Appendix A).

TABLE 24-1 Domperidone vs CYP Enzymes

Drug Name	1A2	2A6	2B6	2C8	2C9	2C18	2C19	2D6	2E1	3A4
Domperidone										Sub

Abbreviations: Sub, substrate of the enzyme; Inh, inhibits the enzyme; Ezi, induces the enzyme

Metabolic inactivation of domperidone requires the presence of microsomal CYP3A4 and thus, inhibition of this enzyme by drugs taken together may raise blood levels of domperidone to possibly exacerbate its adverse effects. (*See* the left-hand column of Table-0 at the 'Introduction' for possible inhibitors of this enzyme.)

METOCLOPRAMIDE

See Chapter 13.

25

Irritable Bowel Syndrome

Irritable bowel syndrome (IBS), also known as intestinal neurosis, refers to a chronic complex disorder in which the enteric nerves that control the intestinal muscles are abnormally active, making the intestines excessively sensitive to foods, stool, and gas. IBS is characterized by nausea, abdominal pain, and bloating. Irregular spastic contractility is also common, causing diarrhea. Other times these nerves are too sluggish, causing constipation.

There is no perfect cure for IBS. However, medications that may possibly be effective in the treatment of IBS include: **alosetron** (Lotronex); (2) **cholestyramine;** (3) **loperamide;** and (4) anticholinergic agents such as **dicyclomine** and **hyoscyamine;** and (5) **tegaserod** (Zelnorm).

ALOSETRON

Alosetron is used for the management of IBS with predominant, severe diarrhea in women.

MECHANISM OF ACTION

The 5-HT3 receptor, a subset of the serotonin receptors, is a nonselective cation channel extensively distributed at neurons in the gastrointestinal tract, whose activation leads to neuronal depolarization to cause pain and diarrhea. Alosetron (Fig. 25-1) is a potent and selective 5-HT3 antagonist to oppose the receptor-mediated pain and diarrhea.

SIDE EFFECTS

Alosetron may cause fast heartbeat; nausea, indigestion, heartburn, and bloody stools; headache; and allergic reactions such as skin rash and itching.

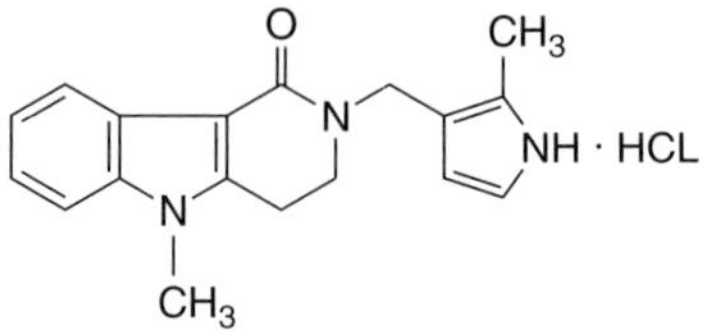

FIGURE 25-1   Molecular structure of alosetron.

DRUG INTERACTIONS

See Table 25-1.

CHOLESTYRAMINE

MECHANISM OF ACTION

Excess bile acid in the intestines due to its malabsorption can lead to diarrhea. Idiopathic bile acid malabsorption is thought to be a cause for chronic diarrhea in IBS. Cholestyramine is an anion-exchange resin that binds bile acids in the intestine in exchange for the chlorine released from the drug molecule. It was demonstrated that cholestyramine is beneficial in diarrhea-predominant IBS.

SIDE EFFECTS

Cholestyramine may cause increased heart rate; abdominal pain, bloating, black stools, and constipation; and headache, dizziness, and drowsiness.

TABLE 25-1 Alosetron vs CYP Enzymes

Drug Name	1A2	2A6	2B6	2C8	2C9	2C18	2C19	2D6	2E1	3A4
Alosetron	Sub+ Inh				Sub					

Abbreviations: Sub, substrate of the enzyme; Inh, inhibits the enzyme; ezi, induces the enzyme

1. Alosetron is mainly processed through hepatic CYP 1A2 and thus, co-administration with drugs that inhibit this enzyme delays its clearance to increase blood levels and adverse effects of alosetron. Those strong inhibitors of CYP 1A2 include ciprofloxacin and fluvoxamine (Floxyfral) (*See* the left-hand column of Table-0 at the 'Introduction' for other possible inhibitors of this enzyme.)

2. Alosetron exerts an inhibitory effect on CYP 1A2 and thus, administration of it in combination with other drugs that require this enzyme for their metabolic clearance may result in their elevated blood levels, exacerbating their adverse effects. (*See* the middle column of Table-0 at the 'Introduction' for possible substrates of the enzyme.)

BOX 25-1

Basic Concepts of Cholestyramine Interactions

Cholestyramine binds to and reduces the intestinal absorption of many drugs taken concomitantly, undercutting their therapeutic effectiveness. To avoid this, give them two hours before or four to six hours after administration of cholestyramine. Those possibly affected drugs include: **calcium preparations; chlorothiazide** and other **thiazide diuretics** (*See* Ω-73 in Appendix A); **loop diuretics** (*See* Ω-49 in Appendix A); **dicumarol; digoxin; fluvastatin; iron preparations; loperamide** (an antidiarrheal agent); **raloxifene** (a drug to treat osteoporosis); **valproic acid** (an antiepileptic drug); and **warfarin** (an anticoagulant).

DRUG INTERACTIONS

See Box 25-1.

Miscellaneous Interactions of Cholestyramine (CSM)

Parentheses below indicate an herb.

CSM ⟷ Ezetimibe: Concurrent use of ezetimibe and cholestyramine decreases the peak serum concentration of ezetimibe to its diminished effect. This is because ezetimibe, though by itself active, is normally absorbed and quickly metabolized to its more active glucuronide form in the liver. Hence, the smaller its amount absorbed, the lesser its effectiveness.

CSM ⟷ (Gotu Kola): As this herb may raise blood levels of cholesterol, it may undermine the cholesterol-lowering effects of such ion-exchange resins as colestipol (Colestid) and cholestyramine (Questran).

CSM ⟷ Vitamins: Co-administration of cholestyramine with vitamins may reduce the gastrointestinal absorption of such vitamins as folic acid, vitamins A, D, E, and K.

LOPERAMIDE

MECHANISM OF ACTION

Loperamide binds to opioid receptors along the wall of the small intestines to decrease activity of the circular and longitudinal muscles, inhibiting their peristalsis and increasing anal sphincter tone. It may also inhibit secretions of fluid and electrolytes to alleviate diarrhea associated with IBS.

SIDE EFFECTS

Loperamide may cause stomach pain or bloating, and constipation; dizziness, drowsiness, and tired feeling; allergic reactions such as skin hives; difficulty in breathing; and swelling of the lips, tongue, or face.

DRUG INTERACTIONS

See Box 25-2.

Miscellaneous Interactions of Loperamide (LPM)

LPM ⟷ Bile Acid Sequestrants: (*See* Ω-28 in Appendix A.) Absorption of loperamide is impaired by combined use with bile acid sequestrants to its diminished therapeutic effectiveness.

LPM ⟷ CYP Isozymes: *See* Table 25-2.

LPM ⟷ Phenothiazines Antipsychotic Drugs: (*See* Ω-58 in Appendix A.) The tendency toward central nervous system (CNS) depression by loperamide can be accelerated by combined use with any member of phenothiazine antipsychotic drugs.

LPM ⟷ Tricyclic Antidepressants: (*See* Ω -76 in Appendix A.) The tendency toward CNS depression by loperamide can be enhanced by combined use with any member of tricyclic antidepressant drugs.

BOX 25-2

Basic Concepts of Loperamide Interactions

Loperamide is a substrate of transporter P-glycoproteins, which efflux the drug. When loperamide is taken concurrently with other drugs that inhibit this transporter, the efflux is blocked to raise the blood levels and adverse effects of loperamide. Those inhibitors of the transporter include: **quinidine** (an antiarrhythmic drug) and **ritonavir** (an anti-HIV drug).

TABLE 25-2 Loperamide vs CYP Isozymes

Drug Name	1A2	2A6	2B6	2C8	2C9	2C18	2C19	2D6	2E1	3A4
Loperamide										Sub

Abbreviations: Sub, substrate of the enzyme; Inh, inhibits the enzyme; Ezi, induces the enzyme
Loperamide requires CYP3A4 for its metabolic processing, and hence, inhibition of this enzyme by other drugs taken concurrently can raise blood levels of loperamide to possibly perk up its adverse effects. (*See* the left-hand column of Table-0 at the 'Introduction' for possible inhibitors of the enzyme.)

ANTICHOLINERGIC AGENTS

Dicyclomine and **hyoscyamine**

Hyoscyamine is the levorotatory isomer of atropine (Fig. 25-2).

MECHANISM OF ACTION

Both dicyclomine and hyoscyamine block the actions of acetylcholine at the parasympathetic sites in the smooth muscle of the small intestine to decrease muscle tone and motility to help relieve spasms of the gastrointestinal tract. They are also quite effective in the treatment of diarrhea.

SIDE EFFECTS

Dicyclomine: It may cause palpitation; dry mouth, nausea, vomiting, constipation, bloated feeling, abdominal pain, and anorexia; urinary retention; impotence; dyskinesia and lethargy; dizziness, lightheadedness, headache, drowsiness,

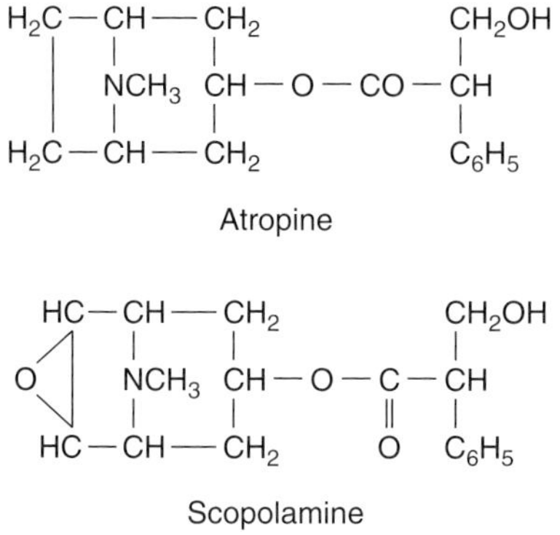

FIGURE 25-2   Molecular structures of atropine and scopolamine.

nervousness, mental confusion, and insomnia; and rare, but severe, allergic reactions such as skin rash, urticaria, and itching.

Hyoscyamine: It may cause tachycardia; dry mouth, nausea, vomiting, bloating, and constipation; difficulty in urination and impotence; ataxia; skin rash; and blurred vision, dizziness, drowsiness, and confusion.

DRUG INTERACTIONS

Dicyclomine: *See* Box 25-3.

Hyoscyamine: *See* Appendix B-15.

Miscellaneous Interactions of Dicyclomine (DCM)

Parentheses below indicate an herb.

DCM ⟷ Alcohol: If ethanol is taken in combination with dicyclomine, additional CNS depressions may ensue.

DCM ⟷ Antiarrhythmic Drugs: (*See* Ω-12 in Appendix A) Dicyclomine, when used in combination, may increase toxicities of other drugs having an anticholinergic side effect, such as type-1 antiarrhythmic drugs.

DCM ⟷ Antiglaucoma Drugs: (*See* Ω-18 in Appendix A.) Dicyclomine tends to elevate intraocular pressure to oppose effectiveness of those drugs that are used to lower intraocular pressure.

DCM ⟷ (Lavender): If lavender (Fig. 25-3 A and B), an herb used to decrease stress in Chinese medicine, is taken in combination with dicyclomine, exaggerated CNS depressions may ensue.

BOX 25-3

Basic Concepts of Dicyclomine Interactions

Dicyclomine is a class of drugs called anticholinergics and thus, concurrent administration with other drugs that also tend to generate an anticholinergic effect may create additive or supra-additive anticholinergic side effects such as tachycardia, dry mouth, nausea, constipation, difficulty in urination, blurred vision, and mental impairment. Examples include: **amantadine** (to treat type-A influenza); **antihistamines** (*See* Ω-19 in Appendix A); **tricyclic antidepressants** (*See* Ω-76 in Appendix A); and authentic **anticholinergic agents** (*See* Ω-14 in Appendix A).

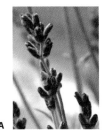
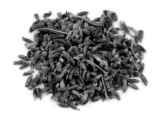

A   B

FIGURE 25-3   A, Lavender flower.
(Attribution: http://www.aromatherapy-at-home.com/lavender-flower-garden.html)
B, Cut and dried flower of lavender.

DCM ⟷ Levodopa: Dicyclomine decreases gastric motility and reduces absorption of levodopa used in combination, to diminish its therapeutic effect.

DCM ⟷ Narcotic Analgesics: (*See* Ω-52 in Appendix A.) Dicyclomine, when used in combination, may increase toxicities of other drugs having an anticholinergic effect, such as narcotic analgesics.

DCM ⟷ Phenothiazine Antipsychotic Drugs: (*See* Ω-58 in Appendix A.) Anticholinergics are frequently used in combination to counter the extrapyramidal side effects of phenothiazines. However, dicyclomine, when used in combination with phenothiazines, can occasionally generate serious additive anticholinergic side effects such as heat stroke, severe constipation, paralytic ileus, and atropine-like psychosis.

TEGASEROD

Tegaserod (Zelnorm) is indicated for the short-term treatment of IBS with constipation.

MECHANISM OF ACTIONS

Tegaserod helps evacuate the bowels by selectively activating 5HT4 receptors present throughout the gastrointestinal tract.

SIDE EFFECTS

Possible side effects by tegaserod include angina pectoris, tachycardia, hypotension; diarrhea, hypovolemia; dizziness and syncope.

DRUG INTERACTIONS

Tegaserod is highly unlikely to inhibit CYP enzymes, and no clinically significant drug interactions have surfaced so far.

26

Intestinal Cramps

Intestinal cramps are due to sudden, spasmodic muscular contractions of the intestines, causing severe pain. Cramps may be caused by hyperactivity of cholinergic neurons to intolerable foods such as wheat, caffeine, and alcohol or to irritable drugs such as aspirin and ibuprofen.

Medications shown effective in the treatment of intestinal cramps include: (1) anticholinergic agents such as **dicyclomine, hyoscyamine,** and **propantheline** (Pro-Banthine); (2) gastric antacids such as **aluminum hydroxide;** and (3) H2 blockers such as **cimetidine, famotidine, nizatidine,** and **ranitidine.**

ANTICHOLINERGIC AGENTS

Dicyclomine, hyoscyamine, and **propantheline**

MECHANISM OF ACTION

Dicyclomine: *See* Chapter 25.

Hyoscyamine: *See* Chapter 25.

Propantheline: Propantheline is used to treat or prevent spasms in the muscles of the gastrointestinal tract, and to reduce GI motility in irritable bowel syndrome. Propantheline blocks the muscarinic receptors at the intestinal smooth muscles to inhibit gastrointestinal propulsive motility and has a direct musculotropic relaxing effect on the smooth muscles to relieve intestinal spasms.

SIDE EFFECTS

Dicyclomine: *See* Chapter 25.

Hyoscyamine: *See* Chapter 25.

Propantheline: Possible side effects of propantheline include irregular heartbeat; dry mouth, constipation, and stomach ache; urinary retention; tremors; flushing; blurred vision; and confusion and drowsiness.

DRUG INTERACTIONS

Dicyclomine: *See* Chapter 25.

Hyoscyamine: *See* Appendix B-15: Interactions of Belladonna Alkaloids.

Propantheline (PPL)

PPL ⟷ Beta Blockers: (*See* Ω-27 in Appendix A.) Propantheline is likely to cause increased heart rate (a positive chronotropic effect) and therefore, when it is taken in combination with a beta blocker, its effect on heart rate may be counteracted.

PPL ⟷ Cefprozil: Propantheline reduces gut motility and when taken together with cefprozil, an antibiotic, the intestinal absorption of cefprozil may be delayed with consequent lowering of the blood concentrations of this drug.

PPL ⟷ Tricyclic Antidepressants: (*See* Ω-76 in Appendix A.) The anticholinergic effects of imipramine, or of other tricyclic antidepressants, may be potentiated by combined use with propantheline, a classic anticholinergic agent.

GASTRIC ANTACIDS

See Chapter 22.

H2 BLOCKERS

See Chapter 22.

27

Constipation

Constipation refers to infrequent bowel movements (fewer than once in three days) with incomplete evacuation of dry, hardened, fecal mass.

Medications shown effective in the treatment of constipation include: (1) **lubiprostone** (Amitiza); (2) bulk cathartics such as **methylcellulose** (Citrucel) and **psyllium** (Metamucil); (3) **docusate sodium** (Colace , Dialose, Surfak); (4) **bisacodyl** (Dulcolax); (5) **sennosides** (Ex-lax, Senna-Lax, Senokot); (6) **magnesium citrate;** and (7) **polyethylene glycol** (*Glycolax*).

LUBIPROSTONE

Lubiprostone (Amitiza) is an orally effective agent to treat chronic idiopathic constipation.

MECHANISM OF ACTION

Lubiprostone activates a voltage-regulated chlorine ion channel (ClC-2) located at the luminal surface of the small intestine to increase secretions of chloride-rich fluid, which in turn promotes gastrointestinal motility to enhance passage of the stool and lessen abdominal bloating and discomfort.

SIDE EFFECTS

Lubiprostone may cause nausea, bloated stomach, and abdominal pain with gas; and headache.

DRUG INTERACTIONS

There is no clinically important interaction reported.

BULK CATHARTICS

Methylcellulose and **psyllium**

BOX 27-1

Basic Concepts of Psyllium Interactions

1. Psyllium can reduce intestinal absorption of other drugs used concurrently to undercut their therapeutic effectiveness. Those affected drugs include: **carbamazepine** (an antiepileptic drug); **digoxin; lithium;** and **tricyclic antidepressants** (*See* Ω-76 in Appendix A).

2. Psyllium has a cholesterol-lowering effect of its own, and when used in combination with other cholesterol-lowering drugs, they may result in additive lowering of cholesterol. Those drugs include: **cholestyramine** and **colestipol.**

MECHANISM OF ACTION

Methylcellulose is a hydrophilic carbohydrate, and psyllium is a fiber commonly used in the treatment of chronic constipation. They are both taken with an ample amount of water (20 grams of each in 250 ml of water). They absorb water, swelling to a bulky substance that distends the wall of the colon to elicit a defecation reflex.

SIDE EFFECTS

Either of them may cause difficulty in swallowing; and intestinal obstruction, nausea, vomiting, abdominal pain, and increased constipation if not taken with enough amount of water.

DRUG INTERACTIONS

Methylcellulose: No serious interactions reported.

Psyllium: *See* Box 27-1.

DOCUSATE SODIUM

MECHANISM OF ACTION

Docusate is an anionic surfactant that works by allowing penetration of water into the hardened fecal mass to soften it, and not by promoting peristaltic activity of the intestine. The onset of laxative effect may require one to two days.

SIDE EFFECTS

It may cause throat irritation and stomach or intestinal cramping.

DRUG INTERACTIONS

Since it is a surfactant, it can increase intestinal absorption of mineral oil and fat-soluble vitamins such as vitamin A, D, E, and K, to lead to their toxicities.

BISACODYL

MECHANISM OF ACTION

It stimulates peristalsis by directly irritating the smooth muscles of the intestine and/or of the intramural plexus of the colon. It also appears to promote secretions of water and electrolytes into the intestinal lumen.

SIDE EFFECTS

Bisacodyl may cause nausea, vomiting, and abdominal cramps; alteration of blood pH; hypocalcemia; and rarely, vertigo.

DRUG INTERACTIONS

Bisacodyl (BCD)

BCD ⟷ Antacids: (*See* Ω-11 in Appendix A.) No antacids should be taken within one hour of taking bisacodyl delayed-release tablets, because the antacids, by increasing the gastric pH, may reduce the resistance of the enteric-coated tablets to let bisacodyl be released prior to reaching the colon, its site of action. The released bisacodyl can cause gastric irritation and dyspepsia.

BCD ⟷ Digoxin: Co-administration of digoxin and bisacodyl resulted in a reduction in blood levels of digoxin. Bisacodyl appears to interfere with absorption of digoxin.

BCD ⟷ Milk: Bisacodyl tablets should not be taken within one hour of taking any milk or dairy products, because milk can dissolve the bisacodyl tablet too quickly before reaching the colon, increasing the incidences of severe stomach cramps and vomiting.

SENNOSIDES

Sennosides are hydroxyanthracene glycosides derived from senna leaves. Senna leaves contain laxative chemicals called sennosides A and B.

MECHANISM OF ACTION

The sennosides are converted by the normal bacteria in the colon into rhein-anthrone, which in turn stimulates production of prostaglandin E2-like material in the colon, a substance that quickens bowel movements and increases fluid secretions by the colon.

SIDE EFFECTS

Sennosides may cause bloating, cramping, rectal irritation, diarrhea, and bleeding; skin rash; and dizziness and weakness. In addition, senna may turn urine brown or brown-black, but this does not usually indicate medical emergency.

DRUG INTERACTIONS

See Box 27-2.

Miscellaneous Interactions of Sennosides (SNS)

SNS ⟷ Vitamin K: Chronic use of sennosides may decrease absorption of vitamin K to enhance the bleeding tendency of such vitamin K antagonists as dicumarol and warfarin.

BOX 27-2

Basic Concepts of Sennoside Interactions

1. Sennosides may cause hypokalemia and hypomagnesemia to quicken cardiac conduction speed, leading to ventricular tachycardia. When a sennoside is taken in combination with other drugs that also tend to cause cardiac arrhythmia, it may lead to life-threatening torsades de pointes. Those drugs having a proarrhythmic tendency include: **amiodarone** (an antiarrhythmic drug); and **dofetilide.** (Note that dofetilide is a specific class-III antiarrhythmic drug usually used to maintain normal sinus rhythm in patients who have been converted to normal sinus rhythm from atrial fibrillation or flutter for longer than 1-week. Its own usual adverse effects include ventricular tachycardia and torsade de pointes.)

2. Chronic use of sennosides tends to cause significant loss of fluid and electrolytes, including sodium and potassium, and concurrent administration of sennosides with other drugs that also tend to cause loss of sodium and potassium may result in an excessive imbalance of blood electrolytes. Examples of other such drugs include: **chlorthalidone** and other **thiazide diuretics** (*See* Ω-73 in Appendix A) and **loop diuretics** (*See* Ω-49 in Appendix A).

MAGNESIUM CITRATE

MECHANISM OF ACTION

Magnesium citrate is poorly or not at all absorbed from the gastrointestinal tract, but withdraws water from tissues and retains water owing to its high osmolarity. This drug stimulates the stretch receptors of the colon to induce evacuating peristalsis.

SIDE EFFECTS

It may cause nausea, bloating, cramping, and diarrhea; and thirst.

DRUG INTERACTIONS

See Appendix B-19: Interactions of Magnesium Salts.

POLYETHYLENE GLYCOL

MECHANISM OF ACTION

Polyethylene glycol is an osmotic laxative that retains water in the colon to soften stool, which subsequently facilitates bowel evacuation.

SIDE EFFECTS

It may cause nausea, abdominal cramping, and diarrhea; and, very rarely, allergic reactions such as skin rash, itching, and swelling of tissues.

DRUG INTERACTIONS

No serious interaction has been reported.

Diarrhea

28

Diarrhea refers to frequent evacuation of watery stools more than three times in one day. Viral and bacterial infections are the most common causes of acute diarrhea.

Medications shown effective in the treatment of diarrhea include: (1) opiate agonists such as **diphenoxylate** and **loperamide** (Imodium); (2) **bismuth subsalicylate**; and to treat traveler's diarrhea, (3) **ciprofloxacin**, **norfloxacin**, or **ofloxacin**.

OPIATE AGONIST

Diphenoxylate and **loperamide**

Both diphenoxylate (Fig. 28-1) and loperamide (Fig. 28-2) are chemically related to morphine, but, unlike morphine, they have no pain-killing effect. Diphenoxylate is often used in combination with atropine, an anticholinergic agent that functions as a universal blocker of all the cholinergic receptors (M-1, M-2 and M-3), to reduce motility of the intestine.

MECHANISM OF ACTION

Both drugs act as opiate receptor agonists by apparently activating the μ-receptors in the submucosal plexus of the intestines that regulates circular

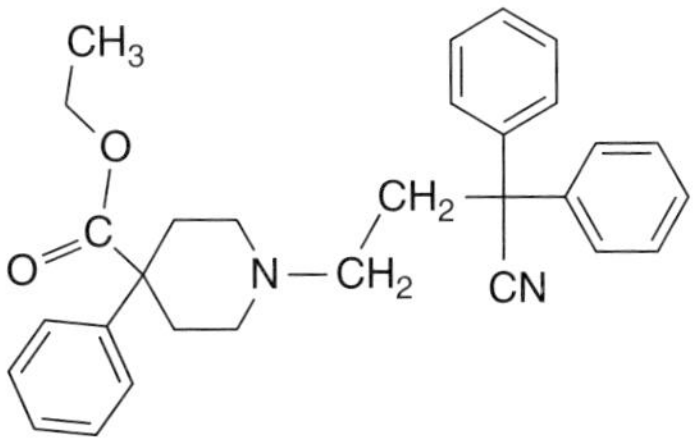

FIGURE 28-1 Molecular structure of diphenoxylate.

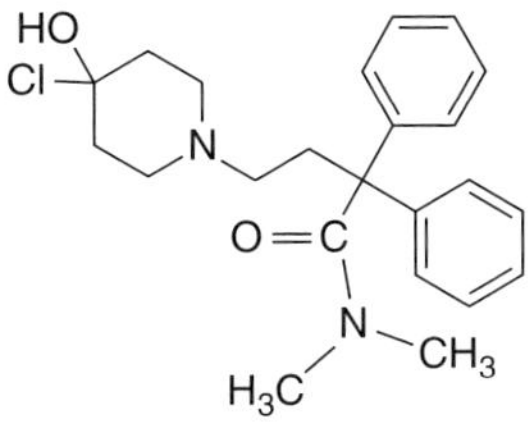

FIGURE 28-2 Molecular structure of loperamide.

muscle contractions, and this receptor activation leads to decreased intestinal peristalsis, constricted sphincters, and enhanced reabsorption of sodium and chloride, reducing the fecal volume.

SIDE EFFECTS

Diphenoxylate: Side effects that may be generated by diphenoxylate include fast or irregular heartbeat; difficulty in breathing or shortness of breath; dry mouth, loss of appetite, nausea, vomiting, and bloating; dry skin; blurred vision; drowsiness or dizziness; and headache. High doses of diphenoxylate may cause euphoria and physical dependency.

Loperamide: Loperamide may cause stomach pain, bloating, and constipation; dizziness, drowsiness, and tired feeling; and allergic reactions such as skin hives.

DRUG INTERACTIONS

Diphenoxylate (DPX)

DPX ↔ Alcohol: Co-administration of diphenoxylate with ethanol may result in deepened central nervous system (CNS) depression.

DPX ↔ Barbiturates: (*See* Ω-24 in Appendix A.) As diphenoxylate has a CNS depressant effect, its action can be potentiated by combined use with a hypnotic barbiturate, such as pentobarbital.

DPX ↔ MAO Inhibitors: (*See* Ω-51 in Appendix A.) Diphenoxylate, as an opioid agonist, can depress functions of the CNS. Don't take it together with an inhibitor of the enzyme MAO, such as isocarboxazid and phenelzine, for otherwise it may cause severe respiratory depression and coma. The exact mechanism behind this observation is not clear.

DPX ↔ Quinidine: Co-administration of diphenoxylate with quinidine may lower the blood levels of quinidine by a mechanism yet to be clarified.

Loperamide: *See* Chapter 25.

BISMUTH SUBSALICYLATE

This drug should be avoided by individuals who are allergic to aspirin. *See* Chapter 22.

QUINOLONE ANTIBIOTICS

Ciprofloxacin, norfloxacin, and **ofloxacin**

To treat traveler's diarrhea (diarrhea caused by eating food or drinking water that contains germs), an antibiotic may be administered for three to five days. Currently, the drugs of choice are fluoroquinolone antibiotics such as ciprofloxacin, norfloxacin, and ofloxacin. Also note that bismuth subsalicylate, mentioned earlier, is effective in the treatment of treat traveler's diarrhea.

MECHANISM OF ACTION

The quinolone antibiotics generate an antibacterial effect by inhibition of DNA gyrase, an essential bacterial enzyme that catalyzes the ATP-dependent introduction of negative super-coiling of double-stranded bacterial DNA, which is required for DNA replication.

SIDE EFFECTS

Any of the quinolone antibiotics may cause nausea and vomiting; jaundice (yellowing of the skin or eyes); seizure (convulsions); allergic reactions such as skin hives; difficulty in breathing; and swelling of the face, lips, tongue, or throat.

DRUG INTERACTIONS

See Appendix B-28: Interactions of Quinolone Antibiotics.

CHAPTER
29

Hemorrhoids

Hemorrhoids refer to enlarged veins in or around the anus that cause pain, itching and sometimes bleeding. The following therapies may reduce the symptoms of itching and bleeding from hemorrhoids: (1) local anesthetic such as **benzocaine, dibucaine** (Nupercainal), and **pramoxine;** (2) glucocorticoids such as **hydrocortisone** ointment (Anusol-HC; Cortifoam); and (3) **phenylephrine** suppositories (Anu-Med, Preparation H).

LOCAL ANESTHETICS

Benzocaine, dibucaine, and pramoxine

MECHANISM OF ACTION
See Chapter 18.

SIDE EFFECTS
Side effects of these local anesthetic agents may include a stinging or tingling sensation at the site of application and allergic reactions such as skin rash.

DRUG INTERACTIONS
No serious drug interactions have been reported.

GLUCOCORTICOIDS

Hydrocortisone

MECHANISM OF ACTION
See Chapter 11.

SIDE EFFECTS

See Chapter 11.

DRUG INTERACTIONS

No serious interactions have been reported.

PHENYLEPHRINE SUPPOSITORY

MECHANISM OF ACTION

Phenylephrine is an alpha-adrenergic agonist that acts directly on its receptors to cause constriction of anal arterioles, leading to local hemostasis in the small vessels of hemorrhoids. It thereby shrivels hemorrhoidal tissues.

SIDE EFFECTS

Phenylephrine is well tolerated when applied topically, but may cause pain in the rectum and, rarely, may it cause allergic reaction such as skin hives and itching.

DRUG INTERACTIONS

Phenylephrine (PEP): It is not known whether other medications will interact with this medication applied topically, but if absorbed extensively from its site of application the following interactions may take place.

PEP ⟷ Antihypertensive Drugs: (*See* Ω-20 in Appendix A.) By causing vasoconstriction phenylephrine may undercut the effectiveness of antihypertensive drugs.

PEP ⟷ MAO Inhibitors: (*See* Ω -51 in Appendix A.) MAO inactivates phenylephrine, and in the presence of an inhibitor of MAO, the pharmacologic effect of phenylephrine may be intensified and prolonged.

PEP ⟷ Tricyclic Antidepressants: (*See* Ω-76 in Appendix A.) Tricyclics block reuptake of norepinephrine, and when used in combination with phenylephrine they may pull together toward excessive sympathomimetic adverse effects.

CHAPTER

30

Erectile Dysfunction (Impotence)

Erectile dysfunction (ED), or impotence, refers to the inability to achieve penile erection or to maintain an erection to participate in sexual activities until achieving ejaculation.

Medications that are shown effective in the treatment of ED include: (1) phosphodiesterase inhibitors such as **sildenafil** (Viagra), **tadalafil** (Cialis), and **vardenafil** (Levitra). And on an experimental basis, **pycnogenol** is a potential long-term remedy to treat ED, but since it is not yet approved by the FDA, it should not be intended to replace any FDA-approved drugs currently in use.

PHOSPHODIESTERASE INHIBIOTRS

Sildenafil, **tadalafil**, and **vardenafil**

MECHANISM OF ACTION

All of them are inhibitors of the enzyme phosphodiesterase-5 that destroys cyclic-GMP, and thus, they accumulate C-GMP, which rapidly relaxes vascular smooth muscles to increase blood flow into the corpus cavernosum of the penis, a mechanism that provides penile erection. Major differences among these three are found with their onset and duration of action, although there is great variation from person to person. The time required after oral administration to reach the maximum plasma concentration for sildenafil is around 50 minutes; for vardenafil around 35 to 50 minutes; and for tadalafil about 120 minutes. (Accordingly, onset of action for both sildenafil and vardenafil is around 10 minutes and tadalafil around 30 minutes.) The elimination half-life of sildenafil is about 4 hours; vardenafil, about 5 hours; and tadalafil is the longest at about 17 to 21 hours. Accordingly, the duration of action of both sildenafil and vardenafil is anywhere between 4 and 12 hours, as compared to tadalafil, which is up to 36 hours.

SIDE EFFECTS

Possible side effects of these drugs include cardiac arrhythmia; upset stomach and nausea; swelling in the hands, ankles, or feet; headache; sudden visual defect; and dizziness and fainting.

DRUG INTERACTIONS

See Box 30-1.

BOX 30-1

Basic Concepts of Sildenafil, Tadalafil or Vardenafil Interactions

Sildenafil, tadalafil, and vardenafil cause peripheral vasodilation, and when any one of them is taken in combination with drugs that lower blood pressure, it may lead to excessive hypotension, causing dizziness. Those drugs include: alpha blockers such as **alfuzosin, doxazosin, tamsulosin,** and **terazosin; amyl nitrite; calcium-channel blockers** (*See* Ω-31 in Appendix A); **sodium nitroprusside** (nitric oxide released from sodium nitroprusside increases levels of c-GMP to cause vasodilation); and **nitroglycerin** (*See* Fig. 2-4) or **isosorbide dinitrate** (Fig. 30-1) (a source of nitric oxide, which causes rapid vasodilation to lower blood pressure).

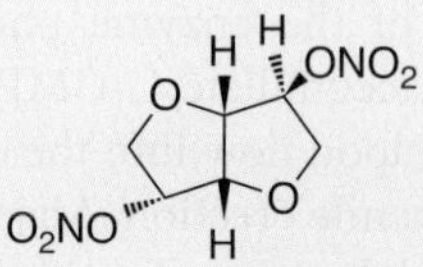

FIGURE 30-1   Molecular structure of isosorbide dinitrate.

TABLE 30-1 ED Drugs vs CYP Enzymes

Drug Name	1A2	2A6	2B6	2C8	2C9	2C18	2C19	2D6	2E1	3A4
Sildenafil	Inh									Sub
Tadalafil										Sub
Vardenafil										Sub

Abbreviations: Sub, substrate of the enzyme; Inh, inhibits the enzyme; Ezi, induces the enzyme

1. All of the above drugs require CYP3A4 for their elimination or inactivation in the intestine and in the liver and thus, inhibition of this enzyme by other drugs can raise the blood levels and potentially exacerbate their adverse. Those strong inhibitors of CYP 3A4 include clarithromycin, indinavir, itraconazole, ketoconazole, nefazodone, nelfinavir, ritonavir, saquinavir, and telithromycin. (*See* the left-hand column of Table-0 at the 'Introduction' for other possible inhibitors of the enzyme.) Ingestion of 500 ml or more a day of grapefruit juice, another inhibitor of CYP3A4, may also inhibit inactivation of these drugs to raise their blood levels and possibly exacerbate their adverse effects.
2. Sildenafil only, among the above, has an inhibitory effect on CYP1A2 and thus, administration of it in combination with drugs that require this enzyme for metabolic clearance may result in elevated blood levels, exacerbating their adverse effects. (*See* the middle column of Table-0 at the 'Introduction' for possible substrates of this enzyme.)

Miscellaneous Interactions of Sildenafil, Tadalafil, or Vardenafil (STV)

STV ⟷ Alcohol: Drinking alcohol can temporarily impair the ability to get an erection. Additionally, alcohol has a mild vasodilating effect that slightly increases the blood-pressure-lowering effect of ED drugs, especially tadalafil, but in most cases the combination is well tolerated.

STV ⟷ CYP Isozymes: *See* Table 30-1.

STV ⟷ Narcotic Analgesics: (*See* Ω-52 in Appendix A.) Because of the possibility of a precipitous fall of blood pressure, use of sildenafil, tadalafil or vardenafil in conjunction with such opioid analgesics as codeine and morphine is contraindicated.

PYCNOGENOL AND ARGININE

Pycnogenol represents a group of plant extracts rich in bioflavonoids (yellowish pigments also referred to as vitamin P, which is considered important to maintaining capillary integrity) and in proanthocyanidins, which are polymeric chains of flavonoids, and in several other phenolic acids. Pycnogenol is obtainable from the bark of the pine (*Pinus maritima*) growing in the southwest coastal region of France. The doses suggested for long term help for ED include 100 mg of pycnogenol taken in combination with 1.5 gram of L-arginine a day for three months. L-arginine is an unusual amino acid in that it is manufactured in the body, but not to a sufficient quantity, and hence, some of it must still be consumed through diet. Thus, it is called a conditionally essential amino acid.

There are some data showing that long term intake of these two in combination may help provide penile erection in otherwise healthy males. Researches have to be directed toward isolating and characterizing the key ingredients of pycnogenol that may provide therapeutic benefits for ED in the future.

MECHANISM OF ACTION

Pycnogenol: Pycnogenol appears to stimulate production of nitric oxide synthase, the enzyme that promotes production of nitric oxide from arginine. Nitric oxide, formerly called endothelium-derived relaxing factor (EDRF), is the substance that activates guanylyl cyclase to lead to accumulation of cyclic-GMP, a rapid vasodilator, whose destruction by phosphodiesterase-5 is blocked by all the current FDA-approved ED drugs.

L-Arginine: L arginine (Fig, 30-2) is the precursor from which nitric oxide (chemically, NO) is formed. Nitric oxide, as mentioned above, can induce vasodilation that allows more blood to flow into the spongy tissue of the penis, bringing about penile erection.

SIDE EFFECTS

Pycnogenol: The most common side effects of pycnogenol include bloating, flatulence, nausea, constipation, and minor stomach discomfort owing to its astringent taste; and headaches and dizziness. It may also lower blood pressure, and rarely cause bleeding, hypercalcemia, and kidney stones.

L-Arginine: If the dose of L-arginine is excessive (above 9 grams a day), it can increase stomach acid to cause or worsen heartburn, ulcers, and may also cause nausea, gastrointestinal discomfort, diarrhea; and thickening of skin. Since L-arginine may lower blood pressure and its safety in pregnant and nursing women and children is not assessed, they are not advised to take supplemental L-arginine. Additionally, arginine may increase blood sugar levels, so its use in diabetics is not recommended.

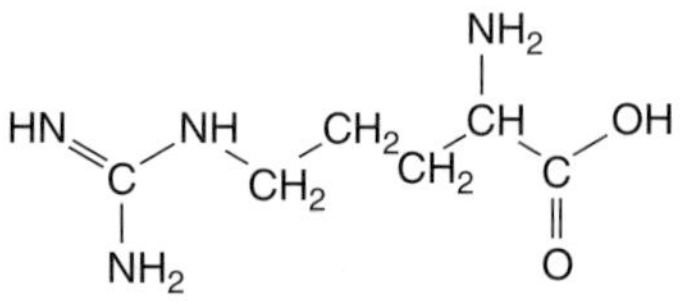

FIGURE 30-2   Molecular structure of arginine.

BOX 30-2

Basic Concepts of Pycnogenol Interactions

Pycnogenol tends to prevent the aggregation of blood platelets, generating a blood thinning effect. Thus, pycnogenol may increase the risk of bleeding when taken with drugs that have a blood thinning effect. Those drugs include: **anticoagulants** (*See* Ω-16 in Appendix A) and **antiplatelet agents** (*See* Ω-22 in Appendix A).

DRUG INTERACTIONS

Pycnogenol

See Box 30-2.

Miscellaneous Interactions of Pycnogenol (PGN)

PGN ⟷ Antihypertensive Drugs: (*See* Ω-20 in Appendix A.) As pycnogenol can lower blood pressure, it may potentiate efficacies of antihypertensive drugs, specifically angiotensin-converting enzyme (ACE) inhibitors, such as benazepril (Lotensin), captopril (Capoten), enalapril (Vasotec), fosinopril (Monopril), lisinopril (Prinivil), moexipril (Univasc), perindopril (Aceon), quinapril (Accupril), ramipril (Altace), and trandolapril (Mavik); or angiotensin receptor (AR) blockers, such as candesartan (Atacand), irbesartan (Avapro), losartan (Cozaar), and valsartan (Diovan).

PGN ⟷ NSAIDs: (*See* Ω-54 in Appendix A.) The bleeding tendency of pycnogenol is increased when taken together with non-steroidal anti-inflammatory drugs (NSAIDs), such as ibuprofen (Motrin, Advil) and naproxen (Naprosyn, Aleve).

PGN ⟷ Oral Hypoglycemic Agents: (*See* Ω-55 in Appendix A.) Pycnogenol may lower blood levels of sugar and hence, an additive effect may be expected when it is used in combination with medications that lower blood sugar such as insulin, glipizide, glyburide, and metformin.

L-Arginine

See Box 30-3.

BOX 30-3

Basic Concepts of L-Arginine Interactions

L-arginine was shown to attenuate secretions of aldosterone from the adrenal cortex either by inhibiting the steroidogenic effects of angiotensin-II or by altering its plasma levels. Accordingly, L-arginine can raise blood levels of potassium, especially in individuals with a liver or kidney disease, and thus, L-arginine used in combination with any drug that raises blood levels of potassium can result in life-threatening hyperkalemia. Those potassium-retainers include: **ACE inhibitors** (*See* Ω-1 in Appendix A) (Note: ACE inhibitors retain potassium that may lead to cardiac conduction blockade, and so use of L-arginine in individuals taking an ACE inhibitor is not recommended); potassium-sparing diuretics such as **amiloride** and **triamterene;** and aldosterone antagonists such as **canrenone** and **spironolactone.**

Miscellaneous Interactions of L-Arginine (AGN)

AGN ⟷ Lysine: Researches have shown that a diet rich in lysine wards off herpes recurrences, whereas a diet rich in arginine can bring on its outbreak to counteract the medical benefits of lysine in the treatment of genital herpes. Hence, individuals with herpes should not take L-arginine, lest it aggravate their symptoms.

AGN ⟷ NSAIDs: (*See* Ω-54 in Appendix A.) Since L-arginine stimulates the production of gastric acid, a member of the NSAIDs such as aspirin or ibuprofen that causes gastric ulcers should not be taken in combination.

CHAPTER

31

Condylomata (Genital Warts)

Condylomata (genital warts, the plural of 'condyloma'), also known as venereal warts, are pathologic growths of small cauliflower-like red lumps in the genital region. The pathogen of this abnormal growth is the human papilloma virus (HPV), a sexually transmitted organism. The warts are painful, contagious, and are the most common sexually transmitted disease (STD). Even if the warts are not visible, HPV can still be passed on to others. To remove genital warts, the following medications may be of help: (1) **podofilox** gel (Condylox); (2) **imiquimod** (Aldara) cream; and (3) **fluorouracil** (Adrucil, Efudex, Fluoroplex) cream.

PODOFILOX

Application of this gel to warts several times over the course of three weeks may cause the warts to shrivel off gradually.

MECHANISM OF ACTION

The exact mechanism of action of podofilox has yet to be fully elucidated, but podofilox functions as a potent inhibitor of cell mitosis, causing necrosis of the genital wart.

SIDE EFFECTS

Frequent side effects of podofilox include burning, blistering, bleeding, scabbing, and severe irritation of treated skin and neighboring tissues. Rarely, it may cause allergic reactions such as skin rash, itching or hives, and swelling of the face, lips, or tongue.

DRUG INTERACTIONS

No serious drug interactions with podofilox are expected. However, it may be wise not to use any other skin products on the same area of the skin.

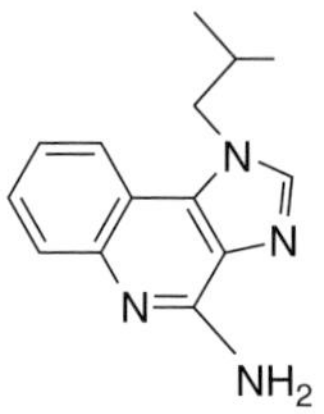

FIGURE 31-1   Molecular structure of imiquimod.

IMIQUIMOD

Imiquimod cream (Fig. 31-1) is used not only to treat external genital or anal warts, but also to treat other skin conditions such as actinic keratosis and certain types of skin cancer.

MECHANISM OF ACTION

Imiquimod does not have a direct antiviral activity, and its mechanism of action in treatment of genital warts is not completely understood. It has been shown that imiquimod stimulates helper-T (TH-1) cells to produce interferon-γ (IFN-γ), which in turn can activate cytotoxic T-lymphocytes. TH-1 cells also stimulate natural killer cells, and activate other immune cells including the macrophages which secrete cytokines such as interferon-α (IFN-α), interleukin-6 (IL-6), and tumor necrosis factor-α (TNF-α). The stimulation of innate and acquired immune responses can ultimately lead to apoptosis of the diseased tissue such as warts and basal cell carcinoma.

SIDE EFFECTS

Possible side effects of imiquimod cream may include skin itching, burning, bleeding, stinging, and induration.

DRUG INTERACTIONS

No clinically significant drug interactions of imiquimod are reported, but the drug may cause increased sensitivity to sunlight, providing a higher risk of sunburn.

FLUOROURACIL

Creams or solutions containing 5-fluorouracil may help kill the cells of genital warts.

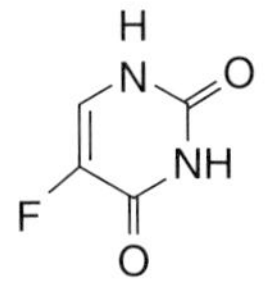

FIGURE 31-2   Molecular structure of fluorouracil.

MECHANISM OF ACTION

Fluorouracil (Fig. 31-2), chemically, is 5-F-uracil, which is converted *in vivo* to 5-dUMP, a false nucleotide that inhibits thymidylate synthase, the enzyme that catalyzes transfer of a methyl group from $N^{5,10}$-CH_2-FH_4 to uracil of deoxyuridine monophosphate (dUMP) (*See* Fig. 77-15), to form thymine, a unique and essential base in the DNA, without which no DNA can be synthesized. Thus, fluorouracil causes death of cells in the genital wart.

SIDE EFFECTS

Side effects of fluorouracil may include skin burning, crusting, redness, pain, soreness, inflammation or irritation, changes in skin color, increased sun sensitivity, and hair loss. Rarely, it may cause allergic reactions such as skin rash and itching; and if extensively absorbed from the site of application, it may cause abdominal pain, bloody diarrhea, vomiting, watery eyes, fever, chills, and insomnia.

DRUG INTERACTIONS

Fluorouracil cream applied topically is unlikely to cause serious interactions. However, if it is absorbed to a great extent, it is possible to generate such interactions as are explained in Chapter 77.

CHAPTER

32

Benign Prostate Hypertrophy

Benign prostate hypertrophy, or benign prostatic hyperplasia (BPH), refers to enlargement or overgrowth of the prostate gland, a gland that surrounds the urethra (tube that drains urine from the bladder to the exterior). The enlargement of the gland may block the otherwise smooth flow of urine. The following medications are effective in symptomatic treatment of BPH: (1) adrenergic alpha blockers such as **alfuzosin** (UroXatral), **doxazosin** (Cardura), **tamsulosin** (Flomax), and **terazosin** (Hytrin); and (2) 5-alpha reductase inhibitors such as **dutasteride** (Avodart) and **finasteride** (Proscar).

ADRENERGIC ALPHA BLOCKERS

Alfuzosin, doxazosin, tamsulosin, and **terazosin**

MECHANISM OF ACTION

All of these alpha blockers relax the neck of the urinary bladder and muscles of the prostate, easing the flow of urine. However, they do not cure the underlying cause of BPH.

SIDE EFFECTS

Possible side effects of these alpha blockers include excessively low blood pressure; runny nose or stuffy nose; priapism (painful, sustained penile erection lasting longer than 4 hours); decreased sex drive; and severe dizziness, drowsiness, fainting, fatigue, and insomnia.

DRUG INTERACTIONS

See Appendix B-2: Interactions of Alpha Blockers.

INHIBITORS OF 5-ALPHA REDUCTASE

Dutasteride (Fig. 32-1) and **finasteride** (Fig. 32-2)

MECHANISM OF ACTION

They inhibit 5-alpha reductase, the enzyme that converts testosterone (Fig. 32-3) to dihydrotestosterone (Fig. 32-4), the hormone more powerfully involved than testosterone in causing hypertrophy of the prostate gland.

SIDE EFFECTS

They may cause decreased sex drive, impotence, and reduced counts of semen per ejaculation.

DRUG INTERACTIONS

No clinically significant drug interactions have been reported. However, *See* Table 32-1.

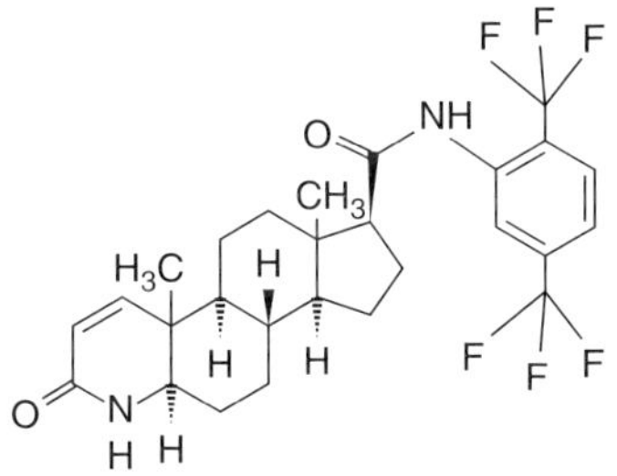

FIGURE 32-1 Molecular structure of dutasteride.

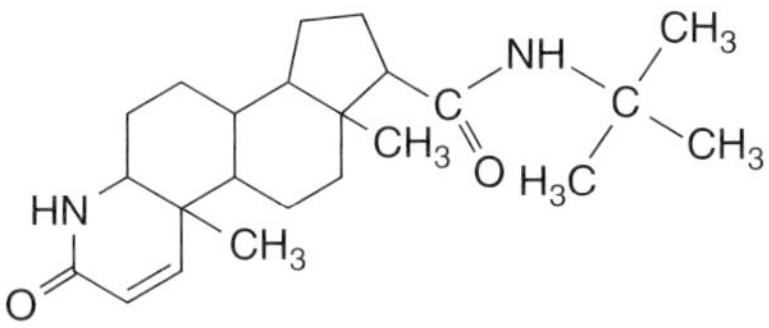

FIGURE 32-2 Molecular structure of finasteride.

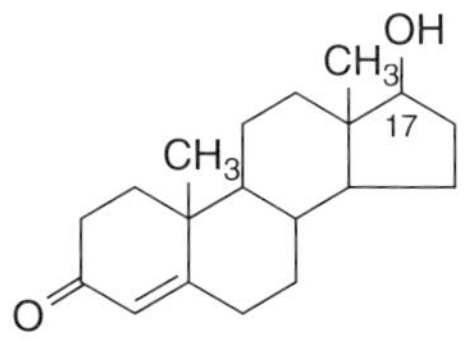

FIGURE 32-3 Molecular structure of testosterone.

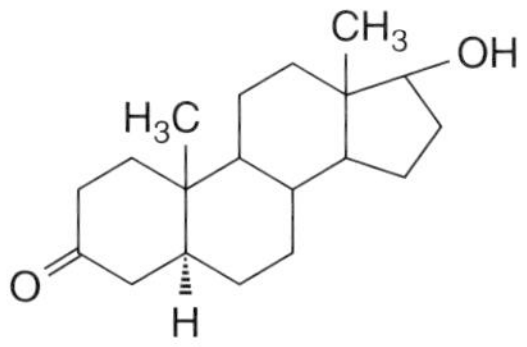

FIGURE 32-4 Molecular structure of dihydrotestosterone.

TABLE 32-1 5-Alpha Reductase Inhibitors vs CYP Isozymes

Drug Name	1A2	2A6	2B6	2C8	2C9	2C18	2C19	2D6	2E1	3A4
Dutasteride										Sub
Finasteride										Sub

Abbreviations: Sub, substrate of the enzyme; Inh, inhibits the enzyme; Ezi, induces the enzyme

Both dutasteride and finasteride require the microsomal enzyme CYP 3A4 for their clearance and thus, inhibition of this enzyme by certain drugs can raise blood levels and potentially exacerbate their adverse effects. Those strong inhibitors of CYP 3A4 include clarithromycin, indinavir, itraconazole, ketoconazole, nefazodone, nelfinavir, ritonavir, saquinavir and telithromycin; and its moderate inhibitors include aprepitant (Emend), erythromycin, fluconazole, grape fruit juice, and verapamil. (*See* the left-hand column of Table-0 at the 'Introduction' for other possible inhibitors of this enzyme.)

Urinary Incontinence

Urinary incontinence (bed-wetting) refers to the inability to control urination, owing either to a failure to accommodate urine in the bladder or to a loss of voluntary control over the sphincter of the urinary bladder. Urination may occur without warning, which is a common problem among children and elderly individuals.

Medications that may possibly be effective in the treatment of urinary incontinence include: (1) anticholinergic agents such as **dicyclomine** (Bentyl), **hyoscyamine** (the levorotary isomer to atropine), **oxybutynin** (Ditropan), and **tolterodine** (Detrol). Since a single pill of tolterodine works for 24 hours to relieve the symptoms, it is the most frequently prescribed drug for urinary incontinence.

ANTICHOLINERGIC AGENTS

Dicyclomine, hyoscyamine (the levo-isomer of atropine) (*See* Fig. 25-2), **oxybutynin** (Fig. 33-1), and **tolterodine** (Fig. 33-2)

MECHANISM OF ACTION

The detrusor muscle of the urinary bladder is contracted by activation of the parasympathetic system, whereas its relaxation is mediated through activation of the sympathetic system via its beta-adrenergic receptors. On the other

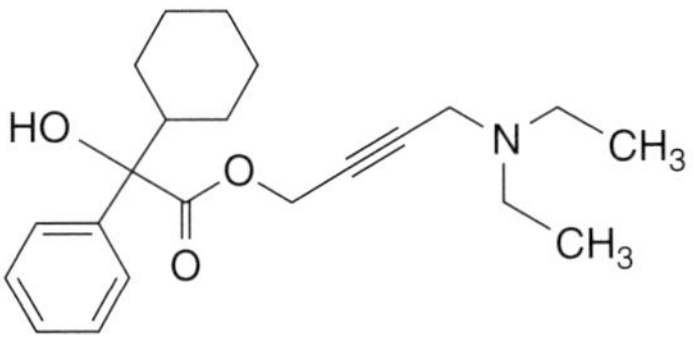

FIGURE 33-1 Molecular structure of oxybutynin.

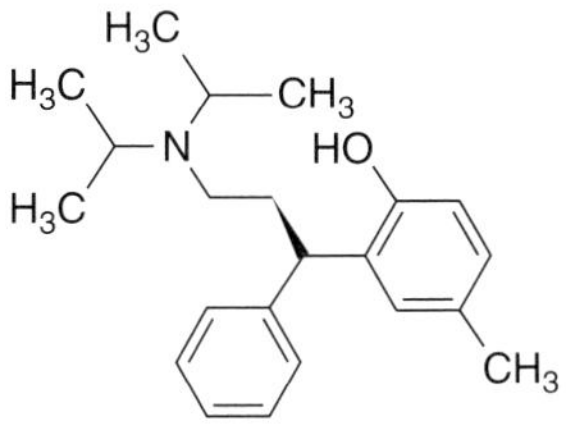

FIGURE 33-2 Molecular structure of tolterodine.

hand, contraction of the internal urethral sphincter of the bladder is mediated through activation of sympathetic alpha receptors, whereas the external urethral sphincter is innervated by the somatic nervous system to allow voluntary control of urination. Therefore, urination normally takes place by simultaneous inhibition of the sympathetic impulses to relax the internal sphincter, and activation of the parasympathetic impulses to contract the detrusor muscle of the bladder. As the muscular wall of the bladder is innervated by cholinergic fibers that release acetylcholine, activation of its receptors will contract the urinary bladder to raise pressure within the bladder, which facilitates urination. Hence, use of anticholinergic drugs, by blocking the effect of acetylcholine on the bladder muscle, relaxes the detrusor muscle of the urinary bladder to dampen the build-up of pressure within the bladder, suppressing the urge to urinate and preventing involuntary urination.

SIDE EFFECTS

Possible side effects of the above-mentioned anticholinergics include fast or irregular heartbeats; dry mouth, nausea, vomiting, stomach pain, loss of appetite, and constipation; hot or dry skin; blurred vision; and drowsiness, dizziness, confusion, headache, and hallucinations.

DRUG INTERACTIONS
Dicyclomine
See Chapter 25.

Hyoscyamine
See Appendix B-15: Interactions of Belladonna Alkaloids.

Oxybutynin
See Box 33-1.

Miscellaneous Interactions of Oxybutynin (OBT)

OBT ⟷ Digoxin: If oxybutynin is taken with digoxin, the blood levels of digoxin may be elevated to increase the risk of cardiac arrhythmia. The mechanism behind this observation is not fully elucidated, but it is known that elimination of digoxin depends heavily on its renal excretions, and oxybutynin impairs urination.

OBT ⟷ Levodopa: Oxybutynin decreases gastric motility to reduce absorption and therapeutic effectiveness of levodopa.

BOX 33-1

Basic Concepts of Oxybutynin Interactions

1. Oxybutynin is an anticholinergic agent, and when taken with drugs that generate anticholinergic effects, excessive, adverse anticholinergic effects such as xerostomia (dry mouth), constipation, heat stroke, blurred vision, hallucinations, drowsiness, and mental impairment may result. Those drugs include: **amantadine** (note: amantadine has a wide range of toxicities including its anticholinergic effects); **clozapine** (an atypical antipsychotic drug having significant anticholinergic activity); **phenothiazine antipsychotic drugs** (See Ω-58 in Appendix A); tricyclic antidepressants (See Ω-76 in Appendix A); and classic **anticholinergic agents** (See Ω-14 in Appendix A).

2. Since oxybutynin has an anticholinergic effect, when it is taken with drugs that work by cholinergic effect, it may counteract the therapeutic effectiveness of the cholinomimetic drugs, which include: **bethanechol** and **pilocarpine**.

Tolterodine

See Box 33-2.

BOX 33-2

Basic Concepts of Tolterodine Interactions

1. Tolterodine is an anticholinergic agent, and when taken with drugs that generate anticholinergic effects, excessive adverse effects may appear, including severe dry mouth, constipation, heat stroke, blurred vision, hallucinations, drowsiness, and mental impairment. Those drugs include: **amantadine** (note: amantadine has a wide range of toxicities including its anticholinergic effects); **anticholinergic agents** (See Ω-14 in Appendix A); **phenothiazine antipsychotic drugs** (See Ω-58 in Appendix A); and **tricyclic antidepressants** (See Ω-76 in Appendix A).

2. Tolterodine has an anticholinergic effect, and when taken with drugs that work by cholinergic effect, it may counteract the therapeutic efficacy of cholinomimetic drugs. Those drugs include: **bethanechol** and **pilocarpine**.

Miscellaneous Interactions of Tolterodine (TTD)

TTD ←→ CYP Isozymes: *See* Table 33-1.

TABLE 33-1 Oxybutynin and Tolterodine vs CYP Enzymes

Drug Name	1A2	2A6	2B6	2C8	2C9	2C18	2C19	2D6	2E1	3A4
Oxybutynin										Sub
Tolterodine								Sub		Sub

Abbreviations: Sub, substrate of the enzyme; Inh, inhibits the enzyme; Ezi, induces the enzyme

1. Dicyclomine and hyoscyamine (not shown) either do not interact with cytochrome P450 isozymes, or their natures of interaction are not as clearly elucidated as other drugs shown in this table.

2. Metabolic clearance of oxybutynin, unlike tolterodine, requires the presence of microsomal CYP3A4 only and thus, inhibition of this enzyme by any other drug taken together may raise blood levels of oxybutynin to possibly exacerbate its adverse effects. Inhibitors of CYP3A4 include clarithromycin, erythromycin, fluconazole, itraconazole, fluoxetine, and ketoconazole. (*See* the left-hand column of Table-0 at the 'Introduction' for other possible inhibitors of this enzyme.)

34

Nephrolithiasis (Kidney Stone)

Nephrolithiasis results from abnormal depositions of minerals such as calcium salts (calcium phosphate and calcium oxalate), uric acid, and cystine in the kidney or at the lower urinary tract. The tendency toward developing kidney stones is related to decreased urine volume or to increased excretions of the stone-forming compounds. These stones may cause excruciating pain, bleeding, and obstruction of urinary flow, which may eventually lead to kidney failure.

Medications that may possibly be effective in the treatment of nephrolithiasis include: (1) diuretic agents such as **hydrochlorothiazide** (Esidrix) and **trichlormethiazide**; (2) **potassium citrate**; and (3) **allopurinol** (Aloprim, Zyloprim), which is to treat nephrolithiasis caused by uric acid crystals.

DIURETIC AGENTS

Hydrochlorothiazide and **trichlormethiazide**

MECHANISM OF ACTION

Both drugs work by inhibition of the electroneutral Na^+-Cl^- reabsorption pump located at the distal renal tubules.

SIDE EFFECTS

Their possible side effects include hypokalemia, hyperuricemia, and hyperglycemia; loss of appetite, nausea, vomiting, and upset stomach; muscle cramps and weakness; and dizziness and lightheadedness.

DRUG INTERACTIONS

See Appendix B-4: Interactions of Thiazide Diuretics.

POTASSIUM CITRATE

MECHANISM OF ACTION

Potassium citrate decreases the formation of calcium oxalate and tends to reduce renal calcium excretions.

SIDE EFFECTS

Potassium citrate may cause irregular heartbeats; nausea, vomiting, abdominal pain, and bloody diarrhea; and muscle weakness.

DRUG INTERACTIONS

Potassium citrate (PCT)

PCT ◆▶ Antihypertensive Drugs: (*See* Ω-20 in Appendix A.) Potassium citrate itself has a powerful effect in lowering blood pressure. If combined with other anti-hypertensive medications, it may further pull down the pressure to an alarming degree.

PCT ◆▶ Digoxin: As potassium citrate slows the impulse conduction speed of the heart; this condition may be aggravated by combined use with certain heart medications such as digoxin, which also slows the conduction.

PCT ◆▶ Potassium-Sparing Diuretics: If potassium citrate is used in combination with a potassium-sparing diuretic, such as amiloride, canrenone, spironolactone, or triamterene, it will further raise the blood levels of potassium, leading toward heart failure.

PCT ◆▶ Quinidine: As potassium citrate slows the impulse conduction speed of the heart, this condition may be aggravated by combined use with certain heart medications, such as quinidine which also slows down the conduction speed.

PCT ◆▶ Salicylates: (*See* Ω-64 in Appendix A.) Potassium citrate makes urine less acidic (elevated pH) to accelerate urinary excretions of acidic drugs, such as aspirin, and other salicylates such as salsalate, to reduce their blood levels and therapeutic effects.

ALLOPURINOL

MECHANISM OF ACTION

Both allopurinol (Fig. 34-1) and its metabolite oxypurinol (or alloxanthine) inhibit xanthine oxidase, the enzyme involved in the formation of uric acid from

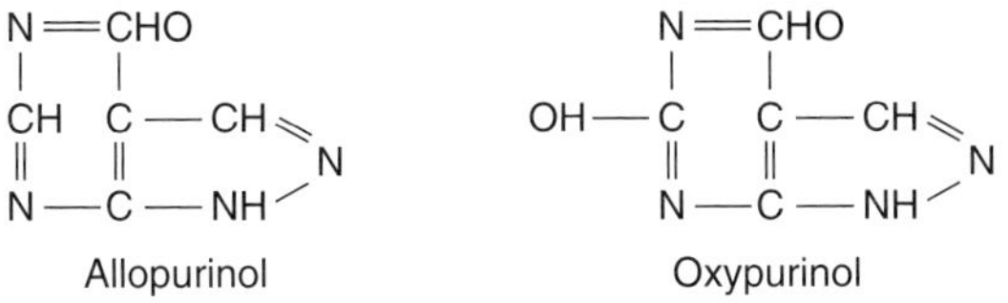

FIGURE 34-1 Molecular structures of allopurinol and oxypurinol.

xanthine, during degradation of the purine bases such as adenine and guanine of both DNA and RNA.

SIDE EFFECTS

Allopurinol may cause nausea and diarrhea; jaundice; bone marrow depression; maculopapular skin rash or erythema multiforme exudativum (Stevens-Johnson syndrome); and fever and chills.

DRUG INTERACTIONS

See Box 34-1.

Miscellaneous Interactions of Allopurinol (APN)

APN ⟷ Captopril: Captopril may cause, as side effects, renal impairment (elevation of urea and creatinine blood levels), maculopapular skin rash, and, rarely, appearance of antinuclear antibodies in the blood. Hence, concomitant use of allopurinol (whose side effects may include Stevens-Johnson syndrome) and captopril may promote the risk of hypersensitivity reactions such as Stevens-Johnson syndrome and granulocytopenia. A similar interaction with other angiotensin-converting enzyme inhibitors is possible.

BOX 34-1

Basic Concepts of Allopurinol Interactions

Allopurinol inhibits the enzyme xanthine oxidase, and when taken concurrently with drugs that require this enzyme for their inactivation, it may elevate their blood levels and toxicities. Those drugs include: **azathioprine** (an immunosuppressant); **didanosine** (an anti-HIV drug); **mercaptopurine** (a drug to treat leukemia); and **theophylline** (a drug to treat chronic bronchitis).

APN ⟷ Chlorpropamide: Allopurinol, when taken together, competes with chlorpropamide, an oral hypoglycemic agent, for excretions through the renal tubules. Hence, their combination may delay elimination of chlorpropamide, increasing its plasma concentrations, and whipping up its adverse effect of hypoglycemia.

APN ⟷ Cyclophosphamide: Allopurinol, when it is taken in combination, may either accelerate hepatic metabolism of cyclophosphamide to generate its cytotoxic metabolites, or decrease renal excretions of cyclophosphamide, to raise its blood levels, provoking its side effect of myelosuppression.

APN ⟷ Penicillins: (*See* Ω-56 in Appendix A.) Concurrent administration of amoxicillin, ampicillin, or penicillin-V with allopurinol substantially increases the incidences of skin rash as compared to patients receiving one of the antibiotics alone. It is not known whether this potentiation of rash is due to allopurinol itself or due to hyperuricemia caused by the above antibiotics.

APN ⟷ Pentostatin: Allopurinol may increase the incidences of skin rash and allergic vasculitis associated with pentostatin, a drug useful to treat acute lymphocytic leukemia.

APN ⟷ Porfirmer: While some photosensitizing agents, such as griseofulvin, tetracyclines, and sulfonamides, could boost the photosensitivity reactions of porfirmer, allopurinol when used in combination can interfere with the photodynamic therapy of porfirmer. Hence, it is best to avoid this combination.

Cystitis/Urethritis

Cystitis is inflammation of the urinary bladder, whereas urethritis is inflammation of the urethra. Urinary tract infections (UTIs) are caused by bacterial infections of the kidneys, the bladder, or the ureter (tube draining urine from the kidneys to the bladder). Cystitis is the most common type of UTI and causes pain, burning, and urinary urgency. Most UTIs are due to the bacteria *Escherichia coli* (*E. coli*).

Medications shown effective in the treatment of lower urinary tract infections include: (1) penicillins such as **amoxicillin** (Amoxil, Trimox, Wymox), and **ampicillin** (Omnipen, Polycillin, Principen, Totacillin); (2) quinolone antibiotics including **ciprofloxacin** (Cipro), **norfloxacin** (Noroxin), and **ofloxacin** (Floxin); (3) the sulfa preparation Septra **(sulfamethoxazole + trimethoprim);** (4) urinary antiseptics like **nitrofurantoin** (Macrobid); and (5) urinary tract analgesics such as **phenazopyridine** (Pyridium).

PENICILLINS

Amoxicillin and **ampicillin**

MECHANISM OF ACTION
See Chapter 12.

SIDE EFFECTS
See Chapter 12.

DRUG INTERACTIONS
See Appendix B-24: Interactions of Penicillins.

QUINOLONE ANTIBIOTICS

Ciprofloxacin, norfloxacin, and ofloxacin

MECHANISM OF ACTION

Quinolones generate their antibacterial effect by inhibiting DNA gyrase, an essential bacterial enzyme which catalyzes the ATP-dependent negative super-coiling of double-stranded bacterial DNA, which is required for DNA replications.

SIDE EFFECTS

Ciprofloxacin and others above may cause nausea, vomiting, diarrhea, and abdominal pain; jaundice (yellowing of the skin or eyes); rarely, nephrotoxicity; headache and restlessness; and allergic reactions such as anaphylactic shock and skin rash are also possible. Ciprofloxacin should be used with caution in patients with seizures, since seizure activities have rarely been reported in patients receiving ciprofloxacin.

DRUG INTERACTIONS

See Appendix B-28: Interactions of Quinolone Antibiotics.

SULFAMETHOXAZOLE WITH TRIMETHOPRIM

MECHANISM OF ACTION

Sulfamethoxazole (Fig. 35-1) is a sulfonamide member that works by interfering with incorporation of para-aminobenzoic acid (PABA) into dihydrofolate, the precursor from which tetrahydrofolate can be formed. Trimethoprim (Fig. 35-2) is a non-sulfonamide drug that works by inhibition of dihydrofolate reductase, the enzyme that catalyzes conversion of dihydrofolate to tetrahydrofolate. As no tetrahydrofolate is formed by this two-drug combination, bacteria cannot synthesize thymine, an essential base required for the synthesis of bacterial DNA, without which the bacteria cannot proliferate.

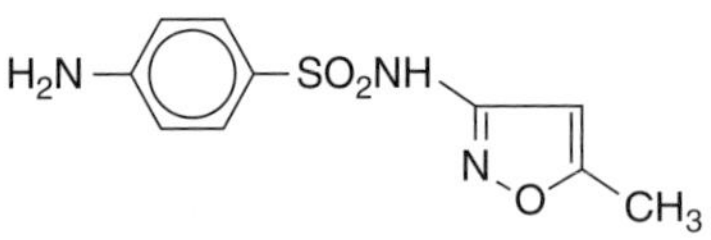

FIGURE 35-1 Molecular structure of sulfamethoxazole.

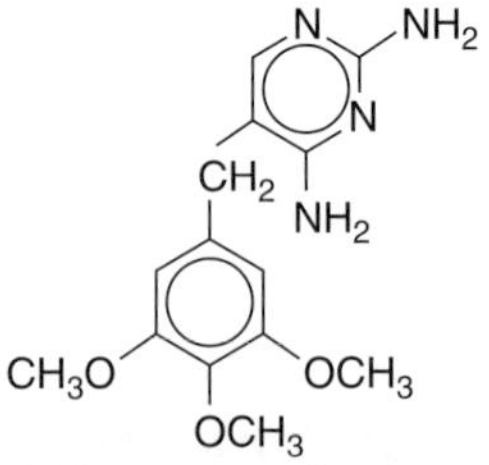

FIGURE 35-2 Molecular structure of trimethoprim.

SIDE EFFECTS

Sulfamethoxazole: This drug may cause nausea, vomiting, and diarrhea; nephrotoxicity, headache, fatigue, and dizziness; and allergic reactions such as difficulty in breathing, swelling of the face, lips, tongue, or throat, and skin hives.

Trimethoprim: It may cause irregular heartbeat; methemoglobinemia; leukopenia, thrombocytopenia, and megaloblastic anemia; nausea, vomiting, stomach upset, and diarrhea; decreased urination (nephrotoxicity); chills, fever, and sore throat; seizures; and allergic reactions such as skin hives and swelling of the face, lips, tongue, or throat.

DRUG INTERACTIONS

See Box 35-1.

Miscellaneous Interactions of Sulfamethoxazole (SMZ)

SMZ ↔ Cyclosporine: If used in combination, sulfamethoxazole can enhance kidney damage caused by cyclosporine.

SMZ ↔ CYP Isozymes: *See* Table 35-1.

SMZ ↔ Digoxin: Co-administration of co-trimoxazole (sulfamethoxazole + trimethoprim) with digoxin may lead to increased plasma levels of the digitalis glycoside enhancing its tendency toward cardiac arrhythmia. Trimethoprim contained in co-trimoxazole is known to decrease renal tubular secretions of digoxin.

BOX 35-1

Basic Concepts of Sulfamethoxazole Interactions

Sulfamethoxazole binds to plasma proteins with high affinity, and when taken with drugs that are bound to the same proteins with a lower affinity, sulfamethoxazole can displace them to increase their free drug concentrations and adverse effects. Those drugs include: **chlorpropamide** (an antidiabetic drug); **methotrexate** (an anticancer drug); **tolbutamide** (an antidiabetic drug; and **warfarin** (an anticoagulant).

TABLE 35-1 Sulfamethoxazole vs CYP Isozymes

Drug Name	1A2	2A6	2B6	2C8	2C9	2C18	2C19	2D6	2E1	3A4
Sulfamethoxazole					Sub+ Inh					

Abbreviations: Sub, substrate of the enzyme; Inh, inhibits the enzyme; Ezi, induces the enzyme

1. Sulfamethoxazole inhibits the liver enzyme CYP 2C9 and thus, co-administration with drugs that require this enzyme for hepatic clearance may raise their blood levels and possibly exacerbate their adverse effects. Those drugs include: phenytoin and warfarin. (*See* the middle column of Table-0 at the 'Introduction' for other substrates of this enzyme.)

2. Hepatic inactivation of sulfamethoxazole requires the presence of microsomal CYP2C9 and thus, inhibition of this enzyme by drugs taken together may raise blood levels and possibly exacerbate the adverse effects of sulfamethoxazole. (*See* the left-hand column of Table-0 at the 'Introduction' for possible inhibitors of this enzyme.)

SMZ ⟷ Pyrimethamine: Co-administration of pyrimethamine, an anti-folate drug, with co-trimoxazole (sulfamethoxazole + trimethoprim), another antifolate preparation, may increase the risk of bone marrow suppressions, megaloblastic anemia, and pancytopenia.

DRUG INTERACTIONS

Miscellaneous Interactions of Trimethoprim (TMP)

TMP ⟷ Antacids: (*See* Ω-11 in Appendix A.) Concurrent administration of trimethoprim and a gastric antacid, such as aluminum hydroxide or magnesium hydroxide, may decrease the intestinal absorption of trimethoprim.

BOX 35-2

Basic Concepts of Trimethoprim Interactions

1. Trimethoprim is an inhibitor of renal cationic secretions, and when this drug is taken with drugs that are secreted through the renal tubules, it may result in their elevated blood levels, inciting their adverse effects. Those drugs include: **aspirin, dofetilide** (an antiarrhythmic drug, which is eliminated in the kidney by cationic secretion route); **methotrexate** (an anticancer drug); **probenecid** (an antigout drug); **procainamide** (an antiarrhythmic drug); **salicylates** (*See* Ω-64 in Appendix A); and **thiazide diuretics** (*See* Ω-73 in Appendix A).

2. Trimethoprim is prone to cause nephrotoxicity as one of its side effects, and concurrent administration with drugs that tend to generate nephrotoxicity may create serious renal dysfunctions. Examples include: **azathioprine** (an immunosuppressant) and **cyclosporine** (an immunosuppressant).

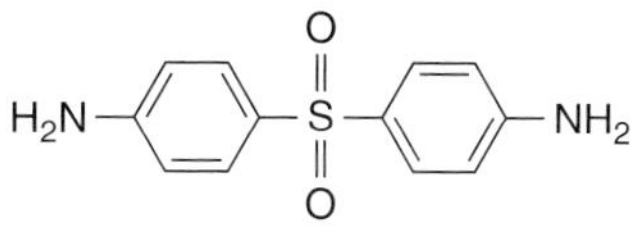

FIGURE 35-3 Molecular structure of dapsone.

TMP ⟷ Dapsone: Dapsone (Fig. 35-3) can induce methemoglobinemia as does trimethoprim and hence, concomitant administration of the two may increase incidences of the hematologic disorder.

TMP ⟷ Phenylbutazone: Trimethoprim, alone or in combination with sulfamethoxazole, decreases the renal secretions of phenylbutazone, to increase its blood levels and toxicities.

TMP ⟷ Phenytoin: Trimethoprim is a selective inhibitor of both CYP2C8 and CYP2C9. Concomitant administration of trimethoprim with phenytoin, an antiepileptic substrate of CYP2C9, causes impaired metabolism of phenytoin to elevate its blood levels and adverse effects.

TMP ⟷ Pyrimethamine: Both pyrimethamine and trimethoprim have an anti-folate activity. Co-administration of them may lead to a severe reduction in normal folate metabolism, resulting in megaloblastic anemia and pancytopenia.

TPM ⟷ Zidovudine: Trimethoprim, when used in combination, may increase the pharmacological effects of zidovudine (AZT), because the former can decrease the renal excretions of the latter.

NIROFURANTOIN

MECHANISM OF ACTION

Nitrofurantoin (*See* Fig. 79-4) is reduced first before inhibiting bacterial enzymes and damaging the bacterial DNA.

SIDE EFFECTS

Nitrofurantoin may cause peripheral neuritis, rarely pancreatitis , and pulmonary interstitial fibrosis. Therefore, use of nitrofurantoin for more than six months is not recommended. Nitrofurantoin may turn urine brownish-black, but this does not amount to a medical emergency.

BOX 35-3

Basic Concepts of Nitrofurantoin Interactions

Renal tubular secretions of nitrofurantoin can be inhibited by uricosuric drugs, resulting in increased serum levels of nitrofurantoin, augmenting its adverse effects; whereas its decreased concentration in the urine is accountable for its weakened effectiveness as a urinary tract antibacterial agent. Those uricosuric drugs include: **probenecid** and **sulfinpyrazone**.

DRUG INTERACTIONS

Miscellaneous Interactions of Nitrofurantoin (NFT)

NFT ⟷ Antacids: (*See* Ω-11 in Appendix A.) Gastric antacids when used in combination may decrease intestinal absorption of nitrofurantoin.

NFT ⟷ Anticholinergic Agents: (*See* Ω-14 in Appendix A.) Combined intake of nitrofurantoin with an anticholinergic drug may result in reduced intestinal absorption of nitrofurantoin.

NFT ⟷ Didanosine: Didanosine is reported to cause fatal or nonfatal pancreatitis, while nitrofurantoin also rarely causes acute pancreatitis. The intake of the two in combination may enhance incidences of such adverse effects.

NFT ⟷ Phenytoin: Concomitant administration of nitrofurantoin and phenytoin has reduced blood levels of phenytoin to undercut its effectiveness in controlling seizures. However, the mechanism behind this observation is yet to be determined.

NFT ⟷ Zalcitabine: Adverse effects of nitrofurantoin include neuropathy. When this drug is taken together with zalcitabine, an anti-HIV drug whose side effects also include peripheral neuropathy, it may foment such symptoms as numbness and burning sensations at the distal extremities.

PHENAZOPYRIDINE

MECHANISM OF ACTION

Phenazopyridine exerts a topical analgesic effect on the mucosa of the urinary tract to reduce the burning and urgency associated with cystitis, but its precise mechanism of action is unknown.

SIDE EFFECTS

Phenazopyridine may cause hemolytic anemia; shortness of breath; stomach pain; blue-purple colored skin; yellow eyes; dizziness, confusion, and headache; skin rash; and swelling of the face, fingers, and feet. Phenazopyridine may turn urine orange-red or orange-brown, but this does not usually amount to a medical emergency.

DRUG INTERACTIONS

There are no known interactions between phenazopyridine and other medications.

36

Urinary Retention

Urinary retention refers to the condition in which urine is held in the bladder due to inability to urinate. Urinary retention is a common complication in patients with benign prostatic hyperplasia. Medications shown effective in the treatment of urinary retention include: (1) **bethanechol** (Duvoid, Urecholine); (2) alpha blockers such as **alfuzosin** (UroXatral), **doxazosin** (Cardura), **tamsulosin** (Flomax), and **terazosin** (Hytrin); and (3) 5-alpha reductase inhibitors such as **dutasteride** (Avodart), and **finasteride** (Proscar).

BETHANECHOL

See Chapter 23.

ALPHA BLOCKERS

Alfuzosin, doxazosin, tamsulosin, and **terazosin**

MECHANISM OF ACTION

All of these drugs relax the neck of the urinary bladder and relax muscles in the prostate to ease urination.

SIDE EFFECTS

Possible side effects of these drugs include excessively low blood pressure; runny nose or stuffy nose; priapism (painful, sustained, penile erection lasting longer than four hours), decreased sex drive; severe dizziness, drowsiness, fainting, fatigue, and insomnia.

DRUG INTERACTIONS

See Appendix B-2: Interactions of Alpha Blockers.

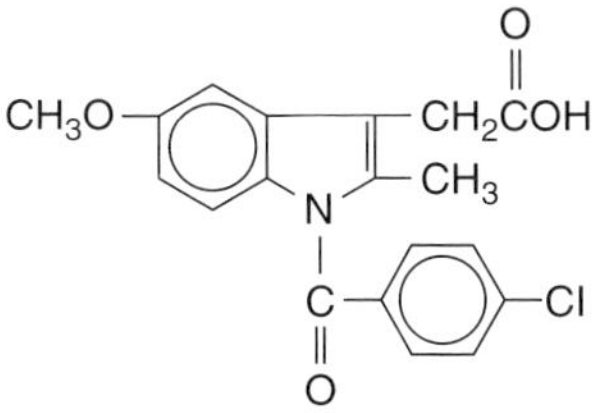

FIGURE 37-2 Molecular structure of indomethacin.

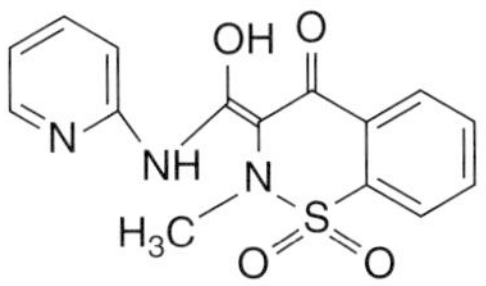

FIGURE 37-3 Molecular structure of piroxicam.

cytochrome P450, which are responsible for the metabolism of many other drugs.

ABR ⟷ Estrogens: (*See* Ω-40 in Appendix A.) Combined use of any of the above bisphosphonates with estrogens, such as found in oral contraceptive pills, can further suppress the bone turnover to benefit patients with osteoporosis.

ABR ⟷ NSAIDs: (*See* Ω-54 in Appendix A.) Risk of gastrointestinal irritation by alendronate, ibandronate, or risedronate may be increased by combined use with any non-steroidal anti-inflammatory drug (NSAID), including aspirin, indomethacin (Fig. 37-2), and piroxicam (Fig. 37-3).

RALOXIFENE

MECHANISM OF ACTION

Raloxifene (Fig. 37-4) belongs to a class of drugs called selective estrogen-receptor modulators (SERM). Raloxifene provides beneficial effects of estrogens on the bone without the negative effects of estrogens on the breast and endometrium. Raloxifene binds to estrogen receptors to produce estrogen-like effects on the bone, reducing its resorption and increasing bone mineral density in postmenopausal women.

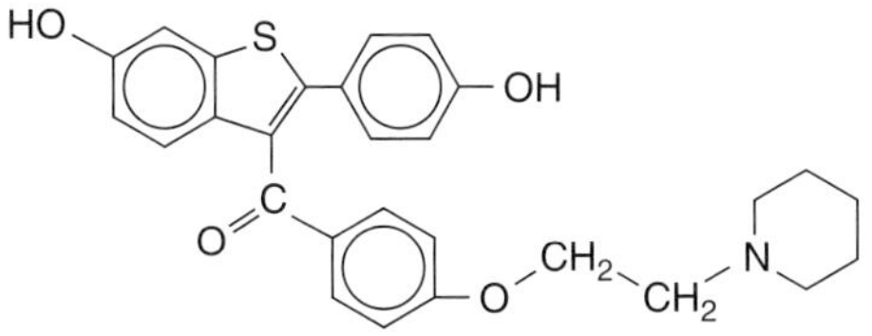

FIGURE 37-4 Molecular structure of raloxifene.

BOX 37-1

Basic Concepts of Raloxifene Interactions

Raloxifene is more than 95% bound to plasma proteins but with low affinity, and when co-administered with drugs that bind to the same proteins with higher affinity, they displace raloxifene to raise its serum levels and to foster its adverse effects. Those high affinity drugs include: **clofibrate** (a cholesterol-lowering drug); **ibuprofen** (an NSAID); **indomethacin** (an NSAID); and **naproxen** (an NSAID).

SIDE EFFECTS

Raloxifene may cause hot flashes with sudden sweating and feelings of warmth; shortness of breath and congestion in the lungs; loss of appetite, nausea, vomiting, upset stomach, and diarrhea; painful urination; joint or muscle pain; swelling of the hands, ankles, or feet; and migraine headaches.

DRUG INTERACTIONS

See Box 37-1.

Miscellaneous Interactions of Raloxifene (RXP)

RXP ⟷ Cholestyramine: Cholestyramine, a cholesterol-lowering resin, adsorbs many drugs, including raloxifene, to reduce their intestinal absorptions.

RXP ⟷ Levothyroxine: When taken together, raloxifene can reduce absorption of levothyroxine (T4), to permit sustained hypothyroidism.

CALCITONIN-SALMON

MECHANISM OF ACTION

This hormone inhibits osteoclastic bone resorption.

SIDE EFFECTS

This drug may cause nausea; nasal irritation and bleeding, runny or stuffy nose; back pain; headache, fainting; and, rarely, allergic reactions such as difficulty in breathing, skin hives, and swelling of the face, lips, tongue, or throat.

DRUG INTERACTIONS

No drug interaction studies have been performed with this drug.

ANABOLIC STEROIDS

Oxandrolone (Fig. 37-5) and testosterone (*See* Fig. 32-3)

MECHANISM OF ACTION

Both of the above anabolic steroids appear to have the ability to directly stimulate collagen synthesis in the bone, thereby facilitating mineralization of the bone by the osteoblasts.

SIDE EFFECTS

Either of the above drugs may cause nausea; painful or prolonged erection and change in sex drive; weight gain; yellowing of the skin or eyes; acne; hair loss; and headache.

DRUG INTERACTIONS

See Box 37-2.

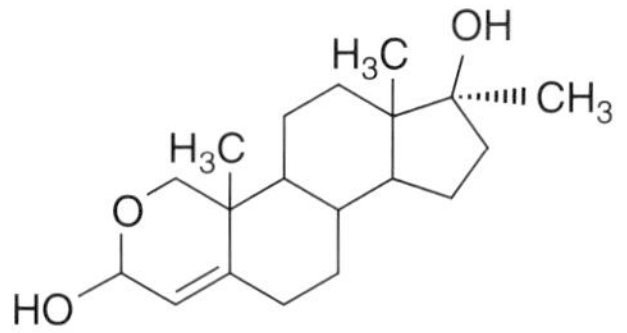

FIGURE 37-5   Molecular structure of oxandrolone.

BOX 37-2

Basic Concepts of Anabolic Steroids Interactions

Anabolic steroids such as testosterone and oxandrolone tend to oppose formation of blood clotting factors, and when either of them is taken with an anticoagulant they may lead to enhanced hemorrhagic episode. Those anticoagulant drugs include: **dicumarol** and **warfarin**.

TABLE 37-1 Anabolic Steroids vs CYP Enzymes

Drug Name	1A2	2A6	2B6	2C8	2C9	2C18	2C19	2D6	2E1	3A4
Oxandrolone					Inh					
Testosterone			Sub							Sub

Abbreviations: Sub, substrate of the enzyme; Inh, inhibits the enzyme; Ezi, induces the enzyme

Oxandrolone, unlike testosterone, exerts an inhibitory effect on the hepatic CYP2C9 and hence, its administration in combination with drugs that require this enzyme for metabolic clearance may elevate blood levels and adverse effects of those substrate drugs. (*See* the middle column of Table-0 at the 'Introduction' for possible substrates of this enzyme.)

Miscellaneous Interactions of Anabolic Steroids (OXT)

OXT ↔ CYP Isozymes: *See* Table 37-1.

OXT ↔ Insulin: Anabolic steroids increase glucose disposal to generate a hypoglycemic activity, which may enhance the hypoglycemic effects of insulin when taken together.

GLUCOSAMINE PLUS CHONDROITIN SULFATE

Taking glucosamine plus chondroitin sulfate everyday for more than one month may help promote the formation of bone cartilage.

MECHANISM OF ACTION

Glucosamine is a form of amino sugar, which *in vivo* is polymerized to glycosaminoglycan, an essential building block of cartilage and the major matrix of bone to which minerals deposit. Glucosamine may increase the rate of formation of new cartilage, and it also appears to inhibit the bone-destructive enzyme collagenase. Chondroitin is chemically composed of repeated chains of N-acetylgalactosamine and glucuronic acid, and is the most abundant glycosaminoglycan in cartilage. Its function is similar to glucosamine.

SIDE EFFECTS

They may induce loss of appetite, stomach pain, nausea, upset stomach, constipation or diarrhea, and flatulence; and skin rash or itching

DRUG INTERACTIONS

See Box 37-3.

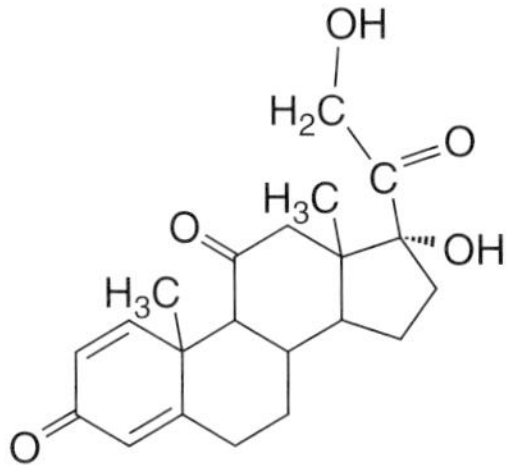

FIGURE 38-1 Molecular structure of prednisone.

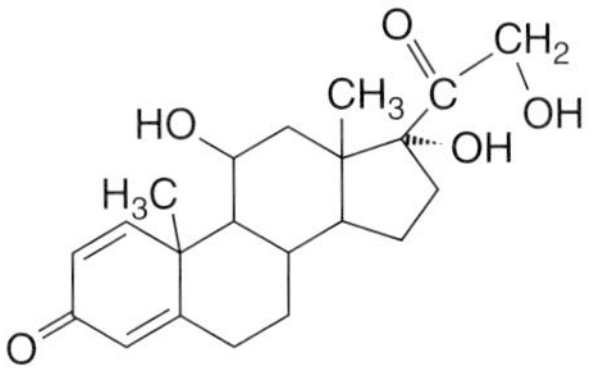

FIGURE 38-2 Molecular structure of prednisolone.

DRUG INTERACTIONS

See Appendix B-20: Interactions of Glucocorticoids.

NSAIDs

Celecoxib, diclofenac, etodolac, ibuprofen, indomethacin, meloxicam, nabumetone, naproxen, piroxicam, and **tenoxicam**. All of these NSAIDs suppress swelling, redness, pain, and inflammation of joints. Ibuprofen is additionally approved as a fever-reducing agent.

MECHANISM OF ACTION

All of the above NSAIDs, except celecoxib, inhibit both cyclooxygenase (COX)-1 and COX-2, the enzymes that catalyze conversion of arachidonic acid, which is released from membrane phospholipids due to inflammatory stimuli, to prostaglandin E (PGE) and leukotrienes. Thus, NSAIDs interfere with the synthesis of PGE and leukotrienes in inflammatory tissues. Celecoxib (Fig. 38-3) is unusual in that it selectively inhibits the enzyme COX-2, which is involved in the formation of inflammatory PGE of the joints, to suppress inflammation of arthritis; and in that it does not inhibit the enzyme COX-1 that contributes to the formation of PGE that protects the mucosal surfaces of the stomach.

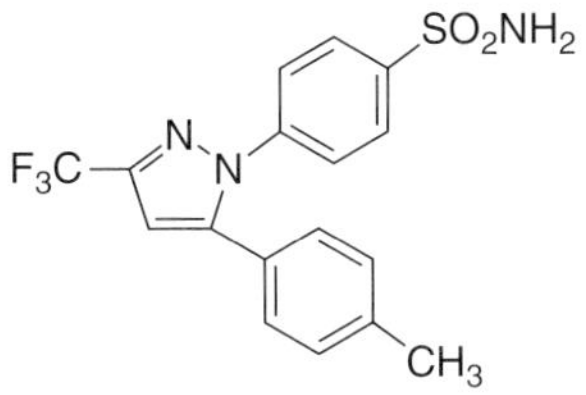

FIGURE 38-3 Molecular structure of celecoxib.

SIDE EFFECTS

NSAIDs may generate the following side effects: difficulty in breathing and wheezing; nausea, vomiting, upset stomach, gas pain, bloating, intestinal bleeding, bloody stool, and heartburn; and jaundice (yellowing of the skin or eyes). Additionally, indomethacin may cause nephrotoxicity, edema, increased blood pressure, and bone marrow depression with seriously low white blood counts, increasing vulnerability to infections. Indomethacin may turn urine blue-green, but this does not usually signal medical emergency.

DRUG INTERACTIONS

See Appendix B-22: Interactions of NSAIDs.

LIDOCAINE

Pain associated with osteoarthritis of the knee may be suppressed by application of a lidocaine patch 5%, which is also used to relieve pain associated with minor cuts; sunburn; poison ivy; hemorrhoids; and shingles.

MECHANISM OF ACTION

Lidocaine is a local anesthetic agent that blocks neuronal sodium channels to interrupt generation and propagation of pain sensations.

SIDE EFFECTS

It may cause redness or swelling at the site of application. If its absorption into the general circulation is extensive, this skin patch may cause irregular heartbeats; nausea and vomiting; blurred or double vision; dizziness or drowsiness; and very rarely allergic reactions such as closing of the throat.

DRUG INTERACTIONS

It is not known whether other medications will interact with this medication applied topically.

Gout

Gout is a form of arthritis (Fig. 39-1) but differs from others in that it is due to deposition of insoluble uric acid crystals (Fig. 39-2) in or around the joint areas, especially of the big toe. Gout usually occurs suddenly and may disappear after one week, but recurrent attacks are common.

Medications that may possibly be effective in the treatment of gout include: (1) **allopurinol** (Aloprim, Zyloprim); (2) **colchicine;** (3) uricosuric agents such as **probenecid** (Benemid, Probalan), and **sulfinpyrazone** (Anturane); and (4) nonsteroidal anti-inflammatory drugs (NSAIDs) such as **ibuprofen** (Advil, Motrin, and others), **indomethacin** (Indocin), and **naproxen** (Aleve, Anaprox, Naprosyn, and others).

ALLOPURINOL

MECHANISM OF ACTION
See Chapter 34.

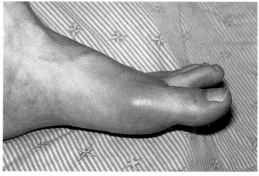

FIGURE 39-1 **Gout.** Reproduced, with permission, from DiPiro JT, Talbert RL, Yee GC, Matzke GR, Wells BG, and Posey LM, eds. *Pharmacotherapy: A Pathologic Approach.* 7th ed. New York, NY: McGraw-Hill; 2008, p 1541.

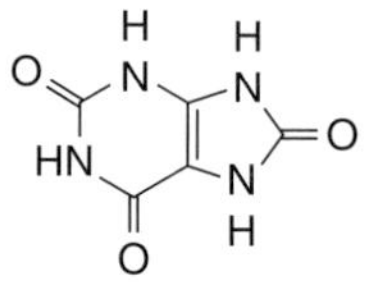

FIGURE 39-2   Molecular structure of uric acid.

SIDE EFFECTS

See Chapter 34.

DRUG INTERACTIONS

See Chapter 34.

COLCHICINE

MECHANISM OF ACTION

Colchicine (Fig. 39-3) binds to tubulin, the microtubular protein monomer, to oppose its polymerization to form microtubules, while allowing their depolymerization, leading to disappearance of the microtubules. This drug thereby inhibits migration to the inflammatory sites of polymorphonuclear leukocytes, which phagocytize urate crystals during which lysosomal enzymes are released, generating an inflammatory response in acute gout.

SIDE EFFECTS

Colchicine may cause nausea, vomiting, and bloody diarrhea; and bone marrow depression with seriously low white blood counts, which increases vulnerability to infections.

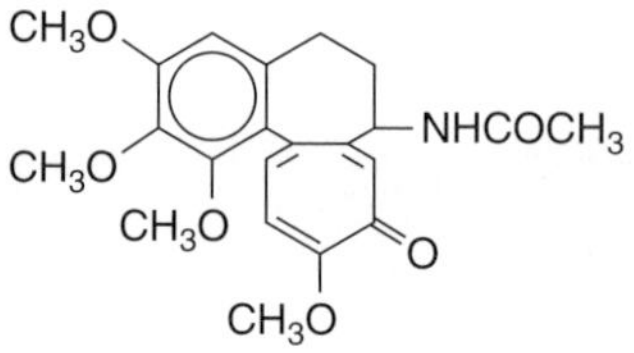

FIGURE 39-3   Molecular structure of colchicine.

TABLE 39-1   Colchicine, Probenecid, and Sulfinpyrazone vs CYP Enzymes

Drug Name	1A2	2A6	2B6	2C8	2C9	2C18	2C19	2D6	2E1	3A4
Colchicine										Sub
Probenecid					Inh		Inh	Inh		
Sulfinpyrazone					Inh					

Abbreviations: Sub, substrate of the enzyme; Inh, inhibits the enzyme; Ezi, induces the enzyme

1. Colchicine requires CYP3A4 for its metabolic clearance and thus, inhibition of this enzyme by certain drugs can raise blood levels of colchicine to possibly exacerbate its adverse effects. Those inhibitors of CYP3A4 include clarithromycin and erythromycin (*See* the left-hand column of Table-0 at the 'Introduction' for other possible inhibitors of this enzyme.)

2. Both probenecid and sulfinpyrazone function as inhibitors of CYP2C9 and thus, co-administration of either of them with drugs that require this enzyme for hepatic clearance may raise their blood levels to possibly exacerbate their adverse effects. (*See* the middle column of Table-0 at the 'Introduction' for possible substrates of the enzyme.)

3. Probenecid also inhibits CYP2C19 and CYP2D6 and thus, co-administration of it with drugs that require these enzymes for their metabolic clearance may result in elevated blood levels of those unmetabolized drugs, exacerbating their adverse effects. (*See* the middle column of Table-0 at the 'Introduction' for possible substrates of these enzymes.)

DRUG INTERACTIONS

See Table 39-1.

URICOSURIC AGENTS

Probenecid (Fig. 39-4) and **sulfinpyrazone** (Fig. 39-5)

These drugs should not be taken by people who have significant kidney disease or who have had a kidney stone.

MECHANISM OF ACTION

They increase urinary excretions of uric acid to lower blood levels of uric acid, facilitating dissolution of tophus (a deposit of crystallized monosodium urate).

SIDE EFFECTS

Both probenecid and sulfinpyrazone may cause shortness of breath; nausea, vomiting, stomach pain, and diarrhea; swelling of the face, fingers, and feet; skin rash; joint pain; and convulsions.

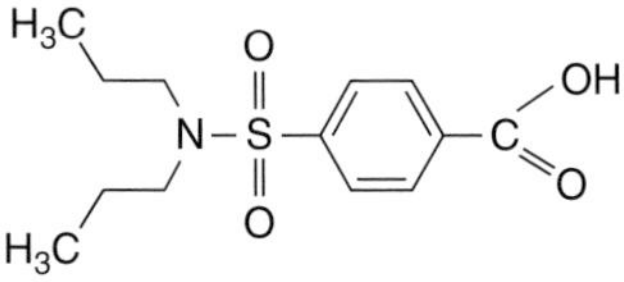

FIGURE 39-4 Molecular structure of probenecid.

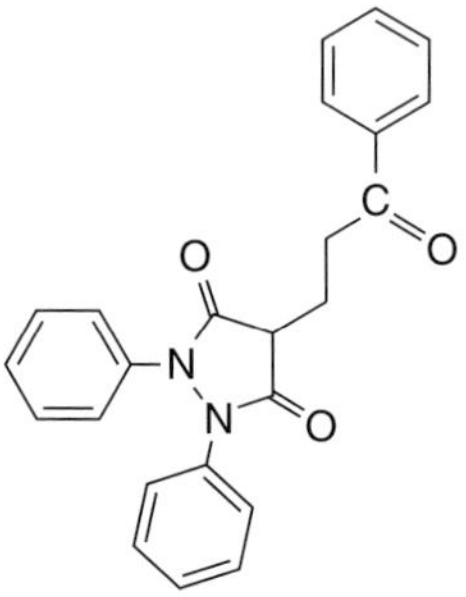

FIGURE 39-5 Molecular structure of sulfinpyrazone.

DRUG INTERACTIONS

Probenecid

See Box 39-1.

Miscellaneous Interactions of Probenecid (PBC)

PBC ⟷ Acyclovir, Famciclovir, Ganciclovir, or Valacyclovir: Renal clearance via active tubular secretions as well as glomerular filtrations is the major route of elimination for acyclovir, to which valacyclovir is converted; and for penciclovir, to which famciclovir is converted; as well as for ganciclovir; and hence, their renal clearance will be reduced by probenecid taken in combination, to raise their plasma levels and adverse effects, especially in the presence of poor kidney functions.

BOX 39-1

Basic Concepts of Probenecid Interactions

Probenecid is an acidic drug (*See* Fig. 39-4) and competes with other acidic drugs taken in combination for renal tubular secretions to interfere with their elimination, raising their blood levels and increasing their adverse effects. Those acidic drugs include: **aspirin; cephalosporin antibiotic drugs** (*See* Ω-32 in Appendix A); **clofibrate** (Fig. 39-6) (it is ethyl ester of clofibric acid, useful to lower blood cholesterol); **diflunisal** (Fig. 39-7) (2′, 4′-difluoro-4-hydroxy-3-biphenylcarboxylic acid useful to relieve pain and to suppress inflammation); **ketorolac** (Fig. 39-8) (a pyrrolizine carboxylic acid derivative, useful to relieve pain and to suppress inflammation); **meropenem** (Fig. 39-9) (an acidic antibiotic drug); **methotrexate** (*See* Fig. 77-14) (an anticancer drug); **mycophenolate**

BOX 39-1 *(continued)*

mofetil (*See* Fig. 55-8) (an immunosuppressant); **penicillamine** (an acidic chelating agent); **penicillins** (*See* Ω-56 in Appendix A); **phenobarbital; thiazide diuretics** (*See* Ω-73 in Appendix A) (weakly acidic drugs); and **tolbutamide** (Fig. 39-10) (an acidic antidiabetic drug).

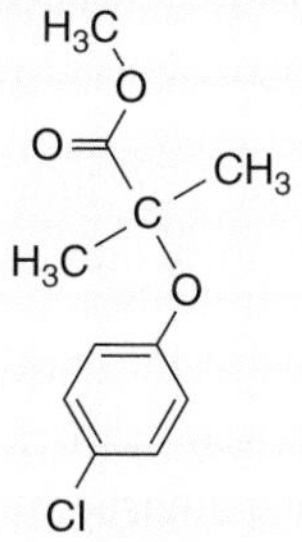

FIGURE 39-6 Molecular structure of clofibrate.

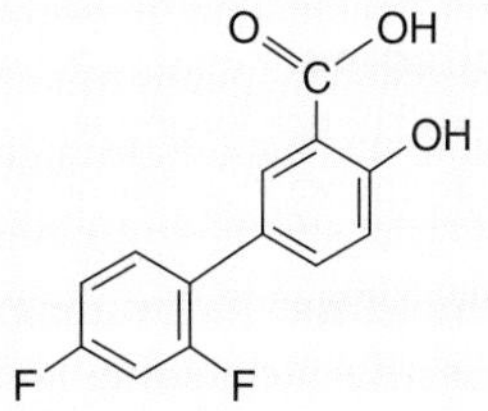

FIGURE 39-7 Molecular structure of diflunisal.

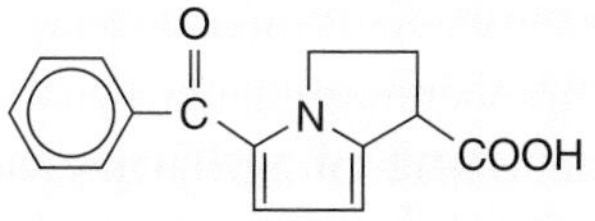

FIGURE 39-8 Molecular structure of ketorolac.

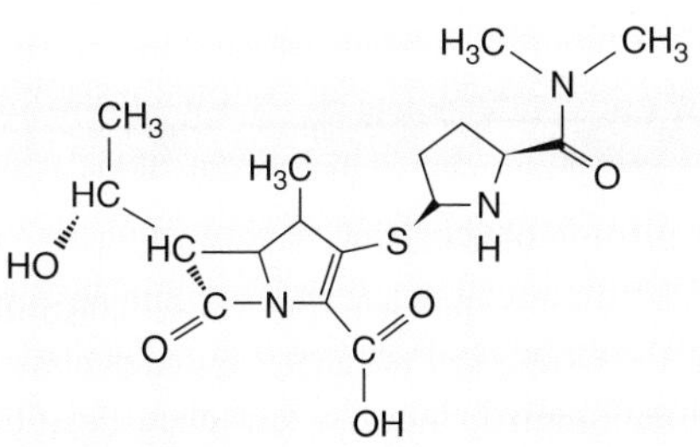

FIGURE 39-9 Molecular structure of meropenem.

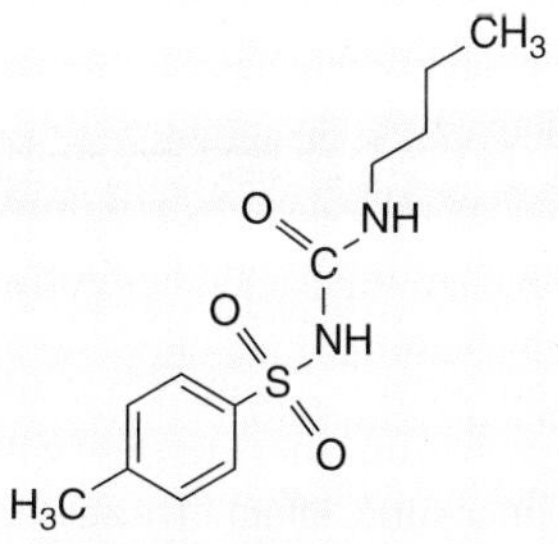

FIGURE 39-10 Molecular structure of tolbutamide.

PBC ⟷ CYP Isozymes: *See* Table 39-1.

PBC ⟷ Hydroxyurea: Hydroxyurea causes temporary impairment of the renal tubular functions, raising the serum uric acid levels to undercut the uricosuric effect of probenecid.

PBC ⟷ Nitrofurantoin: Renal tubular secretions of nitrofurantoin can be inhibited by combined use with a uricosuric drug such as probenecid. The resultant increase in nitrofurantoin serum levels may increase its adverse effects, while its decreased urinary concentrations may lessen its effectiveness as a urinary tract antibacterial agent.

PBC ⟷ Zalcitabine: Renal tubular secretion is the primary route of elimination of zalcitabine and hence, probenecid used in combination can reduce the clearance of zalcitabine to increase its blood levels and toxic effects.

PBC ⟷ Zidovudine: Zidovudine, following its glucuronidation in the liver to become an inactive metabolite, is eliminated from the body primarily by renal excretions. Probenecid, when used in combination, has an inhibitory effect on the glucuronidation and renal excretions of zidovudine, raising its blood levels and adverse effects.

Sulfinpyrazone

See Box 39-2.

Miscellaneous Interactions of Sulfinpyrazone (SFP)

SFP ⟷ CYP Isozymes: *See* Table 39-1.

SFP ⟷ Hydroxyurea: Hydroxyurea causes temporary impairment of renal tubular functions, raising the serum levels of uric acid. When used together

---

BOX 39-2

Basic Concepts of Sulfinpyrazone Interactions

Sulfinpyrazone increases urinary excretions of uric acid, but co-administration with drugs that interfere with the excretion of uric acid can result in a diminished uricosuric effect. Those drugs include: **aspirin (**note: a low dose [less than 2 grams a day] of aspirin can inhibit urinary excretions of uric acid to elevate its blood levels); **bismuth subsalicylate** (a drug to treat traveler's diarrhea); and **salicylates** (*See* Ω-64 in Appendix A).

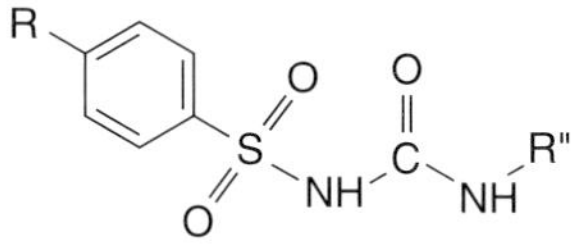

FIGURE 39-11 Molecular structure of sulfonylureas.

with uricosuric agents such as sulfinpyrazone, hydroxyurea can undercut their uricosuric effect, requiring increased doses to become effective.

SFP ⟷ Nitrofurantoin: Renal tubular secretions of nitrofurantoin can be inhibited by combined use with such uricosuric drugs as sulfinpyrazone. The resultant increase in nitrofurantoin serum levels may spur to action its adverse effects, while its decreased urinary concentrations may lessen its effectiveness as a urinary tract antiseptic agent.

SFP ⟷ Tolbutamide: Sulfinpyrazone also increases the plasma concentrations of sulfonylureas (Fig. 39-11), such as tolbutamide, by decreasing their renal excretions; displacing them from serum albumin binding sites; and inhibiting their metabolism by microsomal CYP2C9. The increased serum levels of the sulfonylureas are accountable for the excessive hypoglycemia along with other adverse effects of them.

SFP ⟷ Warfarin: Sulfinpyrazone, an inhibitor of CYP2C9, inhibits metabolism of warfarin, a substrate of CYP2C9, to increase its effects and side effects.

NSAIDs

Ibuprofen, indomethacin, and **naproxen**

Note that aspirin, though a member of the NSAID family, is best avoided because its low doses (less than 2 grams a day) can inhibit, rather than promote, urinary excretions of uric acid to elevate its blood levels to a detrimental effect for gout patients.

MECHANISM OF ACTION

See Chapter 38.

SIDE EFFECTS

See Chapter 38.

DRUG INTERACTIONS

See Appendix B-22: Interactions of NSAIDs.

CHAPTER

40

Myasthenia Gravis

Myasthenia gravis is a neuromuscular disease that presents with decreased muscle strength. It is a chronic disorder in which nicotinic receptors at the neuromuscular junctions are destroyed by autoimmune responses, making it difficult to fully activate the skeletal muscles involved.

Medications shown effective in the treatment of myasthenia gravis include: (1) anticholinesterase agents such as **neostigmine** (Prostigmin) and **pyridostigmine** (Mestinon); (2) glucocorticoids such as **prednisone;** and (3) immunosuppressants such as **azathioprine** (Imuran) and **cyclosporine.**

ANTICHOLINESTERASE AGENTS

Neostigmine (Fig. 40-1) and **pyridostigmine** (Fig. 40-2)

Both are among the most commonly prescribed medications for myasthenia gravis.

MECHANISM OF ACTION

They inhibit cholinesterase, the enzyme that destroys acetylcholine, so as to let acetylcholine, the cholinergic neurotransmitter at the neuromuscular junctions,

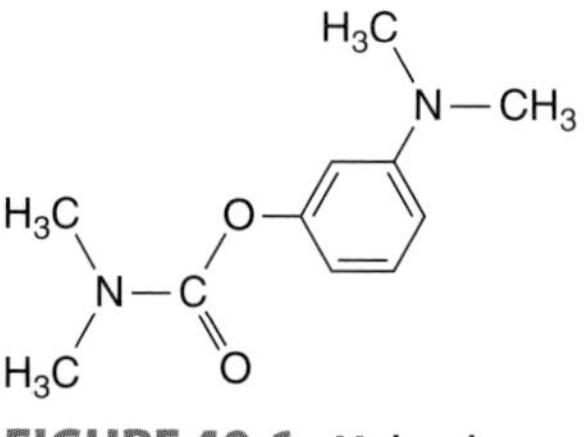

FIGURE 40-1 Molecular structure of neostigmine.

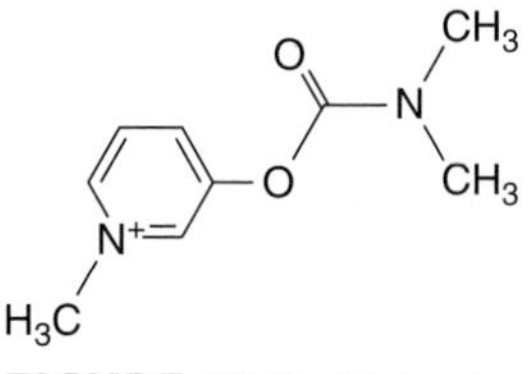

FIGURE 40-2 Molecular structure of pyridostigmine.

228

BOX 41-1

Basic Concepts of SMR (above) Interactions

Carisoprodol, cyclobenzaprine, metaxalone, and **methocarbamol** have anticholinergic properties and when used with drugs that work by cholinomimetic effect, their therapeutic effectiveness may be nullified. Those drugs include: **neostigmine** and **pyridostigmine** (both used to treat myasthenia gravis by accumulation of acetylcholine to activate nicotinic receptors).

with alcohol or other central nervous system (CNS) depressants, any of the drugs mentioned may cause additive CNS depressions.

SMR ↔ CYP Isozymes: *See* Table 41-1.

SMR ↔ Magnesium Hydroxide: Magnesium can cause neuromuscular blockade and can potentiate the effectiveness of the above muscle relaxants.

SMR ↔ MAO Inhibitors: (*See* Ω -51 in Appendix A.) Monoamine oxidase (MAO) plays an important role in the inactivation of cyclobenzaprine (*See* Fig. 47-4), and if this drug is used in combination with any drug that inhibits the enzyme MAO, it may cause a hyperpyretic crisis, severe seizures, and death. Thus, carisoprodol (and probably others above) is warned to not be taken together with an MAO inhibitor within a period of 2 weeks.

TABLE 41-1   Centrally Acting Skeletal Muscle Relaxants vs CYP Enzymes

Drug Name	1A2	2A6	2B6	2C8	2C9	2C18	2C19	2D6	2E1	3A4
Carisoprodol							Sub			
Cyclobenzaprine	Sub							Sub		Sub

Abbreviations: Sub, substrate of the enzyme; Inh, inhibits the enzyme; Ezi, induces the enzyme

1. Metaxalone and methocarbamol (not shown) either do not interact with cytochrome P450 isozymes, or their natures of interaction are not as clearly elucidated as carisoprodol and cyclobenzaprine.

2. Carisoprodol requires CYP2C19 for its clearance and thus, inhibition of this enzyme by any drug taken concomitantly may raise blood levels of carisoprodol to potentially exacerbate its adverse effects. (*See* the left-hand column of Table-0 at the 'Introduction' for possible inhibitors of the enzyme.) On the other hand, inducers of this enzyme taken together can lower blood levels to cause insufficient efficacy of carisoprodol. (*See* the right-hand column of Table-0 at the 'Introduction' for possible inducers of the enzyme.)

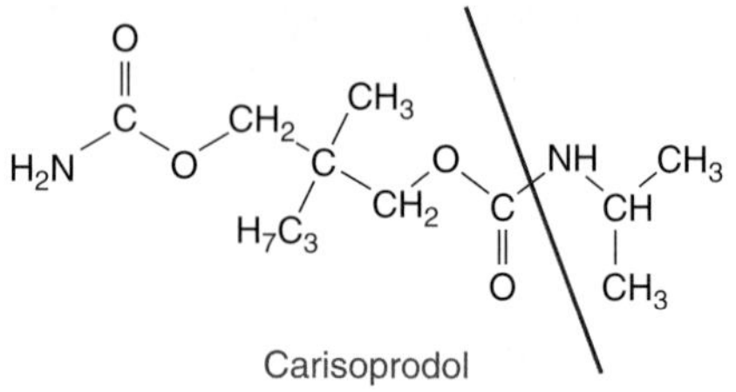

Carisoprodol

FIGURE 41-1   Molecular structure of carisoprodol.

[Carisoprodol (CPD)]

CPD ⟷ CYP Isozymes: *See* Table 41-1.

CPD ⟷ Opioids: Carisoprodol can potentiate the analgesic effects of codeine-like opioids when used in combination. This is because a considerable portion of carisoprodol (Fig 41-1) is metabolized to meprobamate [the $-NH-CH(CH_3)_2$ group of carisoprodol is converted to $-NH_2$ to become meprobamate], a known drug of abuse and dependency that can potentiate analgesic effects. This accounts for the great abuse potential of carisoprodol.

BACLOFEN

MECHANISM OF ACTION

Baclofen (*See* Fig. 13-3) is a gamma-aminobutyric acid (GABA) analog, and activates GABA-B receptors in presynaptic neurons to inhibit the release of acetylcholine, an excitatory neurotransmitter, thereby depressing neuromuscular excitation.

SIDE EFFECTS

Baclofen may generate arrhythmia; nausea and constipation; drowsiness and dizziness; seizure (convulsions); and headache, confusion, and hallucinations.

DRUG INTERACTIONS

See Chapter 13.

TIZANIDINE

Tizanidine (Fig. 41-2), an imidazole derivative, is a muscle relaxant used to treat muscle spasms, cramping, and abnormally enhanced muscle tone.

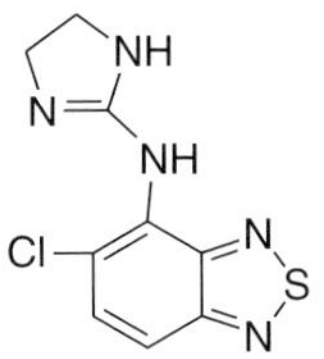

FIGURE 41-2 Molecular structure of tizanidine.

MECHANISM OF ACTION

Tizanidine is a centrally acting alpha-adrenergic agonist that inhibits the release of excitatory amino acids in spinal interneurons, to oppose excitation of motor neurons. It may also facilitate the actions of glycine, an inhibitory transmitter in the CNS neurons.

SIDE EFFECTS

Possible side effects of tizanidine include hypotension and irregular heartbeat; dry mouth and constipation; acute hepatitis; and asthenia (weakness, fatigue and/or tiredness); dizziness and drowsiness; and hallucinations.

DRUG INTERACTIONS

See Box 41-2.

Miscellaneous Interactions of Tizanidine (TZN)

TZN ⟷ Alcohol: Tizanidine is a CNS depressant and may produce additive sedations when taken with other CNS depressants, such as alcohol.

TZN ⟷ CYP Isozymes: *See* Table 41-2.

BOX 41-2

Basic Concepts of Tizanidine Interactions

Tizanidine tends to reduce blood pressure in many people, and when co-administered with drugs that lower blood pressure, they may result in severe hypotension. Those drugs include: **antihypertensive drugs** (*See* Ω -20 in Appendix A), including clonidine, and lisinopril.

TABLE 41-2 Tizanidine vs CYP Isozymes

Drug Name	1A2	2A6	2B6	2C8	2C9	2C18	2C19	2D6	2E1	3A4
Tizanidine	Sub									

Abbreviations: Sub, substrate of the enzyme; Inh, inhibits the enzyme; Ezi, induces the enzyme

The liver enzyme CYP1A2 is required for metabolic clearance of tizanidine and thus, inhibition of this enzyme by drugs taken concomitantly can raise the blood levels and increase the adverse effects of tizanidine. Strong inhibitors of CYP 1A2 include ciprofloxacin and fluvoxamine. (*See* the left-hand column of Table-0 at the 'Introduction' for other possible inhibitors of this enzyme.)

MAGNESIUM CITRATE

MECHANISM OF ACTIONS

Magnesium helps to relax muscle tension and spasm by opposing influx of the calcium ions, which are responsible for exciting nerves to muscle contraction (spasm), into the nerve cells.

SIDE EFFECTS

Side effects of magnesium citrate may include slowing of heartbeat; slow or difficult breathing; nausea and vomiting; unusual tiredness or weakness; double vision; lightheadedness or fainting spells; low body temperature and flushing; and headache. Individuals with high-grade atrioventricular block should be warned not to take magnesium, and individuals with kidney disease should not take more than 3,000 mg per day.

DRUG INTERACTIONS

See Appendix B-19: Interactions of Magnesium Salts.

42

Carpal Tunnel Syndrome

Carpal tunnel syndrome is a disorder caused by increased pressure on the median nerve passing through the carpal tunnel of the wrist. Symptoms include burning pain, numbness, and tingling in the forearm, hands and fingers.

Medications that may be effective in the treatment of early carpal tunnel syndrome include: (1) **cortisone** or **hydrocortisone** and (2) non-steroidal anti-inflammatory drugs (NSAIDs) such as **ibuprofen, ketoprofen,** and **naproxen**.

CORTISONE OR HYDROCORTISONE

MECHANISM OF ACTION

A glucocorticoid such as above has its own specific receptors in cytosol. Binding to those receptors invariably leads to suppression of inflammation, for the receptor-bound glucocorticoid enhances expressions of anti-inflammatory proteins in the nucleus, while suppressing the MAP (mitogen-activated protein) kinases required for proinflammatory gene activation that appears to cause joint degeneration.

SIDE EFFECTS

Possible side effects of these drugs include increased blood pressure; nausea, vomiting, stomach upset, and bloody or black stools; weight gain (more than five pounds in a day or two); acne; moon face (roundness of the face); osteonecrosis (bone death caused by temporary or permanent loss of blood supply to the bone); vulnerability to infections; cataracts or glaucoma; and insomnia.

DRUG INTERACTIONS

Cortisone (CTS) (Fig. 42-1), being inactive, is converted in the liver to its active metabolite hydrocortisone (or cortisol) (Fig. 42-2).

Parentheses below indicate an herb.

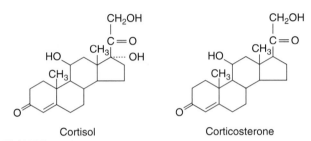

FIGURE 42-1   Molecular structure of cortisone.

Cortisol   Corticosterone

FIGURE 42-2   Molecular structures of cortisol and corticosterone.

CTS ⟷ Anticholinesterase Agents: (*See* Ω-15 in Appendix A.) Cortisone or hydrocortisone, an active metabolite of cortisone, may antagonize the effectiveness of anticholinesterase agents, such as pyridostigmine, in the treatment of myasthenia gravis.

CTS ⟷ CYP Isozymes: *See* Table 42-1.

CTS ⟷ Diuretics: (*See* Ω-49 and Ω-73 in Appendix A.) Both parties have a potassium-depleting effect and they may pull together toward severe hypokalemia, a condition that may aggravate the cardiac arrhythmia caused by digoxin.

CTS ⟷ (Licorice): The glycyrrhizinic acid contained in licorice (Fig. 42-3 A and B), an herb traditionally used in Chinese medicine to treat ulcers and common colds, is hydrolyzed to glycyrrhetic acid that inhibits 11-beta-hydroxysteroid dehydrogenase, the enzyme that converts hydrocortisone (cortisol) to its inactive metabolite cortisone in the liver. Thus, licorice taken with cortisone can elevate blood levels of hydrocortisone (cortisol), enhancing its pharmacologic effects. Therefore, doses of hydrocortisone may have to be reduced to stave off adverse effects.

TABLE 42-1   Cortisone vs CYP Isozymes

Drug Name	1A2	2A6	2B6	2C8	2C9	2C18	2C19	2D6	2E1	3A4
Cortisone										Sub

Abbreviations: Sub, substrate of the enzyme; Inh, inhibits the enzyme; Ezi, induces the enzyme

1. Cortisone requires microsomal enzyme CYP3A4 to form 6-betahydroxycortisone for its metabolic clearance. Thus, an inducer of the CYP 3A4 enzyme such as carbamazepine, phenobarbital, and rifampin can quicken its metabolic clearance, lowering its blood levels and decreasing its therapeutic effectiveness. (*See* the right-hand column of Table-0 at the 'Introduction' for other possible inducers of this enzyme.)

2. As cortisone requires microsomal enzyme CYP3A4 for its metabolic clearance, inhibition of this enzyme by other drugs can raise blood levels of cortisone, possibly exacerbating its adverse effects. Inhibitors of CYP3A4 include: itraconazole and ketoconazole. (*See* the left-hand column of Table-0 at the 'Introduction' for other possible inhibitors of this enzyme.)

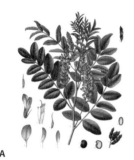
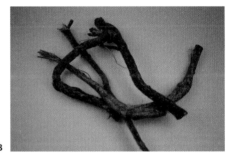

FIGURE 42-3   **A,** Image of licorice leaves in nature. **B,** Cut and dried root of licorice.
(http://www.learnnc.org/lp/multimedia/9824)

CTS ⟷ Oral Hypoglycemic Agents: (*See* Ω-55 in Appendix A.) Cortisone and hydrocortisone can raise blood glucose levels and undercut the effectiveness of antidiabetic drugs such as glipizide and glyburide.

NSAIDs

Ibuprofen (Fig. 42-4), **ketoprofen** (Fig. 42-5), and **naproxen** (Fig. 42-6)

MECHANISM OF ACTION

All of the above NSAIDs inhibit both cyclooxygenase (COX)-1 and (COX)-2, the enzymes that catalyze the conversion of arachidonic acid, which is released from membrane phospholipids due to inflammatory stimuli, to prostaglandin E (PGE) and leukotrienes. Thus, NSAIDs interfere with the synthesis of PGE and leukotrienes in inflammatory tissues.

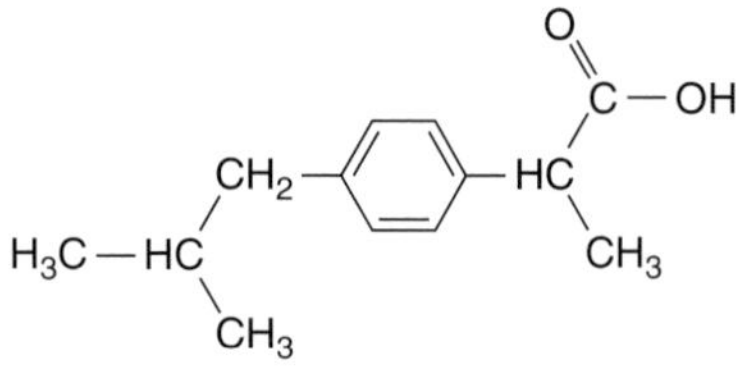

FIGURE 42-4   Molecular structure of ibuprofen.

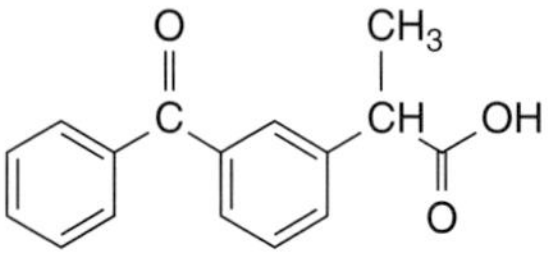

FIGURE 42-5   Molecular structure
of ketoprofen.

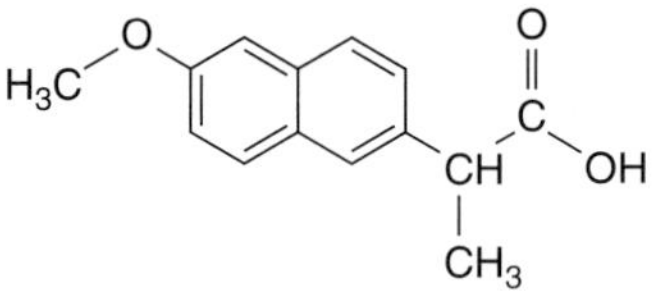

FIGURE 42-6   Molecular structure of
naproxen.

SIDE EFFECTS

Possible side effects include difficulty in breathing and wheezing; nausea, vomiting, upset stomach, gas pain, bloating, intestinal bleeding, and bloody stool; and jaundice (yellowing of the skin or eyes).

DRUG INTERACTIONS

See Appendix B-22: Interactions of NSAIDs.

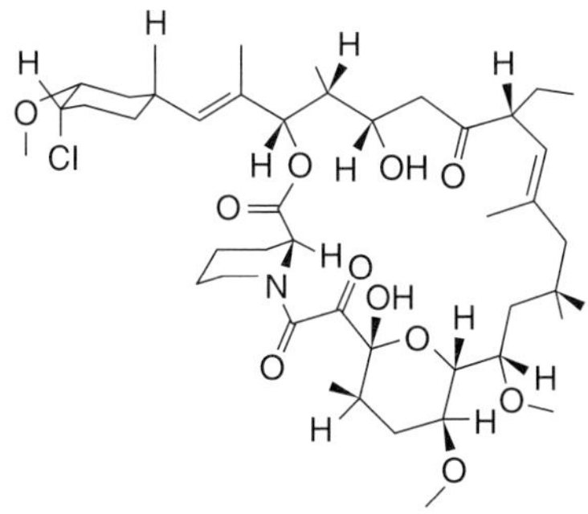

FIGURE 44-2   Molecular structure of pimecrolimus.

result in the interruption of signal transduction in target cells, consequently block-ing the release of cytokines, such as interleukin-2 (IL-2) that cause inflammation, redness, and itching, from the T-cells and the mast cells.

SIDE EFFECTS

Pimecrolimus: It may cause mild burning, stinging, and redness of skin at the site of application; and headache. If any of these effects persist more than a few days, or allergic reactions occurs such as difficulty in breathing, swelling of glands, face, throat, tongue, or lips, seeking medical help is advised.

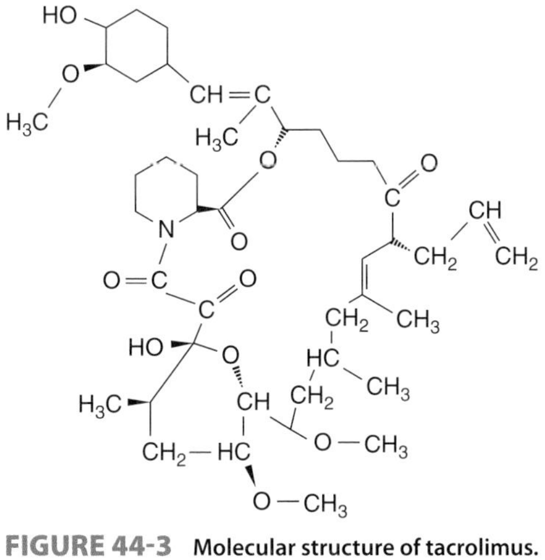

FIGURE 44-3   Molecular structure of tacrolimus.

Tacrolimus: It may heighten the skin's sensitivity to sunlight, causing burning, redness, and itching. Wear clothing to cover skin treated with topical tacrolimus or avoid sunlight and sun lamps. Consulting a health care professional is recommended if any of these serious side effects occur: increased blood pressure; muscle pain; swollen glands; nephrotoxicity; and tremor or tingling of the hands or feet.

DRUG INTERACTIONS

Pimecrolimus: Pimecrolimus is not extensively absorbed into the bloodstream after topical application. Thus, systemic drug interactions are unlikely but cannot be ruled out. The dermatologic adverse effects of alcohol such as facial flushing and skin irritation may be exacerbated by pimecrolimus. Since pimecrolimus, like tacrolimus, is inactivated through hepatic enzyme CYP3A4, inhibitors of this enzyme may elevate blood levels and toxicities of pimecrolimus (*See* Table 44-1).

Tacrolimus: It is not known whether other medications will interact with this medication applied topically, but if it is absorbed extensively from its site of application the interactions outlined in Box 44-1 may take place.

TABLE 44-1 Tacrolimus and Picrolimus vs CYP Enzymes

Drug Name	1A2	2A6	2B6	2C8	2C9	2C18	2C19	2D6	2E1	3A4
Pimecrolimus										Sub
Tacrolimus										Sub+ Inh

Abbreviations: Sub, substrate of the enzyme; Inh, inhibits the enzyme; Ezi, induces the enzyme

1. Metabolic clearance of both pimecrolimus and tacrolimus require the presence of microsomal CYP3A4 and thus, inhibition of this enzyme by any other drug taken concomitantly may raise blood levels of both drugs to possibly exacerbate their adverse effects, such as nephrotoxicity. Inhibitors of CYP3A4 include chloramphenicol. (*See* the left-hand column of Table-0 at the 'Introduction' for other possible inhibitors of this enzyme.)
2. An inducer of CYP3A4 such as rifampin, when used in combination, may quicken elimination of both pimecrolimus and tacrolimus to result in lowered blood levels and therapeutic insufficiency .(*See* the right-hand column of Table-0 at the 'Introduction' for other possible inducers of this enzyme.)
3. Tacrolimus exerts an inhibitory effect on CYP3A4 and thus, administration of it in combination with drugs that require this enzyme for metabolic clearance may result in their elevated blood levels, possibly inciting their adverse effects to surface. Those drugs include: budesonide, felodipine, fluticasone, lovastatin, qunidine, sildenafil (Viagra), simvastain, triazolam, and vardenafil. (*See* the middle column of Table-0 at the 'Introduction' for other possible substrates of this enzyme.)

BOX 44-1

Basic Concepts of Tacrolimus Interactions

Tacrolimus is apt to cause nephrotoxicity as a side effect, and when co-administered with drugs that generate similar side effects, severe renal impairment may ensue. Those drugs include: **azathioprine** (an immunosuppressant); and **cyclosporine** (an immunosuppressant).

Miscellaneous Interactions of Tacrolimus (TLM)

TLM ⟷ Alcohol: Drinking alcohol while using tacrolimus topically may cause the skin or face to feel hot and flushed. Drinking alcohol should be avoided while using this drug.

TLM ⟷ Azole Antifungal Drugs: Since many azole antifungals inhibit the CYP3A4-mediated metabolism of tacrolimus and the activity of P-glycoproteins that efflux tacrolimus, co-administration of azole antifungal drugs with tacrolimus may increase the serum concentration of tacrolimus, resulting in increased effects and toxicities.

TLM ⟷ Clotrimazole: Clotrimazole used in combination may raise serum levels and risks of toxicity of tacrolimus. One possible mechanism of this interaction is that tacrolimus is a strong substrate of CYP3A4 and clotrimazole inhibits this enzyme. However, absorption of clotrimazole from the skin is extremely poor.

TLM ⟷ CYP Isozymes: *See* Table 44-1.

TLM ⟷ Danazol: Danazol used in combination may raise serum levels and the risks of toxicity of tacrolimus. One possible mechanism of this interaction is that tacrolimus is cleared through CYP3A4 and danazol is inhibitory to this enzyme.

TLM ⟷ Live Vaccines: (*See* Ω-48 in Appendix A.) Tacrolimus, an immunosuppressant, may suppress the host's normal responses to vaccines, and may make the body vulnerable to infections from receiving live vaccines. Hence, at least six months should elapse between discontinuation of tacrolimus and receiving vaccination.

TLM ⟷ NSAIDs: (*See* Ω-54 in Appendix A.) Tacrolimus-induced immuno-suppression has nephrotoxic effects, causing a significant fall in the glomerular filtration rate (GFR). NSAIDs, on the other hand, are known to inhibit the production of prostaglandins on which renal blood flow depends. When the two are taken in combination a significant impairment of GFR may take place.

GLUCOCORTICOID

Clobetasol and **triamcinolone**

Both of these drugs are useful to treat inflammation, scaling, and discomfort of skin disorders.

MECHANISM OF ACTION

Clobetasol and triamcinolone have their own specific receptors in cytosol. Binding to those receptors invariably leads to suppression of inflammation, for the receptor-bound glucocorticoid enhances the expression of anti-inflammatory proteins in the nucleus, while suppressing the MAP (mitogen-activated protein) kinases required for proinflammatory gene activation.

SIDE EFFECTS

These two glucocorticoids may cause dryness, burning, redness, shrinking, and loss of the skin color.

DRUG INTERACTIONS

It is not known whether other medications will interact with these medications applied topically.

45

Psoriasis

Psoriasis is a chronic and common autoimmune disease mediated by T-lymphocytes with impaired regulations of skin cell divisions. Psoriatic lesions are often marked by increased levels of tumor necrosis factor (TNF)-alpha. It is characterized by periodic flare-ups of a reddish rash covered by silvery-white scales of dead skin, often located on the surface of the buttocks, ears, elbows, genitals, knees, and scalp. With psoriasis, the abnormally multiplying keratinocytes (immature new skin cells) in the bottom skin layer move to the surface too quickly (in about 4 days instead of the normal 28 to 30 days) to replace the worn-out dead cells. The skin accumulates these premature cells, giving the appearance of red bumpy patches covered with white scales.

Medications that may be effective in the treatment of psoriasis include: (1) immunosuppressants such as **alefacept** (Amevive), **efalizumab** (Raptiva), **etanercept** (Enbrel), and **infliximab** (Remicade); and (2) retinoids such as **acitretin**.

IMMUNOSUPPRESANTS

Alefacept, efalizumab, etanercept, and **infliximab**

These drugs are officially approved by the FDA for treating psoriasis.

MECHANISM OF ACTION

They competitively inhibit binding of TNF-alpha at its receptor sites, so as to stave off inflammatory responses. TNF-alpha, a key cytokine in immune response, can generate inflammation and even apoptosis. TNF-alpha increases the production of pro-inflammatory molecules such as IL-1, IL-6, and IL-8.

SIDE EFFECTS

Alefacept: Its side effects may include pain or swelling at the injection site; nausea; throat inflammation; increased cough; muscle pain; and chills and dizziness.

Efalizumab: The most common adverse reactions of efalizumab are the "first-dose reactions," which include nausea; myalgia; fever; chills; and headache within two days following the first two injections. Other side effects that develop later may include serious infections; arthritis; thrombocytopenia; hemolytic anemia; and even malignancies.

Etanercept: Reactions such as itching, swelling, and redness and pain at the injection site may develop. These reactions occurring in the first month may later subside in frequency, but etanercept, functioning as a competitive inhibitor for binding of TNF-alpha at its receptors, may bring about serious infections such as bronchitis, pneumonia, abdominal abscess, osteomyelitis, and pyelonephritis.

Infliximab: The most common side effects of infliximab include upper respiratory tract infections with cough; nausea, vomiting, and abdominal pain; urinary tract infections; back pain and weakness; skin rash; and fever and headache.

DRUG INTERACTIONS

Immunosuppression caused by these agents may stoke generalized infections from receiving live vaccines. (*See* Ω-48 in Appendix A.) They may also cause a reduced response to vaccines. At least six months separation between these two classes of drugs is recommended.

Etanercept (ETP)

ETP ⟷ Anakinra: Concurrent administration of etanercept (a TNF-alpha blocking agent) and anakinra (an interleukin-1 receptor antagonist) has been associated with increased risk of neutropenia and serious infections without added clinical benefits.

ETP ⟷ Cyclophosphamide: When etanercept was combined with cyclophosphamide in treatment of Wegener granulomatosis, it led to higher incidences of non-cutaneous solid malignant tumors, as compared with cyclophosphamide therapy alone. Thus, it is prudent to hold off combination of the two.

ACITRETIN

Acitretin (Fig. 45-1) is a retinoid, having a structure similar to that of vitamin A (Fig. 45-2) , and is the active metabolite of etretinate (Fig. 45-3), a drug which is usually taken orally once a day with food. Acitretin is the only retinoid approved by the FDA specifically for treatment of psoriasis. This drug reduces redness of the skin, and should be continued until plaques have decreased. (Its maximum benefit may occur in about twelve weeks.) The affected skin may peel off or gradually

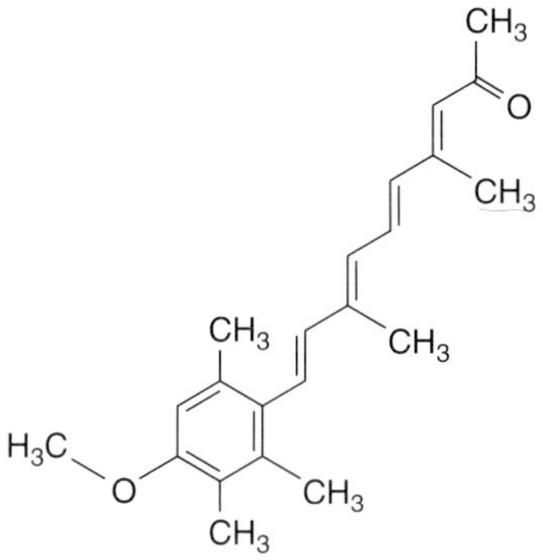

FIGURE 45-1 Molecular structure of acitretin.

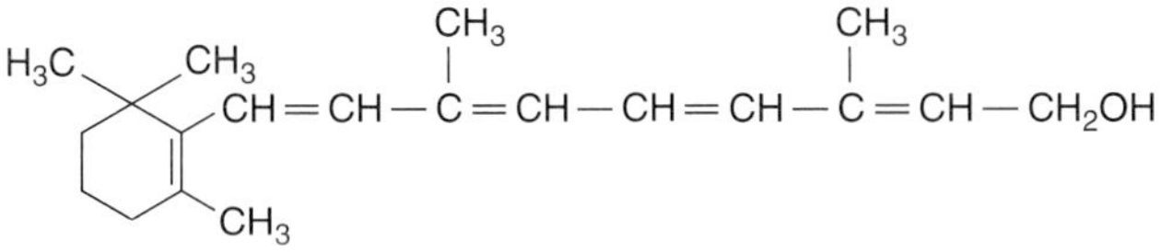

FIGURE 45-2 Molecular structure of vitamin A-1.

clear. However, acitretin is teratogenic, and should always be used in association with oral contraceptives in women of childbearing age.

MECHANISM OF ACTION

The exact mechanism of action of acitretin is unknown, but it is believed to work by competition with retinoic acid for binding to retinoid binding proteins in the cytoplasm of epidermal tissue. This may affect expression of nuclear retinoid receptors, which are important in differentiation of basal keratinocytes and other epidermal cell layers. Accordingly, acitretin appears to reduce the redness, scaling, and plaques by slowing down excessive growth of skin cells, which is causative for

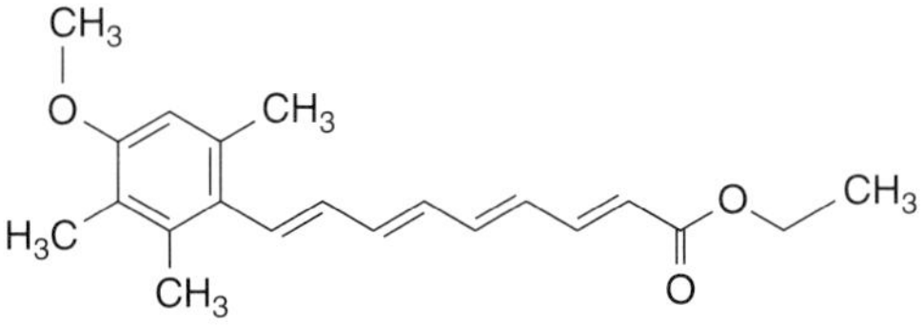

FIGURE 45-3 Molecular structure of etretinate.

the keratinization and thickening of the skin (plaque formation) via intracellular deposition of a specific protein called "psoriasis-associated fatty acid-binding protein."

SIDE EFFECTS

Its side effects may include shortness of breath; pain in the tongue and stomach; diarrhea; cholestatic hepatitis; clumsy or jerky movements; chapped or swollen lips; brittle or weak fingernails or toenails; abnormal skin with loss of eyebrows or eyelashes; increase in intracranial pressure; and either hypoglycemia that may cause visual changes, seizures, and loss of consciousness; or hyperglycemia that may cause extreme thirst and frequent urination. As acitretin may harm the fetus, it should not be taken during pregnancy, and female patients of childbearing age must take contraceptive pills continuously for at least three years after termination of acitretin because this drug lingers in the body.

DRUG INTERACTIONS

Miscellaneous Interactions of Acitretin (ATT)

ATT ⟷ Alcohol: Concurrent use of acitretin with alcohol may lead to the formation of etretinate, a long-acting form of vitamin A, which increases the duration of the teratogenic potential in women. Do not drink alcohol while taking acitretin and for two months after termination of the medicine.

ATT ⟷ Contraceptives (Oral) (*See* Ω-35 in Appendix A.) The effectiveness of progestin-only oral contraceptives (Ovrette, Micronor, Nor-QD), may be undermined by concurrent use of acitretin, to possibly result in contraceptive failure. However, acitretin has not been shown to reduce the effectiveness of oral contraceptives containing both estrogens and progestogens.

ATT ⟷ Methotrexate: Hepatitis caused by acitretin may be aggravated by the hepatotoxic side effects of methotrexate.

BOX 45-1

Basic Concepts of Acitretin Interactions

Acitretin can lower blood sugar even in normal healthy individuals and thus, when co-administered with any antidiabetic drugs, it may lead to excessive hypoglycemia. Those antidiabetic drugs include: **glipizide** and **glyburide**.

ATT ↔ Phenytoin: Since acitretin is extensively bound to blood proteins with high affinity, it may reduce the protein binding of phenytoin to elevate its free drug levels in the blood, exacerbating its adverse effects.

ATT ↔ Tetracycline Antibiotics (*See* Ω-72 in Appendix A.) Because both acitretin and tetracyclines can cause increased intracranial pressure, concurrent use may lead to greater incidences of such adverse effects. Their combined use is contraindicated.

ATT ↔ Vitamin A: Concomitant use of acitretin and vitamin A can potentiate some adverse effects of vitamin A, such as hypervitaminosis A syndrome, which includes pain of the muscles and bones; inflammation of mucous membranes; loss of hair; and elevation of blood triglyceride levels.

TABLE 46-1 Buspirone vs CYP Enzymes

Drug Name	1A2	2A6	2B6	2C8	2C9	2C18	2C19	2D6	2E1	3A4
Buspirone										**Sub**

Abbreviations: Sub, substrate of the enzyme; Inh, inhibits the enzyme; Ezi, induces the enzyme

1. Buspirone requires the presence of microsomal enzyme CYP3A4 for its clearance and thus, inhibition of this enzyme by drugs taken concomitantly can raise blood levels of buspirone to incite its adverse effects. Those strong inhibitors of CYP3A4 include clarithromycin, indinavir, itraconazole, ketoconazole, nefazodone, nelfinavir, ritonavir, saquinavir, and telithromycin; and its moderate inhibitors include aprepitant, erythromycin, fluconazole, grape fruit juice, and verapamil. (*See* the left-hand column of Table-0 at the 'Introduction' for other possible inhibitors of the enzyme.)

2. Oral contraceptives contain estrogens that are at least partially metabolized by cytochrome CYP3A4, as does buspirone. When the two are used in combination, they may compete with each other for the same enzyme for metabolic clearance, and the blood levels of buspirone may be raised, possibly exacerbating its adverse effects. (*See* the middle column of Table-0 at the 'Introduction' for other possible substrates of the enzyme.)

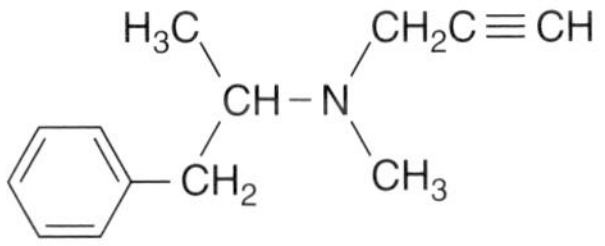

FIGURE 46-4 Molecular structure of selegiline.

lost, to inhibit oxidation of norepinephrine by MAO-A as well, to raise its blood levels and to elevate blood pressure. Thus, do not administer buspirone within 14 days of an inhibitor of MAO-A or MAO-B.

BSP ⟷ Verapamil: Verapamil may increase serum levels and the adverse effects of buspirone. One possible mechanism of this interaction is that buspirone is cleared through CYP3A4 and verapamil is inhibitory to this enzyme.

HYDROXYZINE

MECHANISM OF ACTION

The mechanism for its anti-anxiety effect still remains uncharacterized, since there has been no extensive research made on this drug. However, hydroxyzine, in addition to its antihistaminic effect, has CNS depressant and anticholinergic effects. Its sedative and tranquilizing effects may derive from suppression of subcortical activities in the CNS, rather than from its cortical depressant activities.

SIDE EFFECTS

Hydroxyzine may cause dry mouth and stomach upset; thickening of tracheal secretions; urinary retention (use caution in persons with prostatic hypertrophy); double vision and blurred vision (use caution in patients having narrow-angle glaucoma); and sedation, tiredness, and dizziness.

DRUG INTERACTIONS

See Appendix B-10: Interactions of Antihistamines, First-Generation.

Seasonal Affective Disorder

Seasonal affective disorder (SAD), also known as winter depression, is a form of mental depression that is prevalent in the winter due to lack of sunlight. It usually starts in early winter and ceases in the summer. Symptoms include fatigue, drowsiness, and sadness.

Medications that may possibly be effective in the treatment of SAD include: (1) selective serotonin reuptake inhibitors (SSRIs) such as **fluoxetine** (Prozac), **paroxetine** (Paxil, Seroxat), and **sertraline** (Zolof, Lustral); (2) monoamine oxidase (MOA) inhibitors such as **phenelzine** (*See* Fig. 13-4) (Nardil) and **tranylcypromine** (*See* Fig. 13-5) (Parnate); (3) tricyclic antidepressants such as **amitriptyline** (Elavil), **desipramine** (Norpramin), **doxepin** (Sinequan), **imipramine** (Tofranil), **nortriptyline** (Pamelor), **protriptyline** (Vivactil), and **trimipramine** (Surmontil); and (4) non-tricyclic antidepressant such as **bupropion** (Fig. 47-1) (Wellbutrin XL).

SSRIs

Fluoxetine, paroxetine, and **sertraline**

MECHANISM OF ACTION

Dysfunction of presynaptic serotonergic neurons appears to be responsible for major mental depression. If this theory is correct, then one must normalize synaptic serotonin either by decreasing reuptake of serotonin or by increasing the synthesis

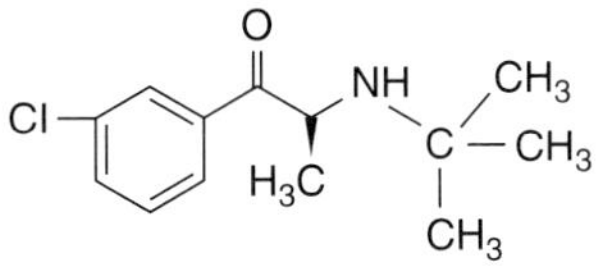

FIGURE 47-1 Molecular structure of bupropion.

of serotonin. However, the exact mechanism for the antidepressant effects of SSRIs remains unclear.

SIDE EFFECTS

Frequent side effects of these drugs include dry mouth, loss of appetite, upset stomach, nausea, and vomiting; sexual impotence, delayed ejaculation (men), and reduced sexual desire (libido); and headache, dizziness, insomnia, and anxiety. SSRIs, including paroxetine (Paxil), can cause akathisia and suicidal tendencies. Exposure to paroxetine in the first trimester of pregnancy may be associated with an increased risk of birth defects, including cardiac septal defect in the newborn where the wall between the right and left sides of the heart is not fully developed.

DRUG INTERACTIONS

See Appendix B-29: Interactions of SSRIs (Selective Serotonin Reuptake Inhibitors).

MAO INHIBITORS

Phenelzine and **tranylcypromine**

MECHANISM OF ACTION

One proposed cause of depression is supersensitive beta adrenoceptors in the thalamus and temporal cortex. Both norepinephrine and serotonin are required for the process of desensitization of the central beta adrenoceptors. Both phenelzine and tranylcypromine, as inhibitors of MAO, can oppose inactivation of norepinephrine and serotonin to let them be accumulated at the beta adrenoceptors, and their continuous presence there can desensitize them.

SIDE EFFECTS

Frequent side effects of these drugs include rapid heartbeat; dry mouth, nausea, vomiting, upset stomach, and constipation; decreased urination; sexual impotence; and headache, lightheadedness, and insomnia. Rarely, they may cause allergic reactions such as skin rash and itching; and swelling of tissues.

DRUG INTERACTIONS

See Box 47-1.

BOX 47-1

Basic Concepts of Phenelzine or Tranylcypromine Interactions

1. Both **phenelzine** (*See* Fig. 13-4) and **tranylcypromine** (*See* Fig. 13-5) possess an MAO inhibitory effect, and when either is co-administered with drugs that have a monoamine structure, such as epinephrine (*See* Fig. 3-5), norepinephrine (Fig. 47-2), and serotonin (*See* Fig. 11-5), requiring the presence of MAO for their inactivation, it can result in accumulation of the unmetabolized drugs, generating adverse effects such as severe headache, hypertensive crisis, and hyperpyrexia. Other drugs that are similarly affected include: **amphetamine** and **levodopa.**

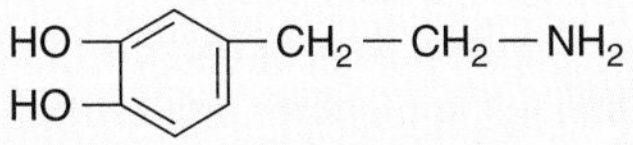

FIGURE 47-2   Molecular structure of norepinephrine.

2. When either **phenelzine** or **tranylcypromine** is co-administered with drugs that accumulate norepinephrine by blocking its neuronal reuptake, it can bring about unsafe symptoms such as hypertensive crisis, hyperthermia, and seizures. Those drugs include: **bupropion** (this antidepressant can release catecholamines and block their reuptake); **carbamazepine** (Fig. 47-3) (an antiepileptic drug whose chemical structure is similar to tricyclic antidepressants, and weakly inhibits neuronal monoamine reuptake); **cyclobenzaprine** (Fig. 47-4) (which has a structure very similar to amitriptyline, and inhibits reuptake of norepinephrine); **dextromethorphan** (Robitussin-DM) (a cough suppressant that inhibits neuronal serotonin reuptake and is not recommended within 14 days of discontinuation of an MAO inhibitor); **maprotiline** (Fig. 47-5) (an antidepressant with a secondary amine structure

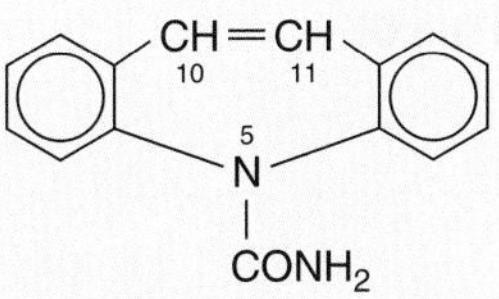

FIGURE 47-3   Molecular structure of carbamazepine.

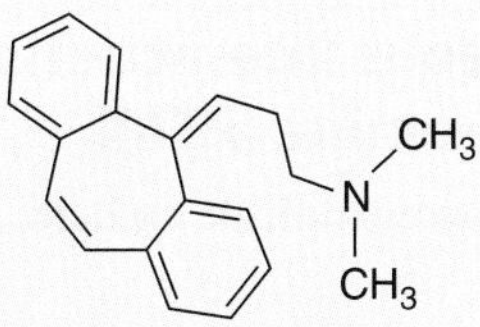

FIGURE 47-4   Molecular structure of cyclobenzaprine.

continued

BOX 47-1 (continued)

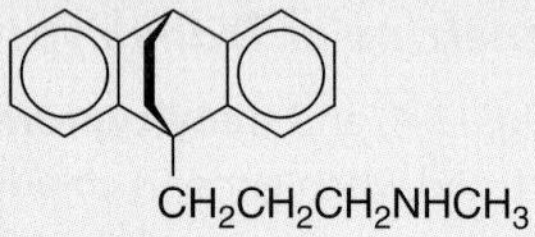

$$CH_2CH_2CH_2NHCH_3$$

FIGURE 47-5 Molecular structure of maprotiline.

that inhibits presynaptic reuptake of catecholamines, and whose combined use with an MAO inhibitor may lead to symptoms such as hypertensive crisis, hyperthermia, mental status changes, and seizures); **meperidine** (Fig. 47 6) (a narcotic analgesic with a tertiary amine structure that increases concentrations of serotonin (5-hydroxytryptamine) and catecholamine in synaptic clefts by inhibiting their neuronal reuptake); **SSRIs** (See Ω-68 in Appendix A) [there have been reports of serious, sometimes fatal reactions (serotonin syndrome) in patients receiving SSRIs in combination with MAO inhibitors]; and **tricyclic antidepressants** (See Ω-76 in Appendix A) (tricyclic antidepressants block reuptake of both norepinephrine and serotonin, whose inactivations can be interrupted by an MAO inhibitor).

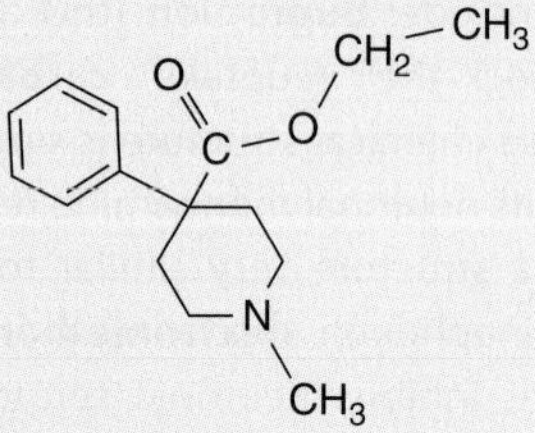

FIGURE 47-6 Molecular structure of meperidine.

Miscellaneous Interactions of Phenelzine or Tranylcypromine (PTM)

Parentheses below indicate an herb.

PTM ⟷ Alcohol: Tyramine, a releaser of norepinephrine, contained in alcoholic drinks such as wine, beer, and lager, may induce a severe hypertensive crisis when taken in combination with an MAO inhibitor such as pargyline, phenelzine, or tranylcypromine.

oxidase (MAO). Therefore, methylphenidate should not be used within 14 days of any MAO inhibitor, in order to avoid a hypertensive crisis.

MPD ⬌ Phenytoin: Methylphenidate may increase blood levels and the pharmacological and adverse effects of phenytoin in some patients. Some suggest that methylphenidate may decrease the metabolism of phenytoin, but it remains unproven.

MPD ⬌ Vasopressors: (*See* Ω-79 in Appendix A.) Since methylphenidate increases blood levels of norepinephrine by blocking its reuptake, intake with any other pressor drugs, such as ergotamine and pseudoephedrine, may further the rise of blood pressure.

ATOMOXETINE

This drug is approved for the treatment of ADHD in both children and adults.

MECHANISM OF ACTION

Atomoxetine works by selectively inhibiting the neuronal reuptake of norepinephrine in the central and peripheral nervous systems. Atomoxetine, unlike amphetamine and methylphenidate, does not appear to increase the availability of dopamine in the brain.

SIDE EFFECTS

Atomoxetine may cause cardiac arrhythmia and high blood pressure that may cause blurred vision or severe headache; other side effects may include dry mouth, decreased appetite and weight loss, upset stomach, nausea, vomiting, and constipation; liver damage; difficulty in urination; decreased libido; dizziness, tiredness, mood swings, and suicidal thoughts or behaviors. Rarely, it may cause allergic reactions such as skin hives and fluid retention.

DRUG INTERACTIONS

Atomoxetine (ATX)

ATX ⬌ Albuterol: Sympathetic activities of atomoxetine can increase blood pressure and heart rate, and its concurrent administration with albuterol, a sympathetic beta-agonist, may further exacerbate the adverse effects of atomoxetine.

ATX ⬌ CYP Isozymes: *See* Table 48-1.

ATX ⬌ Epinephrine: Atomoxetine, when taken with a sympathomimetic drug such as epinephrine or pseudoephedrine, may further the rise of blood pressure.

ATX ⬌ MAO Inhibitors: (*See* Ω-51 in Appendix A.) Co-administration of atomoxetine, a selective norepinephrine reuptake inhibitor, and an MAO inhibitor is contraindicated, for serious, life-threatening adverse effects may ensue. It is recommended to have at least two weeks separation between the two drugs.

ADDERALL XR (AMPHETAMINE + DEXTROAMPHETAMINE)

This preparation may lessen fatigue and increase wakefulness with greater focus. Adderall XR is a long-acting, slow-release mixture of amphetamine and dextroamphetamine.

MECHANISM OF ACTION

This preparation releases both dopamine and norepinephrine in the brain. However, amphetamine is not recommended for children under the age of six because of a risk of toxicity that may outweigh its benefits.

SIDE EFFECTS

The frequent side effects of this preparation include cardiac arrhythmia and severe hypertension; unpleasant taste, dry mouth, diarrhea or constipation; altered libido (sex drive); and severe headache, dizziness, anxiety, confusion, insomnia, and hallucinations. Rarely, this preparation may cause allergic reactions such as swelling of tissues.

DRUG INTERACTIONS

See Box 48-1.

Miscellaneous Interactions of Amphetamine + Dextroamphetamine (ADR)

ADR ⬌ CYP Isozymes: *See* Table 48-2.

ADR ⬌ Dextromethorphan: Avoid co-administration of dextromethorphan with a CNS stimulant such as amphetamine, because it tends to increase incidences of the unfavorable side effects of dextromethorphan, such as impaired judgment and erratic euphoria.

ADR ⬌ Digoxin: Co-administration of amphetamine or dextroamphetamine with digoxin can increase the risk of cardiac arrhythmias caused by the digitalis glycoside.

BOX 48-1

Basic Concepts of Amphetamine + Dextroamphetamine Interactions

1. Both amphetamines are a basic drug (*See* Fig. 3-4), and when either is co-administered with a drug that makes urine alkaline, more of the basic drug is shifted to the nonionized form that is favored for back-diffusion through the renal tubules to return to circulation, raising its blood levels and adverse effects. Such adverse effects include hypertensive crisis, as they can release norepinephrine that causes vasoconstrictions. Those drugs that make urine alkaline include: **acetazolamide** (an antiepileptic drug) and **sodium bicarbonate**.

2. Both amphetamines are a basic drug and when either is co-administered with a drug that makes urine acidic, more of the basic drug is shifted to its ionized form that cannot diffuse back into circulation but is readily excreted in the urine, leading to lowered blood levels and decreased therapeutic effectiveness of the basic drug. Those drugs that make urine acidic include: **ammonium chloride** and **methenamine mandelate** (a urinary tract antiseptic agent).

3. Dopamine released by amphetamine or dextroamphetamine cannot work on its receptors in the presence of other drugs that block dopamine-receptors, to result in the diminished CNS effects of amphetamine and dextroamphetamine. Those dopamine receptor blockers include: **chlorpromazine** (an antipsychotic drug); and **haloperidol** (an antipsychotic drug).

ADR ⟷ MAO Inhibitors: (*See* Ω-51 in Appendix A.) Since both amphetamine and dextroamphetamine are a monoamine, their elimination requires presence of MAO. Thus, combined use with an MAO inhibitor can result in their elevated blood concentrations and toxicities.

TABLE 48-2 Adderall XR vs CYP Isozymes

Drug Name	1A2	2A6	2B6	2C8	2C9	2C18	2C19	2D6	2E1	3A4
Amphetamine								Sub		

Inactivation of both amphetamine and dextroamphetamine in the liver calls for the presence of CYP2D6 and thus, inhibition of this enzyme by another drug can raise the blood levels and adverse effects of these drugs. Those strong inhibitors of CYP2D6 include: bupropion, fluoxetine, paroxetine, and quinidine; and its moderate inhibitors include: duloxetine and terbinafine. (*See* the left-hand column of Table-0 at the 'Introduction' for other possible inhibitors of the enzyme.)

49

Chronic Fatigue Syndrome

Chronic fatigue syndrome refers to a severe, incapacitating fatigue that is continuous or recurring for at least six months, and is characterized by feelings of weariness and tiredness. This debilitating fatigue is not relieved by bed rest, and may be worsened by physical or mental activities.

Medications that may possibly be effective in the treatment of chronic fatigue syndrome include: (1) **modafinil** (Provigil); (2) **bupropion** (Wellbutrin); and (3) monoamine oxidase (MAO)inhibitors such as **selegiline** (l-deprenyl, Eldepryl, Zelapar).

MODAFINIL

Modafinil is a central nervous stimulant, which is useful in alleviating fatigue and promoting wakefulness in daytime sleepiness.

MECHANISM OF ACTION

Modafinil increases the release of norepinephrine and dopamine from the synaptic terminals in the brain. Because dopamine acts on the brain's reward center, modafinil has a potential for abuse, like cocaine and amphetamines. Modafinil was also shown to increase the release of serotonin, to elevate serotonin levels in the brain cortex.

SIDE EFFECTS

Modafinil may cause dry mouth, upset stomach, and heartburn; involuntary shaking of limbs; and headache, anxiety, restlessness, dizziness, and insomnia.

DRUG INTERACTIONS

Modafinil (MDF)

MDF ⟷ CYP Isozymes: *See* Table 49-1.

TABLE 49-1 Modafinil and Selegiline vs CYP Enzymes

Drug Name	1A2	2A6	2B6	2C8	2C9	2C18	2C19	2D6	2E1	3A4
Modafinil	Ezi				Inh		Inh	Sub		Sub+ Ezi
Selegiline	Inh		Sub							

Abbreviations: Sub, substrate of the enzyme; Inh, inhibits the enzyme; Ezi, induces the enzyme

1. Modafinil exerts an inhibitory effect on both CYP2C9 and CYP2C19 and thus, administration in combination with drugs that require these enzymes for their metabolic clearance may result in elevated blood levels, possibly exacerbating their adverse effects. (*See* the middle column of Table-0 at the 'Introduction' for possible substrates of these enzymes.)

2. Selegiline is an inhibitor of CYP1A2 and co-administration with drugs that require this enzyme for hepatic clearance may raise their blood levels to exacerbate their adverse effects. Those drugs include: alosetron, duloxetine, theophylline, and tizanidine. (*See* the middle column of the Table-0 at the 'Introduction' for other possible substrates of the enzyme.)

4. Selegiline is cleared through CYP2B6 in the liver and thus, concurrent administration of it with an inhibitor of this enzyme may raise blood levels of selegiline to exacerbate its adverse effects. Such CYP2B6 inhibitors include: itraconazole and orphenadrine. (*See* the left-hand column of Table-0 at the 'Introduction' for other possible inhibitors of the enzyme.)

MDF ⟷ MAO Inhibitors: (*See* Ω-51 in Appendix A.) Caution is advised when modafinil, a possible releaser of serotonin, is taken with an MAO inhibitor, for it may produce serotonin syndrome, including hypertensive crisis.

MDF ⟷ Phenobarbital: Modafinil is a substrate of hepatic CYP2D6 and CYP3A4; and its co-administration with inducers of such enzymes, like phenobarbital, may quicken its metabolism to result in decreased blood levels with therapeutic failure.

BUPROPION
MECHANISM OF ACTION
Bupropion is an atypical antidepressant. It has an ability to block neuronal reuptake of both norepinephrine and dopamine.

SIDE EFFECTS
Possible side effects of bupropion include dry mouth, nausea, and constipation; and agitation, insomnia, headache, and tremor.

DRUG INTERACTIONS
See Chapter 50.

SELEGILINE

At normal clinical doses selegiline is a selective inhibitor of MAO-B, the enzyme that preferentially oxidizes dopamine. However, if its doses are excessive its selectivity tends to be lost to inhibit MAO-A as well.

MECHANISM OF ACTION

Selegiline, by inhibition of MAO-B, causes increased dopamine levels. It also blocks the reuptake of dopamine and activates dopamine receptors. In addition, selegiline was shown to reduce the production of toxic oxidative free radicals and can protect neurons against a variety of neurotoxins. Selegiline is used in the treatment of mental depression, and also is effective in treatment of chronic fatigue syndrome.

SIDE EFFECTS

Possible side effects of selegiline include tachycardia; difficulty breathing; dry mouth, stomach upset, nausea, heartburn, loss of appetite, and constipation; difficult urination; chest pain and muscle pain; tremors; increased skin sensitivity to sunlight; and dizziness, lightheadedness, severe headache, and hallucinations.

DRUG INTERACTIONS

See Box 49-1.

Miscellaneous Interactions of Selegiline (SLG)

SLG ⟷ CYP Isozymes: *See* Table 49-1.

SLG ⟷ Dextromethorphan: Dextromethorphan tends to accumulate serotonin by inhibiting its neuronal reuptake. When dextromethorphan is used in combination with selegiline, it may increase the risk of serotonin syndrome.

SLG ⟷ MAO Inhibitors: (*See* Ω-51 in Appendix A.) Severe orthostatic hypotension may occur when selegiline, an inhibitor of MAO, is taken with another inhibitor of MAO, probably because dopamine accumulated by selegiline has hypotensive effect.

SLG ⟷ Meperidine: Meperidine, an opioid analgesic drug, inhibits serotonin reuptake to result in increased brain levels of serotonin. When meperidine is taken in combination with selegiline, the interaction may cause muscle rigidity, severe agitation, elevated body temperature, and stupor.

BOX 49-1

Basic Concepts of Selegiline Interactions

MAO-A preferentially deaminates serotonin, epinephrine, and norepinephrine, whereas MAO-B specifically inactivates dopamine. Although selegiline inhibits MAO-B more specifically, its specificity is lost at doses greater than 10 mg a day to inhibit MAO-A as well. Thus, when selegiline is co-administered with drugs requiring MAO–A for their inactivation, it may lead to accumulation of the affected drugs to exacerbate their adverse effects. Those drugs include: **ephedrine**; **norepinephrine** (when its inactivation is opposed by selegiline, it may increase the risk of hypertensive crisis); **pseudoephedrine** (a vasoconstrictor to relieve nasal congestion); and **fluoxetine** (an antidepressant working as a serotonin reuptake inhibitor; its co-administration with selegiline may generate serotonin syndrome); **SSRIs** (*See* Ω-68 in Appendix A); and **tricyclic antidepressants** (when co-administered with a tricyclic antidepressant, such as amitriptyline, which blocks reuptake of norepinephrine and serotonin, selegiline may cause serotonin syndrome).

50 Mental Depression

Mental depression is a common disorder characterized by dispirited mood with feelings of sadness, despair, and loss of interest or pleasure.

Medications that may possibly be effective in the treatment of mental depression include: (1) **duloxetine** (Cymbalta); (2) **venlafaxine** (Effexor XR); (3) selective serotonin reuptake inhibitors (SSRIs) such as **citalopram, escitalopram** (Lexapro), **fluoxetine** (Prozac), **paroxetine** (Paxil CR), and **sertraline** (Zoloft); (4) **trazodone** (Desyrel, Beneficat, Deprax, Desirel, Molipaxin, Thombran, Trazorel, Trialodine, Trittico); (5) **mirtazapine** (Remeron); (6) **bupropion** (Budeprion SR, Wellbutrin XL); and (7) tricyclic antidepressants such as **amitriptyline** (Elavil, Etrafon, Limbitrol, Triavil), **desipramine** (Norpramin), **doxepin** (Adapin, Sinequan), **imipramine, nortriptyline** (Pamelor), **protriptyline** (Vivactil), and **trimipramine** (Surmontil).

DULOXETINE

MECHANISM OF ACTION

Duloxetine (Fig. 50-1) equally blocks reuptake of both serotonin and norepineph-rine in central neurons. Its mechanism of action for treatment of major depression is not fully understood, but there is speculation that it might affect signaling of neurons mediated by serotonin and norepinephrine in the brain.

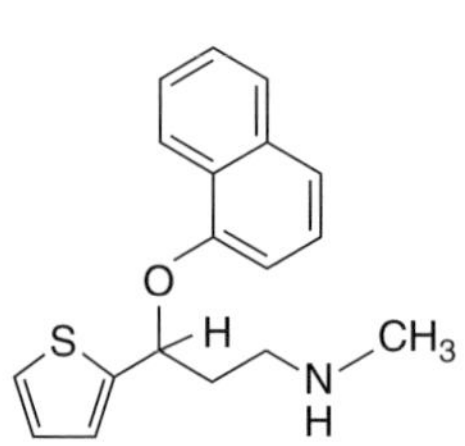

FIGURE 50-1 Molecular structure of duloxetine.

SIDE EFFECTS

Duloxetine may cause tachycardia (rapid heartbeat); nausea, stomach pain, vomiting, and diarrhea; jaundice (yellowing of the skin or conjunctiva); loss of libido; and drowsiness, dizziness, headache, and hallucinations.

DRUG INTERACTIONS

See Box 50-1.

Miscellaneous Interactions of Duloxetine (DXT)

DXT ↔ Alcohol: Avoid taking alcohol with duloxetine. Excessive depression of the central neurons may occur with this combination.

DXT ↔ CYP Isozymes: *See* Table 50-1.

DXT ↔ MAO Inhibitors: (*See* Ω-51 in Appendix A.) Concurrent use of duloxetine and a monoamine oxidase (MAO) inhibitor is contraindicated. If taken together, serotonin accumulated by duloxetine cannot be inactivated, increasing the incidence of serotonin syndrome, whose symptoms include hypertension and tachycardia; and myoclonus, shivering, ataxia; hyperpyrexia and diaphoresis (sweating). It is recommended that duloxetine not be started within 14 days of discontinuation of an MAO inhibitor, or allow at least five days after termination of duloxetine before starting an MAO inhibitor.

DXT ↔ Propafenone: Duloxetine is a strong inhibitor of CYP2D6, and when used in combination, it can increase the serum levels of propafenone, a substrate of CYP2D6, and its incidences of toxicity.

BOX 50-1

Basic Concepts of Duloxetine Interactions

Duloxetine is extensively bound to plasma proteins (>90%), and when co-administered with drugs that also bind to the same plasma proteins with a lower affinity, duloxetine will displace them from the proteins and will raise their blood concentrations and toxicities. Those drugs include: **dicumarol** and **warfarin**.

TABLE 50-1 Duloxetine and Venlafaxine vs CYP Enzymes

Drug Name	1A2	2A6	2B6	2C8	2C9	2C18	2C19	2D6	2E1	3A4
Duloxetine	Sub+ Inh							Sub+ **Inh**		
Venlafaxine							Sub	Sub+ Inh	Sub	Sub+ Inh

Abbreviations: Sub, substrate of the enzyme; Inh, inhibits the enzyme; Ezi, induces the enzyme

1. Duloxetine is an inhibitor of cytochrome CYP1A2 and, to a greater extent, CYP2D6. Thus, co-administration with drugs that require these enzymes for hepatic clearance may cause elevation of blood levels and adverse effects of the affected drugs. Those drugs affected by CYP1A2 inhibition include: alosetron, duloxetine, theophylline, and tizanidine; and those drugs affected by CYP2D6 inhibition include desipramine, nortriptyline, and thioridazine. (*See* the middle column of Table-0 at the 'Introduction' for other possible substrates of these enzymes.)

2. Hepatic clearance of duloxetine depends on both CYP2D6 and, to a greater extend, CYP1A2. Thus, inhibition of these enzymes by any other drug co-administered may raise blood levels of duloxetine to exacerbate its adverse effects. (*See* the left-hand column of Table-0 at the 'Introduction' for possible inhibitors of these enzymes.)

3. Venlafaxine has an inhibitory function on microsomal enzymes CYP3A4 and CYP2D6 and thus, co-administration of venlafaxine with drugs that require these enzymes for clearance may incite elevation of blood levels and adverse effects of the affected drugs. (*See* the middle column of Table-0 at the 'Introduction' for other possible substrates of these enzymes).

VENLAFAXINE

Venlafaxine (Fig. 50-2) is a bicyclic antidepressant drug used mainly to treat major depression and anxiety.

MECHANISM OF ACTION

Venlafaxine mainly inhibits reuptake of norepinephrine and serotonin, but at high doses it weakly inhibits reuptake of dopamine as well. Therefore, venlafaxine accumulates these neurotransmitters in the synapses of mood-affecting neurons in the prefrontal cortex.

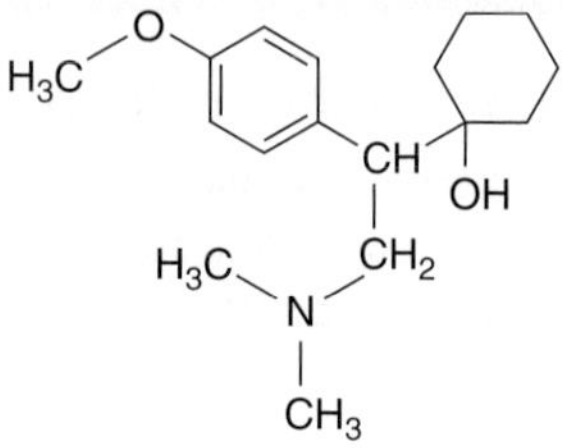

FIGURE 50-2   Molecular structure of venlafaxine.

SIDE EFFECTS

Venlafaxine may cause elevation of blood pressure and intraocular pressure (thus, not for patients with glaucoma); nausea and loss of appetite; and headaches, anxiety, insomnia, drowsiness, and seizures. Venlafaxine is contraindicated in children and young adults because it can increase suicidal thoughts and self-harm.

DRUG INTERACTIONS

See Box 50-2.

Miscellaneous Interactions of Venlafaxine (VFX)

VFX ⬌ Alcohol: If venlafaxine is taken with alcohol or other central nervous system (CNS) depressants, it may cause additive CNS depression. Thus, concurrent use of venlafaxine with alcohol is best avoided.

VFX ⬌ CYP Isozymes: *See* Table 50-1.

VFX ⬌ MAO Inhibitors: (*See* Ω-51 in Appendix A.) The combination of venlafaxine, an inhibitor of serotonin reuptake, with an inhibitor of the enzyme MAO (monoamine oxidase) may lead to the rare, but serious, serotonin syndrome,

---

BOX 50 -2

Basic Concepts of Venlafaxine Interactions

1. Venlafaxine is an neuronal reuptake inhibitor of both serotonin and norepinephrine and thus, when co-administered with drugs that generate similar inhibition of reuptake, they may lead to excessive adverse effect of serotonin and/or of norepinephrine. Those drugs include: **sibutramine** (a drug to treat obesity, that inhibits serotonin reuptake, and when combined with venlafaxine it can lead to serotonin syndrome); **tramadol** (an analgesic that decreases the synaptic reuptake of serotonin and norepinephrine); and **triptans.** (*See* Ω-77 in Appendix A.) (If venlafaxine is used together with a 5-HT$_1$ receptor agonist, such as naratriptan, sumatriptan, or zolmitriptan, the risk of serotonin syndrome is increased.)

2. As venlafaxine may lower the seizure threshold, its co-administration with drugs that also lower the seizure threshold is not recommended. Such drugs include: **bupropion** (an antidepressant); **paroxetine** (an antidepressant); **(St. John's Wort)** (an antidepressant); and **Tramadol** (an analgesic).

which include hypertension and tachycardia; myoclonus, ataxia; hyperpyrexia, and diaphoresis. Hence, do not take them concomitantly within 14 days of each other.

SELECTIVE SEROTONIN REUPTAKE INHIBITORS

Citalopram (Fig. 50-3), **escitalopram** (the S-enantiomer of citalopram which is a mixture of R- and S-enantiomer), **fluoxetine** (Fig. 50-4), **paroxetine** (Fig. 50-5), and **sertraline** (Fig. 50-6).

MECHANISM OF ACTION

Reduced level of serotonin in the brain is thought to cause mental depression. The selective serotonin reuptake inhibitors (SSRIs) bind to the transporters of serotonin re-uptake to selectively prevent its re-uptake, resulting in restoration of serotonin levels in the brain associated with mood control.

SIDE EFFECTS

Frequent side effects of them include dry mouth, loss of appetite, upset stomach, and vomiting; sexual impotence; and headache, insomnia, dizziness, and anxiety.

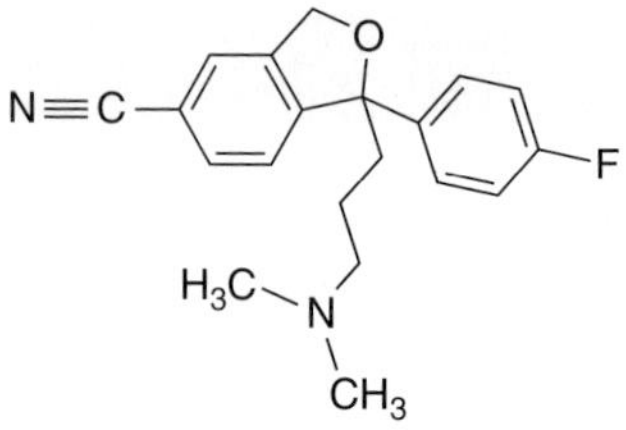

FIGURE 50-3   Molecular structure of citalopram.

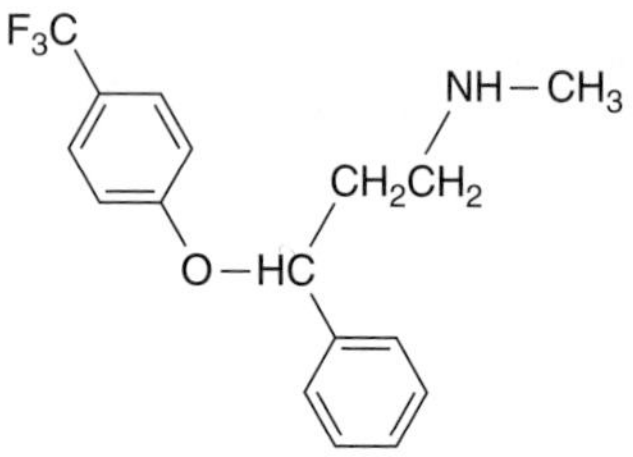

FIGURE 50-4   Molecular structure of fluoxetine.

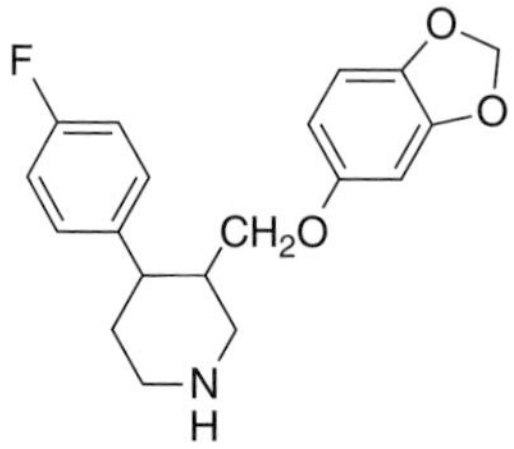

FIGURE 50-5   Molecular structure of paroxetine.

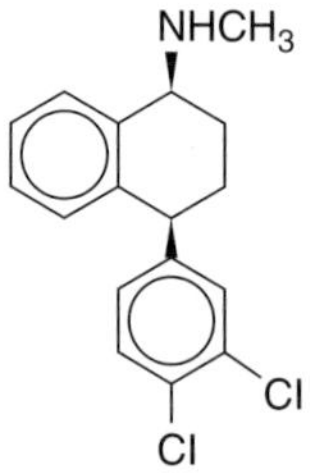

FIGURE 50-6   Molecular structure of sertraline.

DRUG INTERACTIONS

See Appendix B-29: Interactions of Selective Serotonin Reuptake Inhibitors (SSRIs).

TRAZODONE

Though this drug is not a true member of the SSRIs, it shares many of their properties. For instance, its withdrawal symptoms, which occur when trazodone is stopped too quickly, include flu-like symptoms, sensory disturbances, and hyperarousal. To stave off such symptoms, a gradual tapering of its dose over a period of time is recommended.

MECHANISM OF ACTION

Trazodone inhibits reuptake of serotonin, but its difference from authentic SSRIs is that it has far less affinity for the serotonin transporters to block its reuptake than do SSRIs. Further, trazodone is also a serotonin receptor ($5\text{-}HT_2$) antagonist. Some believe that the antidepressant effect of trazodone derives from its antagonistic effect at the $5\text{-}HT_2$ receptor sites, whose activation appears to be abnormally high in dysthymia.

SIDE EFFECTS

Trazodone may cause dry mouth, decreased appetite, stomach pain, nausea, and constipation; muscle aches, tremors, and lack of coordination; tiredness, dizziness, drowsiness, headache, lightheadedness, nervousness, and sleeplessness; and blurred vision. However, the intensity of the anticholinergic effects of trazodone is considerably less than with tricyclic antidepressants. A unique side effect of trazodone is priapism, a prolonged, painful penile erection in the absence of sexual desires.

DRUG INTERACTIONS

See Box 50-3.

Miscellaneous Interactions of Trazodone (TZD)

Parentheses below indicate an herb.

TZD ↔ Alcohol: If Trazodone is taken with alcohol, it may cause amplified CNS depression. Therefore, it is prudent to hold off combination of the two.

TZD ↔ CYP Isozymes: *See* Table 50-2.

BOX 50-3

Basic Concepts of Trazodone Interactions

Though far less active than a typical SSRI, trazodone inhibits neuronal reuptake of serotonin, and when co-administered with drugs that also inhibit the reuptake of serotonin, they may create excessive accumulation of serotonin that may cause serotonin syndrome, which includes myoclonus, CNS irritability, loss of consciousness, and shivering. Those drugs include: **nefazodone** (a SSRI that also has a 5-HT$_2$ antagonistic effect) and pure **SSRIs** (*See* Ω-68 in Appendix A.)

TZD ↔ Digoxin: When digoxin is used with trazodone, the serum levels of digoxin may be elevated by an unknown mechanism.

TZD ↔ MAO Inhibitor: (*See* Ω-51 in Appendix A.) Combination of trazodone with an inhibitor of the enzyme MAO may lead to rare but serious serotonin syndrome, a possibly fatal reaction that includes hypertension; myoclonus and ataxia; and hyperpyrexia. To stave off this mishap do not use them concomitantly within 14 days of each other.

TZD ↔ (St. John's Wort): This herbal antidepressant increases the effects and toxicities of trazodone.

TZD ↔ Triptans: (*See* Ω-77 in Appendix A.) If trazodone is used together with a 5-HT$_1$ receptor agonist, such as naratriptan, sumatriptan, or zolmitriptan, the

TABLE 50-2 Trazodone and Mirtazapine vs CYP Enzymes

Drug Name	1A2	2A6	2B6	2C8	2C9	2C18	2C19	2D6	2E1	3A4
Trazodone								Sub		Sub
Mirtazapine	Sub+ Inh							Sub		Sub

Abbreviations: Sub, substrate of the enzyme; Inh, inhibits the enzyme; Ezi, induces the enzyme

1. Trazodone is metabolized through CYP2D6 and CYP3A4 and thus, inhibition of these enzymes by another drug can raise the blood levels and adverse effects of trazodone. (*See* the left-hand column of Table-0 at the 'Introduction' for possible inhibitors of these enzymes.)

2. Mirtazapine functions as an inhibitor of CYP1A2 and thus, co-administration with drugs that require this enzyme for hepatic clearance may raise their blood levels and exacerbate their adverse effects. Those drugs include: alosetron, duloxetine, theophylline, and tizanidine. (*See* the middle column of Table-0 at the 'Introduction' for other possible substrates of the enzyme.)

incidence of serotonin syndrome become greater, generating such symptoms as muscle weakness, lack of coordination, and hyperreflexia.

MIRTAZAPINE

Mirtazapine (Fig. 50-7) is a tetracyclic antidepressant.

MECHANISM OF ACTION

Mirtazapine, unlike most conventional antidepressants, has no appreciable affinity for the transporters of serotonin, norepinephrine, or dopamine to block their reuptake. Instead, it inhibits the central adrenergic alpha-2 receptors to enhance sympathetic and serotonergic activities. Mirtazapine is referred to as an indirect activator of the 5-HT_{1A} receptors, and increased activation of the central 5-HT_{1A} receptors is deemed accountable for the effectiveness of most antidepressant drugs.

SIDE EFFECTS

Mirtazapine may cause cardiac arrhythmia; dry mouth, constipation; and increase in body weight; and dizziness, drowsiness, and seizure. Rarely, it may cause allergic reactions such as swelling of tissues.

DRUG INTERACTIONS

Mirtazapine (MTZ)

MTZ ↔ Alcohol: Mirtazapine, when taken with alcohol or other CNS depressants, may generate excessive CNS depression.

MTZ ↔ Alpha-2 Activators: (*See* Ω-4 in Appendix A.) Mirtazapine, a central alpha-2 receptor antagonist, may reduce the antihypertensive effects of a central alpha-2 receptor agonist, such as clonidine.

MTZ ↔ CYP Isozymes: *See* Table 50-2.

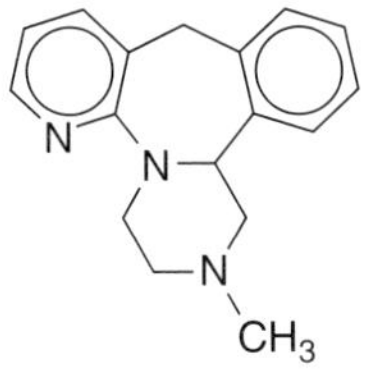

FIGURE 50-7   Molecular structure of mirtazapine.

MTZ ⟷ Diazepam: Concurrent administration of mirtazapine, an inhibitor of CYP1A2, and diazepam, a benzodiazepine antianxiety drug, which though is not a CYP1A2 substrate, may cause a pharmacodynamic interaction that results in impaired physical and mental performances.

MTZ ⟷ MAO Inhibitors: (*See* Ω-51 in Appendix A.) If used with an MAO inhibitor, mirtazapine may precipitate a hypertensive crisis, causing convulsions and possibly fatal results. Do not use mirtazapine within 14 days of starting or stopping therapy with an MAO inhibitor.

BUPROPION

MECHANISM OF ACTION

Bupropion is an atypical antidepressant that acts as a reuptake inhibitor of both norepinephrine and dopamine in central neurons.

SIDE EFFECTS

Possible side effects of bupropion include dry mouth, nausea, and constipation; agitation and tremor; and seizure, headache, and insomnia.

DRUG INTERACTIONS

Bupropion (BPN)

BPN ⟷ Alcohol: Ingestion of alcohol may alter the seizure threshold so as to increase the risk of seizures in patients taking bupropion.

BPN ⟷CYP Isozymes: *See* Table 50-3.

BPN ⟷ Guanfacine: Combined use of bupropion and guanfacine may foster grand mal seizures. However, its interaction mechanism remains unclear.

BPN ⟷ MAO Inhibitors: (*See* Ω-51 in Appendix A.) The side chain of bupropion (*See* Fig. 47-1) is oxidized by MAO to form the meta-chlorobenzoic acid conjugate with glycine, which is then excreted as the major urinary metabolite. Therefore, never take bupropion with an MAO inhibitor, such as phenelzine, another antidepressant drug; or selegiline, an anti-Parkinson drug. It is recommended to discontinue an MAO inhibitor at least 14 days before starting bupropion, otherwise it may engender greater risks of bupropion toxicities.

BPN ⟷ Nicotine: Co-administration of bupropion, a reuptake inhibitor of norepinephrine, with a patch of nicotine, which stimulates sympathetic ganglia and the adrenal medulla to increase blood pressure, may lead to excessive hypertension.

TABLE 50-3 Bupropion vs CYP Isozymes

Drug Name	1A2	2A6	2B6	2C8	2C9	2C18	2C19	2D6	2E1	3A4
Bupropion			Sub					Inh		Sub

Abbreviations: Sub, substrate of the enzyme; Inh, inhibits the enzyme; Ezi, induces the enzyme

1. Bupropion inhibits CYP2D6 and thus, co-administration with drugs that require this enzyme for hepatic clearance may cause elevation of blood levels and adverse effects of those drugs. Those drugs sensitively affected by CYP2D6 inhibition include: desipramine and thioridazine. (*See* the middle column of Table-0 at the 'Introduction' for other possible substrates of the enzyme.)
2. Carbamazepine (an inducer of CYP3A4) may reduce serum levels and the pharmacological effects of bupropion.
3. Ritonavir (an inhibitor of CYP3A4) can increase serum levels of bupropion to increase the risk of its toxicity, symptoms of which include seizures.

TRICYCLIC ANTIDEPRESSANTS

Amitriptyline, desipramine, doxepin, imipramine, nortriptyline, protriptyline (Fig. 50-8), and **trimipramine** (Fig. 50-9)

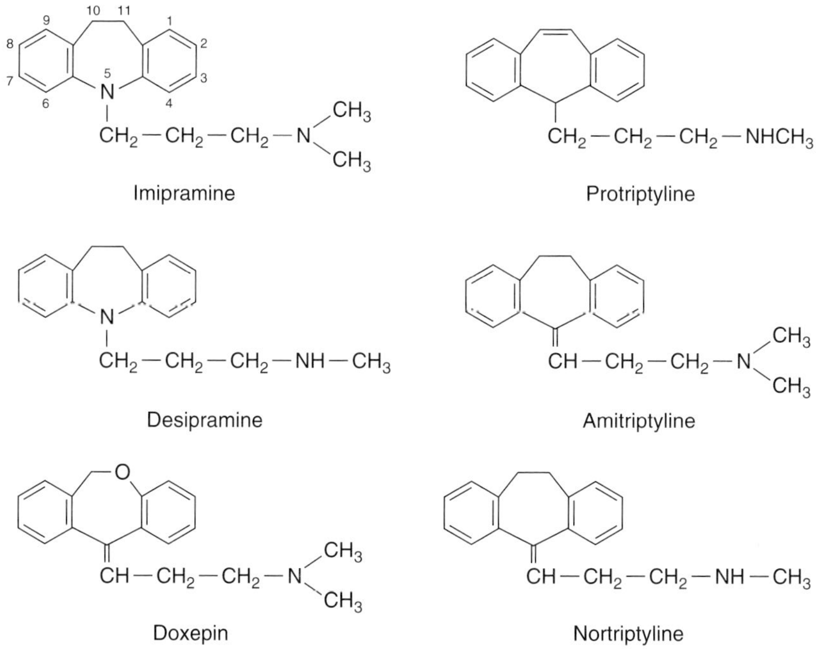

FIGURE 50-8 Molecular structures of tricyclic antidepressants.

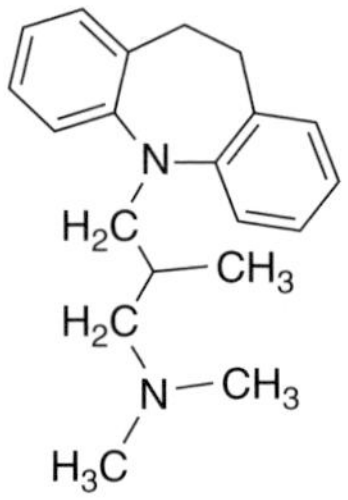

FIGURE 50-9   Molecular structure of trimipramine.

MECHANISM OF ACTION

They act mainly by blocking neuronal reuptake of both serotonin and norepinephrine, causing elevation of their concentrations and enhancing adrenergic and serotonergic neurotransmissions in the brain.

SIDE EFFECTS

Frequent side effects of tricyclic antidepressants include fast or irregular heart rate; dry mouth, nausea, vomiting, and constipation; urinary retention; decreased sex drive and impotence; involuntary muscle movements in the eyes, tongue, jaw, or neck; blurred vision; dizziness, drowsiness, hallucinations, or seizures (convulsions); hostile behaviors; and rarely, allergic reactions such as skin rash and itching. Amitriptyline may turn urine blue-green but this does not usually indicate a medical emergency.

DRUG INTERACTIONS

See Appendix B-31: Interactions of Tricyclic Antidepressants.

Mania

Mania is a mental condition characterized by abnormal elevation of mood and physical hyperactivity. Manic patients often display erratic behaviors such as rapid and pressured speech, risk-taking, and insomnia.

Medications that may be effective in the treatment of mania include: (1) **lithium carbonate** (Cibalith-S, Eskalith, Lithane, Lithobid); (2) **valproic acid** or **divalproex** (Depakote or Depakene); (3) **carbamazepine** (Tegretol, Atretol), and (4) **clozapine** (Clozaril).

LITHIUM CARBONATE

MECHANISM OF ACTION

Its mechanism of action is not well understood, but upon ingestion, lithium carbonate (Li_2CO_3) is widely distributed in the central nervous system (CNS), and decreases the release of norepinephrine. It may also interfere with neuronal signaling by inhibition of inositol monophosphatase, the enzyme required for regeneration of inositol, a key component of the phosphatidyl inositol signaling pathway, which serves as a second messenger of norepinephrine and serotonin. As the level of inositol in the cerebrospinal fluid of mentally depressed patients is low, it is hypothesized that reduction of the brain inositol levels may help to alleviate mania.

SIDE EFFECTS

The frequent side effects of lithium include bradycardia (slowing of heart-beat), hypotension; anorexia (lack of appetite), nausea, vomiting, and diarrhea; glucosuria (presence of glucose in the urine in detectable amounts), and polyuria (a condition characterized by the passage of large volumes of urine—at least 2.5 liters in a 24 hour period in adults); muscle twitching and fatigue; giddiness; tinnitus; blurred vision; and vertigo and confusion. To stave off serious toxicities of lithium, the serum level should not exceed 2.0 mEq/liter.

DRUG INTERACTIONS

See Box 51-1.

Miscellaneous Interactions of Lithium Carbonate (LCB)

LCB ↔ Calcium-Channel Blockers: (*See* Ω-31 in Appendix A.) Similarities exist between the actions of lithium and calcium-channel blockers. Concurrent intake of lithium with a calcium-channel blocker may generate synergistic neurotoxicities, such as ataxia and tremors.

LCB ↔ Carbamazepine: Concomitant use of carbamazepine and lithium may result in neurotoxicity regardless of the therapeutic levels of either drug. One of the drugs may need to be discontinued if signs of neurotoxicity occur such as hyperreflexia, tremor, ataxia, dizziness, lethargy, and muscular weakness.

LCB ↔ COX-2 Inhibitors: (*See* Ω-36 in Appendix A.) Celecoxib, rofecoxib, and valdecoxib have been shown to decrease the renal clearance of lithium to increase its serum levels and toxicity.

LCB ↔ Doxycycline: Doxycycline can impair renal excretion of lithium to increase its serum levels and the risk of its toxicity.

LCB ↔ Haloperidol: Concurrent intake of lithium with haloperidol (Haldol*)* has aroused extrapyramidal symptoms and irreversible brain damage. The mechanism behind this interaction has yet to be elucidated.

BOX 51-1

Basic Concepts of Lithium Carbonate Interactions

When present together, lithium and sodium compete for renal excretion. Thus, when lithium is co-administered with drugs that increase the renal excretion of sodium, the urinary excretion of lithium will be opposed, raising its serum levels and toxicity. Those drugs include: **ACE inhibitors** (*See* Ω-1 in Appendix A) (angiotensin tends to retain sodium and thus, ACE inhibitors such as captopril and enalapril favor urinary excretions of sodium); **angiotensin receptor blockers (ARBs)** such as candesartan and losartan (*See* Ω-10 in Appendix A) (they increase sodium excretions in the urine); **(dandelion)** (an herb that has a diuretic effect, mobilizing sodium for its excretion); **diuretics** (*See* Ω-49 and Ω-73 in Appendix A) (thiazide diuretics and loop diuretics increase renal sodium excretions).

LCB ⟷ Methyldopa: When used in combination, methyldopa appears to reduce renal excretion of lithium, to raise its blood levels and toxicity.

LCB ⟷ Metronidazole: Metronidazole inhibits renal excretion of Lithium, raising its plasma levels and exacerbating its adverse effects.

LCB ⟷ NSAIDs: (*See* Ω-54 in Appendix A.) Concurrent intake of lithium and a non-steroidal anti-inflammatory drug (NSAID) such as indomethacin, phenylbutazone, or piroxicam, tends to impair renal excretion of lithium, elevating its blood levels and toxicity. Therefore, it is recommended not to combine the two.

LCB ⟷ Phenothiazine Antipsychotic Drugs: (*See* Ω-58 in Appendix A.) Co-administration of prochlorperazine or chlorpromazine with lithium may lead to neurological abnormalities such as movement disorders and brain damage.

LCB ⟷ Sodium Bicarbonate: Concurrent intake of lithium with an alkalinizing agent, such as sodium bicarbonate, may increase, by an unknown mechanism, the urinary excretion of lithium, resulting in lowered blood concentrations of lithium with possible therapeutic failure.

VALPROIC ACID OR DIVALPROEX

Divalproex (Fig. 51-1) represents two molecules of valproic acid, and it quickly releases valproic acid (*See* Fig. 55-1) in the gastrointestinal tract.

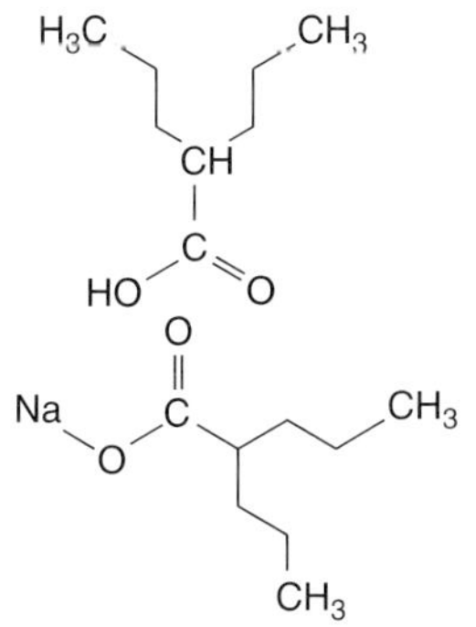

FIGURE 51-1 Molecular structure of divalproex.

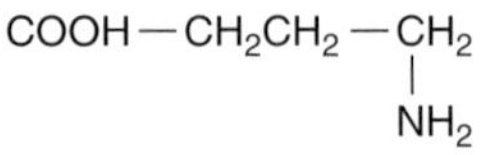

COOH — CH₂CH₂ — CH₂
                    |
                   NH₂

FIGURE 51-2 Molecular structure of GABA.

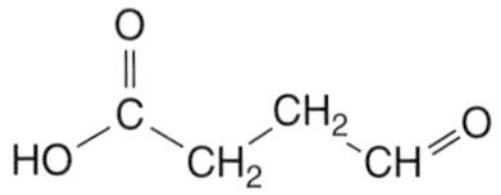

FIGURE 51-3 Molecular structure of succinic semialdehyde.

MECHANISM OF ACTION

The exact mechanism of action of valproic acid or divalproex is unknown, but it is believed that valproic acid released from divalproex elevates brain levels of the inhibitory neurotrasmitter gamma-aminobutyric acid (GABA), because valproic acid can inhibit GABA transaminase, the enzyme that inactivates GABA (Fig. 51-2) by converting it to succinic semialdehyde (Fig. 51-3).

SIDE EFFECTS

Side effects of valproic acid include changes in appetite, heartburn, nausea, vomiting, and stomach pain; jaundice; uncontrollable shaking of a part of the body; back pain; blurred or double vision; and headache, dizziness, drowsiness, and hallucinations. Rarely, it may also cause pancreatitis, and allergic reactions such as skin rash. The use of valproic acid during pregnancy has been associated with fetal abnormalities such as spina bifida and increased bleeding tendency in the mother and the baby. Hence, valproic acid should be used in pregnant women only if its benefits outweigh the risks.

DRUG INTERACTIONS

See Box 51-2.

Miscellaneous Interactions of Valproic Acid (VPA)

VPA ⟷ Alcohol: Valproic acid depresses activity of the CNS. Concurrent administration with alcohol may result in enhanced CNS depressions. Thus, it is prudent to avoid combination of the two.

VPA ⟷ Aspirin: Valproic acid is metabolized by glucuronidation, as is salicylic acid, the major metabolite of aspirin. Competition between the two for glucuronidation by glucuronyl transferase tends to raise blood levels of valproic acid. Furthermore, aspirin displaces valproic acid from its protein binding sites to increase its serum levels and to promote its toxicities.

VPA ⟷ Carbamazepine: Valproic acid inhibits microsomal epoxide hydrolase, the enzyme that converts carbamazepine-10,11-epoxide, the active form of

BOX 51-2

Basic Concepts of Valproic Acid Interactions

1. Valproic acid can either reduce the number of platelets or inhibit aggregation of platelets, to oppose formation of a blood clot, and when co-administered with drugs that generate an anticoagulant effect, excessive bleeding may result. Those drugs include: **anticoagulants** (See Ω-16 in Appendix A); **antiplatelet drugs** (See Ω-22 in Appendix A); and **NSAIDs** (See Ω-54 in Appendix A) (valproic acid can increase the bleeding tendency caused by NSAIDs such as aspirin, ibuprofen [Motrin, Advil], diclofenac [Voltaren, Cataflam, Arthrotec], indomethacin [Indocin], ketorolac [Toradol], nabumetone [Relafen], and naproxen [Naprosyn, Aleve]).

2. Valproic acid is extensively bound to albumin up to 95%, and when co-administered with drugs that are bound to the same protein with lower affinity, valproic acid displaces them to raise their free serum concentrations and adverse effects. Those drugs include: **diazepam** (a benzodiazepine antianxiety drug) and **phenytoin** (an antiepileptic drug).

carbamazepine, to its inactive metabolites. By inhibiting this enzyme, valproic acid raises blood levels of the active metabolite of carbamazepine, prolonging its pharmacologic and adverse effects.

VPA ⟷ Cholestyramine: Cholestyramine (Questran) can reduce the absorption of valproic acid from the intestines. Therefore, valproic acid should be taken at least two hours before or six hours after intake of cholestyramine.

VPA ⟷ CYP Isozymes: See Table 51-1.

VPA ⟷ Diazepam: Divalproex or valproic acid not only displaces diazepam from its binding sites at plasma albumin, but inhibits its metabolism, resulting in increased blood levels and exacerbating the adverse effects of diazepam.

VPA ⟷ Didanosine: Both didanosine and valproic acid have a potential to cause pancreatitis. If taken together they may increase the risk of developing serious damage to the pancreatic tissues.

VPA ⟷ Lamotrigine: Lamotrigine, an anticonvulsant, does not inhibit or induce CYP enzymes, and its major metabolic pathway is via glucuronidation by the enzyme UDP glucuronyltransferase, as are divalproex and valproic acid. When either drug is co-administered with lamotrigine they may compete with

TABLE 51-1 Valproic Acid vs CYP Isozymes

Drug Name	1A2	2A6	2B6	2C8	2C9	2C18	2C19	2D6	2E1	3A4
Valproic Acid					Sub+ Inh		Sub	Inh		Sub

Abbreviations: Sub, substrate of the enzyme; Inh, inhibits the enzyme; Ezi, induces the enzyme

Valproic acid, unlike many other anticonvulsants, does not induce hepatic microsomal enzymes, but rather tends to inhibit the enzyme CYP2C9 and CYP2D6. Therefore, co-administration with drugs that require these enzymes for their hepatic clearance may result in elevation of blood levels and an increase in the adverse effects of those drugs. (See the middle column of Table-0 at the 'Introduction' for possible substrates of these enzymes.)

each other for the same enzyme for elimination, resulting in elevated blood levels of lamotrigine and exacerbating its adverse effects.

CARBAMAZEPINE

MECHANISM OF ACTION

Brain cells generate action potential by opening the voltage-gated sodium channels. However, the sodium channels are quickly closed and inactivated to avoid over-excitation. Carbamazepine is known to stabilize the inactivated state of the sodium channels, causing the brain cells to become less excitable.

SIDE EFFECTS

Possible side effects of carbamazepine include dry mouth, nausea, stomach pain, vomiting, diarrhea, and constipation; jaundice (yellowing of the skin or eyes); bone marrow depression; neurotoxicity (ataxia); blurred vision; and dizziness, drowsiness, confusion, and headache. Rarely, it may also cause allergic reactions such as skin rash and itching. Carbamazepine, in addition, may cause syndrome of inappropriate antidiuretic hormone (SIADH) because it increases the release of ADH (vasopressin).

DRUG INTERACTIONS

See Box 51-3.

Miscellaneous Interactions of Carbamazepine (CZP)

Parentheses below indicate an herb.

CZP ⟷ Alcohol: Avoid taking carbamazepine in combination with alcohol or other CNS depressants, such as a hypnotic drug or an antianxiety drug for they will increase the CNS depressant effects of carbamazepine.

BOX 51-3

Basic Concepts of Carbamazepine Interactions

Absorption of carbamazepine from the gastrointestinal tract is often slow and erratic, and when taken with some drugs, its absorption may be impaired, undercutting its therapeutic effectiveness. Those drugs include: **activated charcoal** (which adsorbs the drug to oppose its absorption) and **psyllium** (a laxative, which absorbs massive amounts of water to expand, and may increase gastric-emptying time and/or decrease small intestinal transit time, to impair absorption of carbamazepine).

CZP ⟷ Clozapine: Carbamazepine, in rare instances, can lead to bone marrow depression, generating aplastic anemia, neutropenia, and/or agranulocytosis. Thus, it is unwise to administer the two together lest it cause additive bone marrow suppression. If concurrent administration is unavoidable, monitor white blood cell counts frequently.

CZP ⟷ CYP Isozymes: *See* Table 51-2.

TABLE 51-2 Carbamazepine vs CYP Isozymes

Drug Name	1A2	2A6	2B6	2C8	2C9	2C18	2C19	2D6	2E1	3A4
Carbamazepine	Ezi			Sub	Ezi		Ezi		Ezi	Sub+ Ezi

Abbreviations: Sub, substrate of the enzyme; Inh, inhibits the enzyme; Ezi, induces the enzyme

1. The formation of carbamazepine-10,11-epoxide, the active metabolite of carbamazepine, is catalyzed mainly by CYP3A4 and, to a lesser degree, by CYP2C8. The active metabolite of carbamazepine in turn is transformed by the microsomal epoxide hydrolase to 10,11-transdiol derivative, which is inactive. Because carbamazepine is an inducer of CYP3A4, high concentrations of carbamazepine in the blood can accelerate its own activation to cause such adverse effects as dizziness, drowsiness, and ataxia. Inducers of CYP3A4 can accelerate formation of carbamzepie-10-11-epoxide, the active form of carbamazepine, to increase its therapeutic and adverse effects. Those inducers of CYP3A4 include felbamate, glucocorticoids, griseofulvin, phenobarbital, phenytoin, rifampin, and topiramate. (*See* the right-hand column of Table-0 at the 'Introduction' for other possible inducers of the enzyme.)

2. Carbamazepine is an inducer of microsomal enzymes such as CYP1A2, CYP2C9, CYP 2C19, CYP2E1, and CYP3A4. Thus, its co-administration with drugs that are eliminated through these enzymes can result in insufficient blood levels and therapeutic efficacies of those drugs. For instance, carbamazepine, an inducer of CYP3A4, can reduce the pharmacologic effects of felodipine, which is mainly cleared through CYP3A4. (*See* the middle column of Table-0 at the 'Introduction' for other possible substrates of these enzymes.)

3. Acetaminophen, when oxidized by CYP1A2 or CYP2E1, generates its hepatotoxic metabolite. Carbamazepine is an inducer of both enzymes and thus, concurrent use of these two drugs may increase the risk of acetaminophen-induced hepatotoxicity.

CZP ↔ Lithium: Both lithium and carbamazepine have neurotoxic activities, and their use in combination may result in neurotoxic symptoms such as tremor, ataxia, lethargy, and hyperreflexia. Discontinuation of this combination is recommended if such symptoms occur.

CZP ↔ MAO Inhibitors: (*See* Ω-51 in Appendix A.) Carbamazepine has a primary amine in its structure (*See* Fig. 47-3) but its inactivation does not involve MAO. However, co-administration of carbamazepine and an MAO inhibitor is contraindicated because potentially fatal reactions may ensue by yet to be defined mechanism. Possible symptoms include hypertensive crisis, hyperthermia, mental status changes, and seizures. Before administration of carbamazepine, any MAO inhibitor should be discontinued for a minimum of 14 days.

CZP ↔ (Valerian): Do not use the herb valerian (Fig. 51-4 A and B), a sedating herb that helps relieve stress, anxiety, and nervousness, together with carbamazepine, whose side effects include blurred vision and confusions. The combination may result in impaired driving skills and ability to operate machinery.

CZP ↔ Valproic Acid: Valproic acid inhibits microsomal epoxide hydrolase (mEH), the enzyme responsible for the breakdown of active carbamazepine-10, 11-epoxide into its inactive metabolites. By inhibiting this mEH, valproic acid accumulates the active carbamazepine-10,11-epoxide to prolong the therapeutic and adverse effects of carbamazepine.

CZP ↔ Vasopressin or Its Analogs: Carbamazepine stimulates the release of vasopressin (an antidiuretic hormone) from the posterior pituitary gland, and can potentiate the effects of vasopressin, lypressin, or desmopressin, when taken in combination.

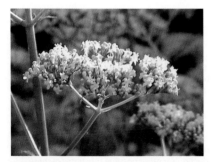

FIGURE 51-4   A, Valerian Flower.
(courtesy of Kurt Stueber, via Wikimedia, at
http://commons.wikimedia.org/wiki/File:Valeriana_
officinalis1.jpg)

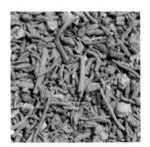

FIGURE 51-4   B, Valerian Root Cut.
(Courtesy of Woodland Herbs Limited,
100 Woodlands Road, Glasgow at
www.woodlandherbs.co.uk)

CLOZAPINE

Clozapine (Fig. 51-5) is classified as an atypical antipsychotic drug, as it is more active within the limbic system than at the striatal dopamine receptors. For this reason, this drug is also relatively free from extrapyramidal side effects. However, because of its potentially lethal side effect of agranulocytosis, it is used to control manic episodes in patients who have not responded to typical antimanic agents.

MECHANISM OF ACTION

Clozapine binds to and blocks dopamine Type-2 (D2)-receptors and serotonin Type-2 ($5HT_2$) receptors. However, its exact mechanism of action for alleviation of mania still remains unclear.

SIDE EFFECTS

Side effects of clozapine include cardiac arrhythmias; agranulocytosis; nausea, vomiting, stomach pain, and constipation; uncontrolled muscle movements; fainting, lightheadedness, and seizures; and rarely, allergic reactions such as swelling of tissues, and skin rash. About one percent of patients taking clozapine develop agranulocytosis, requiring drug cessation. Agranulocytosis causes such symptoms as fever, lethargy, and sore throat.

DRUG INTERACTIONS

See Appendix B-12: Interactions of Atypical Antipsychotic Drugs.

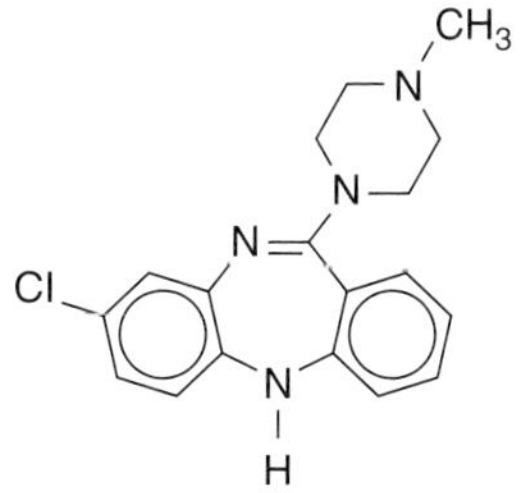

FIGURE 51-5   Molecular structure of clozapine.

52

Psychosis

Psychosis is a manifestation of mental illness characterized by a radically distorted sense of reality in which thinking becomes irrational and is often accompanied by delusions or hallucinations.

Medications that may be effective in the treatment of psychosis include: (1) atypical antipsychotic drugs such as **aripiprazole** (Fig. 52-1) (Abilify), **clozapine** (*See* Fig. 51-5) (Clozaril), **olanzapine** (Fig. 52-2) (Zyprexa), **quetiapine** (Fig. 52-3) (Seroquel), **risperidone** (Fig. 52-4) (Risperdal), and **sertindole** (Fig. 52-5)

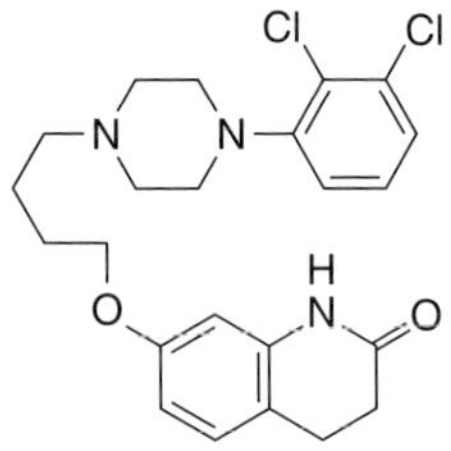

FIGURE 52-1   Molecular structure of aripiprazole.

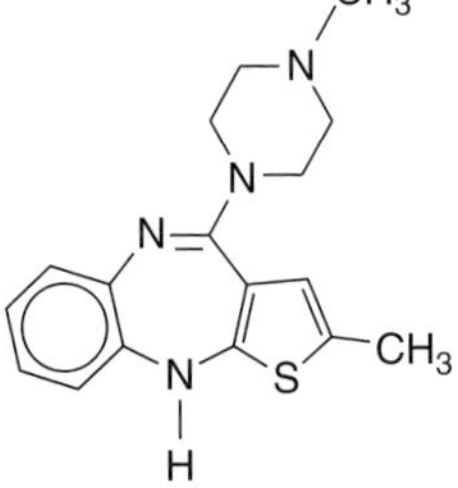

FIGURE 52-2   Molecular structure of olanzapine.

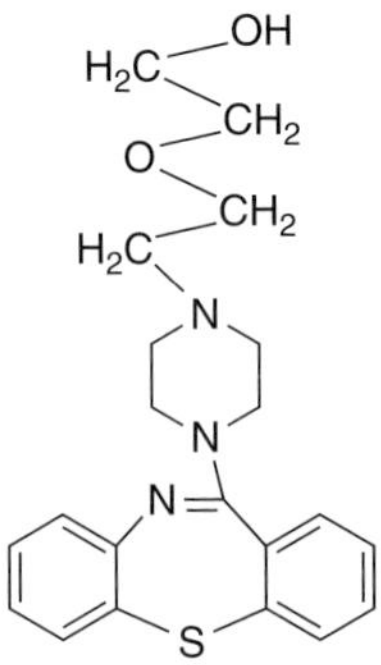

FIGURE 52-3   Molecular structure of quetiapine.

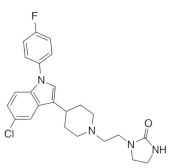

FIGURE 52-4 Molecular structure of risperidone.

FIGURE 52-5 Molecular structure of sertindole.

(Serdolect); and (2) typical traditional phenothiazine antipsychotic drugs such as **chlorpromazine** and **promethazine.**

ATYPICAL ANTIPSYCHOTIC DRUGS

Aripiprazole, clozapine, olanzapine, quetiapine, risperidone, and **sertindole**

MECHANISM OF ACTION

All of the above, except aripiprazole, block both serotonin receptors ($5HT_2$) and dopamine receptors (D2) in the brain. The mechanism of action of aripiprazole is different from the others in that it appears to activate, rather than block, the D2 receptor and the serotonin type $5\text{-}HT_{1A}$ receptor.

SIDE EFFECTS

Common side effects of these drugs include orthostatic hypotension and cardiac arrhythmia; dry mouth, nausea, vomiting, and constipation; agranulocytosis causing fever, lethargy, and sore throat; and extrapyramidal symptoms, though to a lesser degree than by typical phenothiazine antipsychotics, such as muscle stiffness (rigidity), uncontrolled muscle movements (tic-like involuntary movement), and akathisia (an inability to sit still) (note: sertindole appears to be remarkably free from these extrapyramidal symptoms); fainting and lightheadedness; and seizure. Rarely, they may cause allergic reactions such as skin rash and difficulty in breathing.

DRUG INTERACTIONS

See Appendix B-12: Interactions of Atypical Antipsychotic Drugs.

PHENOTHIAZINE ANTIPSYCHOTIC DRUGS

Chlorpromazine and **promethazine**

MECHANISM OF ACTION

The antipsychotic effects of chlorpromazine and promethazine appear to stem from their ability to block the postsynaptic dopamine receptors (type D2) in the mesolimbic system of the brain, including the amygdaloid nucleus and the hippocampus. Their antiemetic effects come from blockade of D2 receptors in the chemoreceptor trigger zone in the medulla; and the extrapyramidal symptoms that are produced as side effects come from blockade of the D2 receptors in the nigrostriatal pathway.

SIDE EFFECTS

Side effects of chlorpromazine and promethazine include dry mouth and constipation; jaundice (yellowing of the skin or eyes); stuffy nose; uncontrollable movements of the tongue, face, lips, arms, or legs; and drowsiness or fainting. Chlorpromazine may turn urine dark, and prochlorperazine turns urine red, but these changes do not indicate medical emergency.

DRUG INTERACTIONS

See Appendix B-25: Interactions of Phenothiazine Antipsychotic Drugs.

Alzheimer Disease

53

Alzheimer disease is a brain illness named after Dr. Alois Alzheimer, a German physician who in 1906 described this disorder, which encompasses a horde of symptoms including progressive memory loss, interference with thought processing, and loss of other mental functions. It is associated with degenerative changes of brain cells. Cholinergic neurons that use acetylcholine as their neurotransmitter are most affected. Alzheimer disease is the most common form of dementia for which there is no known cure.

Medications that may possibly slow the intellectual decline of Alzheimer disease include: (1) cholinesterase inhibitors (or anticholinesterase agents) such as **donepezil** (Fig. 53-1) (Aricept), **galantamine** (Reminyl) (Fig. 53-2), **rivastigmine**

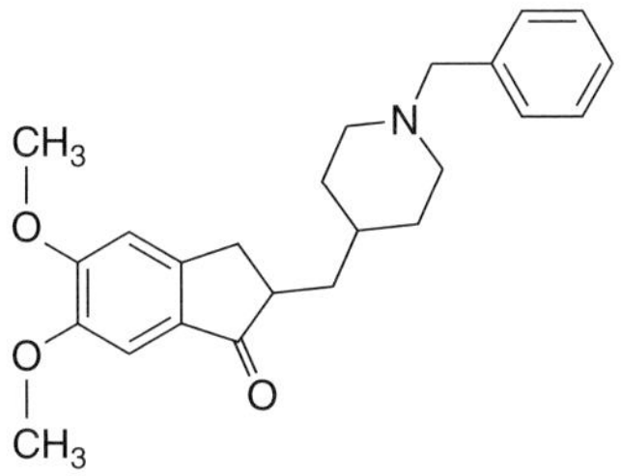

FIGURE 53-1 Molecular structure of donepezil.

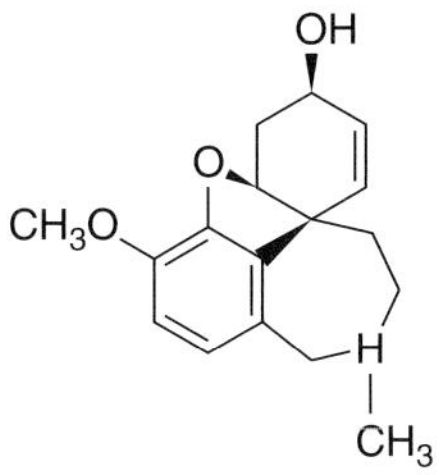

FIGURE 53-2 Molecular structure of galantamine.

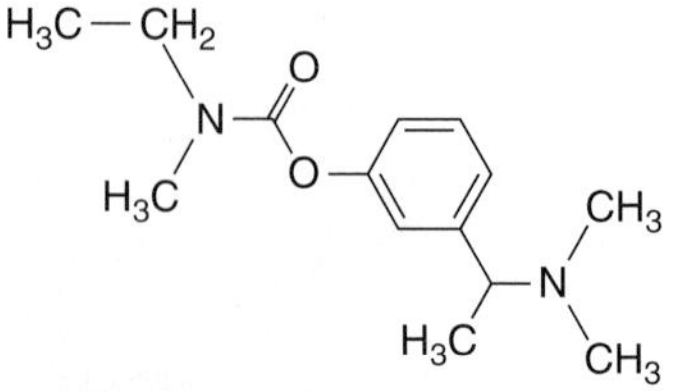

FIGURE 53-3 Molecular structure of rivastigmine.

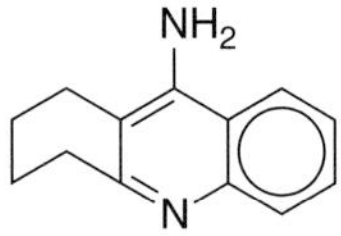

FIGURE 53-4 Molecular structure of tacrine.

(Exelon) (Fig. 53-3), and **tacrine** (Cognex) (Fig. 53-4); and (2) an N-methyl D-aspartate (NMDA) receptor antagonists such as **memantine** (Abixa, Akatinol, Axura, Ebixa, Namenda).

ANTICHOLINESTERASE AGENTS

Donepezil, **galantamine**, **rivastigmine**, and **tacrine**

MECHANISM OF ACTION

The above anticholinesterase agents decrease the activity of acetylcholinesterase, the enzyme that destroys the neurotransmitter acetylcholine (Fig. 53-5) in a number of brain regions in patients with Alzheimer disease. A significant correlation between the inhibition of acetylcholinesterase and an improvement in cognitive function was confirmed. Cholinesterase inhibitors may also increase neurotransmitter release and activate cholinergic receptors in the brain.

SIDE EFFECTS

Possible side effects of these drugs include irregular heartbeat; nausea, vomiting, abdominal pain, diarrhea, and melena (black stools); difficulty in urination; muscle cramps; visual disturbances; and mental depression and insomnia.

DRUG INTERACTIONS

See Box 53-1.

Miscellaneous Interactions of Anticholinesterase Agents (ACA)

ACA ↔ Cholinomimetic Drugs: (*See* Ω-34 in Appendix A.) If one of the above drugs is taken in conjunction with a cholinomimetic drug, such as bethanechol or pilocarpine, or with another cholinesterase inhibitor, such as neostigmine or pyridostigmine, a synergistic cholinergic adverse effect may be generated.

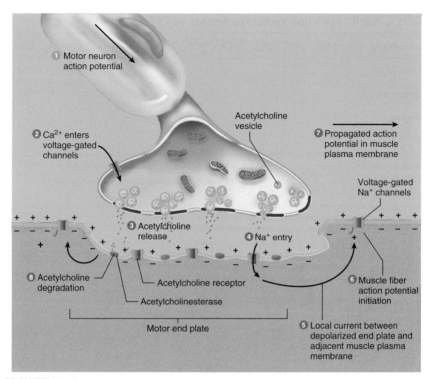

FIGURE 53-5 **Site of action of acetylcholinesterase.** Reproduced, with permission, from Barrett KE, Barman SM, Boitano S, and Brooks HL. *Ganong's Review of Medical Physiology*. 23rd ed. New York, NY: McGraw-Hill; 2010, p 125.

BOX 53-1

Basic Concepts of Anticholinesterase Agent Interactions

All the above cholinesterase inhibitors cause accumulation of acetylcholine in the brain, and when any of them is co-administered with drugs that generate anticholinergic effects in the brain, the therapeutic activities of the above cholinesterase inhibitors may be compromised. Those drugs include: **anticholinergic agents** including atropine and scopolamine (*See* Ω 14 in Appendix A.)

ACA ⟷ CYP Isozymes: *See* Table 53-1.

ACA ⟷ Haloperidol: A parkinsonian syndrome derives from cholinergic dominance over dopaminergic activity in the brain. Tacrine, and possibly others

TABLE 53-1   Anticholinesterase Agents vs CYP Enzymes

Drug Name	1A2	2A6	2B6	2C8	2C9	2C18	2C19	2D6	2E1	3A4
Donepezil								Sub		Sub
Galantamine								Sub		Sub
Tacrine	Sub + Inh									

Abbreviations: Sub, substrate of the enzyme; Inh, inhibits the enzyme; Ezi, induces the enzyme

1. Rivastigmine (not shown), unlike the others listed above, is not significantly metabolized by hepatic microsomal cytochrome (CYP) isoenzymes.
2. Both donepezil and galantamine require CYP2D6 and CYP3A4, and when either is taken together with drugs that inhibit these enzymes their blood levels may rise, exacerbating their adverse effects. (*See* the left-hand column of Table-0 at the 'Introduction' for possible inhibitors of these enzymes.)
3. Tacrine, unlike the others above, is metabolically processed through CYP1A2 and thus, inhibition of this enzyme by other drugs can raise blood levels of tacrine and potentially exacerbate its adverse effects. (*See* the left-hand column of Table-0 at the 'Introduction' for possible inhibitors of the enzyme.)
4. Tacrine, unlike the others above, exerts an inhibitory effect on CYP1A2 and thus, administration in combination with drugs that require this enzyme for metabolic clearance may result in elevated blood levels and an increase in their adverse effects. (*See* the middle column of Table-0 at the 'Introduction' for possible substrates of the enzyme.)

above, by accumulation of acetylcholine, may enhance parkinsonian syndrome caused by haloperidol, an antipsychotic medication that blocks dopamine receptors.

ACA ⟷ Levodopa: Tacrine, and possible others above, may interfere with the effectiveness of levodopa in the treatment of a parkinsonian disease, through cholinergic activities generated by the above drugs.

ACA ⟷ Succinylcholine: All of the above cholinesterase inhibitors including rivastigmine can potentiate and prolong the neuromuscular blocking effects of succinylcholine.

MEMANTINE

MECHANISM OF ACTION

One postulated etiology of Alzheimer disease is dysfunctional glutaminergic neurotransmissions, causing abnormal neuronal excitotoxicity. Memantine binds to the NMDA receptors, a glutamate receptor subfamily, to inhibit the prolonged influx of Ca^{++} ions, which is the basis of neuronal excitotoxicity.

SIDE EFFECTS

Memantine may cause a very low incidence of nausea, vomiting, and diarrhea; cystitis; muscle cramps and tiredness; and dizziness, headache, insomnia, confusion, and hallucinations.

DRUG INTERACTIONS

See Box 53-2.

Miscellaneous Interactions of Memantine (MMT)

MMT ⟷ CYP Enzymes Inhibitors: As memantine is predominantly eliminated through the kidneys, any drug that inhibits the hepatic CYP450 enzyme system is not expected to alter clearance of memantine.

BOX 53-2

Basic Concepts of Memantine Interactions

1. Memantine is a basic drug (Fig. 53-6) that is apt to be nonionized in alkaline pH, and when co-administered with drugs that generate alkaline urine, the nonionized drug diffuses back into circulation to raise its blood levels, exacerbating its adverse effects. Those alkalinizing drugs include: **acetazolamide** (Diamox), a carbonic anhydrase inhibitor, and **sodium bicarbonate.**

2. Memantine is a low-affinity antagonist at the NMDA receptors, activation of which is required for glutaminergic central nervous system (CNS) transmission for memory and sensation of pain. Co-administration of memantine with any other drugs that have an antagonistic effect on the NMDA receptor may result in amplified adverse CNS effects such as profound and long-lasting sedations. Those drugs include: **amantadine** (an antiviral agent); **dextromethorphan** (a cough suppressant), and **ketamine** (an anesthetic agent).

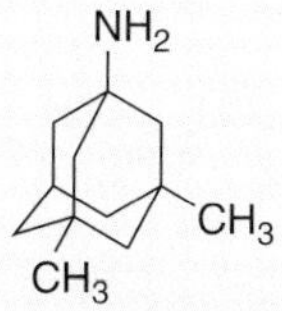

FIGURE 53-6   Molecular structure of memantine.

CHAPTER

54   Memory Impairment

Declining memory is a general trend in advanced age (age-associated memory impairment), for which there is no specific recommendable drug. Current drug therapy aims at treating causes of memory loss, such as diabetes, high cholesterol, thyroid dysfunction, and so forth.

Medications that may possibly be effective in reversing or slowing memory impairment include: (1) **bifemelane,** a gamma-aminobutyric acid (GABA) derivative; (2) **piracetam** (Dinagen, Myocalm, Nebracetam, Nootropil, Qropi) or **oxiracetam**, a piracetam analog, which is more potent than piracetam, requiring a smaller dose; (3) **piribedil** (Trivastal), a dopamine agonist; (4) **ergoloid mesylates** (Hydergine, Gerimal); (5) **idebenone;** and (6) **vinpocetine.**

GABA DERIVATIVE

Bifemelane

MECHANISM OF ACTION

Bifemelane (Fig. 54-1) is a derivative of GABA, an inhibitory brain neurotransmitter. Bifemelane appears to prevent neuronal damage following transient ischemia to the brain. If memory impairment is caused by poor circulation to the brain with insufficient oxygenation in the brain cells, bifemelane may help improve memory.

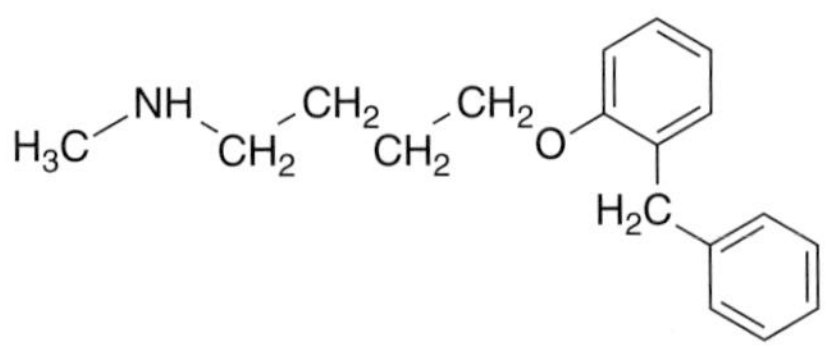

FIGURE 54-1   Molecular structure of bifemelane.

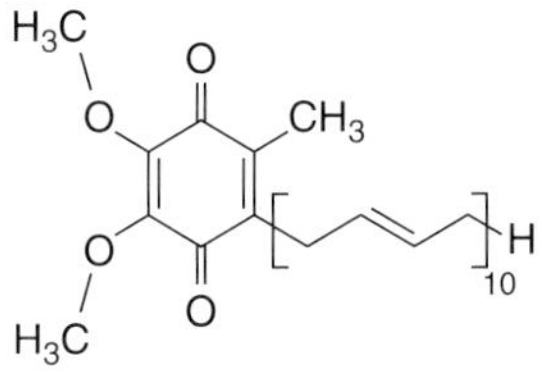

FIGURE 54-3 Molecular structure of CoQ10.

VINPOCETINE

Vinpocetine (Fig. 54-4) is a synthetic ethyl ester of apovincamine, a vinca alkaloid. It aims to relieve cognitive deficits caused by hypoxia and ischemia.

MECHANISM OF ACTION

Vinpocetine was shown to selectively increase brain circulation and oxygenation, without such alteration on systemic circulation. Vinpocetine is a selective inhibitor of a phosphodiesterase that destroys cyclic-GMP and thus, vinpocetine accumulates c-GMP in the vascular smooth muscle to cause vasodilation with consequent reduction of resistance to the cerebral blood flow. If memory impairment is caused by poor circulation with insufficient oxygenation in the brain cells, vinpocetine may help improve memory. Vinpocetine also increases tolerance of the brain toward ischemia and hypoxia, and this drug may prevent neuronal damage following transient ischemia to the brain.

SIDE EFFECTS

Side effects of Vinpocetine may include a temporary drop in blood pressure and facial flushing; dry mouth, indigestion, and nausea; and dizziness, drowsiness, lightheadedness, anxiety, headache, and insomnia.

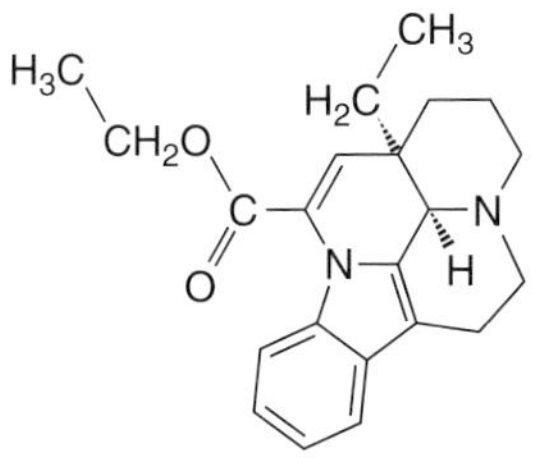

FIGURE 54-4 Molecular structure of vinpocetine.

DRUG INTERACTIONS

As vinpocetine can decrease platelet aggregation, it can potentiate the effects of blood thinning agents to cause excessive bleeding when administered together. Such blood thinners include clopidogrel, dicumarol, ticlopidine, and warfarin. Herbs that would interact similarly include fenugreek, feverfew, garlic, ginger, ginkgo, ginseng, and turmeric (Fig. 54-5 A and B).

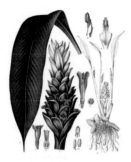

FIGURE 54-5   A, Turmeric Flower.
(http://schools-wikipedia.org/images/609/60977.jpg.htm)

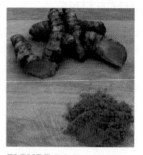

FIGURE 54-5   B, Turmeric Roots.
(Courtesy of Ammini Ramachandran at
http://www.sallybernstein.com/food/columns/
ramachandran/turmeric.htm)

Epilepsy

Epilepsy is a brain disorder in which brain nerve cells fire electrical impulses at a rate up to four times faster than normal. Therefore, epilepsy is characterized by seizures that often manifest as convulsions, and clouded or loss of consciousness, and/or other psychic disturbances.

Medications shown effective in the treatment of epilepsy include: (1) **divalproex** (Depakote); (2) **gabapentin** (Neurontin, Gabarone) or **levetiracetam** (Keppra) or **pregabalin** (3) sodium-channel blockers such as **carbamazepine, lamotrigine** (Lamictal), **oxcarbazepine** (Trileptal), and **phenytoin** (Dilantin); (4) **phenobarbital** or **topiramate** (Topamax); and (5) benzodiazepines such as **clonazepam** and **lorazepam**.

DIVALPROEX

Divalproex (*See* Fig. 51-1) consists of sodium valproate and valproic acid in a 1:1 molar ratio, and sodium valproate is rapidly converted to valproic acid (Fig. 55-1) in the stomach. So, both divalproex and valproic acid produce identical effects, but divalproex is released and absorbed from the intestine more slowly than valproic acid.

MECHANISM OF ACTION

Valproic acid can block the T-type calcium channels as well as the sodium channels in the epileptic brain.

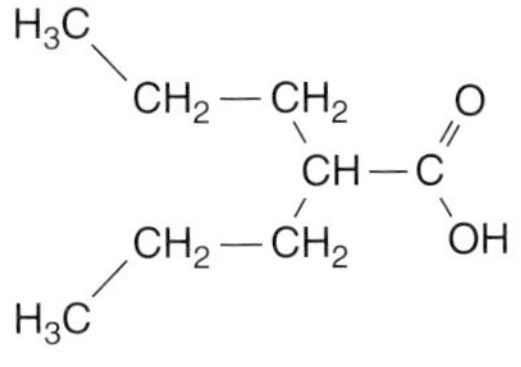

FIGURE 55-1 Molecular structure of valproic acid.

SIDE EFFECTS

Possible side effects include flu symptoms; nausea, vomiting, and stomach pain; jaundice (yellowing of the skin or eyes); tremor; fever and chills; confusion; fainting; and hallucinations.

DRUG INTERACTIONS

See Chapter 51.

GABAPENTIN OR LEVETIRACETAM OR PREGABALIN

Gabapentin and levetiracetam were originally developed to treat epilepsy but currently they are often used to relieve pain of neuropathic origin as well. Pregabalin (Lyrica) is indicated to treat partial seizures.

MECHANISM OF ACTION

Though similar in structure to gamma-aminobutyric acid (GABA), gabapentin (Fig. 55-2) does not bind to GABA receptors in the central nervous system (CNS) or have direct agonistic activity. The exact antiepileptic mechanisms for gabapentin and levetiracetam are unknown, but they appear to modulate presynaptic P/Q-type calcium channel to reduce the release of excitatory neurotransmitters such as glutamic acid (Fig. 55-3) and aspartic acid (Fig. 55-4) in the brain. Pregabalin is a GABA analog and increases brain levels of GABA by increasing in glutamic acid decarboxylase activity.

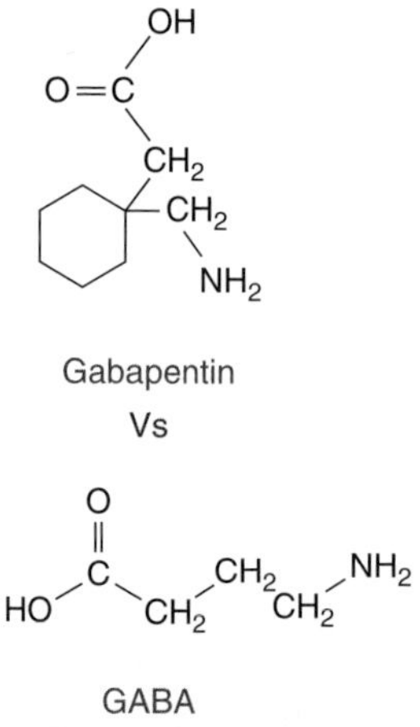

FIGURE 55-2 Molecular structure of gabapentin vs GABA.

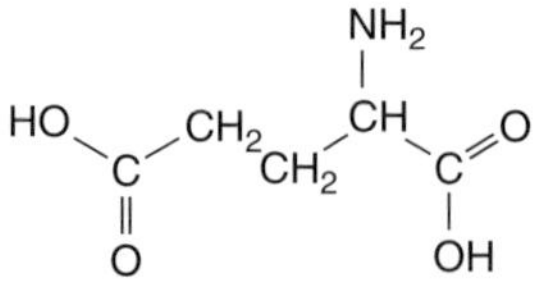

FIGURE 55-3 Molecular structure of glutamic acid.

BOX 55-1 (continued)

methadone (a narcotic analgesic drug and a substrate of CYP2B6 , CYP2C19, and CYP3A4); **naproxen** (an NSAID and a substrate of CYP1A2); **ritonavir** (an anti-HIV drug and a substrate of CYP3A4); **tolbutamide** (an antidiabetic drug and a substrate of CYP2C19); **triazolam** (a hypnotic and a substrate of CYP3A4); and **verapamil** (a drug to lower blood pressure, to treat angina pectoris and cardiac arrhythmia, and a substrate of CYP1A2 and CYP3A4).

2. Phenytoin is extensively (90%) bound to proteins, and when co-administered with drugs that oppose its protein-binding or displace it from its binding sites, it will raise blood levels and increase the adverse effects of phenytoin. Those drugs include: **acitretin** (a drug to treat severe psoriasis that may reduce the protein binding of phenytoin); **mycophenolate mofetil** (Fig. 55-8) (which can decrease protein binding of phenytoin]; and **valproic acid** (which can displace phenytoin from its protein-biding sites).

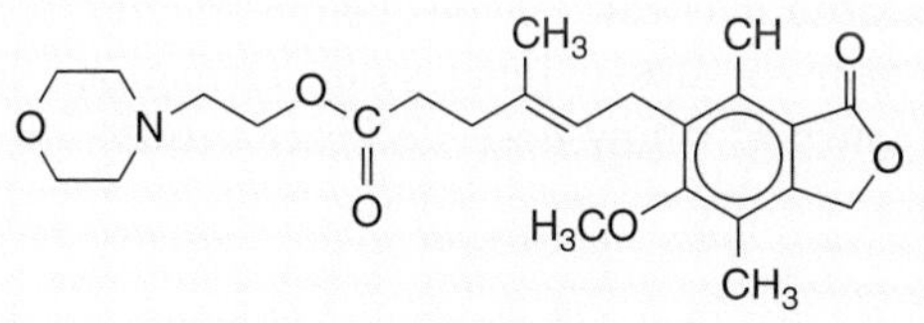

FIGURE 55-8 Molecular structure of mycophenolate mofetil .

PTN ⟷ Thyroid Preparations: (*See* Ω-75 in Appendix A.) Phenytoin, an enzyme inducer, may quicken the metabolism of thyroid hormones, resulting in lowered serum levels of thyroid hormones with consequent relapse of hypothyroidism. Furthermore, phenytoin may also displace thyroid hormones from the sites of thyroxine binding globulin to temporarily elevate blood levels of levothyroxine.

PHENOBARBITAL OR TOPIRAMATE

Phenobarbital is used to treat tonic-clonic seizure and infantile or childhood seizures. Topiramate is mainly used to treat partial seizures.

MECHANISM OF ACTION

Phenobarbital: It binds to the alpha subunit of the $GABA_A$ receptor, a separate site from the binding site for GABA or for benzodiazepine (*See* Fig. 46-2). Phenobarbital thereby potentiates the effect of GABA at its receptor.

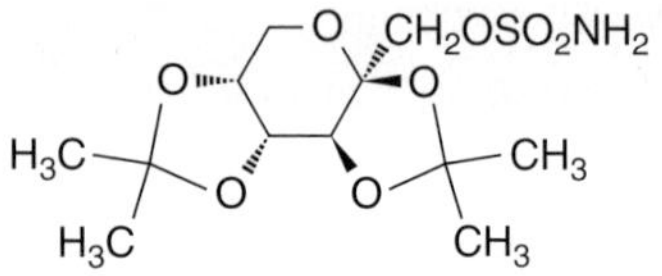

FIGURE 55-9   Molecular structure of topiramate.

Topiramate: It (Fig. 55-9) blocks voltage-dependent sodium channels, and also enhances activity of GABA by binding to one of its subunits.

SIDE EFFECTS

Phenobarbital: Its side effects may include difficulty in breathing and swallowing; upset stomach, vomiting, constipation; severe skin rash; and drowsiness and dizziness.

Topiramate: This drug may cause hypokalemia (rarely); taste changes, loss of appetite; stomach pain or upset; renal stone formation; decreased sweating; flu-like symptoms (such as runny nose; and sore throat); dizziness, drowsiness; and tiredness.

DRUG INTERACTIONS
Phenobarbital (PBT)

PBT ⬌ Alcohol: Phenobarbital may potentiate the CNS depressant effects of alcohol.

PBT ⬌ CYP Enzymes: *See* Table 55-2.

PBT ⬌ Narcotic Analgesics: (*See* Ω-52 in Appendix A.) If a narcotic analgesic is taken with phenobarbital, a deepened CNS depression will result.

PBT ⬌ Probenecid: Probenecid (*See* Fig. 39-4), an acidic drug, competes with phenobarbital (Fig. 55-10), another acidic drug, for renal tubular secretion, interfering with the elimination of phenobarbital.

PBT ⬌ Quinine: About 25% of an administered dose of phenobarbital is cleared by the kidney as unaltered drug, and in patients with severe renal impairment the dose of phenobarbital should be reduced. Quinine, which induces mild renal impairment, may increase the serum levels and adverse effects of phenobarbital.

TABLE 55-2 Phenobarbital vs CYP Enzymes

Drug Name	1A2	2A6	2B6	2C8	2C9	2C18	2C19	2D6	2E1	3A4
Phenobarbital					Sub+		Sub+			
	Ezi	Ezi	Ezi	Ezi	Ezi		Ezi			Ezi

Abbreviations: Sub, substrate of the enzyme; Inh, inhibits the enzyme; Ezi, induces the enzyme

1. Phenobarbital is a potent inducer of several microsomal enzymes including CYP1A2, 2A6, 2B6, 2C8, 2C9, 2C19, and CYP3A4 and thus, co-administration of phenobarbital with drugs that utilize any of these enzymes for clearance may quicken their elimination to possibly lower their blood levels to insufficient therapeutic efficacies: For instance, phenobarbital may quicken elimination of ethinyl estradiol and norethindrone, both substrates of CYP3A4, which are often found in oral contraceptive pills, to result in lowered blood concentrations and potential failure of contraceptive effectiveness. (*See* the middle column of Table-0 at the 'Introduction' for other possible substrates of these enzymes.)

2. Chronic use of phenobarbital, by induction of CYP1A2, may promote oxidation of acetaminophen to generate a metabolite that is hepatotoxic and nephrotoxic.

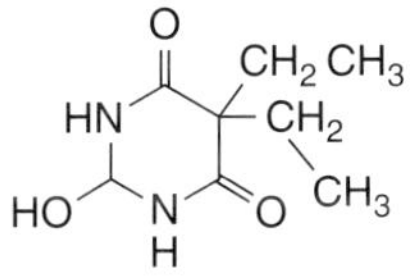

FIGURE 55-10   Molecular structure of phenobarbital.

PBT ⟷ Telithromycin: Concurrent administration of phenobarbital, an inducer of CYP3A4, can quicken elimination of telithromycin, a substrate of CYP3A4, to result in lowered blood levels and insufficient therapeutic efficacy.

Topiramate

See Box 55-2.

BOX 55-2

Basic Concepts of Topiramate Interactions

Topiramate can cause alkaline urine, which may induce kidney stones, and when taken in combination with drugs that also make urine alkaline, it can increase the risk of renal stone formation. Those drugs include: **acetazolamide** and **brinzolamide** (both carbonic anhydrase inhibitors).

TABLE 55-3 Topiramate vs CYP Isozymes

Drug Name	1A2	2A6	2B6	2C8	2C9	2C18	2C19	2D6	2E1	3A4
Topiramate							Sub+ Inh			Sub+ Ezi

Abbreviations: Sub, substrate of the enzyme; Inh, inhibits the enzyme; Ezi, induces the enzyme

1. Though topiramate is not extensively metabolized and is excreted largely through urine, it is a weak inhibitor of CYP2C19 and thus, co-administration with other drugs that require this enzyme for hepatic clearance may raise their blood levels and potentially exacerbate their adverse effects. Those drugs include: mephenytoin and omeprazole. (*See* the middle column of Table-0 at the 'Introduction' for other possible substrates of the enzyme.)

2. Topiramate induces CYP3A4 and thereby increases the metabolic clearance of such estrogens as ethinyl estradiol and mestranol, potentially leading to contraception failure.

Miscellaneous Interactions of Topiramate (TPM)

TPM ⟷ Alcohol: Topiramate can cause CNS depression, and should be used with extreme caution if combined with alcohol or any other CNS depressant.

TPM ⟷ CYP Isozymes: *See* Table 55-3.

TPM ⟷ Diuretics (*See* Ω-49 and Ω-73 in Appendix A.) Hypokalemia (serum potassium level below 3.5 mmol/L) was observed in 0.4% of patients treated with topiramate. Decrease in serum potassium may become excessive when topiramate is taken with potassium-lowering diuretics such as hydrochlorothiazide and loop diuretics.

BENZODIAZEPINES

Clonazepam and lorazepam

Clonazepam is used to treat absence seizures and agoraphobia. Lorazepam is mainly used to suppress status epilepticus.

MECHANISM OF ACTION

They bind to the benzodiazepine-binding site of the GABA receptor complex to interact allosterically with GABA receptors, enhancing activity of the inhibitory neurotransmitter GABA. This effect increases the influx of chloride ions into the neurons to hyperpolarize them, with consequent suppression of neuronal activity in the ascending reticular activating system, the cortex, and the limbic system.

SIDE EFFECTS

Their side effects may include constipation; lack of muscular coordination and speech problems; drowsiness, dizziness, fatigue, and anxiety; and rarely, they may cause allergic reactions.

DRUG INTERACTIONS

See Appendix B-16: Interactions of Benzodiazepines.

CHAPTER

56

Parkinson Disease

Parkinson disease is named after Dr. James Parkinson, an English physician who originally described the symptoms in 1817. The disease is a progressive neurologic disorder characterized by muscle rigidity, pain, tremor, bradykinesia (slow movements), and postural abnormalities. Parkinson disease is caused by degeneration of the substantia nigra (a portion of the brain, literally meaning "dark tissue"), with resultant decrease in brain levels of dopamine. This paucity of dopamine allows the cholinergic output to dominate the central nervous system (CNS), which controls muscle movement.

Medications shown effective in the treatment of Parkinson disease include: (1) **levodopa** (Dopar, Larodopa); (2) anticholinergic medications such as **benztropine** (Cogentin) and **trihexyphenidyl** (Artane, Trihexane); (3) dopamine releasers such as **amantadine** (Symmetrel); (4) dopamine agonists such as **bromocriptine** (Parlodel), **pramipexole** (Mirapex), and **ropinirole** (Requip); and (5) MAO-B inhibitors such as **rasagiline** (Azilect) and **selegiline** (Carbex, Eldepryl).

LEVODOPA

L-dopa (or L-dihydroxyphenylalanine) (Fig. 56-1), if used alone, is quickly converted by dopa decarboxylase to dopamine (Fig. 56-2) in the cytosol outside of the brain. Dopamine thus formed cannot enter the brain to raise its dopamine levels. To prevent this conversion and promote the entry of L-dopa into the brain, L-dopa is always administered in combination with an inhibitor of dopa decarboxylase, such as **carbidopa** (Sinemet) or **benserazide.** Further, since L-dopa

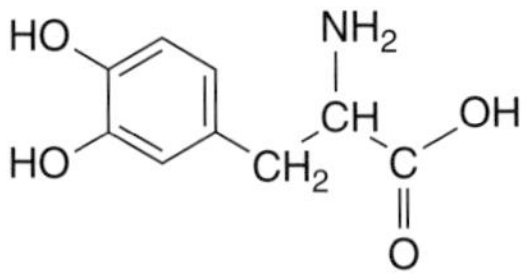

FIGURE 56-1 Molecular structure of DOPA.

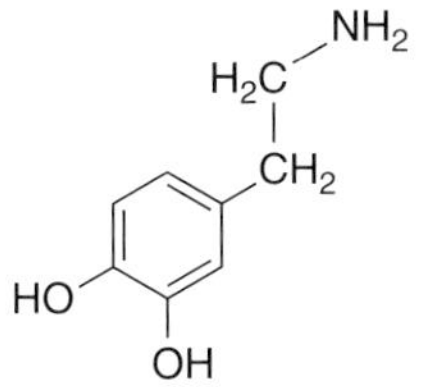

FIGURE 56-2 Molecular structure of dopamine.

can be converted by the enzyme catechol-O-methyltransferase (COMT) to 3-O-methyldopa, which competes with L-dopa to interfere with its transportation into the brain, the so-called COMT inhibitors, such as **entacapone** (Comtan) and **tolcapone** (Tasmar), are also often used in combination.

MECHANISM OF ACTION

L-dopa, once entered into the brain, is converted to dopamine by internal dopa decarboxylase, raising its levels in the substantia nigra.

SIDE EFFECTS

Levodopa + Carbidopa + Entacapone (or **Tolcapone):** The frequent side effects of this combination include altered sense of taste, nausea, and vomiting; increased sweating; dizziness, nervousness, insomnia, and nightmares. Levodopa may turn urine red, but this does not usually indicate medical emergency.

DRUG INTERACTIONS

See Box 56-1.

Miscellaneous Interactions of Levodopa + Carbidopa + Entacapone (or Tolcapone) (LCT)

Parentheses below indicate an herb.

LCT ⟷ Antipsychotic Drugs: Many antipsychotic drugs such as clozapine, haloperidol, olanzapine, and quetiapine block dopamine receptors to offset the antiparkinsonian effect of levodopa. Thus, they should not be used in combination.

LCT ⟷ (Chasteberry): Certain chemicals in chasteberry are known to occupy dopamine receptors in the brain to prevent binding of dopamine to its receptors. Thus, this herb may undercut the therapeutic efficacy of levodopa.

BOX 56-1

Basic Concepts of Levodopa + Carbidopa + Entacapone (or Tolcapone) Interactions

1. Intestinal absorption of levodopa may be impaired by combined intake with drugs that have anticholinergic effects that decrease gastric motility. Those drugs include: **dicyclomine** (an anticholinergic drug useful to relieve GI spasms); **oxybutynin** (an anticholinergic drug to reduce muscle spasms of the bladder and urinary tract); and **phenothiazine antipsychotic agents** (many of them have anticholinergic effects). (*See* Ω-58 in Appendix A.)

2. Levodopa is converted to dopamine to activate dopamine receptors. When co-administered with drugs that generate dopamine-like effects, they may lead to the so-called "L-dopa-induced dyskinesia," characterized by various hyperkinetic movements such as chorea, dystonia, myoclonus; ataxia; and confusion. Those drugs include: **amantadine** (a drug used to treat influenza viral infections); **pergolide** (a dopamine receptor agonist used to treat parkinsonism); **pramipexole** (a dopamine receptor agonist used to treat parkinsonism); and **ropinirole (Requip)** (a dopamine receptor agonist used to treat parkinsonism).

LCT ⟷ Ethaverine: Ethaverine inhibits activity of tyrosine hydroxylase, the enzyme that catalyzes the conversion of tyrosine (Fig. 56-3) to dopa (*See* Fig. 56-1), the precursor of endogenous dopamine (*See* Fig. 56-2). Hence, ethaverine may undermine the production and effectiveness of levodopa, worsening the parkinsonian symptoms.

LCT ⟷ Halothane: Both L-dopa and dopamine have arrhythmogenic potential. The use of halothane, an anesthetic agent, in combination can enhance the cardiac arrhythmias because halothane sensitizes myocardium to the arrhythmogenic effect of the above catecholamines (L-dopa and dopamine).

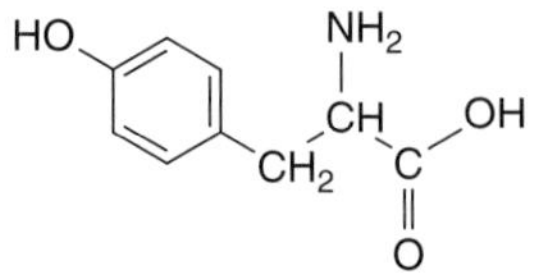

FIGURE 56-3   Molecular structure of tyrosine.

LCT ⟷ Iron Salts: Iron can bind levodopa to reduce its bioavailability and thereby reduce the pharmacologic effects of levodopa. Combination of the two for oral administration is contraindicated.

LCT ⟷ MAO Inhibitors: (*See* Ω-51 in Appendix A.) Concurrent intake of the above preparation with a drug that has an inhibitory effect on the enzyme MAO-A, such as furazolidone (a drug used to treat bacterial and protozoal infections) or linezolid (an antibiotic), may enhance the adverse effects of levodopa, leading to hypertensive crisis for which prompt administration of an alpha blocker such as phentolamine (Regitine) may be of help.

LCT ⟷ Metoclopramide: Metoclopramide may increase intestinal absorption of levodopa to enhance its therapeutic efficacy and adverse effects.

LCT ⟷ Pyridoxine: Pyridoxine (or vitamin B-6) accelerates conversion of L-dopa to dopamine, which is unable to cross the blood-brain barrier to get into the brain, and thereby undercuts the therapeutic effectiveness of levodopa.

LCT ⟷ Tacrine: Concomitant use of levodopa with tacrine, a centrally-acting anticholinesterase agent that accumulates acetylcholine in the brain, may oppose the effectiveness of levodopa via enhanced cholinergic activity over dopaminergic activity.

ANTICHOLINERGIC MEDICATIONS

Benztropine and **trihexyphenidyl**

MECHANISM OF ACTION

The activity of cholinergic neurons is predominant over dopaminergic neurons in parkinsonian patients. Thus, anticholinergic agents are used to treat the cholinergic symptoms of parkinsonism and to suppress dopa-induced extrapyramidal reactions other than tardive dyskinesia.

SIDE EFFECTS

Frequent side effects of these drugs include tachycardia (racing heartbeat); difficulty in breathing; constipation with stomach or intestinal cramps; difficulty in urination; hot, dry skin without sweating; and confusion and hallucination.

DRUG INTERACTIONS

See Box 56-2.

BOX 56-2

Basic Concepts of Benztropine or Trihexyphenidyl Interactions

1. Both benztropine and trihexyphenidyl have anticholinergic effects that delay gastric emptying and therefore, may decrease absorption of some drugs taken in combination. Those potentially affected drugs include: **chlorpromazine** (an antipsychotic agent whose blood levels may fall short to worsen schizophrenic symptoms); **haloperidol** (an antipsychotic agent); and **levodopa** (a drug for Parkinson disease).

2. Both benztropine and trihexyphenidyl have anticholinergic effects. When either is co-administered with other drugs that also generate anticholinergic effects, they may result in excessive anticholinergic symptoms such as dry mouth, constipation, blurred vision, and hyperthermia especially in hot weather. Those drugs include: **amantadine** (a dopamine-releaser that also has an anticholinergic effect); **promethazine** (an antihistamine); and **tricyclic antidepressants** (See Ω-76 in Appendix A). (Note: most of these tricyclic antidepressant drugs have peripheral anticholinergic effects as well).

Miscellaneous Interactions of Benztropine or Trihexyphenidyl (BTP)

BTP ⟷ Digoxin: Digoxin undergoes degradation in gastric juice. Benztropine and, to a lesser extent, trihexyphenidyl may decrease gastric degradation of digoxin and raise the total amount of digoxin absorbed, although they slow gastric emptying of digoxin, delaying its absorption from the small intestine.

BTP ⟷ Galantamine: As galantamine has an inhibitory effect on acetylcholinesterase to accumulate acetylcholine, its concurrent use with these anticholinergic agents may undercut their therapeutic benefits.

BTP ⟷ Tacrine: The therapeutic effectiveness of benztropine and trihexyphenidyl may be counteracted by tacrine, a centrally-acting anticholinesterase agent that accumulates acetylcholine in the brain and a drug useful in the treatment of Alzheimer disease.

AMANTADINE

MECHANISM OF ACTION

Amantadine is known to promote the release of stored dopamine to activate its receptors in the brain.

SIDE EFFECTS

Frequent side effects of amantadine include fast or uneven heartbeat; feeling short of breath; dry nose and mouth; loss of appetite, nausea, and constipation; and muscle tremor; and dizziness.

DRUG INTERACTIONS

See Box 56-3.

Miscellaneous Interactions of Amantadine (AMT)

Parentheses below indicate an herb.

AMT ⟷ Alcohol: Administration of amantadine in combination with alcohol may generate exaggerated CNS depressant effects.

AMT ⟷ (Chasteberry): Certain chemicals in chasteberry occupy dopamine receptors in the brain to prevent dopamine from binding to the receptors. Thus, use of amantadine in combination with this herb might interfere with therapeutic effectiveness of amantadine.

BOX 56-3

Basic Concepts of Amantadine Interactions

1. Amantadine has its own anticholinergic effect, and when co-administered with drugs that also generate an anticholinergic effect, they may lead to excessive anticholinergic symptoms such as dry mouth, constipation, blurred vision, and hyperthermia especially in hot weather. Those drugs include: **benztropine** (a drug to relieve symptoms of Parkinson disease); **dicyclomine** (a drug to relieve spasm of the muscles in the GI tract); **oxybutynin** (an anticholinergic agent useful to reduce muscle spasm of the lower urinary tract); **scopolamine;** and **trihexyphenidyl** (an anticholinergic drug used in the treatment of parkinsonism).

2. Amantadine is a dopamine-releaser, and when co-administered with drugs that accumulate dopamine, they may lead to excessive dopaminergic symptoms such as nausea, vomiting, hypotension, and tachycardia. Those drugs include: **levodopa** and **trihexyphenidyl** (an antiparkinsonian drug of the antimuscarinic class that also blocks dopamine reuptake).

AMT ⟷ Influenza Virus Vaccine: Don't administer the influenza virus vaccine until 48 hours after termination of amantadine therapy, or do not initiate amantadine therapy until two weeks after the influenza virus vaccine is received. Otherwise, it may interfere with amantadine therapy.

AMT ⟷ Levodopa: Amantadine and levodopa used in combination may potentiate dopaminergic side effects or may exacerbate pre-existing dyskinesias, ataxia, and confusion.

AMT ⟷ Quinidine: Quinidine was shown to reduce renal clearance of amantadine by about 30%. Thus, quinidine may increase the serum levels and toxicity of amantadine, including symptoms such as ataxia and confusion.

AMT ⟷ Risperidone: In large overdoses, amantadine causes widening of the QRS complex and prolongation of the Q-T interval, as does risperidone, an atypical antipsychotic drug that has a propensity to cause seizures. When taken in combination, they may cause greater incidences of elongated Q-T interval and seizures.

AMT ⟷ Triamterene: Triamterene, a potassium-sparing diuretic, may reduce glomerular filtration rate and renal plasma flow, to interrupt renal clearance of amantadine, raising its blood levels and incidences of such side effects as dry mouth, dizziness, ataxia, myoclonus, visual hallucination, and confusion.

DOPAMINE AGONISTS

Bromocriptine (Fig. 56-4), **pramipexole** (Fig. 56-5), and **ropinirole** (Fig. 56-6)

MECHANISM OF ACTION

They are synthetic dopamine agonists that can directly activate dopamine receptors in the substantia nigra to mimic the effects of natural dopamine in this part of the brain.

SIDE EFFECTS

Their possible side effects include irregular pulse; shortness of breath with pulmonary infiltrate (especially with bromocriptine); dry mouth, stomach cramps, nausea, and constipation; involuntary muscle movements; dizziness, drowsiness (sudden irresistible urge to sleep), and headache.

DRUG INTERACTIONS

See Appendix B-23: Interactions of Dopamine Agonists.

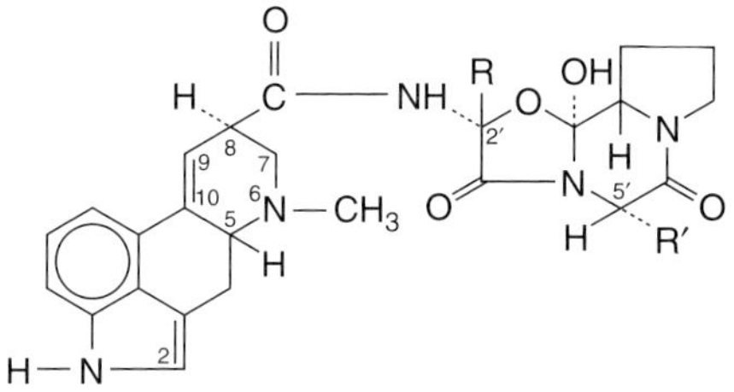

Alkaloid[§]	R(2′)	R′(5′)
Ergotamine	—CH$_3$	—CH$_2$—phenyl
Ergosine	—CH$_3$	—CH$_2$CH(CH$_3$)$_2$
Ergostine	—Ch$_2$CH$_3$	—CH$_2$—phenyl
Ergotoxine group:		
Ergocornine	—CH(CH$_3$)$_2$	—CH(CH$_3$)$_2$
Ergocristine	—CH(CH$_3$)$_2$	—CH$_2$—phenyl
α-Ergocryptine	—CH(CH$_3$)$_2$	—CH$_2$CH(CH$_3$)$_2$

β-Ergocryptine	CH(CH$_3$)$_2$	—CHCH$_2$CH$_3$
		   |
		   CH$_3$

Bromocriptine[¶]	—CH(CH$_3$)$_2$	—CH$_2$CH(CH$_3$)$_2$

FIGURE 56-4   **Molecular structures of ergot alkaloids.** Reproduced, with permission, from Brunton LL, Lazo JS, and Parker KL. *Goodman and Gilman's The Pharmacological Basis of Therapeutics*. 11th ed. New York, NY: McGraw-Hill; 2006, p 310.

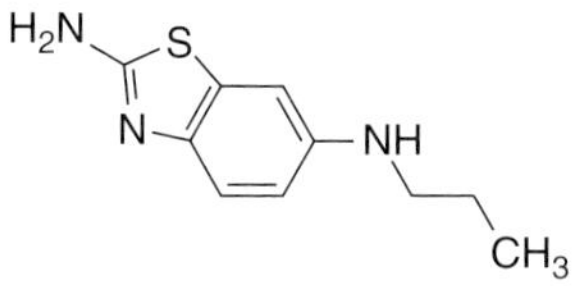

FIGURE 56-5   Molecular structure of pramipexole.

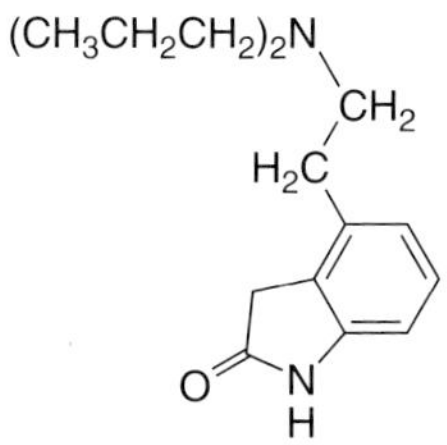

FIGURE 56-6   Molecular structure of ropinirole.

MAO-B INHIBITORS

Rasagiline and **selegiline**

MECHANISM OF ACTION

Dopamine in the brain is oxidatively destroyed mainly by MAO-B (Fig. 56-7). Both selegiline and rasagiline preferentially inhibit this enzyme, opposing the inactivation of dopamine and thereby raising its concentrations in the brain.

SIDE EFFECTS:

Rasagiline: Its side effects include hypotension; dry mouth, vomiting, upset stomach, and constipation; joint pain; hallucinations; and skin rash.

Selegiline: It may cause vomiting, constipation; twitching muscle movements; hallucinations, and seizure. Rarely, it may also cause allergic reactions.

DRUG INTERACTIONS

Rasagiline (RGL)

RGL ⟷ CYP Isozymes: *See* Table 56-1.

RGL ⟷ Selective Serotonin Reuptake Inhibitors (SSRIs): (*See* Ω-68 in Appendix A.) Rasagiline, though it is a relatively selective MAO-B inhibitor, may also oppose, at its high doses, inactivation of serotonin by MAO-A (Fig. 56-8), the serotonin accumulated by any of the SSRIs used in combination, so as to contribute to development of serotonin syndrome.

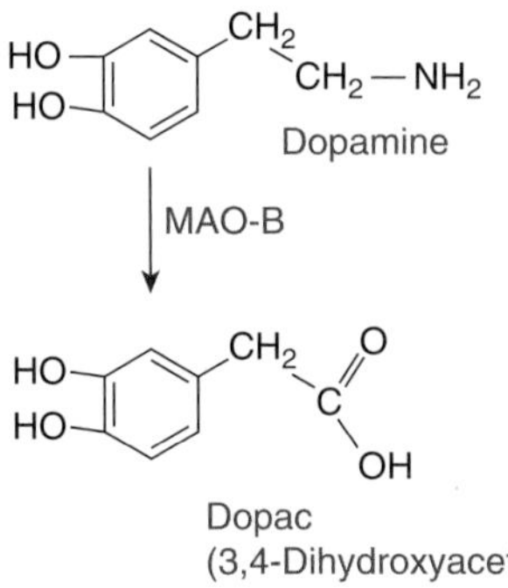

FIGURE 56-7   Molecular structure of DOPAC.

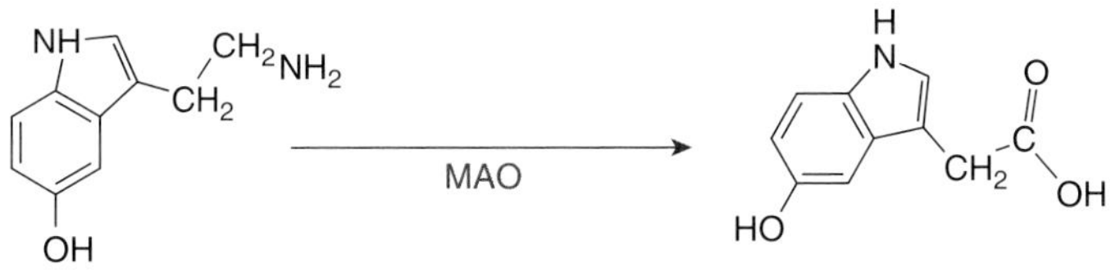

FIGURE 56-8   Serotonin oxidation by MAO.

TABLE 56-1   Rasagiline vs CYP Enzymes

Drug Name	1A2	2A6	2B6	2C8	2C9	2C18	2C19	2D6	2E1	3A4
Rasagiline	Sub									

Abbreviations: Sub, substrate of the enzyme; Inh, inhibits the enzyme; Ezi, induces the enzyme

1. Co-administration of rasagiline, a drug that requires CYP1A2 for its clearance, with a drug that inhibits this enzyme, may result in elevated blood levels of unmetabolized rasagiline, exacerbating its adverse effects. Such inhibitors include ciprofloxacin, mirtazapine, and tranylcypromine. (*See* the left-hand column of Table-0 at the 'Introduction' for other possible inhibitors of this enzyme.)

2. Rasagiline requires CYP1A2 for its metabolic clearance, as do clomipramine and cyclobenzaprine. Co-administration of rasagiline with either of these drugs may cause competition for the same enzyme for clearance, potentially resulting in elevated blood levels of unmetabolized rasagiline that might exacerbate its adverse effects. (*See* the middle column of Table-0 at the 'Introduction' for other possible substrates of the enzyme.)

RGL ⟷ Pseudoephedrine: Rasagiline, a relatively selective MAO-B inhibitor, may also oppose, at its high doses, inactivation of pseudoephedrine by MAO-A, to raise blood levels and incidences of the adverse effects of pseudoephedrine.

Selegiline: *See* Chapter 49.

CHAPTER

57

Vertigo

Vertigo is a type of dizziness, causing a spinning sensation that is due to malfunction of the semicircular canals of the inner ear required for physical balance. Vertigo may also be a symptom of many different illnesses and disorders. It is often associated with nausea, vomiting, and ringing in one or both ears.

Medications that may be effective in the treatment of vertigo include: (1) antihistaminic antiemetics such as **dimenhydrinate** (Dramamine), **meclizine** (Antivert, Bonine), and **promethazine** (Phenergan); (2) **betahistine,** a newer drug often prescribed for vertigo and dizziness; (3) **piracetam** (Nootropil), an analog of gamma-aminobutyric acid (GABA); (4) anticholinergic agents such as **scopolamine** (Transderm-Scop); and (5) **vinpocetine.**

ANTIHISTAMININIC ANTIEMETICS

Dimenhydrinate, **meclizine**, and **promethazine**

MECHANISM OF ACTION

The three most important neurotransmitters in the vestibulo-ocular reflex arc are glutamate, acetylcholine, and GABA. Glutamate is thought to maintain the basic resting tone of the central vestibular neurons, whereas acetylcholine appears to function as an excitatory in its synapses, and GABA, inhibitory. These antihistamines, by virtue of their central anticholinergic effect, may function as vestibular suppressants at the medial vestibular nucleus.

SIDE EFFECTS

Frequent side effects of antihistaminic drugs include cardiac arrhythmia; dry mouth and loss of appetite; jaundice (yellowing of the skin or eyes); urinary retention; goose bumps; blurred vision; chills; and drowsiness, dizziness, confusion, and hallucinations. Promethazine may turn urine blue-green, but this does not usually indicate medical emergency.

DRUG INTERACTIONS

See Appendix B-10 Interactions of Antihistamines, First-Generation.

BETAHISTINE

Betahistine (Fig. 57-1) is a structural analogue of histamine, having a weak agonistic effect at histamine receptor type-H_1, but it is more effective as a potent H_3 receptor antagonist.

MECHANISM OF ACTION

Betahistine, functioning as the H_3 receptor antagonist, promotes the synthesis and release of histamine within the vestibular nuclei. The histamine released appears to dilate blood vessels within the middle ear to reduce endolymphatic pressure by improving the microcirculation, and to decrease activity of the vestibular nuclei.

SIDE EFFECTS

Its side effects may include stomach upset and nausea; chest tightness and worsening of asthma; and headache. Caution is advised in patients with a history of peptic ulcer or with bronchial asthma, as intolerance to betahistine in such patients has been reported.

DRUG INTERACTIONS

Betahistine doesn't cause sedation or drowsiness to impair driving, unlike conventional antihistamines. No drug interactions have been reported between betahistine and conventional antihistamines.

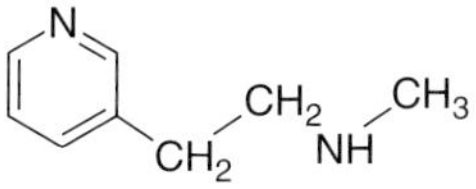

FIGURE 57-1 Molecular structure of betahistine.

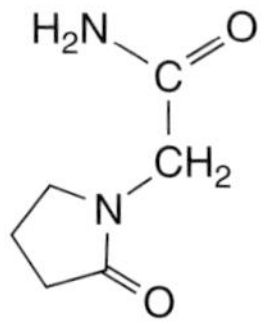

FIGURE 57-2   Molecular structure of piracetam.

PIRACETAM

Piracetam (Fig. 57-2) is an analog of GABA.

MECHANISM OF ACTION

Piracetam was shown effective in vertigo of both central and peripheral origins, but the mechanism by which piracetam exerts its beneficial effect on vertigo is not well established. It is thought that piracetam acts on vestibular and oculomotor nuclei in the brain stem to adjust central control on the genesis of vertigo.

SIDE EFFECTS

Its side effects, though very rare, may include tremor, irritability, agitation; anxiety, nervousness, and insomnia.

DRUG INTERACTIONS

See Chapter 54.

SCOPOLAMINE

MECHANISM OF ACTION

The precise mechanism whereby scopolamine (Fig. 57-3) exerts its effects on vertigo is not well understood but it was shown that scopolamine can decrease the spontaneous firing rate of the vestibular nuclei.

SIDE EFFECTS

Possible side effects of scopolamine, if extensively absorbed from the skin, include irregular or fast heartbeat; dry mouth and constipation; difficulty in urination; dilation of pupils (it may worsen narrow angle glaucoma), blurred vision; and dizziness and drowsiness. Rarely, scopolamine may cause allergic reactions such as skin rash and difficulty in breathing.

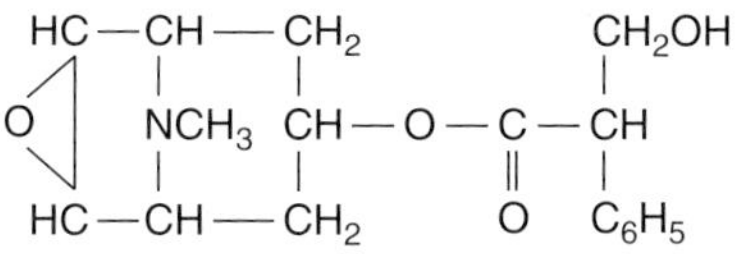

FIGURE 57-3   Molecular structure of scopolamine.

DRUG INTERACTIONS

See Appendix B-15: Interactions of Belladonna Alkaloids.

VINPOCETINE

Vinpocetine, a synthetic ethyl ester of apovincamine, is an alkaloid found in the extract of periwinkle plant (*Vinca major*).

MECHANISM OF ACTION

The precise mechanism by which vinpocetine exerts its beneficial effect on vertigo is not well understood, but vinpocetine is a selective inhibitor of a phosphodiesterase that destroys cyclic-GMP and thus, vinpocetine accumulates c-GMP in the vascular smooth muscle to cause vasodilation with consequent reduction of resistance to cerebral blood flow. By increasing the brain's utilization of oxygen and nutrients such as glucose, vinpocetine increases the cerebral metabolic rate to generate greater amounts of ATP.

SIDE EFFECTS

Possible side effects of vinpocetine include dry mouth and upset stomach; and headache. Avoid using vinpocetine during pregnancy or lactation, due to lack of clinical studies.

DRUG INTERACTIONS

Vinpocetine has a blood-thinning effect that enhances bleeding if taken with an anticoagulant, such as dicumarol or warfarin.

CHAPTER

58

Motion Sickness

Motion sickness refers to symptoms of dizziness, nausea, and vomiting that occur with any disruptive motion that distorts the normal sense of balance. Most often, motion sickness is felt during travel by airplane, automobile, ship, or train.

Medications shown effective in the treatment of motion sickness include: (1) **scopolamine** (Transderm-Scop) patch; and (2) antihistamines such as **dimenhydrinate** (Dramamine), **diphenhydramine** (Benadryl), **meclizine** (Antivert, Bonine), and **promethazine.**

SCOPOLAMINE

A scopolamine patch can be attached behind the ear several hours before travel to prevent nausea and vomiting for up to three days.

MECHANISM OF ACTION

Disorienting motion is thought to activate the hair cells in the vestibular apparatus of the inner ear, which in turn sends neuronal impulses through cholinergic fibers to activate the vestibulocerebellar region of the cerebellum. The acetylcholine thus released diffuses into the cerebrospinal fluid in the fourth ventricle, before reaching and activating the vomiting center within the dorsal brainstem, generating characteristic symptoms of motion sickness. As acetylcholine (Fig. 58-1) is a chemical that mediates emetic messages, scopolamine seems to prevent delivery of these messages to the vomiting center.

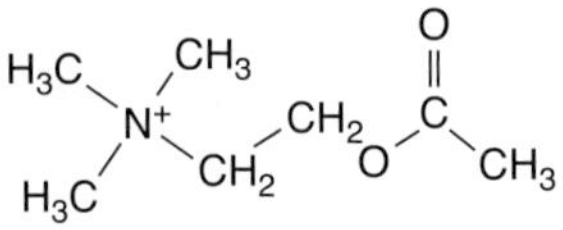

FIGURE 58-1 Molecular structure of acetylcholine.

SIDE EFFECTS

Possible side effects of scopolamine include irregular or fast heartbeat; dry mouth and constipation; difficulty in urination; dry, itchy eyes; dilation of pupils (it may worsen narrow angle glaucoma), blurred vision; and drowsiness. Rarely, scopolamine may cause allergic reactions such as skin rash and swelling of tissues.

DRUG INTERACTIONS

See Appendix B-15: Interactions of Belladonna Alkaloids.

ANTIHISTAMINES

Dimenhydrinate, diphenhydramine, meclizine, and promethazine

MECHANISM OF ACTION

Their mechanism of action for beneficial effect on motion-sickness is not well understood, but it appears that they diminish vestibular stimulation and depress labyrinthine functions. Their action on the medullary chemoreceptive trigger zone may also account for their antiemetic effect.

SIDE EFFECTS

Frequent side effects of these drugs include cardiac arrhythmia; dry mouth and loss of appetite; urinary retention; jaundice (yellowing of the skin or eyes); piloerection (goose bumps) blurred vision; chills; and drowsiness, confusion, and hallucinations.

DRUG INTERACTIONS

See Appendix B-10: Interactions of Antihistamines, First-Generation.

59

Multiple Sclerosis

Multiple sclerosis (MS) is a neurologic autoimmune disorder characterized by gradual destruction of the myelin sheath (insulating layer surrounding nerve fibers) of the brain and spinal cord. This demyelination of neurons leads to patches of hardened tissue in the central nervous system (CNS), which cannot propagate neuronal messages as quickly as they should. This results in partial or complete paralysis of muscles, balance disorders, jerking muscle tremors, deteriorating vision, and other sensations. There is no known cure for MS. Current treatments are aimed at improving the symptoms of this disorder or at modifying the causative immune system to suppress the disease.

Medications that may be effective in the management of MS include: (1) **fampridine (4-aminopyridine)** (Avitrol); (2) **baclofen** (Lioresal); (3) **tizanidine;** (4) **dantrolene;** (5) glucocorticoids such as **methylprednisolone** (Solu-Medrol), **prednisolone,** and **prednisone;** and (6) immunosuppressants such as **interferon beta-1a** (Avonex) and **interferon beta-1b** (Betaseron), which may slow progression of the disease. Another drug to treat relapsing MS is **Glatiramer Acetate** (Copaxone), which is used when interferon-beta therapy is found ineffective or is not well tolerated. Other miscellaneous immune-modifying medications that can be used to suppress the disease include **azathioprine** (Imuran), **cladribine** (Leustatin), **cyclophosphamide** (Cytoxan, Neosar), **cyclosporine, methotrexate** (Methotrexate LPF, Rheumatrex), and **mitoxantrone** (Novantrone).

FAMPRIDINE

Fampridine, or 4-aminopyridine (4-AP) (Fig. 59-1), is a new drug shown to improve visual function and motor skills, relieve fatigue, and improve ability to walk in patients with MS. However, fampridine is a potentially toxic drug with a narrow therapeutic index.

FIGURE 59-1 Molecular structure of 4-aminopyridine.

MECHANISM OF ACTION

4-AP was shown to selectively inhibit voltage-gated K^+ channels involved in regulating membrane potential.

SIDE EFFECTS

It may cause atrial fibrillation; paresthesia; and convulsions.

DRUG INTERACTIONS

There are no clinically important interactions reported.

BACLOFEN

MECHANISM OF ACTION

Baclofen (*See* Fig. 13-3) is a GABA analog that activates GABA-B receptors in presynaptic neurons, inhibiting the release of excitatory acetylcholine. Baclofen relieves skeletal muscle spasticity and pain in patients with MS.

SIDE EFFECTS

Baclofen may generate uneven heartbeat; nausea and constipation; muscle weakness; drowsiness and dizziness; seizure (convulsions); and confusion and hallucinations.

DRUG INTERACTIONS

See Chapter 13.

TIZANIDINE

Tizanidine is a skeletal muscle relaxant.

MECHANISM OF ACTION

Tizanidine is an alpha-2-adrenergic agonist that inhibits the release of excitatory amino acids from presynaptic neurons in the spinal cord, thus reducing motor reflexes through alpha motor neurons. Postsynaptic decreases in neuronal excitation may also occur.

SIDE EFFECTS

Possible side effects of tizanidine include hypotension and irregular heartbeat; dry mouth and constipation; acute hepatitis and asthenia (weakness, fatigue, and/or tiredness); dizziness and drowsiness; hallucinations; and rarely, allergic reactions.

DRUG INTERACTIONS

See Chapter 41.

DANTROLENE

MECHANISM OF ACTION

Dantrolene directly affects the contractile units of skeletal muscle to produce muscle relaxation. It blocks the release of calcium ions from the sarcoplasmic reticulum, limiting its availability for muscle contractions.

SIDE EFFECTS

Dantrolene may cause nausea; hepatotoxicity; general body discomfort and weakness; hyperkalemia; increased sensitivity to sunlight; and dizziness and drowsiness as its side effects. Rarely, dantrolene may cause some allergic reactions.

DRUG INTERACTIONS

Dantrolene (DTL)

DTL ⟷ Estrogens: Hepatotoxicity induced by dantrolene may be caused by an allergic reaction to this drug. Estrogens can cause intrahepatic cholestasis in susceptible women during pregnancy. If used together they may enhance the chance of toxicity.

DTL ⟷ Verapamil: Dantrolene has a tendency to retain potassium, as does verapamil, which tends to reduce transepithelial potassium transport. Concomitant administration of dantrolene and verapamil, a calcium-channel blocker, has caused increased incidence of hyperkalemia, a condition that may cause heart block and myocardial depression.

GLUCOCORTICOIDS

Methylprednisolone, **prednisolone,** and **prednisone**

Though they can suppress inflammation, these steroids do not affect the course of MS over time, but may reduce the duration and severity of attacks in some patients.

MECHANISM OF ACTION

See Chapter 11.

SIDE EFFECTS

See Chapter 11.

DRUG INTERACTIONS

It is not known whether other medications will interact with the above glucocorticoids if applied topically, but since they are taken orally or by injection the following interactions may occur: *See* Appendix B-20: Interactions of Glucocorticoids

IMMUNOSUPPRESSANTS

Interferon beta-1a, interferon beta-1b, azathioprine, cladribine, cyclophosphamide, cyclosporine, glatiramer, methotrexate, and **mitoxantrone**

These drugs may reverse symptoms of MS, but the onset of their action is slow, taking four to eight months; and the MS symptoms recur two to three months after the drugs are discontinued. Glatiramer is reserved to treat relapsing MS, where interferon-beta therapy is found ineffective or not tolerated well. **Mitoxantrone** is an immunosuppressant approved by the FDA for treatment of advanced or chronic MS.

MECHANISM OF ACTION

Multiple sclerosis is an autoimmune, inflammatory, demyelinating disease, which affects the white matter located in the CNS.

The above immunosuppressant can provide a strong anti-inflammatory action. Cyclophosphamide (Fig. 59-2) is a prodrug that is converted by mixed function oxidase enzymes in the liver to its major active metabolite, 4-hydroxycyclophosphamide, and its tautomer, aldophosphamide, which is oxidized by aldehyde dehydrogenase to phosphoramide mustard (Fig. 59-3), which in turn cross-links DNA chains by making a covalent bond between the N-7

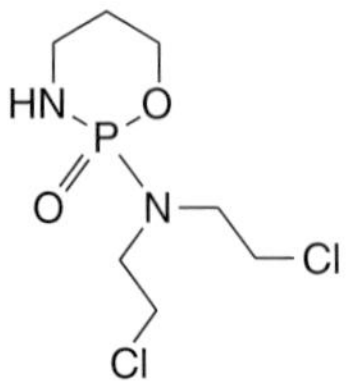

FIGURE 59-2 Molecular structure of cyclophosphamide.

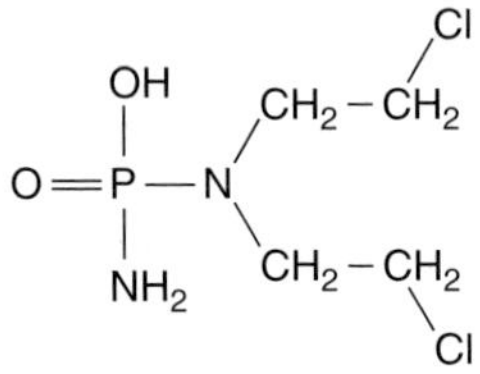

FIGURE 59-3 Molecular structure of phosphoramide mustard.

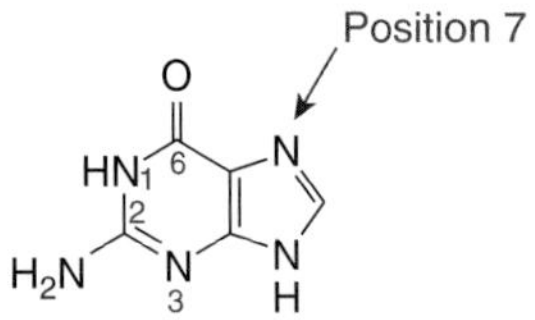

FIGURE 59-4 Molecular structure of guanine.

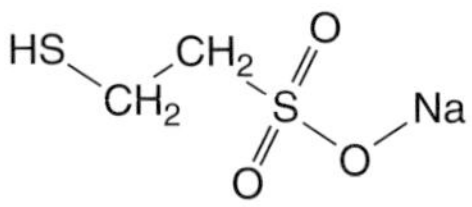

FIGURE 59-5 Molecular structure of mesna.

position of guanine (Fig. 59-4) at one DNA strand and that at the opposite strand as well as that within the same strand (both interstrand and intrastrand cross-linkages). These DNA cross-links lead to cell death. A small proportion of phosphoramide mustard is converted into acrolein (chemically, $CH_2=CH\text{-}CHO$), a toxic substance to the epithelia of the bladder, causing hemorrhagic cystitis, which can be prevented by the use of mesna (Fig. 59-5) or by aggressive hydration.

SIDE EFFECTS

Some patients may experience one or more of the following adverse effects. If the symptoms get worse or a side effect not listed here emerges, a warning to take emergency actions is warranted. The frequent side effects of these drugs include: bone marrow depression, reducing production of white blood cells so as to cause increased risk of life-threatening infections; cardiac dysfunction (cyclophosphamide), congestive heart failure or cardiac necrosis; interstitial pulmonary fibrosis with dyspnea and non-productive coughing and progressive pulmonary fibrosis (cyclophosphamide); tender gums; nausea, vomiting, loss of appetite, and diarrhea; liver toxicity; hemorrhagic cystitis (cyclophosphamide) and other forms of nephrotoxicity such as renal tubular necrosis (azathioprine and cyclosporine); weakness or numbness of limbs; headache, fever, chills, dizziness; blurred vision and seizures; loss of hair; and allergic reactions such as difficulty in breathing; swelling of the face, lips, tongue, or throat; and skin hives.

DRUG INTERACTIONS

Interferon Beta-1a or Interferon Beta-1b: If interferon-beta is taken with agents known to induce hepatotoxicity, such as aldesleukin, the risk of liver injury will be potentiated to cause autoimmune hepatitis, which usually appears in a few months.

Azathioprine: *See* Chapter 40.

Cladribine: There are no known drug interactions with cladribine. However, don't take it with ethanol to avoid irritation in the gastrointestinal tract.

Cyclosporine: *See* Chapter 8.

Cyclophosphamide: *See* Box 59-1.

BOX 59-1

Basic Concepts of Cyclophosphamide Interactions

1. Cyclophosphamide is an inactive prodrug until it is transformed in the liver to 4-hydroxycyclophosphamide, mainly by CYP2B6 and, to a lesser extent, by CYP3A4 (*See* Table 59-1). Thus, co-administration with drugs that inhibit CYP2B6 can oppose activation of cyclophosphamide. Those inhibitors include: **itraconazole** (an antifungal); **orphenadrine** (a drug to relieve pain associated with musculoskeletal injuries); **sertraline** (an antidepressant); and **ticlopidine** (a drug to prevent blood clotting).

2. Cyclophosphamide is highly cytotoxic, and when co-administered with drugs that generate immunosuppression, an additional compromise on immunity may result. Those immunosuppressive drugs include: **aldesleukin** (a drug to treat certain cancers); **cyclosporine** (an immunosuppressant); **etanercept** (a drug to treat rheumatoid arthritis, that, when combined with cyclophosphamide in treatment of Wegener granulomatosis, led to higher incidences of non-cutaneous solid malignancies); and **trastuzumab** (a drug to treat breast cancer). (Note: cardiomyopathy induced by trastuzumab may be enhanced by combined use with cyclophosphamide, whose side effects also include cardiac dysfunction.)

3. Cyclophosphamide has an inhibitory effect on plasma pseudocholinesterases, and its use in conjunction with drugs that are inactivated by these enzymes may prolong their duration of action. Those drugs include: **mivacurium** (a new neuromuscular blocker with a short duration of action, about 30 minutes, due to its rapid hydrolysis by pseudocholinesterases) and **succinylcholine.**

Glatiramer: There is no clinically important interaction elucidated.

Methotrexate: *See* Chapter 77.

Mitoxantrone: *See* Chapter 77.

Miscellaneous Interactions of Cyclophosphamide (CPM)
Parentheses below indicate an herb.

CPM ⟷ Allopurinol: The dose-limiting toxicity of cyclophosphamide is bone marrow suppression, and bone marrow depression has been reported in patients receiving allopurinol as well. When the two are taken together it may increase the incidence of myelosuppression with increased risk of infection.

CPM ⟷ Aminoglycosides Antibiotics: (*See* Ω-7 in Appendix A.) Both cyclophosphamide and aminoglycosides are nephrotoxic, and when used in combination, renal toxicity will be enhanced.

CPM ⟷ Amiodarone: Both cyclophosphamide and amiodarone induce pulmonary toxicity. When taken in combination, severe, sometimes fatal, pulmonary complications may result.

CPM ⟷ (Astragalus): Astragalus (Fig. 59-6), an herb with antibacterial and immune-enhancing action, is thought to counteract the immune-suppressing effect of cyclophosphamide, but the mechanism behind this observation is unknown.

CPM ⟷ Busulfan: Cardiac tamponade, an emergency condition in which fluid accumulates in the pericardium of the heart, has been reported in a small number

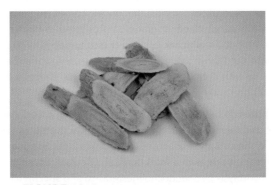

FIGURE 59-6   Cut and dried root of astragalus.

BOX 60-1

Basic Concepts of Insulin Interactions

1. Overdoses of insulin induce hypoglycemia, which in turn triggers activation of the sympathetic system, generating unpleasant symptoms such as anxiety, sweating, tremors, and palpitations. When insulin is co-administered with drugs that block sympathetic transmissions, signs of hypoglycemia caused by overdoses of insulin would be masked. Those drugs include: **beta-adrenergic blockers** (*See* Ω-27 in Appendix A); **alpha-2 activators** such as clonidine (*See* Ω-4 in Appendix A); and **guanethidine,** a ganglionic blocker.

2. The tendency of insulin to cause hypoglycemia can be exacerbated by drugs that tend to lower blood levels of glucose. Those drugs include: **alpha lipoic acid; (bitter gourd)** (*See* Fig. 10-9); **(black cohosh)** (Fig. 60-3) (an herb used for rheumatism and fever in Chinese medicine that is known to stimulate insulin secretions); **(dandelion); (fenugreek)** (Fig. 60-4 A and B) (an herb claimed to

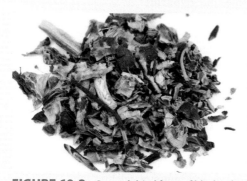

FIGURE 60-3   Cut and dried form of black cohosh.

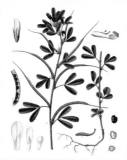

FIGURE 60-4   **A, Partial feature of fenugreek in nature.**
(http://en.wikipedia.org/wiki/File:Koeh-273.jpg)

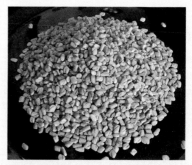

FIGURE 60-4   **B, Seeds of fenugreek.**
(http://en.wikipedia.org/wiki/File:Fenugreek-methi-seeds.jpg)

continued

BOX 60-1 *(continued)*

lower blood glucose, cholesterol, and triglycerides); **(garlic)** (which may increase the release of insulin); **(ginseng);** and **magnesium** (which enhances insulin sensitivity and secretion).

3. Insulin lowers blood glucose levels , but when taken with drugs that raise blood glucose levels, the therapeutic effectiveness of insulin would be compromised. Those drugs include: **glucocorticoids** (*See* Ω-42 in Appendix A) including fludrocortisone; **(gotu kola)**; and **thiazide diuretics** (*See* Ω-73 in Appendix A).

SULFONYLUREAS

Glimepiride, glipizide, and **glyburide**

These drugs are only effective in patients whose pancreas is capable of producing the hormone insulin. Glyburide is often used in combination with metformin, a non-sulfonylurea antidiabetic drug. Glucovance **(glyburide + metformin)** is an example of such a preparation.

MECHANISM OF ACTION

These drugs block the ATP-sensitive potassium channels on the beta cell membrane of the islets of Langerhans to inhibit potassium efflux, which results in prolonged depolarization and influx of calcium ions, which in turn triggers calcium-calmodulin binding and activation of kinases with consequent release of insulin-containing granules by exocytosis.

SIDE EFFECTS

Possible side effects of these sulfonylureas include upper respiratory infections; nausea, vomiting, stomach pain, and diarrhea; hunger feeling; shakiness and cold sweat; and headache and dizziness. Rarely, they may also cause allergic reactions such as skin rash and itching; difficulty in breathing; and swelling of the face, lips, tongue, or throat.

DRUG INTERACTIONS

See Box 60-2.

BOX 60-2

Basic Concepts of Glimepiride, Glipizide and Glyburide Interactions

1. **Glimepiride, glipizide,** and g**lyburide** lower blood glucose levels, but when used with drugs that raise blood glucose levels, the therapeutic value of these drugs may be compromised. Those drugs include: **baclofen** (a drug to treat muscle spasms); **glucocorticoids** (*See* Ω-42 in Appendix A); **(gotu kola); sympathomimetic drugs** including dopamine (*See* Ω-71 in Appendix A); and **thiazide diuretics** (*See* Ω-73 in Appendix A).

2. **Glimepiride, glipizide,** and g**lyburide** are bound extensively to plasma albumin, and when used with drugs that have a higher affinity for binding to the same protein, they will displace these hypoglycemic agents and raise their blood concentrations, causing excessive hypoglycemia. Those drugs include: **non-steroidal anti-inflammatory drugs** (NSAIDs) (*See* Ω-54 in Appendix A): **salicylates** (*See* Ω-64 in Appendix A); and **sulfonamide chemotherapeutics** such as co-trimoxazole **(***See* Ω-70 in Appendix A).

3. The tendency of the above sulfonylureas to cause hypoglycemia can be exacerbated by combined use with drugs that tend to lower glucose blood levels. Those drugs include: **alpha lipoic acid** which increases glucose utilization in muscle cells; **(bitter gourd); (black cohosh)** (an herb that can stimulate insulin secretions); **(dandelion); (Fenugreek); (Garlic)** (which may increase the release of insulin); **(ginseng)** and **magnesium** (which enhances insulin sensitivity and secretion).

4. Overdoses of these sulfonylureas may induce hypoglycemia, which in turn triggers activation of the sympathetic system, generating unpleasant symptoms such as anxiety, sweating, tremor, and palpitations, but when co-administered with drugs that block sympathetic transmissions, it would mask such signs of hypoglycemia. Those drugs include: **beta-adrenergic blockers** (*See* Ω 27 in Appendix A); **alpha-2 activators** including clonidine (*See* Ω-4 in Appendix A); and **guanethidine,** a ganglionic blocker.

Miscellaneous Interactions of Glimepiride, Glipizide, and Glyburide (GPV)

GPV ⟷ Acitretin: Acitretin may influence blood glucose levels, generating either hypoglycemia or hyperglycemia. When taken in combination with an oral hypoglycemic agent such as glyburide, there is a chance that it may enhance hypoglycemia.

GPV ⟷ Alcohol: Alcohol may produce disulfiram-like reactions such as breathlessness, facial flushing, hypotension, and headache.

GPV ⟷ Clarithromycin: Clarithromycin may inhibit the P-glycoprotein transporters that efflux sulfonylureas and thus, may increase the serum concentration and adverse effects of sulfonylureas.

GPV ⟷ CYP Isozymes: *See* Table 60-1.

GPV ⟷ Disopyramide: Disopyramide can decrease the fasting serum glucose levels in men, and its co-administration with oral antidiabetic agents may increase the risk of excessive hypoglycemia.

GPV ⟷ MAO inhibitors: (*See* Ω-51 in Appendix A.) MAO inhibitors enhance the hypoglycemic responses to sulfonylureas. Close monitoring of serum glucose levels is recommended when an MAO inhibitor is added or discontinued.

GPV ⟷ Medroxyprogesterone: Medroxyprogesterone may lead to weight gain, and independently decreases insulin sensitivity. Therefore, use of medroxyprogesterone, a commonly used contraceptive, may worsen glucose tolerance in diabetics and in those with lipodystrophy (disorder of fat metabolism). Hence, monitoring of blood sugar is recommended while taking medroxyprogesterone to avoid severe hyperglycemia.

GPV ⟷ Tetracycline Antibiotics: (*See* Ω-72 in Appendix A.) Tetracyclines induce hypoglycemia, but its mechanism is not clear, even though increased sensitivity to insulin and decreased clearance of insulin have been suggested. When used in combination with sulfonylureas, it may potentiate effects of the sulfonylurea, leading to excessive hypoglycemia.

TABLE 60-1 Sulfonylureas vs CYP Enzymes

Drug Name	1A2	2A6	2B6	2C8	2C9	2C18	2C19	2D6	2E1	3A4
Glimepiride					Sub					
Glipizide					Sub					
Glyburide					Sub					Sub

Abbreviations: Sub, substrate of the enzyme; Inh, inhibits the enzyme; Ezi, induces the enzyme

All of the above drugs are metabolized in the liver by microsomal CYP2C9 and thus, inhibition of this enzyme may raise blood levels to possibly exacerbate their adverse effects such as excessive hypoglycemia. Those strong inhibitors of CYP2C9 include fluconazole. (*See* the left-hand column of Table-0 at the 'Introduction' for other possible inhibitors of the enzyme.)

METFORMIN

In addition to its favorable effect on blood glucose, metformin can lower LDL cholesterol ("bad-cholesterol") and increase HDL cholesterol ("good cholesterol").

MECHANISM OF ACTION

Metformin lowers blood glucose by several different mechanisms. (1) It predominantly inhibits gluconeogenesis from alanine (Fig. 60-5) in the liver; (2) it increases glycolysis in peripheral tissue; and (3) it promotes binding of insulin to its receptor.

SIDE EFFECTS

Metformin may cause nausea, vomiting, abdominal discomfort, indigestion, and diarrhea; muscle weakness; and headache. Metformin seldom causes serious hypoglycemia.

DRUG INTERACTIONS

See Box 60-3.

Miscellaneous Interactions of Metformin (MFM)

MFM ⟷ Alcohol: Avoid drinking alcohol while taking metformin, as alcohol lowers blood sugar and may increase the risk of lactic acidosis caused by metformin.

MFM ⟷ Cephalexin: If cephalexin is co-administered with metformin, the former decreases renal clearance of the latter to raise blood levels and enhance the adverse effects of metformin.

MFM ⟷ CYP Enzymes: Metformin is not metabolized by CYP enzymes in humans but is excreted unchanged in the urine. Thus, CYP inducers or inhibitors are unlikely to influence elimination of this drug.

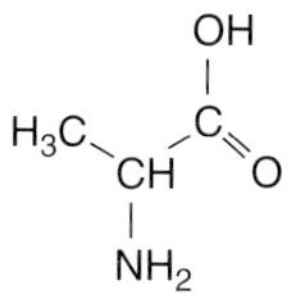

FIGURE 60-5 Molecular structure of alanine.

BOX 60-3

Basic Concepts of Metformin Interactions

1. Metformin can lower blood glucose levels, but when used with drugs that raise blood glucose levels by various mechanisms, the therapeutic value of metformin can be compromised. Those drugs include: **baclofen** (a drug to treat muscle spasms); **glucocorticoids** (*See* Ω-42 in Appendix A); **(gotu kola)**; **sympathomimetic drugs** (*See* Ω-71 in Appendix A); and **thiazide diuretics** (*See* Ω-73 in Appendix A).

2. The ability of metformin to lower blood glucose can be enhanced by combined use with drugs that also lower glucose blood levels. Those drugs include: **alpha lipoic acid** which is known to increase glucose utilization in muscle cells; **(bitter gourd); (black cohosh)** (an herb that can stimulate insulin secretions); **(dandelion); (fenugreek); (garlic)** (which may increase the release of insulin); **(ginseng);** and **magnesium** (which enhances insulin sensitivity and secretion).

MFM ⬌ Nifedipine: Nifedipine, a calcium-channel blocker, appears to enhance the gastrointestinal absorption of metformin, raising its plasma levels as much as 20%, and increasing the chance of developing lactic acidosis.

MFM ⬌ Protein-Bound Drugs: (*See* Ω-60 in Appendix A.) Metformin, unlike the antidiabetic sulfonylureas, is negligibly bound to plasma proteins, and is, therefore, unlikely to interact with highly protein-bound drugs, such as chloramphenicol, salicylates, and sulfonamides.

PPAR-GAMMA ACTIVATORS

Pioglitazone (*See* Fig. 60-1) and **rosiglitazone** (*See* Fig. 60-2) both lower blood glucose levels, but seldom to the point of hypoglycemia.

MECHANISM OF ACTION

They lower blood glucose not by increasing the secretions of insulin but by selective activation of a nuclear receptor group called PPAR-gamma, which modulates transcription of insulin-sensitive genes, resulting in increased tissue sensitivity to the circulating insulin.

SIDE EFFECTS

Their possible side effects include sinus inflammation, respiratory tract infections, and sore throat; muscle aches; and headache. Further, both may exacerbate congestive heart failure and rosiglitazone may cause myocardial ischemia.

BOX 60-4

Basic Concepts of Pioglitazone and Rosiglitazone Interactions

1. Pioglitazone and rosiglitazone can lower blood glucose levels, but when used with drugs that raise blood glucose, their therapeutic effectiveness may be compromised. Those drugs include: **baclofen** (a drug to treat muscle spasm); **glucocorticoids** (*See* Ω 42 in Appendix A); **(gotu kola); sympathomimetic drugs** (*See* Ω-71 in Appendix A); and **thiazide diuretics** (*See* Ω-73 in Appendix A).

2. The ability of pioglitazone and rosiglitazone to lower blood glucose can be enhanced by combined use with drugs that also lower blood glucose levels. Those drugs include: **alpha lipoic acid** which increases glucose utilization in muscle cells; **(bitter gourd); (black cohosh)** (*See* Fig, 60-3) (an herb that can stimulate insulin secretions); **(dandelion); (fenugreek); (Garlic)** (which may increase the release of insulin); **(ginseng);** and **magnesium** (which enhances insulin sensitivity and secretion).

DRUG INTERACTIONS

See Box 60-4.

Miscellaneous Interactions of Pioglitazone and Rosiglitazone (PRZ)

PRZ ⟷ CYP Isozymes: *See* Table 60-2.

PRZ ⟷ Gemfibrozil: Gemfibrozil may raise blood levels and enhance the adverse effects of both pioglitazone and rosiglitazone. One possible mechanism of this interaction is that both pioglitazone and rosiglitazone are at least partially cleared through CYP2C8, and gemfibrozil is inhibitory to this enzyme, opposing their metabolic clearance.

PRZ ⟷ Propranolol: Propranolol interferes with beta-2-mediated glycogenolysis to delay recovery from hypoglycemia rarely caused by pioglitazone or rosiglitazone.

PRZ ⟷ Salicylates (*See* Ω-64 in Appendix A.) Salicylates can lower blood glucose levels by controversial mechanisms, which include: (1) reduced insulin clearance; (2) inhibited gluconeogenesis; and (3) enhanced glycolysis. Thus, the use of salicylates in conjunction with pioglitazone or rosiglitazone may result in an excessive drop in blood sugar.

TABLE 60-2 PPAR-Gamma Activators vs CYP Enzymes

Drug Name	1A2	2A6	2B6	2C8	2C9	2C18	2C19	2D6	2E1	3A4
Pioglitazone				Sub						Sub+ Ezi
Rosiglitazone				Sub+ Inh	Sub					

Abbreviations: Sub, substrate of the enzyme; Inh, inhibits the enzyme; Ezi, induces the enzyme

1. Pioglitazone, but not rosiglitazone, can induce CYP3A4 and co-administration with contraceptive pills containing estrogen may result in contraception failure, because estrogens are a partial substrate of CYP3A4 and are more quickly eliminated by the enzyme inducer pioglitazone.

2. Both pioglitazone and rosiglitazone are metabolized mainly by hepatic CYP2C8 and co-administration with rifampin, an antibiotic and an inducer of CYP2C8, causes a decrease in blood levels of pioglitazone and rosiglitazone, impairing their therapeutic efficacies.

3. Gemfibrozil, an inhibitor of both CYP2C8 and, to a lesser extent, CYP2C9, may inhibit their metabolism to increase the serum concentrations of pioglitazone and rosiglitazone to cause excessive hypoglycemia. (*See* the left-hand column of Table-0 at the 'Introduction' for other possible inhibitors of these enzymes.)

EXENATIDE

Exenatide is injected subcutaneously 30 to 60 minutes before the first and last meal of the day. Exenatide is a 39-amino-acid peptide (COOH-His-Gly-Glu-Gly-Thr-Phe-Thr-Ser-Asp-Leu-Ser-Lys-Gln-Met-Glu-Glu-Glu-Ala-Val-Arg-Leu-Phe-Ile-Glu-Trp-Leu-Lys-Asn-Gly-Gly-Pro-Ser-Ser-Gly-Ala-Pro-Pro-Pro-Ser-NH2) whose treatment was shown to lower blood glucose toward target levels, and to shed body weight. Incidence of mild hypoglycemia by exenatide is low.

MECHANISM OF ACTION

Exenatide generates effects similar to human glucagon-like peptide-1 (GLP-1), by enhancing glucose-dependent insulin secretion and by suppressing glucagon secretion.

SIDE EFFECTS

Possible side effects of exenatide include nausea, vomiting, acid reflux, abdominal pain, and diarrhea; acute pancreatitis (if this is suspected, the drug should be discontinued until pancreatitis is excluded); excessive fall of blood glucose with increased sweating; and headache and nervousness.

DRUG INTERACTIONS

See Box 60-5.

BOX 60-5

Basic Concepts of Exenatide Interactions

1. Exenatide may slow the gastric emptying of other drugs which are absorbed mainly from the intestine, impairing their absorption, lowering their plasma concentrations, and compromising their therapeutic value. Those affected drugs include: **acetaminophen; lovastatin; ciprofloxacin; levofloxacin;** and **ofloxacin.**

2. Overdoses of exenatide may induce hypoglycemia, which in turn triggers activation of the sympathetic system to generate such unpleasant symptoms as anxiety, sweating, tremor, and palpitations. When exenatide is co-administered with drugs that block sympathetic transmission, it would mask such signs of hypoglycemia. Those drugs include: **beta-adrenergic blockers** (*See* Ω-27 in Appendix A); **alpha-2 activators** (*See* Ω-4 in Appendix A); and **guanethidine,** a ganglionic blocker.

3. The tendency of exenatide to cause hypoglycemia can be exacerbated by other drugs that tend to lower blood glucose levels. Those drugs include: **alpha lipoic acid; (bitter gourd); (black cohosh)** (an herb that can stimulate insulin secretion); **(dandelion); (Fenugreek); (Garlic)** (which may increase release of insulin); **(ginseng);** and **magnesium** (which enhances insulin sensitivity and secretion).

4. Exenatide lowers blood glucose levels, but when taken with drugs that raise blood glucose levels, the therapeutic effectiveness of exenatide may be compromised. Those drugs include: **glucocorticoids** (*See* Ω-42 in Appendix A); **(gotu kola);** and **thiazide diuretics** (*See* Ω-73 in Appendix A).

CHAPTER

61

Diabetes Insipidus

Diabetes insipidus is a chronic endocrine disease. Central diabetes insipidus is caused by lack of vasopressin secretion, often caused by damage to the hypothalamus or pituitary gland. Nephrogenic diabetes insipidus is caused by failure of the kidneys to respond to existing vasopressin. Vasopressin, also known as antidiuretic hormone (ADH), is required to reabsorb water from urine in the kidneys. Thus, diabetes insipidus is characterized by a tremendous increase in urine volume—up to 20 liters a day instead of about 1.5 liters a day—and therefore, by intense thirst.

Medications shown effective in the treatment of diabetes insipidus include: (1) **desmopressin** or **vasopressin** for central (or pituitary) diabetes insipidus; and (2) **hydrochlorothiazide** for nephrogenic diabetes insipidus.

DESMOPRESSIN OR VASOPRESSIN

MECHANISM OF ACTION

Both desmopressin and vasopressin bind to V_2 receptors coupled to G_s proteins, activating the adenylate cyclase system. This results in increased permeability to water at the distal convoluted tubules and collecting tubules of the kidneys, which allows increased water reabsorption with a consequently smaller volume of concentrated urine excreted.

SIDE EFFECTS

Their side effects may include upset stomach, pain in the external genital area (in women); stuffy or runny nose; reddening of the skin; and headache.

DRUG INTERACTIONS

Unlike desmopressin, which has a prolonged antidiuretic action but with little pressor effect, vasopressin has a strong vasopressor effect, and its combined intake with a ganglionic blocker may markedly increase sensitivity to its pressor effect.

HYDROCHLOROTHIAZIDE

Hydrochlorothiazide is administered only for nephrogenic diabetes insipidus and is taken with a low-sodium diet. Hydrochlorothiazide reduces the volume of water lost in the urine, but not down to normal levels.

MECHANISM OF ACTION

The aquaporin-2 (AQP2) channel in the renal collecting duct principal cells is regulated by vasopressin, and expression of the AQP2 gene is increased during such conditions as pregnancy and congestive heart failure. Mutations of this channel are thought responsible for nephrogenic diabetes insipidus. Hydrochlorothiazide, though its precise mechanism to reduce urine volume in diabetes insipidus remains unclear, is thought to up-regulate both this water channel and the Na transporters at the distal renal tubules, which are regulated by the hormone aldosterone.

SIDE EFFECTS

Side effects of hydrochlorothiazide may include thirst, loss of appetite, stomach pain, vomiting, and diarrhea; muscle weakness; and dizziness and headache.

DRUG INTERACTIONS

See Appendix B-4: Interactions of Thiazide Diuretics.

CHAPTER

62

Addison Disease

Addison disease (hypoadrenocorticism) is an endocrine disorder caused by insufficient productions of corticosteroid hormones, such as cortisol and aldosterone, in the adrenal cortex.

Medications shown effective in the treatment of Addison disease include: (1) a combination of glucocorticoids, such as **cortisone** + **hydrocortisone** (Cortef) and (2) **fludrocortisone.**

CORTISONE PLUS HYDROCORTISONE

Injection of adrenocorticotropic hormone (ACTH) may promote normal synthesis of corticosteroids in the adrenal gland. However, oral intake of a combination of cortisone + hydrocortisone (Cortef) is often used instead. Administration of these drugs must usually be continuous for life as Addison disease may be due to irreparable adrenal damage. It is important for the individual with Addison disease to always carry a medical identification card showing the type of medications and doses needed in case of an emergency for the patient.

MECHANISM OF ACTION

Cortisone (*See* Fig. 42-1) is activated through hydrogenation of its 11-keto-group to become active cortisol (*See* Fig. 42-2), whose other name is hydrocortisone. By replenishing the deficient corticosteroid produced in Addison disease, this replacement therapy can ameliorate symptoms of the disease.

SIDE EFFECTS

Side effects of this combined medication may include increased blood pressure; nausea, vomiting, and stomach upset; weight gain (more than five pounds in a day or two); bloody or black stools; acne; moon face (roundness of the face); osteonecrosis (bone death owing to poor blood supply to the bone), which is a common and dose-limiting adverse event of glucocorticoids; vulnerability to infections; cataracts or glaucoma; and nervousness and insomnia.

DRUG INTERACTIONS

See Appendix B-20: Interactions of Glucocorticoids.

FLUDROCORTISONE

Fludrocortisone (Fig. 62-1) is a synthetic adrenocortical steroid that is indicated as partial replacement therapy for primary and secondary adrenocortical insufficiency in Addison disease. It has very powerful mineralocorticoid, as well as some glucocorticoid activity, and can ameliorate many symptoms of Addison disease. This drug must usually be continued for life, as Addison disease may be due to irreparable damage to the adrenal cortex.

MECHANISM OF ACTION

Fludrocortisone binds to the mineralocorticoid receptor (aldosterone receptor) at the distal tubules of the kidney, to enhance reabsorption of sodium in exchange for potassium excreted into the urine. Its action on glucose metabolism is similar to that of hydrocortisone.

SIDE EFFECTS

Its side effects may include irregular or absent menstrual periods; easy bruising; thrombophlebitis; stomach ulcer and vomiting; swelling of the face, lower legs, or ankle; muscle weakness; and headache, dizziness, and insomnia.

DRUG INTERACTIONS

See Box 62-1.

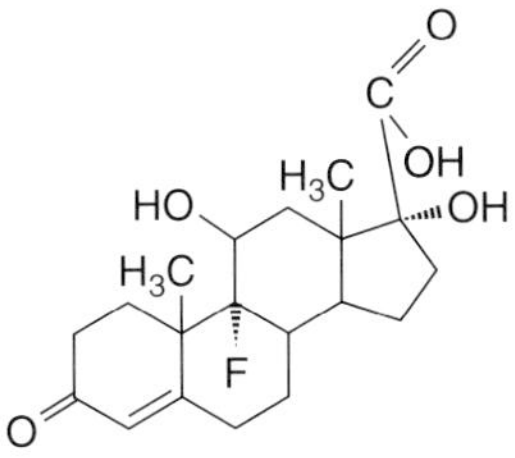

FIGURE 62-1 Molecular structure of fludrocortisone.

BOX 62-1

Basic Concepts of Fludrocortisone Interactions

1. Fludrocortisone loses potassium in exchange for retaining sodium and thus, combination of this drug with drugs that also lose potassium can lead to excessive hypokalemia, a condition that may spawn cardiac arrhythmia. Such potassium-lowering agents include: **acetazolamide** (a drug useful to treat glaucoma and epileptic seizures); **adrenergic beta-2 agonists** such as albuterol (Ventolin, Proventil), metaproterenol (Alupent), pirbuterol (Maxair), and terbutaline (note: they induce uptake of potassium (K^+) into tissue cells and may be effective in treatment of hyperkalemia); **amphotericin** (an antifungal drug); **loop diuretics** (*See* Ω-49 in Appendix A); **theophylline** (which by itself causes a slight decrease in blood potassium concentration); and **thiazide diuretics** including chlorthalidone (*See* Ω-73 in Appendix A).

2. Fludrocortisone may cause hypercoagulability to oppose the effects of anti-coagulants taken in combination. Examples include: **dicumarol** (note: people taking fludrocortisone in combination with dicumarol should have their blood clotting time (INR) regularly monitored) and **warfarin**.

Miscellaneous Interactions of Fludrocortisone (FCT)

FCT ⟷ Antihypertensive Drugs: (*See* Ω-20 in Appendix A.) Fludrocortisone has a mineralocorticoid effect that retains sodium and fluid to undercut the effectiveness of antihypertensive drugs used in combination.

FCT ⟷ CYP Isozymes: *See* Table 62-1.

TABLE 62-1 Fludrocortisone vs CYP Enzymes

Drug Name	1A2	2A6	2B6	2C8	2C9	2C18	2C19	2D6	2E1	3A4
Fludrocortisone										Sub

Abbreviations: Sub, substrate of the enzyme; Inh, inhibits the enzyme; Ezi, induces the enzyme

Fludrocortisone requires microsomal enzyme CYP3A4 for its clearance and thus, inhibition of this enzyme by other drugs can raise blood levels of fludrocortisone to possibly exacerbate its adverse effects. Those strong inhibitors of CYP3A4 include: clarithromycin, indinavir, itraconazole, ketoconazole, nefazodone, nelfinavir, ritonavir, saquinavir, and telithromycin. (*See* the left-hand column of Table-0 at the 'Introduction' for other possible inhibitors of the enzyme.)

FCT ⟷ Digoxin: Fludrocortisone loses potassium in exchange for retaining sodium, and can lead to hypokalemia, a condition that can aggravate cardiac arrhythmia caused by digoxin.

FCT ⟷ Insulin: Fludrocortisone can increase blood sugar levels to undermine the blood sugar-lowering effects of insulin.

FCT ⟷ Live Vaccines: (*See* Ω-48 in Appendix A): Fludrocortisone may decrease the body's immune response, causing serious infections by live vaccines. Such live vaccines include: measles, mumps, rubella, polio, typhoid, yellow fever, and vari-cella-zoster. Therefore, these vaccines should not be administered to people taking fludrocortisone.

FCT ⟷ Midodrine: Midodrine, a drug useful in the treatment of symptom-atic orthostatic hypotension, may increase serum levels of fludrocortisone and intraocular pressure to result in glaucoma. The exact mechanism behind these observations remains unclear.

FCT ⟷ NSAIDs: (*See* Ω-54 in Appendix A.) Both fludrocortisone and most NSAIDS, such as aspirin, ibuprofen, and naproxen, tend to cause stomach ulcer and bleeding. When used in combination they may lead to increased incidence of such adverse effects.

FCT ⟷ Oral Hypoglycemic Agents: (*See* Ω-55 in Appendix A.) Fludrocorti-sone may increase blood sugar levels and oppose the blood sugar-lowering effect of oral antidiabetic drugs, such as glipizide and glyburide.

63

Cushing Disease

Cushing disease (hypercortisolism) is a disorder caused by excessive secretions of adrenocorticotropic hormone (ACTH) from the pituitary gland or by excessive secretions of cortisol from an adrenal tumor. This results in elevated blood levels of cortisol with signs of overactivity of the adrenal gland (Fig. 63-1). Too much cortisol can result in muscle wasting, bone loss, slow or impaired wound healing, and a weakened immune system. Treatment of Cushing disease depends on the precise cause of the disease. The only way to "cure" Cushing disease is to remove the adrenal tumor.

Medications that may be effective in suppressing symptoms of Cushing disease include: (1) **ketoconazole;** and (2) **metyrapone.**

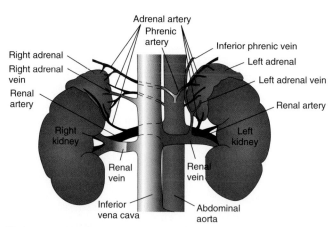

FIGURE 63-1 **Adrenal gland.** Reproduced, with permission, from Gums JG, Anderson S. Adrenal gland disorders, In: DiPiro JT, Talbert RL, Yee GC, Matzke GR, Wells BG, Posey LM. (eds). *Pharmacotherapy: A Pathophysiologic Approach.* 7th ed. New York: McGraw-Hill, 2008, p 1266.

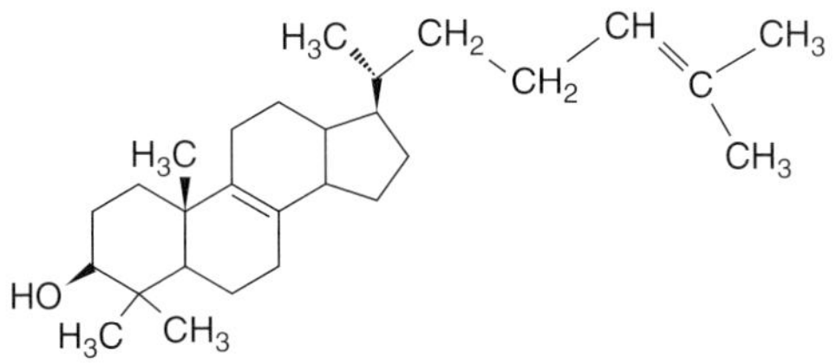

FIGURE 63-2   Molecular structure of lanosterol.

KETOCONAZOLE

MECHANISM OF ACTION

Ketoconazole works by inhibition of the cytochrome P450 (CYP) -dependent enzyme 14-alpha-demethylase, which is involved in the synthesis of lanosterol (Fig. 63-2), a precursor for cholesterol synthesis. Cholesterol, in turn, is required for synthesis of cortisol and many other steroidal hormones in the adrenal cortex. Therefore, ketoconazole inhibits the biosynthesis of many steroids in the adrenal cortex.

SIDE EFFECTS

Side effects of ketoconazole may include abnormalities in blood cell counts, low blood pressure, and shock; nausea, vomiting, and abdominal pain; impotence; fatigue; skin rash and itching; and dizziness and headache. Rarely, it may cause allergic reactions as well.

DRUG INTERACTIONS

See Appendix B-14: Interactions of Antifungal Drugs.

METYRAPONE

This is a drug that is used in the long-term management of pituitary-dependent adrenal hyperplasia (Cushing disease).

MECHANISM OF ACTION

Metyrapone (Fig. 63-3) inhibits hydroxylation at position C-11 in the biosynthesis of glucocorticoids in the adrenal cortex. As a consequence, metyrapone lowers blood levels of both cortisol and corticosterone.

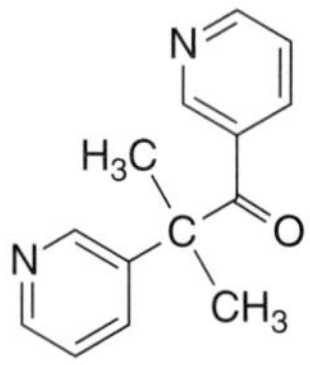

FIGURE 63-3   Molecular structure of metyrapone.

SIDE EFFECTS

Metyrapone may cause stomach pain, nausea, and vomiting; dizziness and drowsiness; and headache. Rarely, it may cause allergic reactions as well.

DRUG INTERACTIONS

Metyrapone (MTP)

MTP ◀▶ Acetaminophen: Metyrapone inhibits the glucuronidation of acetaminophen, allowing its oxidation through hepatic CYP1A2 and CYP2E1, and thereby generating its toxic metabolite to cause hepatic necrosis.

MTP ◀▶ Phenytoin: Metyrapone has complex influences on the hepatic CYP enzymes. Metabolism of metyrapone itself seems accelerated by phenytoin, an inducer of many hepatic CYP enzymes, including CYP1A2, 2B6, 2C19, and 3A4. Therefore, an increased dose of metyrapone may be required to obtain its desired effects when taken with phenytoin.

Hyperthyroidism

Hyperthyroidism is an endocrine disorder caused by an overactive thyroid gland manufacturing an excess amount of thyroid hormones. A high level of thyroid hormones generates uncomfortable symptoms such as tachycardia, irritability, constipation, and heat intolerance.

Medications shown effective in the treatment of hyperthyroidism include: (1) thioamides such as **methimazole** (Tapazole, Thiamazole) and **propylthiouracil** (PTU); (2) **sodium iodide (NaI^{131})**; and (3) **propranolol** (Inderal).

THIOAMIDES

Methimazole (Fig. 64-1) and **propylthiouracil** (Fig. 64-2)

MECHANISM OF ACTION

These thioamides inhibit biosynthesis of thyroid hormones by blocking the iodination of tyrosine, probably via inactivation of the enzyme thyroid peroxidase; and by inhibition of the coupling reaction required to form thyronine.

SIDE EFFECTS

Possible side effects of thioamides include leukocytopenia, unusual bleeding (anti-vitamin K activity) or bruising; loss of taste, upset stomach, and vomiting;

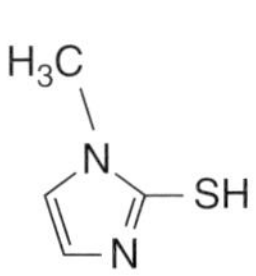

FIGURE 64-1 Molecular structure of methimazole.

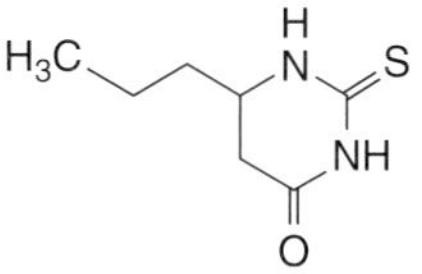

FIGURE 64-2 Molecular structure of propylthiouracil.

BOX 64-1

Basic Concepts of Methimazole or Propylthiouracil Interactions

Both **methimazole** and **propylthiouracil** have an anti-vitamin K activity, and when either is co-administered with drugs that also generate an anticoagulant effect, excessive bleeding may result. Those drugs include: **dicumarol** and **warfarin**.

sore throat; yellowing of the skin or eyes; joint and muscle pain; fever and chills; and drowsiness, dizziness, and headache. Rarely, they may cause allergic reactions as well.

DRUG INTERACTIONS

See Box 64-1.

Miscellaneous Interactions of Methimazole or Propylthiouracil (MPT)

MPT ⟷ CYP Isozymes: *See* Table 64-1.

MPT ⟷ Digoxin: Serum digoxin levels may increase when hyperthyroid patients become euthyroid by the use of either drug. Thus, a reduced dosage of the digitalis glycoside is needed to stave off the cardiac arrhythmia caused by digoxin.

MPT ⟷ Phenothiazine Antipsychotic Drugs: (*See* Ω-58 in Appendix A.) Both antithyroid drugs and phenothiazines have been reported to cause agranulocytosis. Concurrent use may increase this risk.

TABLE 64-1 Methimazole vs CYP Enzymes

Drug Name	1A2	2A6	2B6	2C8	2C9	2C18	2C19	2D6	2E1	3A4
Methimazole	Inh									

Abbreviations: Sub, substrate of the enzyme; Inh, inhibits the enzyme; Ezi, induces the enzyme

1. Propylthiouracil (not shown) does not interact with CYP isozymes.
2. Methimazole inhibits CYP1A2. Thus, co-administration with drugs that require this enzyme for metabolic clearance may result in elevated blood levels and enhanced adverse effects of them. (*See* the middle column of Table-0 at the 'Introduction' for possible substrates of the enzyme.)

SODIUM IODIDE (NaI^{131})

MECHANISM OF ACTION

With oral administration of NaI^{131} (4 to 10 millicurie), the radioisotope incorporates itself into thyroglobulin and emits beta-radiation to destroy hyperactive thyroid tissue. Normal thyroidal function may be obtained in a few months, but excessive destruction of the gland can lead to hypothyroidism later.

SIDE EFFECTS

It may cause palpitation; cough; blood in the urine or stool; muscle pain and uncontrollable movements; dry or red (erythema) skin; changes in menstrual periods; hypothyroidism; fatigue and headache; and rarely, it may cause allergic reactions.

DRUG INTERACTIONS

No clinically significant interactions have been reported.

PROPRANOLOL

MECHANISM OF ACTION

Hyperthyroidism generates symptoms similar to those generated by activation of the sympathetic nervous system, such as tremors, palpitations, heat intolerance, and nervousness; and all these symptoms could be prevented by a beta-adrenergic blocker. Thus, propranolol can offer prompt relief of the adrenergic symptoms of hyperthyroidism.

SIDE EFFECTS

Side effects of propranolol may include bradycardia, nausea, stomach pain, and loss of appetite; jaundice; and rarely, allergic reactions such as skin hives and swelling of tissues.

DRUG INTERACTIONS

See Appendix B-1: Interactions of Beta Blockers.

CHAPTER

65

Hypothyroidism

Hypothyroidism refers to a medical condition in which the thyroid gland is unable to manufacture or release a sufficient amount of thyroid hormones from the gland. Since thyroid hormones influence heart rate, metabolism, physical growth, and mental development, an insufficient supply of these hormones can affect many aspects of physical health.

Medications shown effective in the treatment of hypothyroidism include: (1) synthetic thyroid hormones such as **levothyroxine** (Levothroid, Levoxyl, Synthroid), **liothyronine** (Cytomel), or **liotrix** (Thyrolar) which is a 4:1 mixture of levothyroxine sodium and liothyronine sodium by weight; (2) naturally derived thyroid hormones such as **armour thyroid;** and (3) **thyrotropin alfa** (Thyrogen).

LEVOTHYROXINE OR LIOTHYRONINE

Most people with hypothyroidism will take either of the above medications for the rest of their lives.

MECHANISM OF ACTION

These synthetic forms of thyroid hormones mimic biological effects of natural endogenous hormones, to alleviate symptoms of hypothyroidism.

SIDE EFFECTS

Their side effects may include hot flashes and sweating; increased appetite; and insomnia and headache. And rarely, they may cause allergic reactions.

DRUG INTERACTIONS

See Box 65-1.

BOX 65-1

Basic Concepts of Levothyroxine or Liothyronine Interactions

1. Some drugs may bind to the above thyroid hormones in the gut to decrease their absorption and therapeutic effects. Those drugs include: **aluminum hydroxide** (a gastric antacid) and **attapulgite** (a drug to treat diarrhea); **calcium carbonate; cholestyramine; raloxifene** (Evista) (a drug for osteoporosis that was reported to interfere with absorption of thyroid hormone); and **sucralfate** (a drug to treat active duodenal ulcers whose administration should be separated by at least 8 hours from intake of thyroid hormones).

2. By increasing the catabolism of vitamin K-dependent blood clotting factors, levothyroxine and liothyronine enhance the effects of drugs that work by blocking the availability of the active form of vitamin K. The combination may cause excessive bleeding unless the dose is reduced. Those drugs include: **dicumarol** and **warfarin**.

Miscellaneous Interactions of Levothyroxine or Liothyronine (LLL)

LLL ↔ Alpha Lipoic Acid: Alpha lipoic acid is known to interfere with the conversion of T_4 [tetraiodothyronine (or thyroxine), a less potent thyroid hormone] to T_3 (triiodothyronine, a more potent thyroid hormone), so as to compromise biological activity of thyroid hormones.

LLL ↔ Amiodarone: Amiodarone (*See* Fig. 4-4) has iodine in its molecule, and can alter thyroidal function to induce hypothyroidism or hyperthyroidism. Therefore, monitoring thyroid function is recommended while taking amiodarone.

LLL ↔ Barbiturates: (*See* Ω-24 in Appendix A.) Any barbiturate may increase the hepatic metabolism of levothyroxine, requiring its increased dose to be therapeutically effective.

LLL ↔ Carbamazepine: Carbamazepine, an inducer of many CYP enzymes, can quicken metabolism of thyroid hormones, to reduce the serum concentrations and therapeutic value of the thyroid medications.

LLL ↔ Digoxin: Serum levels of digoxin may be reduced in hyperthyroidism or in patients receiving the above drugs. The mechanism is uncertain, but it has been suggested that changes in glomerular filtration rate may be accountable for lowering digoxin serum levels.

LLL ⟷ Estrogen: Estrogens increase serum concentrations of thyroxine-binding globulin, to increase the bound thyroxine and to decrease the free, therapeutically effective thyroxine. Hypothyroid patients may not be able to compensate for this interaction, requiring an increased dose of thyroxine.

LLL ⟷ Ketamine: Overdose symptoms of the above thyroid preparations include hypertension and tachycardia, which is also true for ketamine. When used in combination, a greater incidences of such adverse effects may result.

LLL ⟷ Ritonavir: Ritonavir increases glucuronyl transferase activity, the enzyme involved in the metabolism (conjugation) of levothyroxine, lowering its blood levels with consequent insufficiency of therapeutic effect.

LLL ⟷ Sertraline: Thyroid hormones are primarily eliminated by the kidneys, and sertraline appears to increase their elimination, tending to cause hypothyroidism. Therefore, the therapeutic effectiveness of levothyroxine may be compromised by administration with sertraline

ARMOUR THYROID

Armour thyroid is a naturally derived thyroid hormone made from desiccated porcine thyroid gland. It provides both levothyroxine (T_4) (or tetraiodothyronine) (Fig. 65-1) and L-triiodothyronine (T_3) (Fig. 65-2).

MECHANISM OF ACTION

This thyroid hormone, derived from hog, mimics the biological effects of human endogenous hormone to alleviate symptoms of hypothyroidism.

SIDE EFFECTS

This preparation may cause irregular heartbeat; changes in appetite and weight, diarrhea, and vomiting; excessive sweating; tremors; nervousness; and allergic reactions.

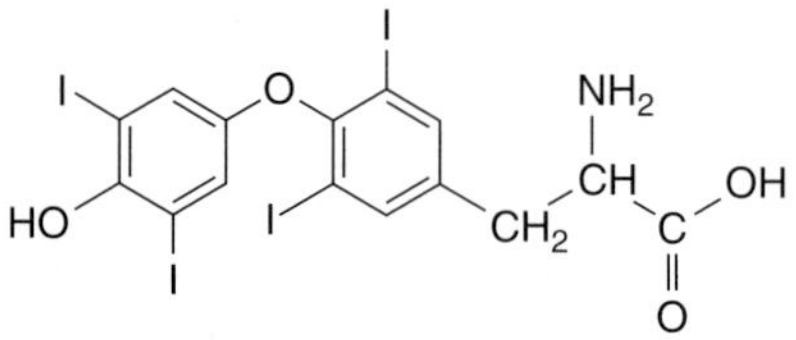

FIGURE 65-1 Molecular structure of tetraiodothyronine (or thyroxine).

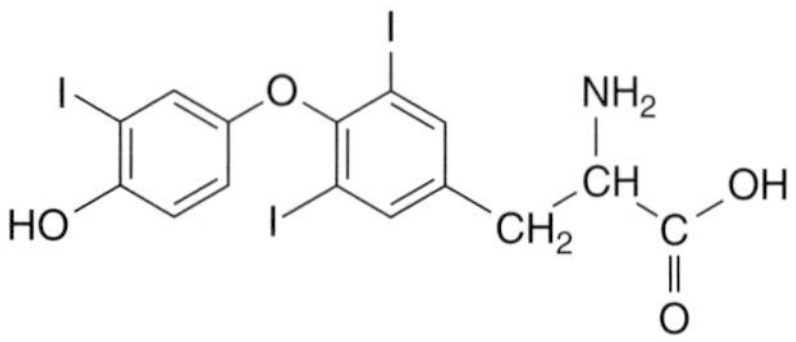

FIGURE 65-2 Molecular structure of triiodothyronine.

DRUG INTERACTIONS

See Chapter 65.

THYROTROPIN ALFA

MECHANISM OF ACTION

This drug binds to the receptors for TSH (thyroid stimulating hormone) at thyroid cells to stimulate iodine uptake, and to stimulate the synthesis and release of both T_3 and T_4.

SIDE EFFECTS

Its side effects may include nausea, vomiting, fatigue, and headache.

DRUG INTERACTIONS

No serious or clinically important interaction have been reported.

CHAPTER

66

Hypogonadism/ Infertility

Hypogonadism refers to subnormal function of the gonads, resulting in diminished ability to produce sex hormones. This may be due to an insufficient influence of gonadotrophic hormones from the pituitary gland or diseases affecting the gonads.

Infertility is defined as an inability to conceive despite regular sexual activity during the time of ovulation, for at least one full year.

Medications shown effective in the treatment of hypogonadism and/or infertility include: (1) **human menopausal gonadotropin (hMG or Menotropins)** (Repronex, Pergonal); (2) **follicle-stimulating hormone (FSH)**; (3) **human chorionic gonadotropin (hCG)** (Ovidrel, Pregnyl); (4) **gonadotropin-releasing hormone analogues**; and (5) **clomiphene.**

HUMAN MENOPAUSAL GONADOTROPIN

Human menopausal gonadotropin is obtained from the urine of postmenopausal women, and consists of FSH and luteinizing hormone (LH). It may be injected subcutaneously.

MECHANISM OF ACTION

This drug binds to cell surface receptors to activate adenylate cyclase to generate c-AMP, which in turn stimulates the growth of follicles and eggs in the ovaries, leading to ovulation.

SIDE EFFECTS

Possible side effects of this medication include abdominal pain and hyperstimulation syndrome such as ovarian enlargement with multiple gestations. Side effects of its long-term treatment (greater than six weeks) include hot flushes, vaginal dryness, and bone loss.

DRUG INTERACTIONS

It is not known whether other medications will interact with this medication.

FOLLICLE STIMULATING HORMONE

This drug may be injected intramuscularly.

MECHANISM OF ACTION

FSH, by binding to its hormone-specific receptors, promotes development of multiple follicles in ovulatory women; and in the anovulatory infertile women, FSH promotes folliculogenesis to lead to ovulation in the presence of LH that triggers ovulation itself.

SIDE EFFECTS

Its possible side effects include rapid heart rate; nausea, vomiting, diarrhea, and flatulence (gas); muscle or joint weakness or aching; swelling or tingling in the arm or leg (which may indicate presence of a blood clot); and dizziness and headache. FSH may develop ovarian hyperstimulation syndrome (OHSS) with symptoms such as breast tenderness and spotting or menstrual changes.

DRUG INTERACTIONS

It is not known whether other medications will interact with this medication.

HUMAN CHORIONIC GONADOTROPIN (hCG)

This drug is a glycoprotein injected intramuscularly.

MECHANISM OF ACTION

HCG has functions similar to those of LH. HCG promotes growth of the corpus luteum, which otherwise involutes at the end of each ovarian cycle, and causes the granulosa cells of the corpus luteum to secrete even greater quantities of both estrogens and progesterone. These secretions enable the endometrium to proliferate, preventing menstruation during pregnancy. If the corpus luteum is removed during the first trimester of pregnancy, it usually entails abortion.

SIDE EFFECTS

Its possible side effects include stomach pain, bloating, indigestion, nausea, and vomiting; rapid weight gain; headache; and rarely, allergic reactions such as skin rash and itching; difficulty in breathing; and swelling of the face, lips, tongue, or throat.

DRUG INTERACTIONS

It is not known whether other medications will interact with this medication.

GONADOTROPIN-RELEASING HORMONE ANALOGUES

These drugs, also known as GnRH analogues, include **leuprolide** (Lupron) and **nafarelin** (Synarel), both of which are synthetic peptides with effects similar to the natural hypothalamic GnRH. They are administered by intramuscular injection.

MECHANISM OF ACTION

GnRH analogues interact with the GnRH receptors in the pituitary gland to stimulate the release of its gonadotropins, namely FSH and LH, which in turn may lead to ovulation. However, continuous presence of these drugs at the receptors desensitizes the receptors and allows the pituitary gland to stop producing LH, which in turn stops ovulation. Based on this, GnRH analogues are now often used to prevent a premature LH surge, which occurs in anywhere between 5 and 20% of women undergoing controlled stimulation of ovaries, such as by menotropins. GnRH analogues are also used for women requiring *in vitro* fertilization (IVF) in order to achieve pregnancy. Since a premature LH surge brings about spontaneous ovulation, wherein the ovarian follicles rupture prematurely and the eggs (immature oocytes) are lost in the pelvic cavity before harvesting them on a predictable schedule. GnRH analogues stop spontaneous LH surges and premature ovulation in most case (about 90%).

SIDE EFFECTS

Possible side effects of GnRH analogues include hot flashes, vaginal dryness, decreased libido, muscle pain, night sweats, headaches, and insomnia.

DRUG INTERACTIONS

It is not known whether other medications will interact with GnRH analogues.

CLOMIPHENE

MECHANISM OF ACTION

Clomiphene has a weak estrogenic effect but functions as an antiestrogen. It competes with the more potent endogenous estrogens for binding to cytosol receptors in the hypothalamus, and once bound clomiphene removes negative feedback from the endogenous estrogen, to permit the release of GnRH from the hypothalamus, which in turn allows the pituitary gland to release more FSH and LH, both of which stimulate the growth of an ovarian follicle containing an egg, eventually leading to ovulation. Clomiphene is used to treat infertility in non-ovulating women if the failure to ovulate is due to lack of gonadotropin secretions.

SIDE EFFECTS

Its possible side effects include fast, irregular, or pounding heartbeat; difficulty in breathing; dry mouth, nausea, vomiting; severe muscle stiffness; drowsiness; seizures; and headache.

DRUG INTERACTIONS

It is not known whether other medications will interact with this medication.

67 Menstrual Dysfunction

Menstrual dysfunction is characterized by an erratic, disruptive menstrual cycle. Menstrual irregularities may manifest as dysmenorrhea (painful menstruation), dysfunctional uterine bleeding, oligomenorrhea (fewer than nine menstrual periods in a year), or amenorrhea (no menstrual periods for three or more months).

Medications that may be effective in the treatment of menstrual dysfunction include: (1) **danazol** (Danocrine); (2) **bromocriptine** (Parlodel), and (3) **progestogens** in oral contraceptives. Progestogens shown effective in the treatment of dysfunctional uterine bleeding include: **desogestrel, drospirenone, etonogestrel, levonorgestrel, norelgestromin, norethindrone, norgestimate,** and **norgestrel.** Long-acting progesterone therapy in the form of **medroxyprogesterone** (Depo-Provera) will stop dysfunctional uterine bleeding in most patients.

DANAZOL

Danazol (or 17-alpha-ethinyl testosterone) (Fig. 67-1) is a synthetic androgen.

MECHANISM OF ACTION

Danazol is used to treat severe primary menorrhagia (excessive bleeding with regular menstrual cycles), for up to six months. Danazol inhibits the release of both follicle-stimulating hormone (FSH) and luteinizing hormone (LH) from the pituitary gland, and thereby suppresses growth of ovarian follicles and secretions

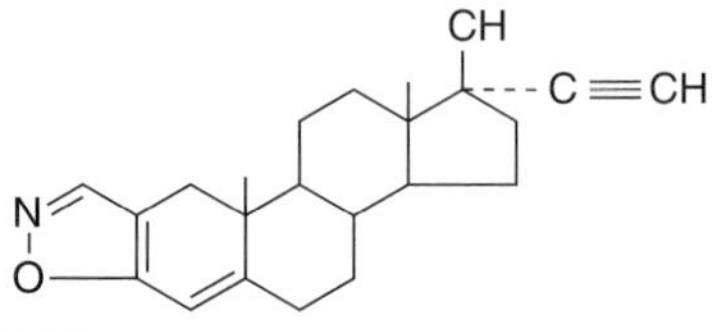

FIGURE 67-1   Molecular structure of danazol.

of estrogen from the follicles. Thus, danazol creates a hypoestrogenic state with 70% to 80% decrease in loss of menstrual blood. This suppressive action is reversible, as ovulation and cyclic bleeding usually returns within two to three months following discontinuation of danazol.

SIDE EFFECTS

Possible side effects of danazol include weight gain; deepening of the voice; fluid retention in the hands or feet; hirsutism (abnormal hair growth); weight gain; acne; visual changes; hot flashes and lack of menstruation; and dizziness and headache.

DRUG INTERACTIONS

Danazol (DNZ)

DNZ ⟷ Anisindione: Danazol reduces the amount of vitamin K available for blood clotting, and may increase the anticoagulant effect of anisindione.

DNZ ⟷ CYP Isozymes: *See* Table 67-1.

DNZ ⟷ Oral Contraceptives: It is recommended to avoid concurrent use of oral contraceptives (containing estradiol, ethinyl estradiol, norethindrone, and medroxyprogesterone) with danazol since there is a theoretical risk that danazol may compete for the same receptors for estrogens, progestogens, and androgens, altering their therapeutic effectiveness.

TABLE 67-1 Danazol and Bromocriptine vs CYP Enzymes

Drug Name	1A2	2A6	2B6	2C8	2C9	2C18	2C19	2D6	2E1	3A4
Danazol										Inh
Bromocriptine	Inh									Inh+ Sub

Abbreviations: Sub, substrate of the enzyme; Inh, inhibits the enzyme; Ezi, induces the enzyme

1. Danazol exerts an inhibitory effect on CYP3A4 and thus, administration with drugs that require this enzyme for metabolic clearance may result in elevated blood levels and increased incidence of adverse effects. Such drugs include: buspirone, cyclosporine, lovastatin, and tacrolimus. (*See* the middle column of Table-0 at the 'Introduction' for other possible substrates of this enzyme.)

2. Bromocriptine functions as an inhibitor of both CYP1A2 and CYP3A4 and thus, administration with drugs that require these enzymes for their hepatic clearance may raise blood levels and possibly exacerbate their adverse effects. (*See* the middle column of Table-0 at the 'Introduction' for possible substrates of these enzymes.)

3. Bromocriptine requires microsomal enzyme CYP3A4 for its metabolism and thus, inhibition of this enzyme by another drug may raise blood levels and exacerbate the adverse effects of bromocriptine. (*See* the left-hand column of Table-0 at the 'Introduction' for possible inhibitors of this enzyme).

BROMOCRIPTINE

Bromocriptine (*See* Fig. 56-4), a semisynthetic ergot alkaloid (a lysergic acid derivative), is indicated in the treatment of secondary amenorrhoea due to elevation of prolactin.

MECHANISM OF ACTION

Bromocriptine is a direct-acting dopaminergic agonist. It activates postsynaptic D2 receptors in the hypothalamus to inhibit the release of prolactin from the pituitary gland. Since excessive levels of prolactin can suppress secretions of FSH and GnRH to cause hypogonadism and amenorrhea, bromocriptine can bring about regular ovulations and normal menstruations.

SIDE EFFECTS

Possible side effects of bromocriptine include irregular heart rate; dizziness caused by low blood pressure in the first few days; shortness of breath; stomach ulcers or bleeding, nausea, vomiting, and constipation; involuntary movements; persistent headache and vision changes; and sudden attack of sleepiness (exercise caution when driving).

DRUG INTERACTIONS

See Box 67-1.

Miscellaneous Interactions of Bromocriptine (BCT)

Parentheses below indicate an herb.

BCT ↔ Alcohol: Dizziness and drowsiness can be made worse by drinking alcohol, endangering safety during driving.

BOX 67-1

Basic Concepts of Bromocriptine Interactions

The therapeutic effectiveness of Bromocriptine, a dopamine agonist, may be counteracted by dopamine antagonists. Those include: **chlorpromazine; haloperidol; metoclopramide** (a drug to treat heartburn due to gastroesophageal reflux); and **pimozide** (a drug to suppress severe motor tics in Tourette disorder).

BCT ⟷ (Chasteberry): Chemicals in chasteberry can occupy dopamine receptors in the brain to prevent bromocriptine from interacting with the receptors, opposing its therapeutic effectiveness.

BCT ⟷ CYP Isozymes: *See* Table 67-1.

BCT ⟷ Isometheptene: Concurrent use of bromocriptine with isometheptene, a migraine drug that constricts blood vessels and increases heart rate via release of norepinephrine, may result in hypertension and ventricular tachycardia.

BCT ⟷ (Sage): The hypotensive property of sage may potentiate the blood pressure-lowering effect of bromocriptine.

PROGESTOGENS

Progestogens contained in oral contraceptives are effective in the treatment of menorrhagia (excessive uterine bleeding at the expected intervals of the menstrual cycle).

MECHANISM OF ACTION

One important function of progesterone is to enrich the endometrium to support an implanted fertilized egg. If no implantation took place, secretions of progesterone from the corpus luteum decline to cause breakdown of the endometrium, resulting in menstruation. Excessive menstrual bleeding can be predictably suppressed within three days by use of progestogens such as norethindrone (Norlutate) and medroxyprogesterone (Provera). Progestogens treat dysfunctional uterine bleeding not only by controlling the acute bleeding but also by establishing normal ovulatory cycles.

SIDE EFFECTS

The progestogens may induce nausea, stomach upset, and cramping; jaundice (yellowing of the skin or eyes); breast tenderness; swelling in the hands, ankles, or feet; hirsutism; sudden headache, drowsiness, or dizziness; and darkened patches of skin (sunscreen ointment may help minimize this effect).

DRUG INTERACTIONS

See Appendix B-26: Interactions of Progesterone or Progestogens.

68 Menopausal Symptoms

Menopause is medically defined as the lack of menstruation for 12 consecutive months due to lack of secretion of female sex hormones, namely estrogens and progesterone. Menopausal symptoms include hot flashes, extreme sweating, vaginal dryness, water retention, weight gain, mood swings, headaches, anxiety, insomnia, and mental depression.

Medications that may be effective in the treatment of menopausal symptoms include: (1) **estradiol cypionate** injection or **estradiol transdermal** patch (Vivelle-DOT); (2) Prempro **(conjugated estrogens + medroxyprogesterone)** or **progesterone** (Prometrium); and (3) **paroxetine** (Paxil or Seroxat).

ESTRADIOL

Estradiol (Fig. 68-1) is prescribed for symptomatic treatment of the usual symptoms associated with menopause, such as hot flashes and vaginal dryness.

MECHANISM OF ACTION

Estrogens increase secretions from the cervix to alleviate vaginal dryness and promote growth of the inner lining of the uterus (endometrium). Estrogens prevent up-regulation of the calcitonin gene-related peptide (CGRP) receptor that mediates vasorelaxation and hot flashes.

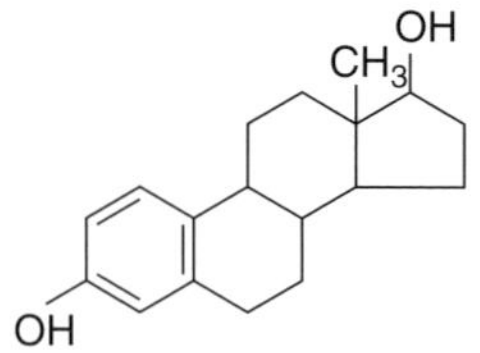

FIGURE 68-1   Molecular structure of estradiol.

SIDE EFFECTS

Side effects of estradiol may include nausea and vomiting; jaundice; water retention (swollen hands, feet, breasts or ankles); abnormal vaginal bleeding; headache, dizziness; and allergic reactions such as difficulty in breathing, and skin hives.

DRUG INTERACTIONS

Estradiol (ETD)

Parentheses below indicate an herb.

ETD ⟷ Anticoagulants: (*See* Ω-16 in Appendix A.) Estradiol decreases antithrombin-III activity to increase levels of fibrinogen, promoting blood coagulation and opposing the effectiveness of anticoagulants.

ETD ⟷ (Black Cohosh): This herb has an estrogen-like effect and may, probably by competition, interfere with the action of estrogens in birth control pills.

ETD ⟷ Cholesterol-Lowering Drugs: (*See* Ω-33 in Appendix A.) Estradiol may increase plasma levels of HDL-cholesterol ("good" cholesterol) and triglycerides, while decreasing the blood levels of LDL-cholesterol ("bad" cholesterol), promoting the effects of the cholesterol-lowering drugs.

ETD ⟷ CYP Isozymes: *See* Table 68-1.

ETD ⟷ Insulin: Estradiol was shown to increase tissue sensitivity to insulin, which may be beneficial in patients having elevated blood glucose levels and taking an antidiabetic agent.

TABLE 68-1 Estradiol vs CYP Enzymes

Drug Name	1A2	2A6	2B6	2C8	2C9	2C18	2C19	2D6	2E1	3A4
Estradiol	Sub Inh				Sub					Sub

Abbreviations: Sub, substrate of the enzyme; Inh, inhibits the enzyme; Ezi, induces the enzyme

1. Estradiol is mainly metabolized by CYP3A4, and, at high concentration, also by CYP1A2 and CYP2C9. Therefore, inducers of these enzymes such as carbamazepine, phenobarbital, phenytoin, rifampin, and St. John's wort may quicken its elimination, resulting in lowered blood levels and insufficient therapeutic effectiveness. (*See* the right-hand column of Table-0 at the 'Introduction' for other inducers of these enzymes.)

2. Estradiol has an inhibitory effect on CYP1A2. Therefore, administration in combination with drugs that require this enzyme for metabolic clearance may result in elevated blood levels, exacerbating their adverse effects. (*See* the middle column of Table-0 at the 'Introduction' for possible substrates of this enzyme.)

ETD ⟷ (Licorice): Estrogens can cause weight gain due to fluid retention. Licorice contains glycyrrhizin, which can produce effects similar to aldosterone, such as sodium retention, hypertension, and loss of potassium. Ingestion of oral contraceptives containing estrogens together with licorice may make women more vulnerable to hypertension, potassium loss, and fluid retention.

ETD ⟷ NSAIDs: (*See* Ω-54 in Appendix A.) Estradiol can cause water retention and thus, special care should be taken when estradiol is administered with drugs that cause fluid retention, such as NSAIDs.

ETD ⟷ Vasodilators: (*See* Ω-78 in Appendix A.) At high doses estradiol is known to cause weight gain due to fluid retention. Special care should be taken when estradiol is administered with drugs that cause fluid retention, including such vasodilators as hydralazine.

MEDROXYPROGESTERONE (PREMPRO) OR PROGESTERONE

Progesterone (Fig. 68-2) is used to protect the uterine lining in women on estrogen replacement therapy. Estrogens, if used alone in postmenopausal period, increase the risk of endometrial hyperplasia (abnormal proliferation of the uterine lining) that may be conducive to uterine cancer. Taking estrogens with progesterone is known to lower the risk of developing this cancer. Oral contraceptive pills are another form of hormone therapy to treat irregular vaginal bleeding for women in perimenopause.

MECHANISM OF ACTION

At menopause, estrogen levels drop about 50%, but a more drastic drop of progesterone occurs to create a severe imbalance of these two important sex hormones. The hormonal imbalance by estrogen dominance may trigger many menopausal symptoms. Therefore, transdermal progesterone cream alone will significantly improve vasomotor symptoms in perimenopause.

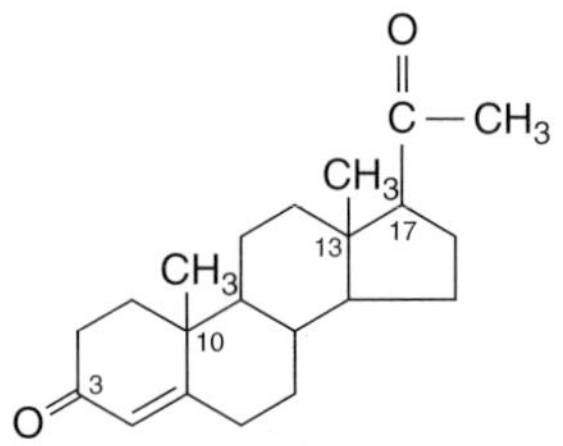

FIGURE 68-2   Molecular structure of progesterone.

SIDE EFFECTS

Prempro: This preparation may cause nausea, vomiting, bloating, and stomach pain; jaundice; abnormal vaginal bleeding; and headache, confusions, and dizziness. Rarely, it may cause allergic reactions such as difficulty in breathing; swelling of the face, lips, tongue, or throat; and skin hives and itching.

Progesterone: It may cause pounding heartbeat; nausea, diarrhea, and stomach pain; jaundice; muscle pain; and dizziness, headache, and confusions. It may also cause allergic reactions such as difficulty in breathing and swelling of tissues.

DRUG INTERACTIONS

Estrogen: *See* Chapter 67.

Progesterone: *See* Appendix B-26: Interactions of Progesterone or Progestogens.

PAROXETINE

MECHANISM OF ACTION

Paroxetine is a selective serotonin reuptake inhibitor (SSRI) used to treat mental depression. Its mode of action for treating hot flashes is unknown, but paroxetine appears to raise plasma levels of BDNF (brain-derived neurotrophic factor), a protein supporting the survival of existing neurons and generating new neurons. BDNF also appears to support survival of endothelial cells of blood vessels, possibly contributing to suppression of hot flashes.

SIDE EFFECTS

Frequent side effects of paroxetine include dry mouth, loss of appetite, upset stomach, nausea, and vomiting; sexual impotence; and headache, insomnia, dizziness, and anxiety.

DRUG INTERACTIONS

See Appendix B-29: Interactions of SSRIs (Selective Serotonin Reuptake Inhibitors).

CHAPTER

69

Breast Engorgement

Breast engorgement refers to a condition in which the mammary glands are over-filled with milk, blood, or other fluid. The engorged breast is swollen, hard, and painful. Breast engorgement usually starts with the onset of lactation (day two to five after parturition).

Medications that may be effective in the treatment of breast engorgement include: (1) **cabergoline** (Dostinex); (2) **bromocriptine**; (3) **azithromycin**; and (4) cephalosporin antibiotics such as **cefuroxime and cephalexin.**

CABERGOLINE

MECHANISM OF ACTION

Cabergoline is a long-acting dopamine receptor agonist that activates D2 receptors in the hypothalamus to inhibit prolactin secretion from the anterior pituitary gland.

SIDE EFFECTS

Possible side effects of cabergoline include orthostatic hypotension; nausea, vomiting, and constipation; tingling, fatigue, or numbness of limbs; swelling of feet or ankles; and headache, dizziness, and drowsiness.

DRUG INTERACTIONS

Cabergoline (CBG)

CBG ⟷ Haloperidol: Haloperidol (Fig. 69-1) is a dopamine antagonist that may counteract the dopamine-agonistic effect of cabergoline.

CBG ⟷ Macrolides: (*See* Ω-50 in Appendix A.) Cabergoline is known to be metabolized by CYP3A4, and bioavailability of cabergoline was increased two to four times by use with macrolide antibiotics such as clindamycin or erythromycin, both of which inhibit CYP3A4.

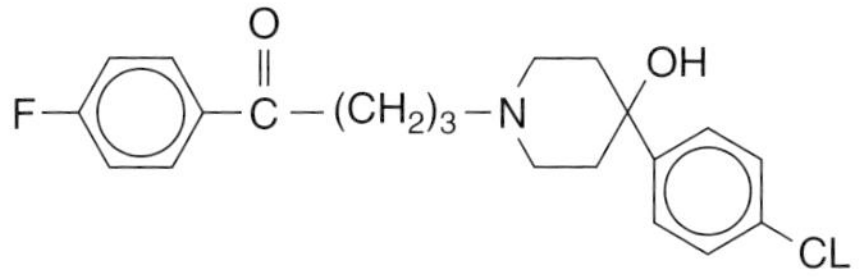

FIGURE 69-1   Molecular structure of haloperidol.

CBG ⟷ Metoclopramide: Cabergoline inhibits the release of prolactin, whereas metoclopramide tends to increase it. Therefore, combination of the two may compromise therapeutic value.

CBG ⟷ Phenothiazine Antipsychotic Drugs: (*See* Ω-58 in Appendix A.) Cabergoline is a dopamine agonist, whereas phenothiazine antipsychotic drugs have dopamine antagonistic properties. Thus, their co-administration may diminish their therapeutic efficacy.

BROMOCRIPTINE

Bromocriptine is a drug originally approved for use in the treatment of postpartum breast engorgement.

MECHANISM OF ACTION

Secretion of prolactin from the anterior pituitary gland is inhibited by dopamine produced in the tuberoinfundibular dopamine neurons of the hypothalamus. Bromocriptine is a synthetic dopamine agonist that can directly activate dopamine receptors to mimic effects of natural dopamine in the brain, thus suppressing excessive secretions of milk to reduce post-partum breast engorgement.

SIDE EFFECTS

Its possible side effects include hypotension and irregular pulse; shortness of breath; dry mouth, stomach cramps, nausea, and constipation; involuntary movements; and dizziness, drowsiness (sudden irresistible urge to sleep), and headache.

DRUG INTERACTIONS

See Appendix B-23: Interactions of Dopamine Agonists.

AZITHROMYCIN

Breast engorgement is conducive to development of lactation mastitis (inflammation of the milk ducts with mild fever from germ invasion), usually in one to two weeks postpartum. Azithromycin, an erythromycin derivative, may help suppress proliferation of the infecting germs.

MECHANISM OF ACTION

Azithromycin binds to the 50S subunit of the bacterial ribosome to inhibit peptidyl transferase, the enzyme required for elongation of the bacterial peptide chain.

SIDE EFFECTS

Possible side effects of azithromycin include uneven heartbeat; nausea, vomiting, stomach pain, and bloody diarrhea; dizziness, tiredness, and headache; and rarely, such allergic reactions as skin hives and swelling of tissues.

DRUG INTERACTIONS

See Appendix B-13: Interactions of Macrolide Antibiotics.

CEPHALOSPORIN ANTIBIOTICS

Cefuroxime and **cephalexin**

Use of a cephalosporin antibiotic, such as cefuroxime or cephalexin, may help treat lactation mastitis.

MECHANISM OF ACTION

Their mechanism of antibacterial action is identical to that of penicillin antibiotics. *See* Chapter 12.

SIDE EFFECTS

The possible side effects of the above cephalosporin antibiotics include nausea, vomiting, bloody diarrhea, and stomach pain; muscle ache; nephrotoxicity; headache, dizziness, and convulsions; and allergic reactions such as difficulty in breathing; swelling of the face, lips, tongue, or throat, and skin hives.

DRUG INTERACTIONS

See Appendix B-17: Interactions of Cephalosporins.

70

Hyperemesis Gravidarum

Hyperemesis gravidarum (literally, excessive vomiting in pregnant women, or morning sickness) is a severe form of nausea and vomiting in the morning during the first trimester of pregnancy. It is characterized by persistent vomiting, weight loss, and dehydration. Nausea is thought to result from increased estrogen levels. The onset of nausea is as early as one month of pregnancy, and tends to taper off by month four.

Medications that may be effective in the treatment of morning sickness include: (1) **ondansetron** (Zofran); (2) **hydroxyzine** (vistaril); (3) **metoclopramide** (Reglan); and (4) **promethazine** (Phenergan).

ONDANSETRON

See Chapter 20.

HYDROXYZINE

MECHANISM OF ACTION

The exact mechanism of action by which hydroxyzine works to suppress hyperemesis gravidarum is not clear, but the chemoreceptor trigger zone has an abundance of both H_1 receptors and acetylcholine receptors; and hydroxyzine is an H_1 receptor antagonist and has an anticholinergic effect as well.

SIDE EFFECTS

Hydroxyzine may cause dry mouth; difficulty in breathing; abnormal muscle movements in the eyes, jaw, or neck; tremors; dizziness, drowsiness, blurred vision, headache, confusion, convulsions; and rarely, allergic reactions such as skin hives and itching.

DRUG INTERACTIONS

See Appendix B-10: Interactions of Antihistamines, First-Generation.

METOCLOPRAMIDE

Metoclopramide, 10 mg taken orally four times a day, 30 minutes before each meal and at bed time, was found effective in controlling hyperemesis gravidarum.

MECHANISM OF ACTION

The exact mechanism of action by which metoclopramide works to suppress hyperemesis gravidarum is not clear, but the chemoreceptor trigger zone at the base of the fourth ventricle has numerous dopamine receptors (type D_2), serotonin receptors (type 5-HT_3), and acetylcholine receptors, and metoclopramide blocks both dopamine receptors and serotonin receptors (at higher doses) in the chemoreceptor trigger zone.

SIDE EFFECTS

Possible side effects of metoclopramide include fast heartbeat; nausea, dry mouth, and diarrhea; muscle stiffness, spasms, and involuntary trembling movements of the eyes, face and limbs (like in Parkinson disease); sweating; and dizziness, drowsiness, headache, anxiety, restlessness, and insomnia.

DRUG INTERACTIONS

See Chapter 13.

PROMETHAZINE

Promethazine (Fig. 70-1) is a phenothiazine with antihistaminic activity. Promethazine is one of the most frequently used medications to treat hyperemesis gravidarum.

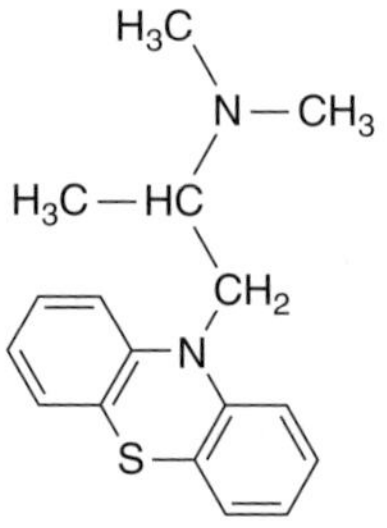

FIGURE 70-1   Molecular structure of promethazine.

MECHANISM OF ACTION

The exact mechanism of action by which promethazine works to suppress hyperemesis gravidarum is not clear, but promethazine has strong anticholinergic and antihistaminic effects (competitively blocks histamine type H_1 receptors) and also blocks, although weakly, dopamine type D_2 receptors in the neurons of the central nervous system (CNS).

SIDE EFFECTS

Side effects of promethazine may include cardiac arrhythmia, bruising, or bleeding; breathing difficulty; dry mouth, sore throat, stomach pain, and constipation; jaundice (yellowing of the skin or eyes); urinary infrequency; joint pain, and dyskinesia; weight gain; and increased sensitivity to light, ringing in the ears, dizziness, drowsiness, convulsions, and hallucinations.

DRUG INTERACTIONS

See Appendix B-25: Interactions of Phenothiazine Antipsychotic Drugs.

CHAPTER

71

Algesia (Physical Pain)

Algesia (physical pain) refers to localized sensations of suffering, such as pricking, stabbing, burning, throbbing, and aching caused by a noxious stimulus associated with disease or injury. Physical pain arises from stimulation of specific nerve endings that carry pain impulses to the brain. Untreated chronic pain may herald irritability, hopelessness, depression, and anger. Cephalalgia (headache) refers to pain or discomfort in the region of the head or neck. Primary headaches, not associated with any underlying diseases, include tension headache, migraine, and cluster headache.

Tension headache is caused by muscle strain. Migraine usually affects only one side of the head, arousing intense pain that could last more than several hours. Cluster headache, which usually originates near an eye and spreads to the facial area, also generates intense pain but lasts somewhere between thirty minutes and three hours, with attacks recurring several times during the same day or night (in clusters), for several weeks or months.

Medications shown effective in the treatment of headache include: (1) **acetaminophen** (Tylenol); (2) NSAIDs (non-steroidal anti-inflammatory drugs) such as **aspirin, ibuprofen** (Advil, Motrin, and others), and **naproxen;** (3) opioid analgesics such as **codeine, fentanyl, hydrocodone, methadone** (Methadose), **morphine,** and **oxycodone** (OxyContin); (4) **tramadol** (Ultracet, Ultram); (5) triptans such as **almotriptan** (Axert), **naratriptan** (Amerge), **rizatriptan**

(Maxalt), **sumatriptan** (Imitrex), and **zolmitriptan** (Zomig); (6) **ergotamine** (Cafergot, Ergomar); and (7) **topiramate** (Topamax).

ACETAMINOPHEN

Acetaminophen is used alone, or in combination with a barbiturate or with trama-dol: For instance, Fioricet **(acetaminophen + butalbital +caffeine),** and Ultracet [**acetaminophen + tramadol**], respectively.

MECHANISM OF ACTION

The analgesic action of acetaminophen remains poorly understood, but it app-ears that acetaminophen converts the active form of oxidized COX-1 and COX-2 to the inactive reduced form of those enzymes. Therefore, this drug is more effective under a condition where hydrogen peroxide concentration is low, such as in the central nervous system (CNS), and poorly effective in a condition where hydrogen peroxide concentration is high, such as in an inflammatory tissue. This may explain why acetaminophen is not an effective agent to treat inflammatory diseases such as arthritis and gout.

SIDE EFFECTS

Acetaminophen: Possible side effects of acetaminophen include nausea, bloat-ing, and upset stomach; jaundice (yellowing of the skin or eyes) and hepatotoxicity (overdoses only); renal impairment (overdoses only); and rarely, allergic reactions such as swelling of tissues.

Fioricet **(Butalbital + Acetaminophen + Caffeine):** Possible side effects of this preparation include shortness of breath; abdominal pain, nausea, and vomiting; and dizziness, drowsiness, and lightheadedness.

Ultracet **(Acetaminophen + Tramadol):** This preparation may cause weakened cardiac contractility; nausea, vomiting, constipation, and loss of appetite; sweat-ing; dizziness, drowsiness, and convulsions (seizures); and rarely, allergic reactions such as skin hives.

DRUG INTERACTIONS

Parentheses below indicate an herb.

Acetaminophen

See Chapter 18.

MECHANISM OF ACTION

All the above opioid drugs mainly bind to and activate opioid mu receptors that are located on presynaptic neuronal cell membranes mostly in the periaqueductal gray region and the substantia gelatinosa at the dorsal horns of the spinal cord. Activation of the mu receptors causes not only analgesia, euphoria, sedation, and miosis, but also fall of blood pressure, respiratory depression, nausea, and constipation. Activation of the mu receptors dulls neuronal excitability, probably by causing the release of gamma-aminobutyric acid (GABA) which opposes the release of excitatory neurotransmitters, or by opening the G protein-gated potassium channel, enhancing the efflux of potassium ions, to cause hyperpolarization that impedes conduction of the pain impulse toward the thalamus, providing the so-called supraspinal analgesia. The opioids also bind to and activate the kappa receptors in the spinal cord to decrease influx of calcium ions and thereby impede the release of substance P, an algesic (or pain-producing) substance, providing the so-called spinal anesthesia, sedation, and miosis.

SIDE EFFECTS

Opioids may generate one or more of the following adverse effects. If the symptoms get worse or a side effect not listed here emerges, taking emergency action is warranted. The frequent side effects of the above narcotic drugs include slowing of heartbeat; difficulty in breathing (a common side effect of narcotic analgesics is constipation and respiratory depression); nausea, vomiting, and stomach pain; dizziness, confusion, and convulsions; and allergic reactions such as skin hives and swelling of tissues.

DRUG INTERACTIONS

See Appendix B-32: Interactions of Opioid Analgesics.

TRAMADOL

Tramadol (*See* Fig. 71-4) is a synthetic opioid but its chemical structure is quite different from that of authentic opioids. Tramadol is indicated for the management of moderate to moderately severe pain, and is often used in combination with acetaminophen.

MECHANISM OF ACTION

The mode of analgesic action of tramadol is poorly understood, but it appears that it weakly binds to the mu-opioid receptor and inhibits reuptake of norepinephrine and serotonin to exert influences on the noradrenergic and serotonergic systems. Tramadol has less potential for respiratory depression than do authentic narcotic pain-killers.

BOX 71-1

Basic Concepts of Tramadol Interactions

1. Tramadol produces CNS depression such as coma, seizure, nausea, vomiting, and respiratory depression at large doses, although to a lesser extent than morphine; and when co-administered with drugs that also generate a CNS depressant effect, excessive neuronal depression may result. Those drugs include: **alcohol; antihistamines** (*See* Ω-19 in Appendix A); **barbiturates; benzodiazepine antianxiety drugs** (*See* Ω-26 in Appendix A); **chloral hydrate; phenothiazine antipsychotic drugs** (*See* Ω-58 in Appendix A); and **tricyclic antidepressants** (*See* Ω-76 in Appendix A).

2. Tramadol inhibits the synaptic reuptake of serotonin and norepinephrine, and when co-administered with drugs that also inhibit reuptake of serotonin or that activate serotonin receptors, serotonin syndrome may results. Symptoms include: hypertension, renal failure, hyperthermia (body temperature as high as 104°), diaphoresis (sweating), myoclonus (intermittent tremors or twitching), delirium, and seizure. Those drugs include: **SSRIs** (*See* Ω-68 in Appendix A); **triptans** including rizatriptan and sumatriptan (serotonin receptor agonists acting on the most abundant 5-HT1D receptors) (*See* Ω-77 in Appendix A); and **venlafaxine** (an antidepressant that inhibits the synaptic reuptake of serotonin and norepinephrine).

SIDE EFFECTS

Tramadol may cause nausea, loss of appetite, and constipation; sweating; dizziness and drowsiness; convulsions; and allergic reactions.

DRUG INTERACTIONS

Tramadol is a prodrug which has to be oxidatively activated by CYP2D6. Thus, tramadol is ineffective with low CYP2D6 activity.

Miscellaneous Interactions of Tramadol (TMD)

Parentheses below indicate an herb.

TMD ⟷ Benzodiazepine Antianxiety Drugs: (*See* Ω-26 in Appendix A.) If tramadol is taken with a benzodiazepine antianxiety drug such as diazepam, an alarming CNS depression may ensue, causing severe respiratory depression.

TMD ⟷ CYP Isozymes: *See* Table 71-2.

TABLE 71-3 Ergotamine vs CYP Enzymes

Drug Name	1A2	2A6	2B6	2C8	2C9	2C18	2C19	2D6	2E1	3A4
Ergotamine										Sub+ Inh

Abbreviations: Sub, substrate of the enzyme; **Inh**, inhibits the enzyme; Ezi, induces the enzyme

1. Elimination of ergotamine requires the microsomal CYP3A4 and thus, inhibition of this enzyme by other drugs can raise blood levels and enhance the adverse effects of ergotamine, such as ergotism with serious vasospasm. Those strong inhibitors of CYP3A4 include: clarithromycin, indinavir, itraconazole, ketoconazole, nefazodone, nelfinavir, ritonavir, saquinavir, and telithromycin. (*See* the left-hand column of Table-0 at the 'Introduction' for other possible inhibitors of the enzyme.)

2. Ergotamine is an inhibitor of the microsomal CYP3A4 and thus, co-administration with drugs that require this enzyme for clearance may raise their blood levels and possibly exacerbate their adverse effects. Those drugs include: alfentanil, budesonide, buspirone, cyclosporine, ergotamine, felodipine, fentanyl, fluticasone, lovastatin, pimozide, quinidine, saquinavir, sildenafil (Viagra), simvastatin, sirolimus, tacrolimus, triazolam, and vardenafil. (*See* the middle column of Table-0 at the 'Introduction' for other possible substrates of this enzyme.)

TOPIRAMATE

Topiramate is an anticonvulsant indicated in the treatment of epilepsy and migraine. Topiramate is occasionally used in the treatment of chronic pain as well.

MECHANISM OF ACTION

Topiramate appears to potentiate $GABA_A$-evoked influx of chloride ions to facilitate hyperpolarization, which helps suppress the paroxysmal neuronal discharge involved in algesia.

SIDE EFFECTS

Topiramate may cause hypokalemia; taste changes and loss of appetite; stomach pain or upset, nausea, and diarrhea; renal stone formation; decreased sweating; flu-like symptoms such as numbness or tingling of the skin, runny nose, and sore throat; dizziness, and drowsiness; and tiredness.

DRUG INTERACTIONS

See Chapter 55.

72

Pyrexia (Fever)

Pyrexia (fever) refers to a rise in body temperature above 104° F. Fever causes sweating and body water loss. Therefore, drinking plenty of fluids helps prevent dehydration and allows the body to rid itself of the fever. If the temperature is above normal (98.6° F) but below 102° F, fever has a beneficial effect by helping fight germs that cause infections.

Fever may be combated by the following medical treatments: (1) **acetaminophen** (Tylenol); (2) **aspirin**; and (3) **ibuprofen** (Advil, Motrin, Medipren, Nuprin).

ACETAMINOPHEN

The WHO recommends that acetaminophen, rather than aspirin, be given to children with fever, for aspirin is thought to generate Reye syndrome in that age group. Therefore, acetaminophen is the most commonly used drug to treat fever in children.

MECHANISM OF ACTION

The mode of action whereby acetaminophen reduces fever is debatable. However, it is shown that endogenous pyrogens generated by leukocytes increase production of prostaglandin E (PGE), which jacks up the thermostat set-point at the thermocontrol center (preoptic area of the anterior hypothalamus). It is believed that acetaminophen inhibits the enzyme cyclooxygenase (COX-3) (a tissue-specific COX with the highest expressions in the brain) to block the synthesis of PGE, thereby returning the set-point to normal, allowing heat dissipation by peripheral vasodilation and sweating. All of these effects are mediated through activation of the parasympathetic system.

SIDE EFFECTS

Acetaminophen may cause nausea, bloating, and upset stomach; jaundice (yellowing of the skin or eyes) and hepatotoxicity (overdoses only); renal impairment (overdoses only); headache, dizziness, and nervousness; and rarely, allergic reactions such as swelling of tissues.

DRUG INTERACTIONS

See Chapter 18.

ASPIRIN

Aspirin should not be given to infants and children younger than 16 because of the risk of Reye syndrome, a life-threatening neurological disorder.

MECHANISM OF ACTION

The acetyl group of aspirin (Fig. 72-1) acetylates and irreversibly inhibits COX-1 and modifies the enzymatic activity of COX-2, and thereby blocks the synthesis of PGE by endogenous pyrogens. The thermocontrol set-point raised by PGE cannot be sustained without continuous synthesis of PGE and therefore, is now allowed to return back to normal. This results in heat dissipation by peripheral vasodilation and sweating, all mediated through activation of the parasympathetic system.

SIDE EFFECTS

Aspirin may cause gastric pain, nausea, and vomiting; ringing in the ears; and rarely, allergic reactions such as skin rash and itching; difficulty in breathing; and swelling of the face, lips, tongue, or throat.

DRUG INTERACTIONS

See Box 72-1.

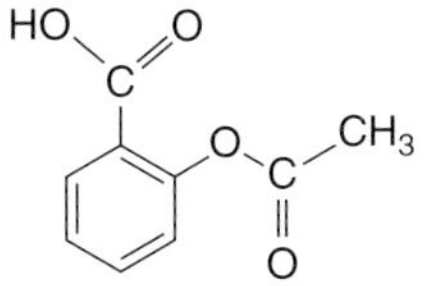

FIGURE 72-1   Molecular structure of aspirin.

BOX 72-1

Basic Concepts of Aspirin Interactions

1. Aspirin irreversibly inhibits the enzyme COX-1 so as to oppose synthesis of thromboxane within platelets, generating its antiplatelet effect. When co-administered with drugs that generate a bleeding tendency, excessive hemorrhage with prolongation of prothrombin time may result. Those drugs include: **anticoagulants** including Enoxaparin, a low molecular weight heparin (*See* Ω-16 in Appendix A); **(chamomile)** (Fig. 72-2 A and B) (a sedating herb that has anti-inflammatory effect, contains coumarins that have an anticoagulant effect); **clopidogrel** (a potent oral antiplatelet agent that binds to and inhibits the ADP receptors on the platelet cell membrane so as to block activation of the glycoprotein IIb/IIIa pathway that leads to platelet aggregation); **eptifibatide** (blocks the platelet glycoprotein IIb/IIIa receptor, the binding site for fibrinogen); **(ginkgo biloba)** (an herb reported to cause bleeding complications); **glucocorticoids** (*See* Ω-42 in Appendix A) (known to cause peptic ulcer bleeding); **(hawthorn)** (an herb that inhibits synthesis of thromboxane to facilitate bleeding); **NSAIDs** (*See* Ω-54 in Appendix A) (all of the NSAIDs ,with possible exception of celecoxib, meloxicam, and nabumetone, can inhibit platelet aggregation by binding reversibly to platelet enzyme COX); **omega-3 fatty acids** (intake of three grams or more in one day may increase the risk of bleeding); **thrombolytic agents** (*See* Ω-74 in Appendix A);

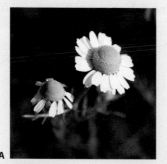
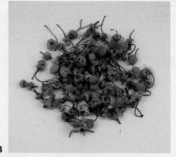

A   **B**

FIGURE 72-2   **A, Partial feature of chamomile in nature. B, Chamomile (cut & dried flowers).**

(Attribution: Fir0002/Flagstaffotos at http://www.google.com/imgres?imgurl=http://upload.wikimedia. org/wikipedia/commons/7/7f/Chamomile_flowers.jpg&imgrefurl=http://commons.wikimedia.org/wiki/ File:Chamomile_flowers.jpg&usg=__UGsTdG_M70IOP1XpVQylqZ8abNw=&h=1184&w=1600&sz=179&hl= en&start=2&um=1&itbs=1&tbnid=_Q4IkIjFj5QjzM:&tbnh=111&tbnw=150&prev=/images%3Fq%3DCham omile,%2BWikimedia%26um%3D1%26hl%3Den%26sa%3DG%26tbs%3DIsch:1, Permission is granted to copy, distribute and/or modify this image under the terms of the *GNU Free Documentation License*)

TABLE 73-1   GABA Activators vs CYP Enzymes

Drug Name	1A2	2A6	2B6	2C8	2C9	2C18	2C19	2D6	2E1	3A4
Eszopiclone										Sub
Zaleplon										Sub
Zolpidem										Sub

Abbreviations: Sub, substrate of the enzyme; Inh, inhibits the enzyme; Ezi, induces the enzyme

1. All three require microsomal CYP3A4 for their metabolic clearance. Therefore, inhibition of this enzyme by another drugs can raise their blood levels and enhance their adverse effects. Those strong inhibitors of CYP 3A4 include: clarithromycin, indinavir, itraconazole, ketoconazole, nefazodone nelfinavir, ritonavir, saquinavir, and telithromycin. (*See* the left-hand column of Table-0 at the 'Introduction' for other possible inhibitors of the enzyme.)

2. As all three require microsomal CYP3A4 for their metabolic clearance, co-administration with an inducer of this enzyme, such as rifampin, can quicken their elimination to decrease their blood levels and undercut their therapeutic efficacies. (*See* the right-hand column of Table-0 at the 'Introduction' for other possible inducers of the enzyme.)

ANTIHISTMINES

Diphenhydramine and **doxylamine**

MECHANISM OF ACTION

Both diphenhydramine (*See* Fig. 20-1) and doxylamine are ethanolamine antihistamines that can cross the blood-brain barrier to generate drowsiness and mental impairment. They decrease sleep onset latency and prolong duration of sleep. However, their exact mechanism of action remains elusive, though they are known to generate central anticholinergic effects.

SIDE EFFECTS

Their side effects may include dry mouth; difficulty in urination and enlarged prostate gland; and fatigue, headache, and dizziness.

DRUG INTERACTIONS

See Appendix B-10: Interactions of Antihistamines, First-Generation.

BENZODIAZEPINE SEDATIVES

Diazepam, estazolam, lorazepam, temazepam, and **triazolam**

MECHANISM OF ACTION

Their precise mechanism of action to treat insomnia is debatable, but the BDZs bind to their specific subunit at the GABA/BZD receptor complex to allosterically enhance the effects of GABA, including opening of the chloride channels to generate hyperpolarization of the post-synaptic membrane of the CNS, thus making the membrane less likely to generate action potential in response to excitatory external stimuli.

SIDE EFFECTS

Some patients may experience one or more of the following adverse effects. If the symptoms get worse or a side effect not listed here emerges, taking emergency actions is warranted. Possible side effects include: dry mouth, nausea, and vomiting; diarrhea; difficulty in urination (less frequent than usual or no urination); muscle twitching and tremors; hyperactivity, agitations, and hostility; drowsiness and tiredness; aggressive behavior; and rarely, allergic reactions such as skin rash and itching. Further, they have a potential to develop physical dependency.

DRUG INTERACTIONS

See Appendix B-16: Interactions of Benzodiazepines.

CHAPTER

74

Pregnancy

Pregnancy refers to the consecutive events of an egg being fertilized by a sperm, implanted in the lining of the uterus, and developing from an embryo into a fetus. It culminates in the delivery of a baby. While pregnancy is usually desired to procure offspring, there are circumstances in which the pregnancy may be unwanted or even undesirable.

Medications shown effective in the prevention of pregnancy include: (1) **estrogen + progestogen;** (2) **medroxyprogesterone** (Cycrin, Provera); and (3) **mifepristone** (RU-486).

ESTROGEN + PROGESTOGEN

One of the following oral contraceptive pills containing one estrogen and one progestogen may be effective to prevent undesired pregnancy: (1) **ethinyl estradiol + desogestrel** (Apri, Kariva); (2) **ethinyl estradiol + drospirenone** (Yasmin 28); (3) **ethinyl estradiol + etonogestrel** (NuvaRing); (4) **ethinyl estradiol + levonorgestrel** (Aviane, Trivora-28); (5) **ethinyl estradiol + norelgestromin** (Ortho Evra); (6) **ethinyl estradiol + norethindrone** (Estrostep Fe, Necon 1/35); (7) **ethinyl estradiol + norgestimate** (Fig. 74-1) (Ortho Tri-Cycle, Sprintec, Trinessa, Tri-Sprintec); (8) **ethinyl estradiol + norgestrel** (Fig. 74-2) (Low-Ogestrel); and (9) **ethinyl estradiol + etonogestrel** (Fig. 74-3) (NuvaRing).

Emergency contraception (EC) refers to drugs used to prevent pregnancy after unprotected intercourse. Emergency contraception, however, should not be considered a primary means of contraception because of higher incidences of adverse effects. The EC pills, in fact, are effective when taken shortly before, or within 72 hours after, coitus. The sooner they are taken, the higher the success rates. One medication for this purpose is the Yuzpe regimen (1 mg of norgestrel + 0.1 mg of ethinylestradiol) taken within 72 hours of unprotected intercourse, and then another identical dose 12 hours later, having up to 95% success rate. However, this method is now superseded by taking a single dose of 1.5 mg of levonorgestrel within 72 hours after coitus, or alternatively, taking 0.75 mg and repeating the dose 12 hours later. Ulipristal (Ella), a second-generation selective progesterone receptor modulator (SPRM), is a newer emergency contraceptive

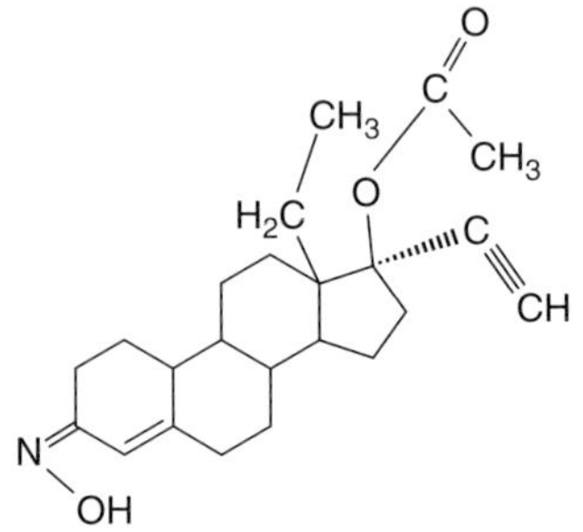

FIGURE 74-1   Molecular structure of norgestimate.

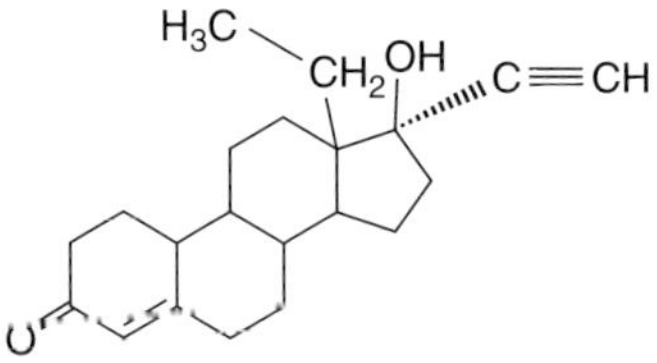

FIGURE 74-2   Molecular structure
of norgestrel.

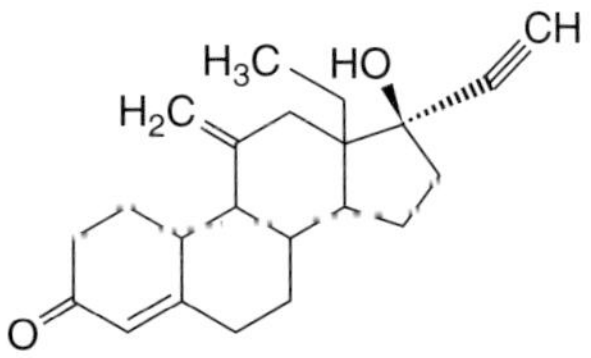

FIGURE 74-3   Molecular structure
of etonogestrel.

approved by the FDA in 2010. If taken within 120 hours of an unprotected coitus, ulipristal may provide about 60% contraception. Though chemically similar to mifepristone, which is considered a first-generation SPRM, ulipristal seems to work more by inhibition or delay of ovulation to prevent pregnancy, whereas mifepristone seems to work mainly by altering endometrium to induce abortion in pregnancies.

MECHANISM OF ACTION

The estrogens at high doses found in the regular contraceptive pills inhibit the release of gonadotropins such as follicle stimulating hormone (FSH) to prevent development of ovarian follicles. Thus, ovulation is avoided and there is no egg to fertilize. The progestogens are added to make the endometrium unsuitable for implantation of a fertilized egg, and to ensure that the withdrawal bleeding (upon discontinuation of the pills) will be quick in onset and short in duration, similar to natural menstruation.

SIDE EFFECTS

Ethinyl Estradiol: Side effects of ethinyl estradiol may include elevation of blood pressure and mid-cycle (breakthrough) bleeding or spotting; nausea, vomiting, and abdominal cramps; change in sexual desire; and headache.

Progestogens: Possible side effects of progestogens found in contraceptive pills may include changes in vaginal bleeding (such as spotting, or breakthrough bleeding); shortness of breath; fainting; chest pain, nausea, and vomiting; jaundice (yellowing of the eyes or skin); breast tenderness or enlargement; edema with swelling of the hands and feet; slurred speech; vision changes; dizziness; and rarely, allergic reaction such as skin rash.

DRUG INTERACTIONS
Ethinyl Estradiol
See Box 74-1.

Miscellaneous Interactions of Ethinyl Estradiol (ETD)
Parentheses below indicate an herb.

ETD ⟷ Anticoagulants: (Refer to Ω-16 in Appendix A.) Estrogens decrease antithrombin-III activity and increase levels of fibrinogen and fibrinogen activity,

---

BOX 74-1

Basic Concepts of Ethinyl Estradiol Interactions

1. A known pathway of elimination of ethinyl estradiol is sulfation in the gastro-intestinal wall, and when ethinyl estradiol is co-administered with a drug that also undergoes sulfation, they may compete with each other for this same process, potentially resulting in increased bioavailability of ethinyl estradiol. Those drugs include: **acetaminophen** and **ascorbic acid.** Ascorbic acid (or vitamin C) is converted to ascorbic acid-2-sulfate, which has no biological activity in humans.

2. Ethinyl estradiol is absorbed from the small intestine to reach its peak serum concentration in about two hours. The absorbed drug enters the liver to undergo metabolism by CYP3A4, and its metabolite and some intact ethinyl estradiol are excreted into the bile, and then get reabsorbed via enterohepatic circulation to provide a second peak concentration in the blood several hours later. This enterohepatic circulation is blocked by combined intake of some antibiotics, leading to reduced therapeutic effectiveness. Those drugs include: **cephalosporin antibiotics** (*See* Ω-32 in Appendix A) (note: it is believed that these antibiotics decrease bacterial hydrolytic enzymes required for regen-erating parent estradiol in the gastrointestinal tract); **penicillins** including amoxicillin, ampicillin, and penicillin-V (*See* Ω-56 in Appendix A); and **tetracycline antibiotics** (*See* Ω-72 in Appendix A).

to promote blood coagulation and oppose the therapeutic effectiveness of anticoagulants.

ETD ⟷ (Black Cohosh): This herb has an estrogen-like effect, interfering with the actions of hormonal medications, including estradiol, in contraceptive pills.

ETD ⟷ (Chasteberry): Certain chemicals in chasteberry are known to occupy dopamine receptors in the brain to prevent binding of dopamine to its receptor. Chasteberry appears to shift estrogen levels down and progesterone levels up, and this hormonal imbalance may interfere with the effectiveness of ethinyl estradiol as an oral contraceptive.

ETD ⟷ Cholesterol-Lowering Drugs: (*See* Ω-33 in Appendix A.) Estradiol may increase plasma levels of HDL-cholesterol ("good" cholesterol) and decrease blood levels of LDL-cholesterol ("bad" cholesterol) to enhance the beneficial effect of cholesterol-lowering drugs.

ETD ⟷ CYP Isozymes: *See* Table 74-1.

ETD ⟷ Dantrolene: Both dantrolene and estrogen can generate hepatotoxicity. Estrogens may cause intrahepatic cholestasis in susceptible women during pregnancy. Concomitant use may increase the chance of hepatotoxicity, especially in the elderly

ETD ⟷ Didanosine: Estrogens can cause hypertriglyceridemia, which rarely can lead to pancreatitis. Didanosine is associated with reports of fatal and nonfatal pancreatitis. The likelihood of developing pancreatitis may be increased when the two are used in combination.

ETD ⟷ Insulin: Estrogens are known to increase the sensitivity of tissues to insulin, which may be beneficial in patients with elevated blood glucose levels taking an antidiabetic agent.

ETD ⟷ (Licorice): Licorice has an aldosterone-like effect to retain fluid, as do estrogens. When the two are taken together, it may make women more vulnerable to hypertension, potassium loss, and fluid retention.

ETD ⟷ NSAIDs: (*See* Ω-54 in Appendix A.) Estradiol in high doses is known to cause water retention, as do most NSAIDs. Special care should be taken when an estrogen is administered with other drugs that also cause fluid retention.

ETD ⟷ Ropinirole: Elimination of ropinirole is believed to be mostly due to hepatic oxidation through CYP1A2 rather than renal clearance. Clearance of

TABLE 74-1 Ethinyl Estradiol and Medroxyprogesterone vs CYP Enzymes

Drug Name	1A2	2A6	2B6	2C8	2C9	2C18	2C19	2D6	2E1	3A4
Ethinyl Estradiol										Sub+ Inh
Medroxyprogesterone										Sub

Abbreviations: Sub, substrate of the enzyme; Inh, inhibits the enzyme; Ezi, induces the enzyme

1. Hepatic inactivation of ethinyl estradiol is mainly via CYP3A4. Therefore, inducers of this enzyme by other drugs can lower blood levels of ethinyl estradiol to compromise its therapeutic effectiveness, possibly resulting in contraceptive failure. Those inducers of CYP3A4 include carbamazepine, phenobarbital, rifampin. and the herb St. John's wort. (*See* the right-hand column of Table-0 at the 'Introduction' for other possible inducers of the enzyme).
2. Ethinyl estradiol has a CYP3A4 inhibitory effect. Thus, co-administration with drugs that require this enzyme for their metabolic clearance may result in elevated blood levels, exacerbating their adverse effects. (*See* the middle column of Table-0 at the 'Introduction' for possible substrates of this enzyme.)
3. Medroxyprogesterone requires microsomal enzyme CYP3A4 for its metabolic clearance, and when taken in combination with another drug that induces this enzyme, such as St John's wort, it may quicken clearance of medroxyprogesterone to lead to therapeutic insufficiency, possibly bringing about contraception failure. (*See* the right-hand column of Table-0 at the 'Introduction' for other possible inducers of this enzyme.)

ropinirole may be decreased in some patients taking ethinyl estradiol. The mechanism of action is unclear, but one possibility is that estradiol is inhibitory to hepatic enzyme CYP1A2.

ETD ⟷ Thyroid Preparations: (*See* Ω-75 in Appendix A.) Estrogens increase the serum concentration of thyroxine-binding globulin to decrease the amount of unbound free thyroxine. Hypothyroid patients cannot compensate for this, and may require an increased dose of thyroxine.

ETD ⟷ Vasodilators: (*See* Ω-78 in Appendix A.) Estrogens in high doses are known to cause weight gain due to their fluid retention. Special care should be taken when estrogens are administered with drugs that also cause fluid retention, including vasodilators such as hydralazine.

Progestogens in Contraceptives: *See* Appendix B-26: Interactions of Progesterone or Progestogens

MEDROXYPROGESTERON

Medroxyprogesterone (Fig. 74-4) is a synthetic progestogen used without an estrogen combined. Its oral preparation is available, but Depo-Provera is for injection into a muscle, whereas Depo-subQ Provera 104 is for injection under the skin. One injected dose may provide effective birth control for three months.

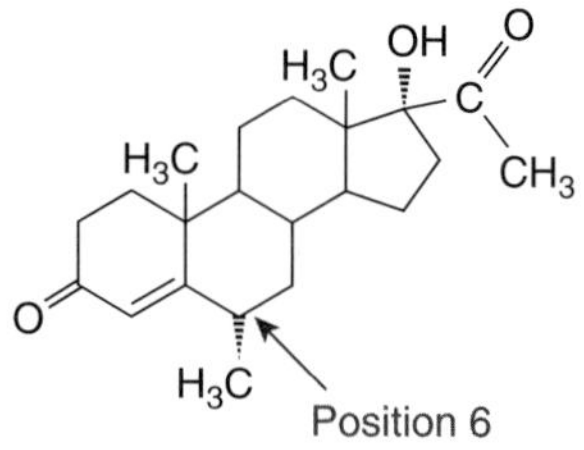

FIGURE 74-4   Molecular structure of medroxyprogesterone (6-methylated progesterone).

MECHANISM OF ACTION

Long term administration of medroxyprogesterone blocks the synthesis of luteinizing hormone in the pituitary gland, probably by negative feedback, thereby preventing maturation of ovarian follicles and ovulation.

SIDE EFFECTS

Its side effects may include blood clots (cigarette smokers are more vulnerable to blood clotting), breakthrough bleeding (menstruation-like bleeding in the middle of the menstrual cycle), vaginal spotting and changes in menstrual flow; sudden shortness of breath; nausea and stomach pain; jaundice; numbness or pain in the arm or leg; rarely, breast tenderness and leakage of liquid from the nipple; skin reactions including hives and acne; and severe headache. As medroxyprogesterone can cause birth defects, it should not be used during pregnancy.

DRUG INTERACTIONS

Medroxyprogesterone (MDP)

MDP ↔ Azole Antifungal Drugs: (*See* Ω-23 in Appendix A.) The contraceptive efficacy of medroxyprogesterone may occasionally be compromised by co-administration with an azole antifungal drug, such a fluconazole, itraconazole, or ketoconazole. The reason for this effect is not known, as it may happen despite of the fact that the antifungal drugs tend to oppose metabolic clearance of medroxyprogesterone to slightly raise its serum level.

MDP ↔ CYP Isozymes: *See* Table 74-1.

MDP ↔ Oral Hypoglycemic Agents: (*See* Ω-55 in Appendix A.) Medroxyprogesterone may lead to weight gain and decreased tissue sensitivity to insulin. Therefore, medroxyprogesterone taken alone is more likely to develop diabetic symptoms than oral contraceptive pills containing both estrogen and progestogen;

and may worsen glucose tolerance in diabetics and in those with lipodystrophy (disorder of fat metabolism). Accordingly, monitoring blood sugar is recommended to avoid severe hyperglycemia in such patients.

MIFEPRISTONE

Mifepristone (Fig. 74-5) is a synthetic steroid useful as an abortifacient to terminate intrauterine pregnancy up to 49 days. It was once called RU-486, a code name of its manufacturer, the Roussel-Uclaf pharmaceutical company in France. If mifepristone does not cause a complete abortion (fetal death), a surgical intervention may be required.

MECHANISM OF ACTION

In the presence of endogenous progesterone, mifepristone acts as a competitive antagonist to induce decidual breakdown of the uterus, resulting in detachment of the blastocyst.

SIDE EFFECTS

Its possible side effects include fast heartbeat; nausea, vomiting, and diarrhea; uterine bleeding and cramping; and dizziness and fatigue.

DRUG INTERACTIONS

Mifepristone (MFS)

MFS ◄► Carbamazepine: Mifepristone requires CYP3A4 for its metabolism, and carbamazepine is an inducer of this enzyme. Therefore, carbamazepine, when used in combination, can quicken clearance of mifepristone to lower its blood concentration and therapeutic efficacy. Other similar inducers include: rifampin and St. John's wort (See the right-hand column of Table-0 at the 'Introduction' for other possible inducers of this enzyme).

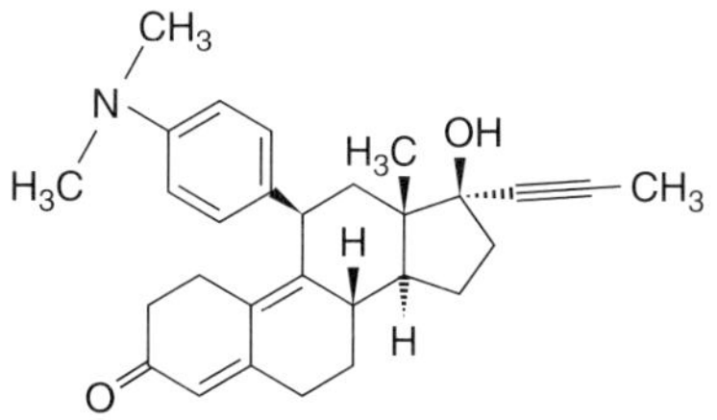

FIGURE 74-5   Molecular structure of mifepristone.

MFS ⟷ Erythromycin: Mifepristone requires CYP3A4 for its metabolism, whereas erythromycin is an inhibitor of this enzyme. Therefore, erythromycin can impede clearance of mifepristone to elevate its blood concentration and enhance its adverse effects. Similar inhibitors include itraconazole and ketoconazole. (*See* the left-hand column of Table-0 at the 'Introduction' for other possible inhibitors of this enzyme.)

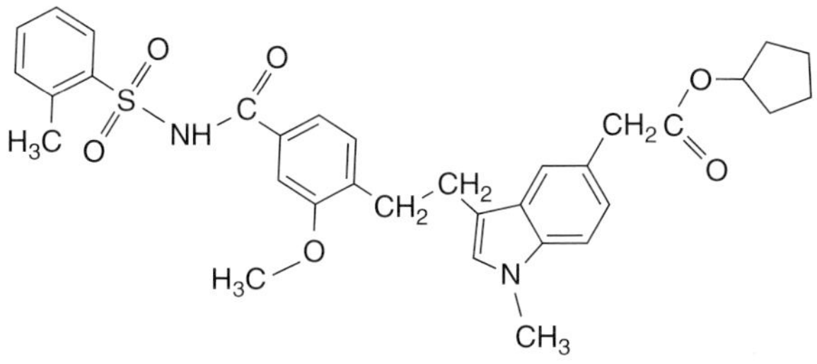

FIGURE 75-3   Molecular structure of zafirlukast.

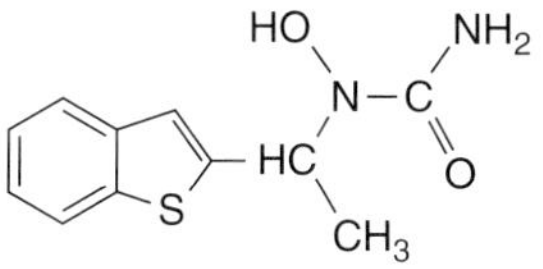

FIGURE 75-4   Molecular structure of zileuton.

zafirlukast (Fig. 75-3) work by blocking the receptors for leukotrienes, and are useful in treatment of allergic inflammation caused by leukotrienes.

Zileuton: Zileuton (Fig. 75-4) is a selective inhibitor of 5-lipoxygenase, the enzyme that converts arachidonic acid to various inflammatory leukotrienes.

SIDE EFFECTS

Montelukast or **Zafirlukast:** Their side effects may include cough; stomach upset or pain; muscle weakness; and dizziness, insomnia, and headache.

Zileuton: Its side effects may include nausea, stomach pain, and constipation; chest pain; jaundice (yellowing of the skin or eyes); fatigue, or muscle aches; drowsiness, and dizziness; and allergic reactions such as skin rash and itching

DRUG INTERACTIONS

Montelukast: *See* Chapter 15.

Zafirlukast: *See* Table 75-1.

Zileuton: *See* Table 75-1.

TABLE 75-1   Zafirlukast and Zileuton vs CYP Enzymes

Drug Name	1A2	2A6	2B6	2C8	2C9	2C18	2C19	2D6	2E1	3A4
Zafirlukast	Inh				Sub+ Inh					Inh
Zileuton	Sub+ Inh									Sub+ Inh

Abbreviations: Sub, substrate of the enzyme; Inh, inhibits the enzyme; Ezi, induces the enzyme

1. Zafirlukast is cleared through CYP2C9. Thus, inhibition of this enzyme by other drugs taken may raise blood levels of zafirlukast to possibly exacerbate its adverse effects. (*See* the left-hand column of Table-0 at the 'Introduction' for other possible inhibitors of the enzyme.)

2. Zafirlukast is an inhibitor of hepatic enzymes CYP1A2, CYP2C9, and CYP3A4. Therefore, co-administration with drugs that require these enzymes for hepatic clearance, such as warfarin, may raise their blood levels, possibly inciting their adverse effects. (*See* the middle column of Table-0 at the 'Introduction' for other possible substrates of these enzymes.)

3. Zileuton functions as a moderate inhibitor of the liver enzyme CYP1A2 and a weak inhibitor of CYP3A4. Thus, co-administration with drugs that require these enzymes for hepatic clearance may raise their blood levels and exacerbate their adverse effects. (*See* the middle column of Table-0 at the 'Introduction' for possible substrates of these enzymes.)

GLUCOCORTICOIDS

Beclomethasone, budesonide, dexamethasone, flunisolide, fluorometholone, fluticasone, mometasone, prednisolone, prednisone, and **triamcinolone**

Nasal sprays of beclomethasone, budesonide, flunisolide, fluticasone, mometasone, and triamcinolone help suppress allergic inflammatory responses, such as nasal stuffiness and itchy or runny nose. These nasal sprays are the most effective treatment for allergy symptoms caused by hay fever or pets. Other eye drops of glucocorticoids, useful to treat severe allergic conjunctivitis caused by hay fever, generating such symptoms as red, watery, and itchy eyes, include dexamethasone, fluorometholone, prednisolone, and prednisone.

MECHANISM OF ACTION
See Chapter 11.

SIDE EFFECTS
See Chapter 11.

DRUG INTERACTIONS
It is not known whether other medications will interact with any of the above glucocorticoids applied topically, but if taken orally or absorbed extensively

from the site of application, these interactions may occur. *See* Appendix B-20: Interactions of Glucocorticoids.

ANTIHISMTAINES

First-generation antihistamines include: **brompheniramine, chlorpheniramine, clemastine, diphenhydramine, doxylamine, hydroxyzine, pyrilamine,** and **triprolidine;** second-generation antihistamines include: **azelastine, cetirizine, fexofenadine,** and **loratadine.** Azelastine is an antihistamine spray approved to treat nasal symptoms caused by seasonal allergens or by environmental irritants.

MECHANISM OF ACTION

When allergens enter the body, they are recognized by IgE antibodies in the basophils, which release the inflammatory substance histamine to generate allergic symptoms such as severe skin rash, itching, hives, swelling of tissues, and airway obstruction, through activation of H_1 receptors. All of the above antihistamines block histamine receptor type H_1 to oppose histamine-induced allergic reactions.

SIDE EFFECTS

First-Generation Antihistamines: Some patients may experience one or more of the following adverse effects. If the symptoms get worse or a side effect not listed here emerges, taking emergency action is warranted. The frequent side effects of these oral antihistamines include cardiac arrhythmia; dry laryngeal mucosa with irritation; dry mouth, loss of appetite, upset stomach, increase risk of acid reflux to cause reflux laryngitis, vomiting, and constipation; difficulty in urination; dizziness, anxiety, hallucinations, and drowsiness which is especially prominent with brompheniramine, chlorpheniramine (Chlor-Trimeton), clemastine (Tavist), diphenhydramine (Benadryl), doxylamine, and pyrilamine.

Second-Generation Antihistamines: Their possible side effects include dry mouth, nausea, vomiting, and diarrhea; weakness, fatigue, dizziness, and headache. Sleepiness is far less likely than with the first-generation antihistamines, and allergic reactions are rather unlikely.

DRUG INTERACTIONS

First-Generation Antihistamines: *See* Appendix B-10: Interactions of Antihistamine, First-Generation.

Second-Generation Antihistamines: *See* Appendix B-11: Interactions of Antihistamine, Second-Generation.

MAST CELL STABILIZERS

Emedastine, olopatadine, and **cromolyn sodium**

Both emedastine and olopatadine are relatively selective H_1 antagonists (antihistamines) as well as conjunctival mast cell stabilizers, useful as drops to inhibit eye itching and redness. Cromolyn sodium, on the other hand, is not an antihistamine but a mast cell stabilizer useful mainly to prevent allergic symptoms. All these mast cell stabilizers are capable of keeping a person free from allergic symptoms associated with hay fever, such as sneezing, itchy or runny nose, sinus congestion, and postnasal drip.

MECHANISM OF ACTION

They interrupt transmembrane calcium influx in pulmonary mast cells to prevent degranulation of the mast cell, induced by allergens bound to IgE on the surface of the mast cell membrane (Fig. 75-5), and thereby block the release of histamine and SRS-A, preventing attack of allergic symptoms.

SIDE EFFECTS

Emedastine or **Olopatadine:** Some patients may experience one or more of the following adverse effects. If the symptoms get worse or a side effect not listed here emerges, taking emergency action is warranted. The frequent side effects of these drugs include: rhinitis with nasal burning or stinging; pharyngitis, sinusitis; dry mouth, bitter taste, nausea; keratitis with blurred vision; dizziness, drowsiness, and headache.

Cromolyn Sodium: Its side effects may include nasal irritation and sneezing; unpleasant taste; and drowsiness and headache.

DRUG INTERACTIONS

No convincing evidence exists that any of these drugs applied topically would interact with any other drugs to a serious consequence.

NAPHAZOLINE

MECHANISM OF ACTION

When applied as eye drops to conjunctiva, naphazoline is thought to directly stimulate the alpha-adrenergic receptor of the sympathetic nervous system, to constrict small arterioles of conjunctiva to relieve conjunctival congestion and redness.

A

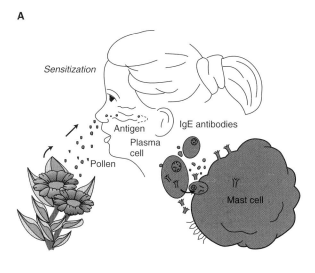

B

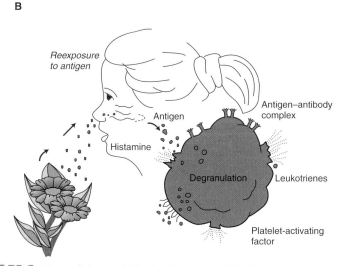

FIGURE 75-5   Mast cell degranulation by allergen sensitization. Reproduced, with permission, from May JR, Smith PH. Allergic rhinitis, In: DiPiro JT, Talbert RL, Yee GC, Matzke GR, Wells BG, Posey LM. (eds). *Pharmacotherapy: A Pathophysiologic Approach.* 7th ed. New York: McGraw-Hill, 2008, p 1566.

SIDE EFFECTS

It is not known whether naphazoline may generate any serious side effects when applied topically other than eye irritation, but if it is absorbed extensively from its site of application the following adverse effect may ensue: slow heartbeat; nausea;

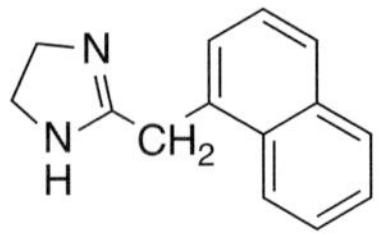

FIGURE 75-6   Molecular structure of naphazoline.

increased sweating; blurred vision and dilated pupils; and dizziness, nervousness, and headache. Use of naphazoline in infants and children can result in serious CNS depression, leading to coma and marked reduction in body temperature.

DRUG INTERACTIONS

It is not known whether other medications will interact with this medication applied topically, but if it is absorbed extensively from its site of application the following interactions may take place.

Naphazoline (NPZ)

NPZ ⟷ MAO Inhibitors: (*See* Ω-51 in Appendix A.) Co-administration of naphazoline (Fig. 75-6) with an MAO inhibitor, such as phenelzine, can cause a hypertensive crisis.

NPZ ⟷ Sympathomimetic Drugs: (*See* Ω-71 in Appendix A.) Exercise caution when using naphazoline with another sympathomimetic drug, such as phenylephrine, to avoid exacerbating adverse effects such as cardiac arrhythmia and hypertension.

AMPHETAMINE OR DEXTROAMPHETAMINE

Amphetamine and dextroamphetamine are both short-term appetite suppressants. However, amphetamines are not often recommended for use in the treatment of obesity, due to their strong potential for abuse and dependency.

MECHANISM OF ACTION

Their anti-obesity mechanism of action is not settled, but their postulated mechanisms include: (1) increase in energy expenditure by promoting muscular activities and (2) increase in the release of norepinephrine from the central noradrenergic neurons to activate the "satiety center" in the ventro-medial portion of the hypothalamus, suppressing food appetite.

SIDE EFFECTS

Some patients may experience one or more of the following adverse effects. If the symptoms get worse or a side effect not listed here emerges, taking emergency actions is warranted. The frequent side effects of these drugs include: cardiac arrhythmia and severe hypertension; dry mouth; altered libido (sex drive); severe headache, dizziness, anxiety, confusion, insomnia, and hallucinations. Rarely, they may cause allergic reactions such as swelling of tissues.

DRUG INTERACTIONS

See Chapter 48.

77

Cancer

The American Cancer Society defines cancer as a group of diseases characterized by abnormal growth and spread of atypical cells. The two main characteristics of cancer are: (1) uncontrolled growth of malignant tumor cells mutated from normal tissues; and (2) their ability to invade and metastasize (extend from the original site to distant sites). If the spread of a tumor is not controlled, the tumor may prevent normal functions of vital organs, culminating in damage and death of the organs.

The most common cancers causing human death are: (A) lung cancer; (B) brain cancer; (C) Hodgkin lymphoma; (D) non-Hodgkin lymphoma; (E) liver cancer; (F) kidney cancer; (G) thyroid cancer; (H) skin cancer; (I) leukemia; (J) breast cancer; (K) cervical cancer; (L) uterine cancer; (M) ovarian cancer; (N) choriocarcinoma; (O) testicular cancer, and (P) prostate cancer.

Cancer may be treated by surgery, radiation, and/or chemotherapy. Chemotherapy is usually given in cycles—a period of drug treatment is followed by a drug-free period in order to allow some time for the body to recover from the toxic effects of the chemotherapeutic agents, such as bone marrow depression, which make the host vulnerable to invasion by infectious agents. Chemotherapeutic treatments for each of the above cancers are explored below in sequential order.

LUNG CANCER

Small cell lung cancer is an aggressive type of cancer with a high tendency toward early regional and distant metastases. Medications that may be effective in the treatment of this type of lung cancer include: (1) **etoposide** (Etopophos, Vepesid) and (2) **topotecan** (Hycamtin); and medications that may possibly be effective in the treatment of non-small cell lung cancer include: (3) **docetaxel** (Taxotere); (4) **gemcitabine** (Gemzar); (5) **paclitaxel** (Taxol); (6) **porfirmer** (photofrin); and (7) **vinorelbine** (Navelbine).

ETOPOSIDE

Etoposide (Fig. 77-1) is also known as podophyllotoxin.

MECHANISM OF ACTION

Etoposide exerts its anticancer effect by inhibiting the enzyme topoisomerase, which ultimately leads to irreparable breakage of the cellular DNA.

SIDE EFFECTS

Its side effects may include hypotension; nausea, vomiting, anorexia, abdominal pain, and diarrhea; hepatocellular necrosis; amenorrhea; alopecia (hair loss); bone marrow suppression; and acute anaphylactoid reactions.

DRUG INTERACTIONS

See Box 77-1.

Miscellaneous Interactions of Etoposide (ETS)

ETS ◆▶ Cyclosporine: Cyclosporine can increase the serum level and toxicity risk of etoposide. One possible mechanism of this interaction is that etoposide

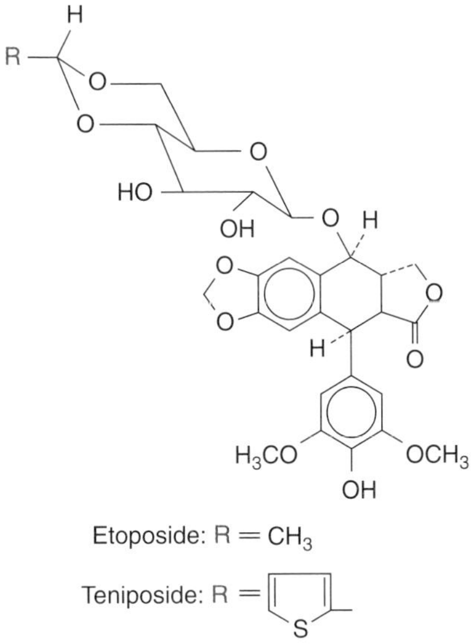

Etoposide: R = CH₃

Teniposide: R =

FIGURE 77-1 Molecular structures of etoposide and teniposide.

BOX 77-1

Basic Concepts of Etoposide Interactions

Etoposide is apt to cause bone marrow depression as a side effect, and when co-administered with drugs that generate a similar side effect, additive hematologic toxicities such as neutropenia and anemia may result. Those drugs include: **chloramphenicol** (an antibiotic) and **zidovudine** (a reverse transcriptase inhibitor, approved as the first anti-HIV drug in the United States that has bone marrow depression as its most severe adverse reaction).

is at least partially cleared through CYP3A4 and cyclosporine can inhibit this enzyme.

ETS ⟷ CYP Isozymes: *See* Table 77-1.

ETS ⟷ Live Vaccines: (*See* Ω-48 in Appendix A.) Patients with bone marrow depression caused by etoposide may develop generalized infections from receiving live vaccines. Therefore, at least six months separation between the two is recommended.

ETS ⟷ Warfarin: Etoposide does not inhibit warfarin metabolism, but it may displace warfarin from its protein binding sites and increase the hypoprothrombinemic effect of warfarin, causing excessive bleeding.

TOPOTECAN

MECHANISM OF ACTION

Topotecan (Fig. 77-2) inhibits topoisomerase-1, the important enzyme in DNA transcription.

TABLE 77-1 Etoposide vs CYP Isozymes

Drug Name	1A2	2A6	2B6	2C8	2C9	2C18	2C19	2D6	2E1	3A4
Etoposide	Sub			Inh					Sub	Sub

Abbreviations: Sub, substrate of the enzyme; Inh, inhibits the enzyme; Ezi, induces the enzyme

Etoposide exerts an inhibitory effect on CYP2C8. Therefore, administration in combination with drugs that require this enzyme for metabolic clearance may result in their elevated blood levels, possibly exacerbating their adverse effects. (*See* the middle column of Table-0 at the 'Introduction' for possible substrates of the enzyme.)

TABLE 77-3 Paclitaxel vs CYP Isozymes

Drug Name	1A2	2A6	2B6	2C8	2C9	2C18	2C19	2D6	2E1	3A4
Paclitaxel				Sub						Sub

Abbreviations: Sub, substrate of the enzyme; Inh, inhibits the enzyme; Ezi, induces the enzyme

1. Ketoconazole, inhibitor of CYP3A4, may inhibit the metabolism of paclitaxel to increase its serum concentration and exacerbate its adverse effects. (*See* the left-hand column of Table-0 at the 'Introduction' for other possible inhibitors of the enzyme.)

2. Both paclitaxel and doxorubicin (not shown) are substrates for the enzyme CYP3A4. When used in combination, they may compete with each other for clearance, consequentially raising blood levels of doxorubicin and amplifying its adverse effects. (*See* the middle column of Table-0 at the 'Introduction' for possible substrates of the enzyme.)

Miscellaneous Interactions of Paclitaxel (PTX)

PTX ⟷ Cisplatin: If paclitaxel is used with cisplatin, whose toxicity includes renal failure, the renal clearance of paclitaxel may be impaired to cause elevated serum levels and hematologic toxicity.

PTX ⟷ CYP Isozymes: *See* Table 77-3.

PTX ⟷ Live Vaccines: (*See* Ω-48 in Appendix A.) Patients with bone marrow depression caused by paclitaxel may develop generalized infections from receiving live vaccines. Therefore, at least six months separation between the two is recommended.

PTX ⟷ Stavudine: Concomitant use of stavudine, an anti-HIV drug, with paclitaxel may increase the risk of developing peripheral neuropathy.

PTX ⟷ Trastuzumab: Concomitant use of trastuzumab, a breast cancer drug, with paclitaxel may increase the serum concentration of trastuzumab, likely by reducing the clearance of trastuzumab through the reticuloendothelial system.

PORFIRMER

MECHANISM OF ACTION

Porfirmer, after intravenous injection, is selectively distributed and maintained in superficial tumor cells, whereas normal cells can get rid of most of the porfirmer within a couple of days. When exposed to a 630 nanometer laser light after two days, porfirmer is activated to generate cytotoxic free oxygen radicals that damage tumor cell mitochondrial and intracellular membranes. As the laser light is a low-power light, it does not normally burn or cause significant pain during the procedure. Porfirmer is particularly useful to treat esophageal cancer.

SIDE EFFECTS

Possible side effects of porfirmer include nausea, vomiting, and constipation; increased skin photosensitivity or eye discomfort (patients must stay out of sunlight or ultraviolet light following treatment); dizziness and insomnia; and rarely, difficulty in breathing.

DRUG INTERACTIONS

There have been no formal interaction studies of porfirmer with any other drugs. However, its combined use with doxorubicin or mitomycin appears to enhance the tumoricidal efficacy of porfirmer. Concomitant use of it with other photo-sensitizing agents, such as tetracyclines, phenothiazines, griseofulvin (Grifulvin V, Grisactin), and fluoroquinolone antibiotics (Fig. 77-5), may increase the risk of photosensitivity.

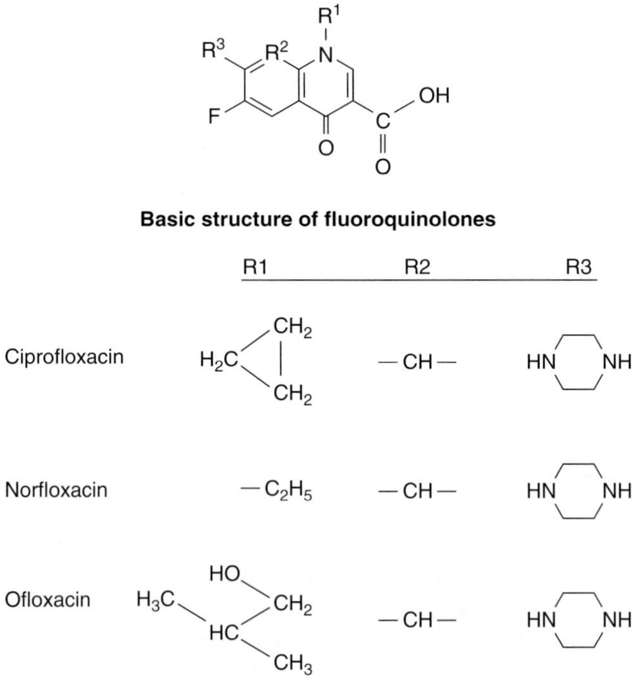

Basic structure of fluoroquinolones

	R1	R2	R3
Ciprofloxacin	H_2C with CH_2 / CH_2	$-CH-$	HN NH
Norfloxacin	$-C_2H_5$	$-CH-$	HN NH
Ofloxacin	H_3C , HO , CH_2 , HC , CH_3	$-CH-$	HN NH

FIGURE 77-5   Molecular structure of fluoroquinolones.

Miscellaneous Interactions of Procarbazine (PCZ)

PCZ ↔ Alcohol: Procarbazine, if taken with alcohol, may cause disulfiram-like alcohol intolerance reactions, including nausea, headache, flushing, palpitations, and fall of blood pressure. Therefore, it is prudent to avoid combination of the two.

PCZ ↔ Chloramphenicol: Procarbazine causes bone marrow depressions, as does chloramphenicol. Concomitant use may cause additive, severe hematologic toxicities.

PCZ ↔ CYP Isozymes: *See* Table 77-5.

PCZ ↔ Digoxin: Procarbazine was shown to reduce the intestinal absorption of digoxin, thus lowering its blood levels and causing therapeutic insufficiency.

PCZ ↔ Live Vaccines: (*See* Ω-48 in Appendix A.) Patients with immunosuppression from procarbazine may develop generalized infections from administration of live vaccines. At least six months should elapse between discontinuation of procarbazine and receiving vaccination.

PCZ ↔ Levamisole: Levamisole is known to cause agranulocytosis, leucopenia, and thrombocytopenia. Therefore, concomitant use of levamisole with procarbazine may increase the risk of such adverse effects.

PCZ ↔ Methotrexate: Procarbazine was shown to delay renal secretion of methotrexate. Therefore, co-administration of procarbazine and methotrexate can increase methotrexate-induced nephrotoxicity. Allow at least 72 hours separation between the last dose of procarbazine and initiation of methotrexate.

PCZ ↔ Phenothiazine Antipsychotic Drugs: (*See* Ω-58 in Appendix A.) Procarbazine can generate nystagmus and ataxia as side effects, as do most phenothiazine antipsychotic drugs. Concurrent use of procarbazine and a phenothiazine may result in aggravation of such extrapyramidal symptoms.

TEMOZOLOMIDE

Temozolomide is used for the treatment of recurrent astrocytoma, or glioblastoma multiforme, an aggressive brain tumor.

MECHANISM OF ACTION

Temozolomide (Fig. 77-8) is not active until it is converted at physiologic pH to its active form, MTIC [*3-methyl-(triazen-1-yl)imidazole-4-carboxamide*], that has an

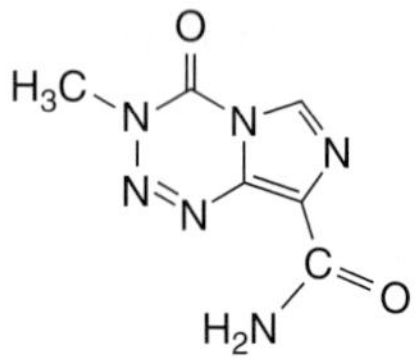

FIGURE 77-8   Molecular structure of temozolomide.

ability to methylate DNA most often at the N7 (or N at position 7) or O6 (or O at position 6) of guanine in DNA (*See* Fig. 59-4). Therefore, this drug functions as a DNA alkylating agent that opposes DNA replication.

SIDE EFFECTS

Its side effects may include peripheral edema; upper respiratory tract infections, dyspnea, and cough; sinusitis; stomatitis, abdominal pain, anorexia; increased urinary frequency; arthralgia; myalgia; ataxia; alopecia; bone marrow depressions; blurred vision; and confusion.

DRUG INTERACTIONS

No clinically important interactions have been reported.

HODGKIN LYMPHOMA

Medications that may be effective in the treatment of Hodgkin lymphoma include: (1) a four-drug combination called **ABVD,** which contains **doxorubicin** (Adriamycin), **bleomycin, vinblastine** (Velban), and **dacarbazine;** and (2) **etoposide** (VePesid) taken in conjunction with steroids.

ABVD

Doxorubicin + bleomycin + vinblastine + dacarbazine

MECHANISM OF ACTION

Doxorubicin: The exact mechanism of action of doxorubicin (Fig. 77-9) is unknown, but it seems to work in the following ways: (1) it intercalates itself into the DNA strands to prevent synthesis of DNA and RNA in the cells; (2) it appears

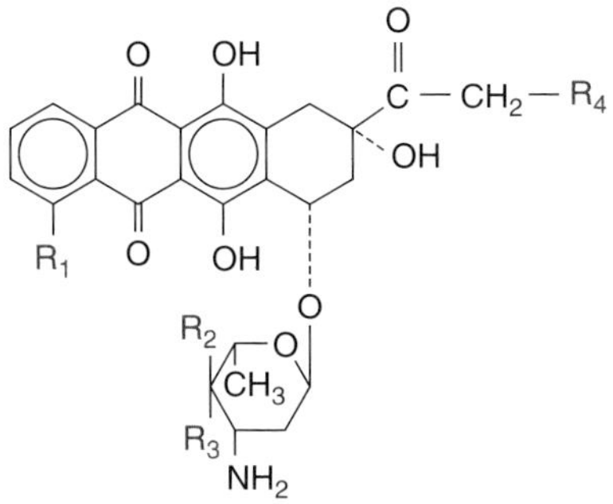

	Doxorubicin	Daunorubicin	Epirubicin	Idarubicin
$R_1 =$	OCH_3	OCH_3	OCH_3	H
$R_2 =$	H	H	OH	H
$R_3 =$	OH	OH	H	OH
$R_4 =$	OH	H	OH	H

FIGURE 77-9 Molecular structures of doxorubicin and analogs.

to inhibit the enzyme topoisomerase-II involved in DNA replication; and (3) it is reduced to doxorubicinol, during which free radicals are generated to damage the DNA strands.

Bleomycin: Bleomycin is a glycopeptide antibiotic that chelates divalent iron and then binds to DNA to form an Fe^{++}-bleomycin-DNA complex. During oxidation of this complex, H^+ ions are released to interact with oxygen, generating superoxide radicals that damage phosphodiesterase bondage of DNA and result in breakdown of the DNA strands.

Vinblastine: Vinblastine inhibits microtubule formation in tumor cells to arrest their mitosis in metaphase.

Dacarbazine: Dacarbazine (Fig. 77-10) is an imidazole carboxamide derivative having a structural similarity to certain purines and can function as an alkylating agent, which prevents replications of DNA strands.

SIDE EFFECTS

Doxorubicin: Possible side effects of doxorubicin include irregular heartbeat (a cardiac toxicity); shortness of breath; mouth ulcer, nausea, vomiting, and diarrhea; painful passing of red colored urine, lasting for about 24 hours (the drug

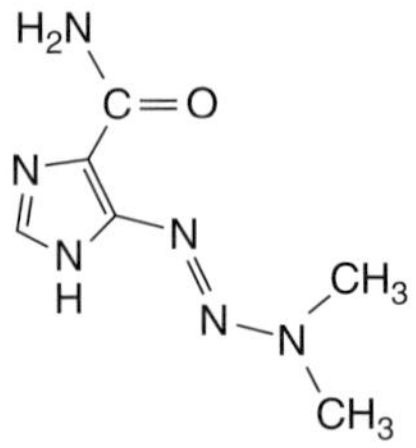

FIGURE 77-10   Molecular structure of dacarbazine.

itself is red in color and the change of urine color is nothing to worry about); fever or chills; hair loss; bone marrow depression; darkened or sun-sensitive skin; and coma and seizure. Doxorubicin must only be slowly injected intravenously, and intramuscular (IM) or subcutaneous (SC) injections should be avoided.

Bleomycin: Its side effects may include pulmonary fibrosis that reduces oxygen diffusion in the lungs, causing dyspnea; vomiting, and loss of weight; hyperkeratosis (thickening of skin layers); and allergic reactions which may include chills and fever. However, bleomycin is virtually free from causing bone marrow depression, unlike most anticancer drugs.

Vinblastine: Its side effects may include hypertension; acute bronchospasm; pharyngitis; vesiculation of the mouth; amenorrhea; loss of semen; bone or jaw pain; loss of deep tendon reflexes; alopecia; bone marrow suppression; and increased photosensitivity.

Dacarbazine: Its side effects may include nausea, and vomiting; myalgia and facial paresthesia; alopecia; bone marrow suppression; flu-like syndrome; and urticarial rashes.

DRUG INTERACTIONS
Bleomycin
No clinically serious drug interaction reported.

Dacarbazine
There is no clinically important interaction reported.

Doxorubicin (DXR)
DXR ⟷ Azithromycin: It appears that azithromycin inhibits binding of doxorubicin to its efflux P-glycoproteins (P-gp), thus preventing its efflux, raising its

Prednisone: Prednisone is a glucocorticoid that produces its anticancer effect by inhibiting the synthesis of essential proteins in tumor cells, and by opposing proliferation of T-lymphocytes.

SIDE EFFECTS

Cyclophosphamide: Side effects of cyclophosphamide may include congestive heart failure and cardiac necrosis; interstitial pulmonary fibrosis; nausea, vomiting, and diarrhea; hemorrhagic cystitis and renal tubular necrosis; amenorrhea; alopecia; and bone marrow suppression.

Doxorubicin: *See* earlier in this chapter.

Vincristine: *See* earlier in this chapter.

Prednisone: Its side effects may include elevated blood pressure; retention of sodium and fluid; weight gain; loss of potassium; muscle weakness; growth retardation in children; slowed healing of cuts and bruises; acne; skin rash; glaucoma and cataract; worsening of diabetes; euphoria; and insomnia.

DRUG INTERACTIONS

Cyclophosphamide: *See* Chapter 59.

Doxorubicin: *See* earlier in this chapter.

Vincristine: *See* earlier in this chapter.

Prednisone: *See* Appendix B-20: Interactions of Glucocorticoids.

LIVER CANCER

Medications that may be effective in the treatment of live cancer include: (1) **cisplatin;** (2) **methotrexate;** and (3) **doxorubicin** (Adriamycin).

CISPLATIN

MECHANISM OF ACTION

Cisplatin (Fig. 77-13) is an inorganic compound, with a chemical name of cis-diamminedichloroplatinum (DDP), which induces its cytotoxic properties

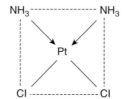

FIGURE 77-13   Molecular structure of cisplatin.

through alkylating to nuclear DNA and subsequent interference with normal transcription and/or replication of DNA.

SIDE EFFECTS

Possible side effects of cisplatin include tachycardia; cough or shortness of breath; nausea and vomiting; marked elevations in blood urea nitrogen (BUN) and creatinine due to renal toxicity (lots of fluid can prevent this); painful urination; pain and swelling of the limbs and loss of balance; tinnitus or loss of high frequency hearing (this usually gets better on its own); blurred visions; dizziness; bone marrow depression; and rarely, anaphylactic-like allergic reactions.

DRUG INTERACTIONS

See Box 77-5.

Miscellaneous Interactions of Cisplatin (CPT)

CPT ⟷ Aldesleukin: Cisplatin may cause severe kidney problems. Aldesleukin, a recombinant IL-2, is rapidly metabolized to its composite amino acid, requiring elimination via renal tubules and glomerular filtration. Therefore, concurrent use of cisplatin and aldesleukin may increase blood levels and incidence of hypersensitivity reactions to the metabolites of aldesleukin, including hypotension, difficulty in breathing, erythema, pruritus, and swelling of tissues.

CPT ⟷ Live Vaccines: (*See* Ω-48 in Appendix A.) Patients whose immunity is compromised by cisplatin may develop generalized infections by receiving live vaccines. At least six months should be allowed between discontinuation of cisplatin and live vaccination.

CPT ⟷ Loop Diuretics: (*See* Ω-49 in Appendix A.) Cisplatin is capable of causing ototoxicity as a side effect. Combined use with a loop diuretic, especially ethacrynic acid, may increase the incidence of ototoxicity (temporary or permanent deafness).

BOX 77-5

Basic Concepts of Cisplatin Interactions

1. Cisplatin is apt to cause nephrotoxicity as a side effect, and when co-administered with drugs that tend to cause nephrotoxicity, a severe life-threatening renal impairment may result. Those drugs include: **aminoglycosides antibiotics** (*See* Ω-7 in Appendix A) (which may cause nephrotoxicity, ototoxicity, and neuromuscular blockade) and **azathioprine** (an anticancer drug, which is not directly nephrotoxic but can cause allergic interstitial nephritis).

2. Cisplatin is apt to cause moderate and transient bone marrow depression in up to 30% of patients, and when co-administered with drugs that generate bone marrow depression, a severe depression of blood cell count may result, generating symptoms such as fever of 101° F, chills, unusual fatigue, and easy bruising and bleeding. Those drugs include: **methotrexate** (an anticancer drug); **paclitaxel** (an anticancer drug); **topotecan** (an anticancer drug); and many other anticancer drugs (*See* Ω-13 in Appendix A).

CPT ↔ Vinorelbine: If vinorelbine is used with cisplatin, whose side effects include renal toxicity, the excretion of vinorelbine may be delayed, raising its serum levels and incidence of toxicities, including granulocytopenia.

CPT ↔ Zalcitabine: Zalcitabine, an anti-HIV agent whose side effects include frequent and disabling peripheral neuropathy, is mainly cleared through glomerular filtration and, to a lesser extent, renal tubular secretion. Concomitant use with cisplatin, a nephrotoxic drug, may bring about increased serum levels and risk of peripheral neuropathies from zalcitabine.

METHOTREXATE

MECHANISM OF ACTION

Methotrexate (Fig. 77-14) inhibits dihydrofolate reductase, the enzyme required for conversion of dihydrofolate to tetrahydrofolate (*See* Fig. 8-1), without which thymine, the unique base of DNA, cannot be formed from uracil. Thus, the drug blocks synthesis of DNA and suppresses lymphocyte proliferation.

SIDE EFFECTS

Its possible side effects include lowered white blood cells (WBC); pneumonitis and pulmonary edema; dry, non-productive coughing; nausea, vomiting, upset

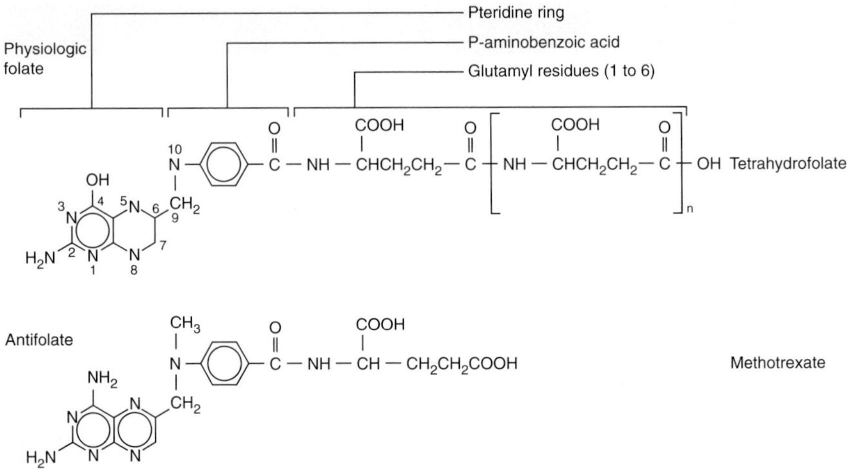

FIGURE 77-14   **Methotrexate vs tetrahydrofolate.** Reproduced, with permission, from Brunton LL, Lazo JS, and Parker KL. *Goodman and Gilman's The Pharmacological Basis of Therapeutics.* 11th ed. New York, NY: McGraw Hill; 2006, p 1337.

stomach, and diarrhea; bloody stool; nephrotoxicity with bloody urine; hepatotoxicity; weakness or numbness of limbs; blurred vision; bone marrow suppression; headache, fever, chills, dizziness, drowsiness, and seizures; and allergic reactions such as skin hives and swelling of tissues.

DRUG INTERACTIONS

See Box 77-6.

Miscellaneous Interactions of Methotrexate (MTX)

Parentheses below indicate an herb.

MTX ⟷ Aldesleukin: Both aldesleukin and methotrexate are highly toxic to organs and tissues. Aldesleukin may cause heart failure and cardiac arrhythmia; and lung congestion with shortness of breath. Methotrexate is harmful to the liver, kidneys, and bone. Therefore, concurrent use can increase toxicity to the above organs and tissues of the body.

MTX ⟷ Amiodarone: Side effects of both methotrexate and amiodarone may include interstitial pneumonitis, alveolitis, and pulmonary edema. If used in combination, the risk of pulmonary toxicity is bound to rise. Further, the use of amiodarone for more than two weeks appears to impair metabolism of

BOX 77-6

Basic Concepts of Methotrexate Interactions

1. Methotrexate is partially bound to serum albumin and can be displaced by certain drugs with a higher affinity for binding. Once displaced, the blood concentrations and toxicities of methotrexate are bound to rise. Those drugs include: **salicylates** (*See* Ω-64 in Appendix A) including **aspirin; phenylbutazone** (an anti-inflammatory drug); **phenytoin** (an antiepileptic drug); and **sulfamethoxazole** (a chemotherapeutic agent).

2. Methotrexate causes liver fibrosis and cirrhosis after prolonged use, and when co-administered with drugs that generate hepatotoxicity, increased incidence of abnormal liver function may result. Those drugs include: **acitretin** (a retinoid, useful in the treatment of psoriasis where other treatments have failed, with hepatotoxicity as a side effect); **azathioprine** (an immunosuppressant); **leflunomide** (an anti-arthritis drug that has hepatotoxicity as a side effect); **retinoids** (*See* Ω-63 in Appendix A); and **sulfasalazine** (an anti-inflammatory drug that has hepatotoxicity as a side effect).

3. The active secretion of methotrexate in the kidney may be interrupted by combined intake of some other drugs, resulting in its elevated serum levels and toxicities. Those drugs include: **non-steroidal anti-inflammatory drugs (NSAIDs)** (*See* Ω -54 in Appendix A) (especially ibuprofen and naproxen); **omeprazole;** 3.3) **penicillins** (*See* Ω-56 in Appendix A); **probenecid** (a drug to treat gout); **salicylates** (*See* Ω-64 in Appendix A); and **trimethoprim** (an antibiotic).

methotrexate, raising its blood levels and incidence of side effects such as ulcerated skin lesions.

MTX ⟷ Cisplatin: Renal clearance of methotrexate involves a complex process consisting of glomerular filtration, tubular reabsorption, and tubular secretion; whereas cisplatin, which is mainly cleared via tubular secretion, produces cumulative nephrotoxicities such as renal tubular dysfunction and decline in glomerular filtration rate. Therefore, combined use may raise blood levels and incite toxicities of methotrexate.

MTX ⟷ CYP Substrate: Methotrexate is not considerably metabolized by hepatic CYP isozymes. Thus, its therapeutic effectiveness and toxicity are not much affected by combined intake of any inducers or inhibitors of cytochrome enzymes.

MTX ↔ Digoxin: Methotrexate treatment causes damage to the rapidly dividing cells, such as epithelial cells in the intestine, especially of the upper small intestine, and diminishes the cell renewal and replacement to lead to ulceration of the cells, which in turn causes malabsorption of digoxin, accounting for the lowered blood level and therapeutic insufficiency of digoxin.

MTX ↔ Doxycycline: Renal clearance of methotrexate involves glomerular filtration, tubular secretion, and tubular reabsorption, whereas doxycycline is eliminated in the urine, largely unchanged, via glomerular filtration, and also in the feces via biliary secretion. When used in combination, doxycycline may raise the serum levels and incite toxicities of methotrexate, such as bone marrow depression.

MTX ↔ (Echinacea): Some of the alkaloids found in echinacea may be harmful to the liver. Thus, it should not be taken with any drugs that are known to be toxic to the liver, such as methotrexate.

MTX ↔ Live Vaccines: (*See* Ω-48 in Appendix A.) Patients with bone marrow depression caused by methotrexate may develop generalized infections from receiving live vaccines. Therefore, at least six months separation between the two is recommended.

MTX ↔ NSAIDs: (*See* Ω-54 in Appendix A.) Renal clearance of methotrexate is impaired when taken in combination with NSAIDs such as ibuprofen and naproxen, resulting in increased blood levels and toxicities of methotrexate.

MTX ↔ Procarbazine: Renal impairment is suspected behind the observation that procarbazine increases methotrexate-induced nephrotoxicity. Allow at least 72 hours separation between the last dose of procarbazine and initiation of methotrexate.

MTX ↔ Teniposide: Teniposide is weakly bound to plasma proteins, and can be displaced by concurrent administration of methotrexate, elevating its blood levels and inciting its adverse effects.

MTX ↔ Theophylline: Microsomal CYP isozymes such as CYP1A2 and CYP2E1 in the liver are involved in the metabolism of theophylline, whereas methotrexate, though it is not metabolized considerably via hepatic CYP isozymes, has the potential to cause hepatotoxicity and interrupt clearance of theophylline. Therefore, concurrent administration may raise blood concentrations of theophylline and lead to CNS excitation and cardiac arrhythmia.

MTX ↔ Zidovudine: Both methotrexate and zidovudine possess hematologic toxicities such as neutropenia and anemia. Hence, their combined use may result in additive bone marrow depression.

DOXORUBICIN

See earlier in this chapter.

KIDNEY CANCER

Medications that may be effective in the treatment of kidney cancer include: (1) **everolimus** (Afinitor), (2) **sorafenib tosylate** (Nexavar); and (3) **sunitinib malate** (Sutent).

EVEROLIMUS

Everolimus is to be taken once daily by the oral route, as a new approach to renal cancer treatment.

MECHANISM OF ACTION

The mammalian target of rapamycin (mTOR) is a multi-domain protein and a protein kinase that controls tumor cell division and blood vessel growth. The TOR is inhibited by the immunosuppressant drug rapamycin. Everolimus, a derivative of sirolimus, is also known to inhibit the protein mTOR to delay progression of metastatic renal cancer.

SIDE EFFECTS

Side effects of everolimus include pneumonitis, dyspnea, and cough; stomatitis, abdominal pain, and diarrhea; fatigue and dehydration; hypercholesterolemia; hypertriglyceridemia; hyperglycemia; and anemia.

DRUG INTERACTIONS

See Table 77-8.

SORAFENIB TOSYLATE

MECHANISM OF ACTION

A critical step in the growth of a tumor is its ability to form new blood vessels (tumor angiogenesis) to establish an independent blood supply through which the tumor cells receive nutrients and remove waste products. To proliferate, the cancerous tumor cells first release molecules that send signals to surrounding normal host tissue, activating certain genes to make proteins that encourage

TABLE 77-8 Everolimus, Sorafenib, and Sunitinib vs CYP Enzymes

Drug Name	1A2	2A6	2B6	2C8	2C9	2C18	2C19	2D6	2E1	3A4
Everolimus										Sub
Sorafenib					Inh		Inh			Sub
Sunitinib										Sub

Abbreviations: Sub, substrate of the enzyme; Inh, inhibits the enzyme; Ezi, induces the enzyme

1. Everolimus, sorafenib, and sunitinib are all metabolized by the microsomal enzyme CYP3A4. Thus, inhibition of this enzyme by other drugs may raise blood levels of these drugs and possibly exacerbate their adverse effects. (*See* the left-hand column of Table-0 at the 'Introduction' for possible inhibitors of the enzyme.)
2. Sorafenib, unlike everolimus and sunitinib, has some inhibitory effects on both CYP2C9 and CYP2C19. Therefore, administration in combination with drugs that require these enzymes for hepatic clearance may raise their blood levels and possibly incite their adverse effects. For instance, S-warfarin is mainly cleared through CYP2C9 and hence, concurrent administration with sorafenib may elevate blood levels of warfarin to increase the risk of bleeding. Further, the international normalized ratio (INR) should be measured prior to and monitored at least weekly during warfarin administration to avoid excessive bleeding. (*See* the middle column of Table-0 at the 'Introduction' for possible substrates of these enzymes.)

growth of new blood vessels. Receptor tyrosine kinases (RTK) are endothelial cell surface receptors for vascular endothelial growth factor, platelet-derived growth factor, and fibroblast growth factor, all having important roles in tumor angiogenesis. This newly approved drug, sorafenib tosylate, belongs in the group known as tyrosine kinase inhibitors, and it works by disruption of the angiogenesis process in the tumors.

SIDE EFFECTS

Side effects of sorafenib tosylate include elevation of blood pressure; mouth soreness and diarrhea; skin redness and pain and callus-like formations on the palms of the hands or soles of the feet; skin rash; and fatigue.

DRUG INTERACTIONS

See Table 77-8.

SUNITINIB MALATE

MECHANISM OF ACTION

Sunitinib is another new drug belonging in the group known as tyrosine kinase inhibitors, which work by disruption of the angiogenesis process in the tumors.

SIDE EFFECTS

Side effects of sunitinib include high blood pressure and bleeding (most commonly mild nosebleeds); mouth irritation, altered taste, nausea, and diarrhea; temporary skin discoloration (tan-like appearance); and weakness and fatigue.

DRUG INTERACTIONS

See Table 77-8.

THYROID CANCER

Medications that may be effective in the treatment of thyroid cancer include: (1) **doxorubicin** (Adriamycin) and (2) **cisplatin.**

DOXORUBICIN

See earlier in this chapter.

CISPLATIN

See earlier in this chapter.

SKIN CANCER

Medications that may possibly be effective in the treatment of skin cancer include: (1) **fluorouracil** (Efudex, Fluoroplex [5FU]) and (2) **imiquimod** (Aldara).

FLUOROURACIL

This drug is most often used to treat non-melanoma skin cancer. It is available as cream or lotion, applicable directly to the skin.

MECHANISM OF ACTION

5-fluorouracil inhibits thymidylate synthase, the enzyme that catalyzes methylation of uracil of uridine to form thymine of thymidine (Fig. 77-15), the unique base of DNA. As no thymine is formed, no DNA can be synthesized, stopping proliferation of the cancer cells.

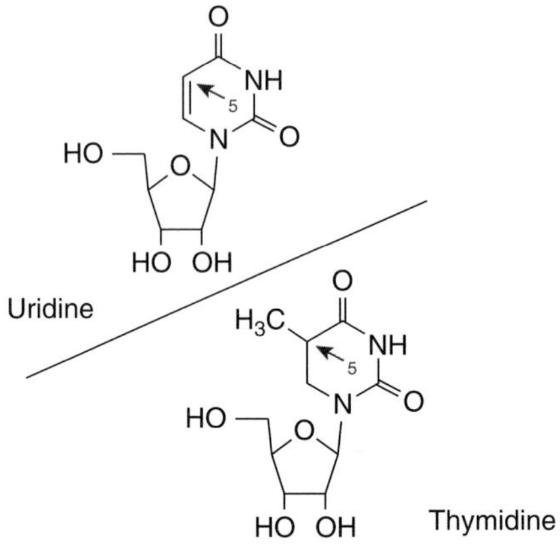

FIGURE 77-15   Molecular structures of uridine and thymidine.

SIDE EFFECTS

5-fluorouracil cream applied topically may cause side effects such as skin irritation, burning, itching, tenderness, changes in the skin color, hair loss at the application site, and increased sun sensitivity.

DRUG INTERACTIONS

It is not known whether other medications will interact with this medication applied topically, but if absorbed extensively from its site of application the following interactions may take place.

Fluorouracil (FUR)

FUR ⟷ Bone Marrow Depressants: (*See* Ω-29 in Appendix A.) Concomitant use of fluorouracil with other drugs known to cause bone marrow suppression should be avoided, lest it cause additive toxicities.

FUR ⟷ CYP Isozymes: *See* Table 77-9.

FUR ⟷ Hydroxyurea: If hydroxyurea, which generates neurotoxicities such as confusion, convulsions, dizziness, and hallucination, is used with fluorouracil, which possesses neurotoxicities such as confusion, cognitive disturbance, and repeated seizures, there is an increased potential for such adverse effects.

FUR ⟷ Live Vaccines: (*See* Ω-48 in Appendix A.) Patients with bone marrow depression caused by fluorouracil may develop generalized infections from

TABLE 77-9   Fluorouracil vs CYP Isozymes

Drug Name	1A2	2A6	2B6	2C8	2C9	2C18	2C19	2D6	2E1	3A4
Fluorouracil					Inh					

Abbreviations: Sub, substrate of the enzyme; Inh, inhibits the enzyme; Ezi, induces the enzyme

Fluorouracil is an inhibitor of the liver enzyme CYP2C9. Therefore, co-administration with drugs that require this enzyme for hepatic clearance may raise blood levels and exacerbate their adverse effects. Those sensitively affected drugs include: phenytoin and warfarin. (*See* the middle column of Table-0 at the 'Introduction' for other possible substrates of this enzyme.)

receiving live vaccines. Thus, at least six months separation between the two is recommended.

FUR ⟷ Zidovudine: Both fluorouracil and zidovudine possess hematological toxicities such as neutropenia and anemia. Therefore, their combined use may result in additive bone marrow depression.

IMIQUIMOD

This drug is effective in the treatment of superficial basal cell carcinoma (Fig. 77-16) and various cutaneous neoplasms. It is available as a cream or lotion, applicable directly to the skin.

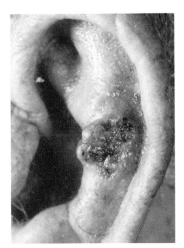

FIGURE 77-16   Basal cell carcinoma. Reproduced, with permission, from Sober AJ, Tsao H, Washington CV. Cancer of the skin. In: Fauci AS, Braunwald E, Kasper DL, et al, eds. *Harrison's Principles of Internal Medicine.* 17th ed. New York, NY: McGraw-Hill, 2008:546.

MECHANISM OF ACTION

This drug functions as an immune response modifier with potent antiviral and antitumor properties. Imiquimod stimulates the production of cytokines such as interferon-alpha, tumor necrosis factor (TNF)-alpha, IL-6, and IL-12 to enhance immune reactions to skin cancer.

SIDE EFFECTS

Its side effects include hard or thickened skin, skin redness, peeling, flaking, itching/burning, and swelling. In the event of flu-like symptoms such as fever and muscle ache, remove the medication by washing the area with mild soap and water before promptly seeking medical help.

DRUG INTERACTIONS

This drug applied to the affected area is not well absorbed. Therefore, there is little chance for it to interact with other drugs.

LEUKEMIA

Medications that may be effective in the treatment of leukemia include: (1) **busulfan** (Busulfex, Myleran); (2) **fludarabine** (Fludara); (3) **gemtuzumab ozogamicin** (Mylotarg); (4) **idarubicin** (Idamycin); (5) **mitoxantrone** (Novantrone); and (6) **teniposide** (Vumon).

BUSULFAN

MECHANISM OF ACTION

Busulfan (Fig. 77-17) is an alkylating agent that appears to alkylate DNA to inhibit both DNA replication and RNA transcription.

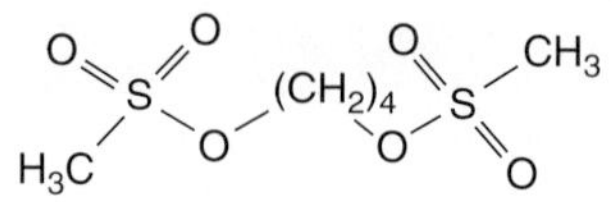

FIGURE 77-17   Molecular structure of busulfan.

SIDE EFFECTS

Its side effects may include tachycardia, hypertension, thrombosis; cough, and dyspnea; rhinitis, pharyngitis; nausea, vomiting; cholestatic jaundice; bone marrow depression; and skin rash and itching.

DRUG INTERACTIONS

Busulfan (BSF)

BSF ⟷ Acetaminophen: Since busulfan is partially eliminated via conjugation with glutathione, co-administration with acetaminophen, whose oxidized metabolite is also conjugated with glutathione for detoxification, may result in impaired clearance of busulfan.

BSF ⟷ Chloramphenicol: Chloramphenicol may cause severe hematologic toxicities, and its use in combination with busulfan may cause additive bone marrow suppression.

BSF ⟷ Cyclophosphamide: Cardiac tamponade (an emergency condition in which fluid accumulates in the pericardium of the heart) occurs, though uncommonly, in patients treated with busulfan, as well as in thalassemic patients given cyclophosphamide prior to bone marrow transplant. When used in combination they may cause increased incidence of such alarming effects.

BSF ⟷ CYP Isozymes: *See* Table 77-10.

TABLE 77-10 Busulfan and Teniposide vs CYP Enzymes

Drug Name	1A2	2A6	2B6	2C8	2C9	2C18	2C19	2D6	2E1	3A4
Busulfan										Sub
Teniposide					Inh		Sub+ Inh			Sub

Abbreviations: Sub, substrate of the enzyme; Inh, inhibits the enzyme; Ezi, induces the enzyme

1. The primary metabolism of busulfan is via the microsomal enzyme CYP3A4 and thus, inhibition of this enzyme by other drugs can delay its elimination to raise its blood levels and incite toxicity. Those strong inhibitors of CYP3A4 include: clarithromycin, indinavir, itraconazole, ketoconazole, nefazodone, nelfinavir, ritonavir, and saquinavir. (*See* the left-hand column of Table-0 at the 'Introduction' for other possible inhibitors of this enzyme.)
2. Teniposide is an inhibitor of both CYP2C9 and CYP2C19. Thus, co-administration with drugs that require these enzymes for hepatic clearance may raise their blood levels and possibly exacerbate their adverse effects. (*See* the middle column of Table-0 at the 'Introduction' for possible substrates of these enzymes.)

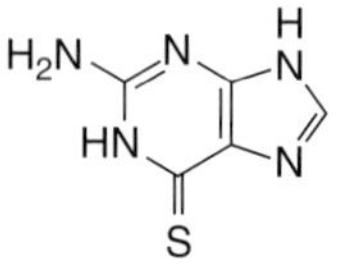

FIGURE 77-18   Molecular structure of thioguanine.

BSF ⬌ Live Vaccines: (*See* Ω-48 in Appendix A.) Patients with bone marrow depression caused by busulfan may develop generalized infections from receiving live vaccines. Therefore, at least six months separation between the two is recommended.

BSF ⬌ Thioguanine: 6-thioguanine (Fig. 77-18) can cause chronic hepato-toxicity and portal hypertension. Continuous co-administration of busulfan and thioguanine for treatment of chronic myelogenous leukemia has caused higher incidence of portal hypertension, esophageal varices, and hepatotoxicity (or abnormal liver function).

FLUDARABINE

MECHANISM OF ACTION

Fludarabine (Fig. 77-19) is phosphorylated to fludarabine triphosphate, which in-hibits several intracellular enzymes important in DNA replication, such as DNA polymerase and DNA ligase-1.

SIDE EFFECTS

Its side effects include deep venous thrombosis; dyspnea, pneumonia, and cough; nausea, vomiting, and anorexia; dysuria and hematuria; myalgia, arthralgia,

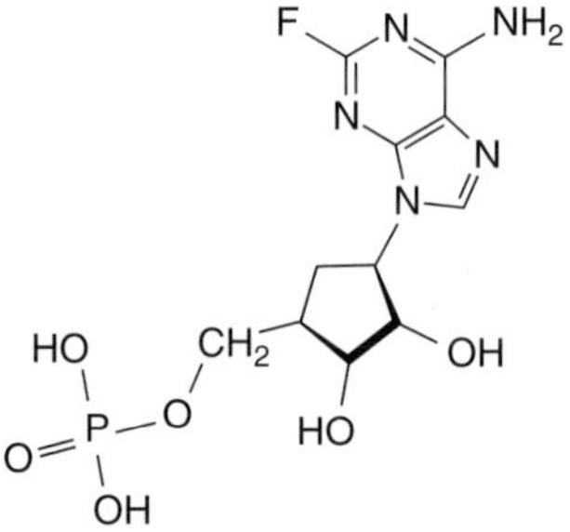

FIGURE 77-19   Molecular structure of fludarabine.

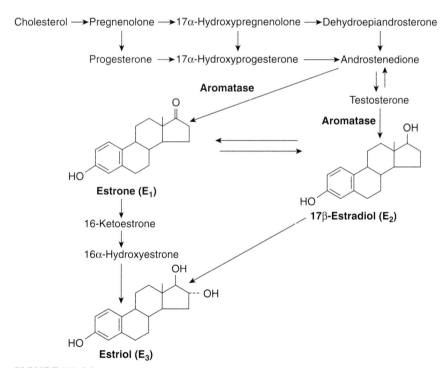

FIGURE 77-22 Molecular structure of letrozole.

MECHANISM OF ACTION

All these drugs work by inhibition of aromatase, the enzyme involved in the synthesis of estrogen from androgen (Fig. 77-23). Thus, all of them block the synthesis of estrogen to treat estrogen-dependent breast cancer.

FIGURE 77-23 **Aromatase site of action.** Reproduced, with permission, from Barrett KE, Barman SM, Boitano S, and Brooks HL. *Ganong's Review of Medical Physiology*. 23rd ed. New York, NY: McGraw-Hill; 2010, p 416.

TABLE 77-12 Aromatase Inhibitors vs CYP Enzymes

Drug Name	1A2	2A6	2B6	2C8	2C9	2C18	2C19	2D6	2E1	3A4
Anastrozole	Inh			Inh	Inh					Inh
Exemestane										Sub
Letrozole		Sub+ Inh					Inh			Sub

Abbreviations: Sub, substrate of the enzyme; Inh, inhibits the enzyme; Ezi, induces the enzyme

1. Anastrozole is inhibitory on several CYP isozymes as shown above, while exemestane is not. Thus, administration of anastrozole in combination with drugs that require those enzymes for metabolic clearance may result in elevated blood levels, inciting their adverse effects. (*See* the middle column of Table-0 at the 'Introduction' for possible substrates of those enzymes.)

2. Metabolic clearance of exemestane requires the presence of microsomal CYP3A4. Therefore, inhibition of this enzyme by other drugs may raise blood levels of exemestane to exacerbate its adverse effects. (*See* the left-hand column of Table-0 at the 'Introduction' for possible inhibitors of this enzyme.)

SIDE EFFECTS

Frequent side effects of these drugs include hot flashes; nausea, vomiting, diarrhea or constipation, and abdominal pain; vaginal bleeding; vulvar itching; increased sweating; swelling of the legs or feet; lightheadedness, dizziness, confusion, and mental depression; and anxiety and insomnia.

DRUG INTERACTIONS

See Table 77-12.

CAPECITABINE

Capecitabine is a prodrug that is metabolically converted to 5-Fluorouracil, its active form.

MECHANISM OF ACTION

Capecitabine (Fig. 77-24) is an orally active prodrug that is first converted to 5'-deoxy-5- fluorouridine, which in turn undergoes hydrolysis in the liver and tissues to form a selectively tumor-activated cytotoxic moiety, 5-fluorouracil (*See* Fig. 31-2), which in turn is converted in the body to a false nucleotide, 5-F-deoxyuridine monophosphate (5-F-dUMP) to inhibit the enzyme thymidylate synthase, which catalyzes transfer of the methyl group from $N^{5,10}$-CH_2-FH_4 to the uracil of dUMP to convert its uracil to thymine. Thus, capecitabine causes the death of cancer cells by blocking the formation of thymine, which is essential for DNA synthesis.

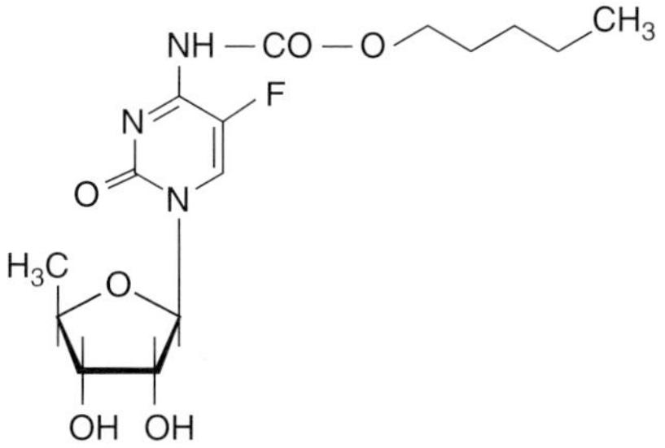

FIGURE 77-24 Molecular structure of capecitabine.

SIDE EFFECTS

Its side effects include mouth ulcer, nausea, vomiting, body aches and weakness; bone marrow suppression; itchy skin; dizziness, and insomnia.

DRUG INTERACTIONS

Capecitabine (CPB)

CPB ⟷ Leucovorin: Deaths from severe necrotizing enterocolitis, diarrhea, and dehydration have been reported in elderly patients receiving leucovorin and 5-fluorouracil for treatment of colorectal carcinoma. Leucovorin can increase the serum levels of 5-fluorouracil to which capecitabine, a prodrug, is converted, inciting its toxicity.

CPB ⟷ Chloramphenicol: Chloramphenicol may cause severe hematologic toxicity, and its use with capecitabine, which is also known to cause bone marrow suppression, may lead to additive adverse effects.

CPB ⟷ CYP Isozymes: *See* Table 77-13.

CPB ⟷ Live Vaccines: (*See* Ω-48 in Appendix A.) Patients with bone marrow depression caused by capecitabine may develop generalized infections from receiving live vaccines. Therefore, at least six months separation between the two is recommended.

CPB ⟷ Zidovudine: Zidovudine therapy has been associated with neutropenia and anemia. Concurrent use with capecitabine, which also causes bone marrow suppression, may result in additive hematologic toxicity.

TABLE 77-13 Capecitabine vs CYP Enzymes

Drug Name	1A2	2A6	2B6	2C8	2C9	2C18	2C19	2D6	2E1	3A4
Capecitabine					Inh					

Abbreviations: Sub, substrate of the enzyme; **Inh**, inhibits the enzyme; Ezi, induces the enzyme

Capecitabine is converted to 5-fluorouracil, its active form, which has an inhibitory effect on hepatic enzyme CYP2C9. Thus, co-administration with phenytoin, an antiepileptic drug, or with S-warfarin, an oral anticoagulant, which are both mostly metabolized via CYP2C9, can impair their clearance, raising their blood levels and inciting their toxicities. (See the middle column of Table-0 at the 'Introduction' for other possible substrates of this enzyme.)

DOCETAXEL OR PACLITAXEL

(See Fig. 77-4.)

MECHANISM OF ACTION

Both drugs bind to the beta-subunit of tubulin to promote abnormal polymerization of tubulin into stable nonfunctional microtubule bundles, useless for mitosis. Therefore, both drugs function as antimitotic agents. The binding affinity of docetaxel for the beta-tubulin subunit is slightly greater than that of paclitaxel (relative potency of 1.9 versus 1.0).

SIDE EFFECTS

The frequent side effects of these drugs include irregular heartbeat; low WBC counts to increase the chance of acquiring infections (with signs of infection such as fever and chills); severe stomach pain, vomiting, and black or bloody stool; swelling of the hands; muscle or joint pain; temporary hair loss; excessive tearing; fatigue; severe headache; and symptoms of a serious allergic reaction such as skin rash, itching, swelling, and difficulty in breathing.

DRUG INTERACTIONS

Docetaxel: The microsomal enzyme CYP3A4 is called for the metabolic processing of both docetaxel, and itraconazole, an antifungal drug. When the two are taken together competition for the same enzyme may develop, resulting in elevated blood levels of unmetabolized docetaxel that may exacerbate its adverse effects.

Paclitaxel: See earlier in this chapter.

EPIRUBICIN

MECHANISM OF ACTION

Epirubicin (*See* Fig. 77-9) is a stereoisomer of doxorubicin, and its exact mechanism of action is not clear. It appears that the drug, by intercalating the DNA, inhibits the synthesis of DNA, RNA, and proteins to generate antimitotic and cytotoxic activities.

SIDE EFFECTS

Its side effects may include nausea, vomiting, and hair loss; and bone marrow depression.

DRUG INTERACTIONS

It is not known whether other medications will interact with this medication with clinical significance.

GOSERELIN

MECHANISM OF ACTION

Goserelin is a 10-amino acid synthetic analog of gonadotropin releasing hormone (GnRH) that initially increases the secretions of gonadotropins from the pituitary gland, but upon continuous administration for four weeks or longer, it desensitizes the pituitary receptors to result in diminished secretion of gonadotropins, which in turn reduces production of estrogen to help treat estrogen-dependent breast cancer.

SIDE EFFECTS

Its side effects include rapid heart rate; hot flashes; stomach upset; difficulty in urination; reduced sexual desire; tenderness of breasts; weight gain; fever and chills; headache; and symptoms of allergic reactions such as breathing difficulty, skin rash, hives, and itching.

DRUG INTERACTIONS

No clinically serious interaction has been reported.

SELECTIVE ESTROGEN RECEPTOR MODULATORS

Both **tamoxifen** and **toremifene** belong in the group called selective estrogen receptor modulators (SERMs). They have antiestrogenic properties on certain tissues and weak estrogen-like effects on other tissues. For instance, both drugs have an antiestrogenic effect on the estrogen-dependent breast tumor, but have an estrogen-like effect on the bones to enhance bone mineralization, mimicking the beneficial effects of estrogen.

MECHANISM OF ACTION

Toremifene (Fig. 77-25) is a close analogue of tamoxifen (Fig. 77-26) with a similar mechanism of action, and is used to prevent or treat estrogen-dependent breast cancer. Both tamoxifen and toremifene compete with endogenous estrogens for binding to the cytoplasmic estrogen receptors, depleting the availability of the cytosolic receptors and thereby opposing proliferation of estrogen-dependent breast tumors.

SIDE EFFECTS

Tamoxifen: Its side effects include hypercalcemia; blood-clots in the lungs; abnormal vaginal bleeding; shortness of breath; chest pain; loss of balance; cancer of the uterine lining (due to activation of estrogen receptors in the uterus); and confusion.

Toremifene: Its side effects include irregular heartbeat; hot flashes and flushing; hypercalcemia; nausea, vomiting; vaginal bleeding; muscle pain; change in vision; hallucinations; and allergic reactions such as skin rash and hives; difficulty in breathing.

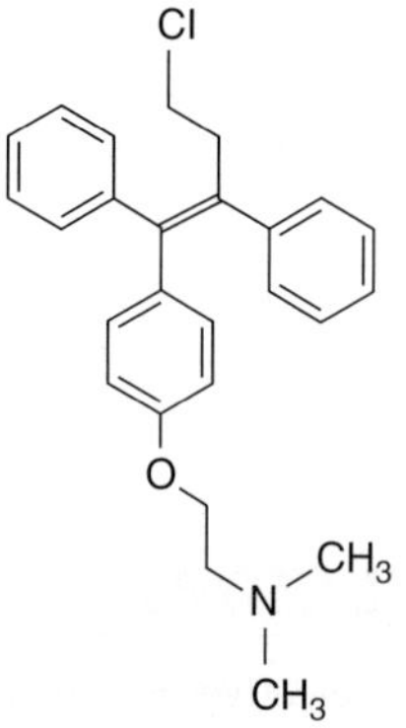

FIGURE 77-25   Molecular structure of toremifene.

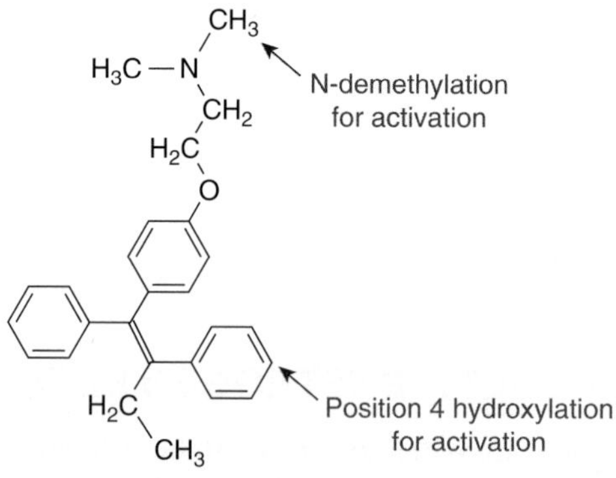

FIGURE 77-26   Molecular structure of tamoxifen.

receiving live vaccines. Therefore, at least six months separation between the two is recommended.

IFM ⬌ Warfarin: Ifosfamide requires multiple CYP enzymes, including CYP2C8, CYP2C9, and CYP3A4, to form 4-hydroxyifosfamide, its active metabolite. The microsomal CYP2C9 is also involved in elimination of S-warfarin, while CYP3A4 is involved in elimination of R-warfarin. Therefore, when ifosfamide is taken with warfarin, the two may compete for the same enzyme—ifosfamide for its activation and warfarin for its elimination. This could raise blood levels of warfarin to exacerbate its adverse effects, such as excessive internal bleeding.

CISPLATIN

See earlier in this chapter.

FLUOROURACIL

See Chapter 31.

UTERINE CANCER

Medications that may be effective in the treatment of uterine cancer include: (1) **carboplatin** (Paraplatin) or **cisplatin;** (2) **paclitaxel;** and (3) **doxorubicin.**

CARBOPLATIN OR CISPLATIN
MECHANISM OF ACTION
Both drugs alkylate guanine in the DNA strands to interfere with normal transcription and/or DNA replication, to cause eventual cell death.

SIDE EFFECTS
Carboplatin: Its side effects may include rapid or irregular heartbeat; breathing difficulty; nausea, vomiting; flue-like symptoms such as fever and chills; hair loss; bone marrow suppression; and very rarely, allergic reaction such as skin rash and itching, which may occur within minutes of administration. Epinephrine (Adrenalin), corticosteroids, and antihistamines may alleviate such symptoms.

Cisplatin: *See* earlier in this chapter.

DRUG INTERACTIONS

Carboplatin: The adverse effects of nephrotoxicity by compounds such as an aminoglycoside antibiotic may be potentiated by combined use with carboplatin; and concomitant use of carboplatin and stavudine, an anti-HIV drug, may result in increased risk of peripheral neuropathy.

Cisplatin: *See* earlier in this chapter.

PACLITAXEL

See earlier in this chapter.

DOXORUBICIN

See earlier in this chapter.

OVARIAN CANCER

Medications that may be effective in the treatment of ovarian cancer include (1) **altretamine** (Hexalen); (2) **carboplatin** (Paraplatin) or **cisplatin** (Platinol); (3) **doxorubicin liposomal** (Doxil); (4) **paclitaxel** (Taxol); and (5) **irinotecan** (Camptosar) or **topotecan** (Hycamtin).

ALTRETAMINE

MECHANISM OF ACTION

The mechanism of action of altretamine is not fully understood, but it is thought that it may inhibit DNA and RNA synthesis by selectively inhibiting incorporation of uridine and thymidine into the strands of DNA and RNA. Some metabolites of altretamine can also form covalent adducts with such macromolecules as DNA, but the relevance of these reactions to anticancer activity remains unclear.

SIDE EFFECTS

Its side effects may include rapid heartbeat; unusual bleeding or bruising; and loss of appetite; tingling of the hands or feet (neurotoxicity); muscle weakness; moderate bone marrow depression with leucopenia; mental confusion; dizziness; and fever and chills.

TABLE 77-16 Altretamine vs CYP Enzymes

Drug Name	1A2	2A6	2B6	2C8	2C9	2C18	2C19	2D6	2E1	3A4
Altretamine			Sub							

Abbreviations: Sub, substrate of the enzyme; Inh, inhibits the enzyme; Ezi, induces the enzyme

Altretamine is metabolized by CYP 2B6. Therefore, inhibition of this enzyme by other drugs can raise blood levels of altretamine to possibly exacerbate its adverse effects. Drugs that inhibit CYP2B6 include: clopidogrel, itraconazole, orphenadrine, sertraline, and ticlopidine. (*See* the left-hand column of Table-0 at the 'Introduction' for other possible inhibitors of this enzyme.)

DRUG INTERACTIONS

Altretamine (ALM)

ALM ⟷ Chloramphenicol: Chloramphenicol may cause severe hematologic toxicity, and its use in combination with altretamine, which is known to cause mild bone marrow suppression, may lead to additive hematologic depression.

ALM ⟷ CYP Isozymes: *See* Table 77-16.

ALM ⟷ Live Vaccines: (*See* Ω-48 in Appendix A.) Patients with bone marrow depression caused by altretamine may develop generalized infections from receiving live vaccines. Therefore, at least six months separation between the two is recommended.

ALM ⟷ MAO Inhibitors: (*See* Ω-51 in Appendix A.) Altretamine, also known as hexamethylmelamine (Fig. 77-28), has a tertiary amine structure, and is well-absorbed following oral administration. It then undergoes extensive demethylation in the liver to generate metabolites such as pentamethylmelamine and tetramethylmelamine. Use of altretamine in the presence of an MAO inhibitor, such as phenelzine and tranylcypromine, may cause severe orthostatic hypotension.

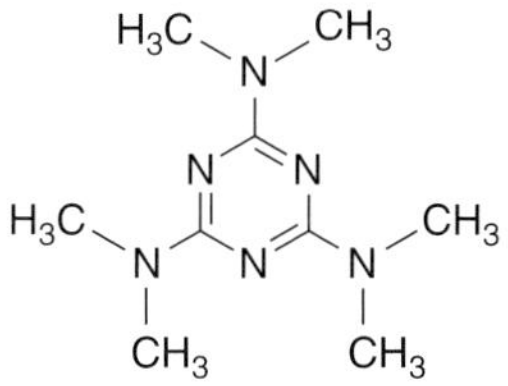

FIGURE 77-28 Molecular structure of altretamine.

ALM ⬌ Pyridoxine: Concurrent administration of altretamine with pyridoxine is not recommended because, though pyridoxine reduces the neurotoxicity of altretamine, it also reduces its anticancer effectiveness. The mechanism behind this observation is yet to be fully elucidated.

ALM ⬌ Zidovudine: Zidovudine therapy has caused anemia and neutropenia, and when used in combination with altretamine, it may result in additive hematologic toxicity.

CARBOPLATIN OR CISPLATIN

MECHANISM OF ACTION

The mechanism of action of carboplatin (Fig. 77-29) is very similar to that of cisplatin. They alkylate guanine in the DNA strands to interfere with normal transcription and/or replication of DNA, to eventually cause death of the tumor cells.

SIDE EFFECTS

Carboplatin: Its side effects may include rapid or irregular heartbeat; breathing difficulty; nausea, vomiting; flu-like symptoms such as fever and chills; hair loss; bone marrow suppression; and very rarely, allergic reaction such as bronchoconstriction and skin rash and itching which may occur within minutes of administration. Epinephrine, corticosteroids, and antihistamines may alleviate such symptoms.

Cisplatin: *See* earlier in this chapter.

DRUG INTERACTIONS

Carboplatin: The renal toxicity of an aminoglycoside antibiotic may be potentiated by combined use with carboplatin.

Cisplatin: *See* earlier in this chapter.

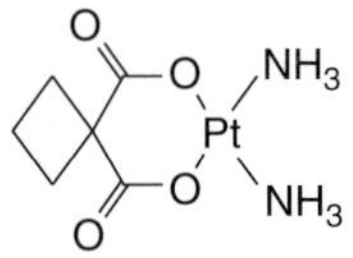

FIGURE 77-29 Molecular structure of carboplatin.

BOX 77-9

Basic Concepts of Vincristine Interactions

1. P-gp is a membrane-bound protein that utilizes energy driven from hydrolysis of ATP to efflux many exogenous compounds including some drugs. Vincristine is one of those substrate drugs, and that is why when co-administered with other drugs that inhibit this transporter protein, the efflux (or elimination) of vincristine is blocked to raise its serum concentration and toxicities. Those P-gp inhibitory drugs include: **cyclosporine** (an immunosuppressant); **nifedipine;** and **verapamil.**

2. Vincristine can cause peripheral neuropathy, and when taken in combination with drugs that generate similar neuropathy, additive peripheral neuritis may result. Those drugs include: **didanosine** (an oral anti-HIV drug); and **zalcitabine** (an anti-HIV drug, also known as ddC [dideoxycytidine]).

concentrations and inciting its adverse effects, such as neuropathy. To minimize this toxicity, vincristine should be given 12-24 hours before intake of asparaginase.

VCS ⟷ CYP Isozymes: *See* Table 77-18.

VCS ⟷ Digoxin: Vincristine may cause atrophy of intestinal villi, and can reduce the absorption of digoxin, undercutting its therapeutic effectiveness.

TABLE 77-18 Vincristine vs CYP Isozymes

Drug Name	1A2	2A6	2B6	2C8	2C9	2C18	2C19	2D6	2E1	3A4
Vincristine										Sub + Inh

Abbreviations: Sub, substrate of the enzyme; Inh, inhibits the enzyme; Ezi, induces the enzyme

1. Vincristine requires the microsomal enzyme CYP3A4 for its inactivation. Thus, inhibition of this enzyme by other drugs can raise blood levels of vincristine to potentially exacerbate its adverse effects. Those strong inhibitors of CYP3A4 include: clarithromycin, indinavir, itraconazole, ketoconazole, nefazodone, nelfinavir, ritonavir, saquinavir, and telithromycin. (*See* the left-hand column of Table-0 at the 'Introduction' for other possible inhibitors of the enzyme.)

2. Vincristine exerts an inhibitory effect on CYP3A4. Co-administration with drugs that require this enzyme for metabolic clearance may result in their elevated blood levels and possibly incite their adverse effects. (*See* the middle column of Table-0 at the 'Introduction' for possible substrates of the enzyme.)

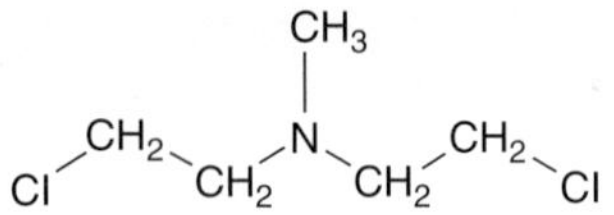

$$\text{Cl} \diagdown \overset{\displaystyle CH_2}{} \diagup \underset{\displaystyle CH_2}{} \diagdown \overset{\displaystyle CH_3}{\underset{\displaystyle N}{|}} \diagup \underset{\displaystyle CH_2}{} \diagdown \overset{\displaystyle CH_2}{} \diagup \text{Cl}$$

FIGURE 77-31   Molecular structure of mechlorethamine.

VCS ⟷ Mitomycin: The pulmonary toxicity of mitomycin may be increased by combined use with vincristine, which also causes severe bronchospasm, leading to acute dyspnea.

CYCLOPHOSPHAMIDE

MECHANISM OF ACTION

Cyclophosphamide (*See* Fig. 59-2) is a cyclic phosphamide ester of mechlorethamine (Fig. 77-31), and functions as an alkylating agent that prevents cell division by cross-linking DNA strands and interrupting DNA synthesis.

SIDE EFFECTS

Its side effects may include congestive heart failure and cardiac necrosis; interstitial pulmonary fibrosis; nausea, vomiting, and diarrhea; hemorrhagic cystitis and renal tubular necrosis; amenorrhea; alopecia; and bone marrow suppression.

DRUG INTERACTIONS

See Chapter 59.

CISPLATIN

See earlier in this chapter.

TESTICULAR CANCER

Medications that may be effective in the treatment of testicular cancer include: (1) **cisplatin** (Platinol); (2) **etoposide** (Etopophos, Vepesid); and (3) **ifosfamide** (Ifex).

CISPLATIN

See earlier in this chapter.

ETOPOSIDE

See earlier in this chapter.

IFOSFAMIDE

See earlier in this chapter.

PROSTATE CANCER

Since prostate tumors require the presence of testosterone to grow, reducing the production of testosterone often works well in preventing further growth and metastasis of the cancer. Medications that may be effective in the treatment of prostate cancer include: (1) **goserelin** (Zoladex) or **leuprolide** (Lupron); (2) **flutamide;** and (3) **estramustine** (Emcyt).

GOSERELIN OR LEUPROLIDE

Both goserelin and leuprolide work by opposing production of testosterone. Both drugs are used to treat advanced prostate cancer.

MECHANISM OF ACTION

Goserelin is a 10-amino acid synthetic analog of gonadotropin-releasing hormone, whose subcutaneous injection initially increases the release of gonadotropins from the pituitary gland, but upon continuous administration for four weeks or longer, desensitizes the pituitary receptors to result in diminished release of gonadotropin required for the production of testosterone. **Leuprolide**, on the other hand, is a 9-amino acid peptide synthetic analog of natural hypothalamic gonadotropin-releasing hormone, having a greater potency and longer duration of action than the natural hormone. Subcutaneous injection once daily initially stimulates the release of gonadotropins, but its continuous administration for more than two weeks will desensitize the pituitary receptors, resulting in diminished release of gonadotropin, which is required for the production of testosterone. (This is why it is called chemical castration.)

SIDE EFFECTS

Their possible side effects include rapid heart rate; hot flashes and night sweats; breathing difficulties; nausea and vomiting; difficulty in urination; bone pain; weight gain; reduced sexual desire; and headache and nervousness.

DRUG INTERACTIONS

There has been no convincing evidence that these drugs would interact with any other drugs to cause serious consequences.

FLUTAMIDE

MECHANISM OF ACTION

Flutamide (Fig. 77-32) works by inhibiting testosterone binding at its target receptors.

SIDE EFFECTS

Its possible side effects include easy bleeding or bruising; diarrhea, nausea, and loss of appetite; sexual impotence; hot flashes; and muscle weakness.

DRUG INTERACTIONS

See Table 77-19.

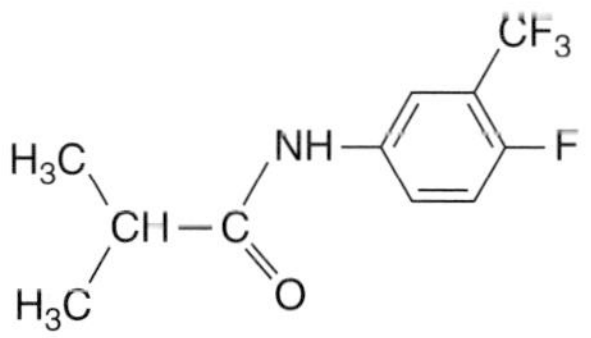

FIGURE 77-32   Molecular structure of flutamide.

TABLE 77-19   Flutamide vs CYP Enzymes

Drug Name	1A2	2A6	2B6	2C8	2C9	2C18	2C19	2D6	2E1	3A4
Flutamide	Sub+ Inh									Sub

Abbreviations: Sub, substrate of the enzyme; Inh, inhibits the enzyme; Ezi, induces the enzyme

Since flutamide exerts an inhibitory effect on CYP1A2, co-administration of this drug with others that require this enzyme for metabolic clearance may result in their elevated blood levels, possibly exacerbating their adverse effects. (*See* the middle column of Table-0 at the 'Introduction' for possible substrates of this enzyme.)

ESTRAMUSTINE

MECHANISM OF ACTION

Estramustine is a chemotherapeutic agent often used to treat prostate cancer, which became resistant to the hormonal treatments discussed earlier. Estramustine (Fig. 77-33) is a derivative of estradiol linked to nitrogen mustard-carbamate, which functions as an alkylating antineoplastic agent. Its mechanism of action is unclear—unlike other alkylating agents, it does not directly damage DNA.

SIDE EFFECTS

Possible side effects of estramustine include easy bruising or bleeding; breathing difficulty; stomach pains, and dark stool; dark urine; jaundice; weakness; chest pain; and swelling of the ankles or feet.

DRUG INTERACTIONS

Co-administration with aldesleukin, a recombinant IL-2 having an inhibitory effects on tumor growth, may increase toxicities such as congestive heart failure, pleural effusion, pulmonary edema; hematuria; and bone marrow depression.

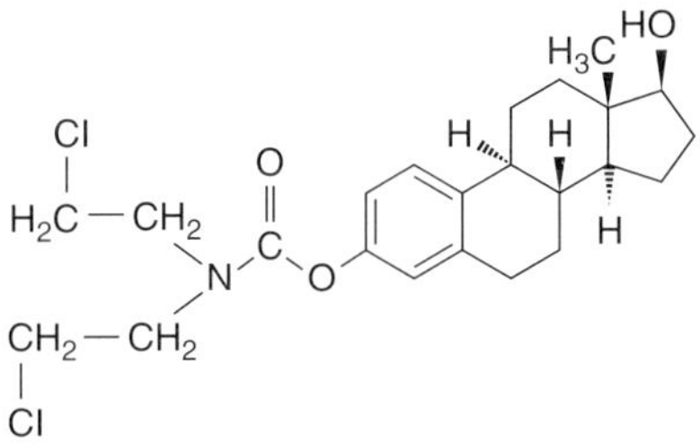

FIGURE 77-33 Molecular structure of estramustine.

78 Systemic Infections by Viruses

This chapter is divided into sections on (A) herpes infections, (B) influenza infections, and (C) human immunodeficiency virus (HIV) infections.

◼ HERPES INFECTIONS

Herpes infections, such as cold sores and genital herpes, are diseases caused by herpes viruses. Though there are eight different types of herpes viruses that can infect humans, *Herpes simplex* virus (HSV) type-1 and type-2 are the most important. HSV-1 usually causes cold sores. HSV-2, mostly causing genital herpes, is a sexually transmitted viral infection whose symptoms vary from person to person, but may include fever and itching or tingling in the genital area.

There is no medication that can eradicate herpes viruses from the body, but some antiviral drugs can reduce their severity, duration, and frequency of attack. Medications shown effective in the treatment of herpes infections include: (1) **acyclovir** or **valacyclovir** (Valtrex); and (2) **penciclovir** or **famciclovir**.

ACYCLOVIR OR VALACYCLOVIR

Valacyclovir (Fig. 78-1) is an inactive prodrug that is almost completely converted by deesterification to active acyclovir (Fig. 78-2). Thus, valacyclovir and acyclovir have similar drug interactions. Both are available for oral intake and for topical application. Valacyclovir has better bioavailability after oral administration.

MECHANISM OF ACTION

Acyclovir, to which valacylovir converts, is phosphorylated by viral thymidine kinase to its triphosphate form, which in turn inhibits the viral enzyme DNA polymerase, inhibiting DNA replications required for the virus to proliferate.

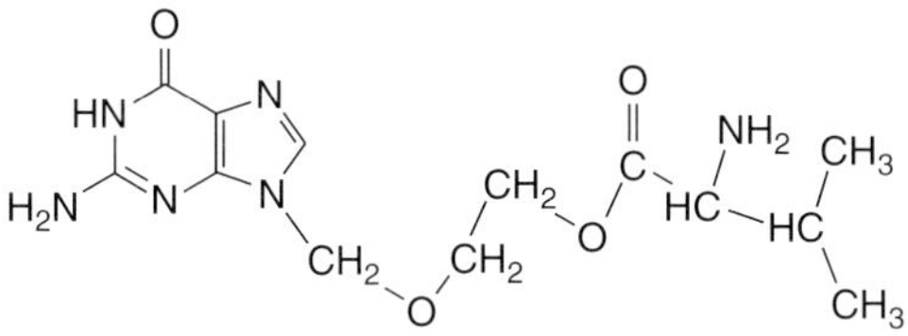

FIGURE 78-1 Molecular structure of valacyclovir.

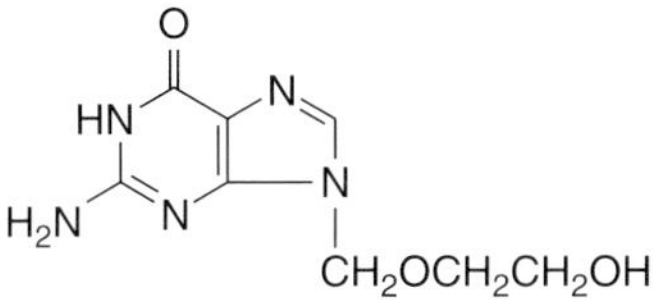

FIGURE 78-2 Molecular structure of acyclovir.

SIDE EFFECTS

Frequent side effects of these drugs include diarrhea, and stomach pain; renal failure; headache and lightheadedness, and allergic reactions such as difficulty in breathing; swelling of the face, lips, tongue, or throat; and skin hives.

DRUG INTERACTIONS
Acyclovir or valacyclovir (AFV)

AFV ⟷ Aminoglycoside Antibiotics: (*See* Ω-7 in Appendix A.) Co-administration of acyclovir or valacyclovir with an aminoglycoside antibiotic such as gentamicin may increase the likelihood of nephrotoxicity.

AFV ⟷ CYP Isozymes: *See* Table 78-1.

AFV ⟷ Mycophenolate Mofetil: If co-administered with mycophenolate mofetil, they may compete for renal tubular secretions, resulting in increased concentrations of acyclovir especially in patients with renal dysfunction.

AFV ⟷ NSAIDs: (*See* Ω-54 in Appendix A.) Co-administration with ibuprofen or other NSAIDs may result in renal insufficiency or acute renal failure, either by decreasing the elimination of acyclovir and valacyclovir or by inhibiting the synthesis of prostaglandin, which is important for renal circulation.

TABLE 78-1 **Acyclovir and Valacyclovir vs CYP Isozymes**

Drug Name	1A2	2A6	2B6	2C8	2C9	2C18	2C19	2D6	2E1	3A4
Acyclovir	Inh									
Valacyclovir	Inh									

1. Both acyclovir and valacyclovir can inhibit CYP1A2. Therefore, co-administration of either with other drugs that require CYP1A2 for hepatic clearance may raise their blood levels and possibly exacerbate their adverse effects. Those drug affected by CYP1A2 inhibition include: acetaminophen, amitriptyline, imipramine, and thioridazine. In fact, acyclovir was shown to decrease clearance of theophylline (a substrate of CYP1A2), increasing its blood levels and inciting its toxicity. (*See* the middle column of Table-0 at the 'Introduction' for other possible substrates of this enzyme.)
2. Neither acyclovir, famciclovir (not shown), nor valacyclovir is significantly metabolized by any CYP enzymes. Therefore, interactions with any CYP inhibitor or inducer must be insignificant.

AFV ⟷ Probenecid: Renal clearance of acyclovir or valacyclovir is reduced by probenecid, raising their plasma levels and inciting their adverse effects. The risk of side effects due to this interaction may be increased in the presence of impaired renal function.

PENCICLOVIR OR FAMCICLOVIR

Famciclovir (Fig. 78-3) is an inactive prodrug of penciclovir (Fig. 78-4). Famciclovir has better bioavailability than penciclovir, when taken orally. Famciclovir is available as an oral tablet and a topical cream; whereas penciclovir, because of poor absorption when given orally, is available only as a topical cream used to treat recurrent cold sores on the lips and face.

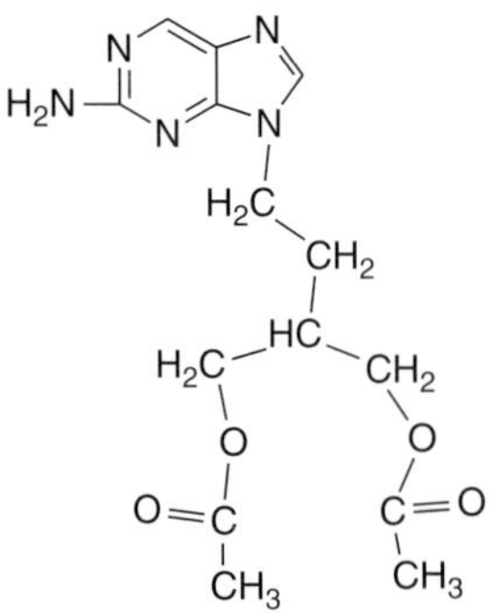

FIGURE 78-3 Molecular structure of famciclovir.

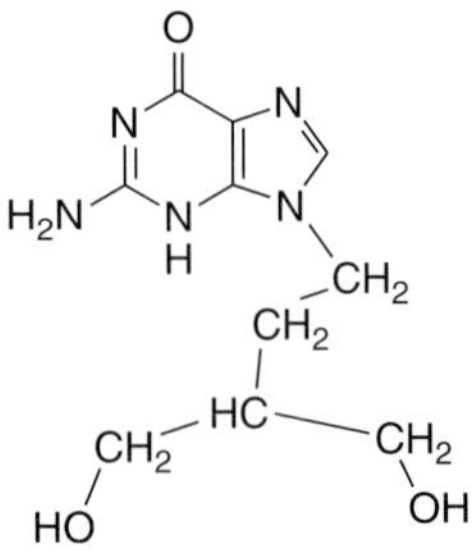

FIGURE 78-4 Molecular structure of penciclovir.

MECHANISM OF ACTION

Penciclovir, to which famciclovir converts, is phosphorylated by viral thymidine kinase to its triphosphate form, which inhibits the viral enzyme DNA polymerase. This mechanism inhibits DNA replication so the virus cannot proliferate.

SIDE EFFECTS

At the site of application, penciclovir may cause skin rash, redness, irritation or numbness. If absorbed, it may cause change in sense of smell, and headache. If swelling of the mouth or throat occurs, seek medical assistance.

Frequent side effects associated with oral intake of famciclovir include flatulence, nausea, vomiting, skin rash, fatigue, confusion, and headache; serious but rare side effects include reduced counts of white blood cells (WBC).

DRUG INTERACTIONS

It is not known whether famciclovir or penciclovir applied topically interact with other drugs to generate serious consequences. Both drugs, famciclovir in particular may generate these interactions after oral administration.

Penciclovir or famciclovir (PFV)

PFV ⟷ Digoxin: Famciclovir may increase serum levels of digoxin by unknown mechanism, but this interaction will not lead to serious consequences in most cases.

PFV ⟷ Probenecid: Probenecid interferes with the renal elimination of famciclovir, raising its blood levels and inciting its adverse effects.

PFV ⟷ Theophylline: Theophylline interferes with elimination of famciclovir from the body. Since CYP enzymes do not play an important role in the metabolism of famciclovir, and the plasma elimination rate of penciclovir, to which famciclovir converts, decreases linearly with a reduction in renal function (the principal route of elimination of both penciclovir and 6-deoxy penciclovir is renal), it appears that theophylline interferes with renal excretion of penciclovir.

INFLUENZA INFECTIONS

Influenza is a respiratory infection caused by several influenza viruses, which are classified as Type-A, B, and C. Type-A is the most common in causing seasonal flu epidemics each year, and the most feared of the three. Type-B can also cause epidemics, but the disease runs a milder course than Type-A. Type-C viruses have never spurred a large scale epidemic and usually generate mild respiratory infections similar to the common cold.

Medications shown effective in the treatment of influenza virus include: (1) **oseltamivir** (Tamiflu) and (2) **rimantadine** (Flumadine).

OSELTAMIVIR

MECHANISM OF ACTION

This drug works by inhibition of neuraminidase, the viral enzyme without which infective viral particles clump and cannot be released to freshly infect other healthy host cells. However, oseltamivir (Fig. 78-5) is a prodrug that is activated by human carboxylesterase-1, a broad spectrum serine hydrolase (or serine esterase), involved not only in drug metabolism, such as the hydrolysis of both heroin and cocaine, but also in inactivation of organophosphate nerve toxins.

SIDE EFFECTS

Side effects of oseltamivir may include nausea, vomiting, and diarrhea; pink eye; and ear infections.

DRUG INTERACTIONS

Oseltamivir has to be converted by a serine hydrolase located in the liver to its active oseltamivir carboxylate. However, if this drug is taken with a live attenuated influenza vaccine, it may interfere with the effectiveness of this drug, probably because the influenza viruses in circulation may change their antigenicity due to presence of the live attenuated influenza vaccine. Thus, avoid taking a live attenuated influenza vaccine within two weeks before or 48 hours after administration of oseltamivir. Activation of oseltamivir by human carboxylesterase-1 is inhibited by clopidogrel, an antiplatelet agent.

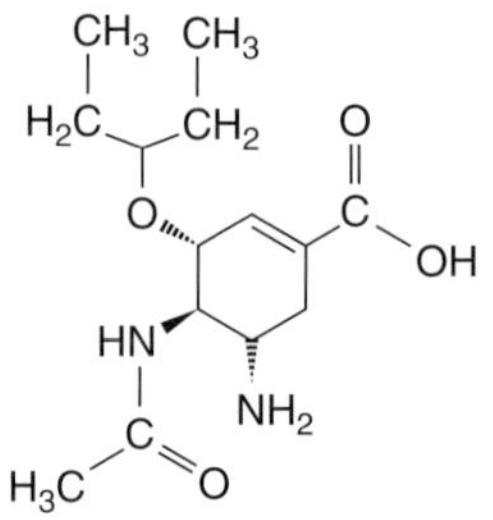

FIGURE 78-5   Molecular structure of oseltamivir.

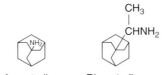

FIGURE 78-6 Molecular structures of amantadine and rimantadine.

RIMANTADINE

Rimantadine is a structural analog of amantadine (Fig. 78-6) to be taken orally to treat, or rarely to prevent, influenza virus-A infections. Rimantadine is almost completely absorbed from the GI tract and metabolized in the liver, so little of it is excreted in the urine. Thus, rimantadine is the preferred drug in patients with renal impairment, and unlike amantadine this drug seldom produces prominent CNS side effects.

MECHANISM OF ACTION

Rimantadine and amantadine both appear to block viral penetration into host cells, thus preventing viral uncoating and subsequent replication.

SIDE EFFECTS

Possible side effects include dry mouth, nausea, vomiting, and loss of appetite; and dizziness and insomnia.

DRUG INTERACTIONS

It is not known whether other medications will interact with this drug to generate a clinically significant outcome.

HIV INFECTIONS

HIV infections will eventually progress to acquired immune deficiency syndrome (AIDS), a deadly, sexually transmitted disease that incapacitates the body's ability to fight off foreign pathogens. Detectable antibodies to HIV rarely appear in the blood immediately after HIV infection, as it normally takes several weeks to several months for the antibodies to develop. Acute HIV infection generates a flu-like syndrome characterized by fever, sore throat, headache, skin rash, and lymphadenopathy (swollen glands).

There is no cure for AIDS at this time. Several treatments are available that can delay progression of the disease for many years, and improve the quality of life for those who have developed symptoms. These drugs include: (1) nucleo-side reverse transcriptase (RT) inhibitors such as **abacavir** (ABC), **didanosine** (Videx), **emtricitabine** (Emtriva), **lamivudine** (Epivir, 3TC), **stavudine** (Zerit, d4T), **tenofovir** (Viread), and **zidovudine** (Retrovir), formerly called azidothy-midine (AZT); (2) so-called non-nucleoside RT inhibitors such as **delavirdine** (Rescriptor), **efavirenz** (Sustiva), and **nevirapine** (Viramune); (3) protease inhibitors such as **amprenavir** (Agenerase), **atazanavir** (Reyataz), **fosamprenavir** (Lexiva), **indinavir** (Crixivan), **lopinavir** (which is usually used in combination with Ritonavir), **nelfinavir** (Viracept), **ritonavir** (Norvir), **saquinavir** (Invirase, Fortovase), and **tipranavir** (Aptivus); and (4) **enfuvirtide** (*Fuzeon*), a fusion inhibitor.

NUCLEOSIDE RT INHIBITORS

These include **Abacavir, didanosine, emtricitabine, lamivudine, stavudine, tenofovir,** and **zidovudine.** There are also combination pills such as Combivir (**lamivudine + zidovudine**) and Truvada (**emtricitabine + tenofovir**).

MECHANISM OF ACTION

All of these drugs are false nucleosides (Fig. 78-7) that are converted by host thymidine kinase to their triphosphate forms, which are chemically aberrant and cannot be served for the formation of the phosphodiester linkages needed for synthesis of the DNA chain. Therefore, they interfere with the proper function of reverse transcriptase, the enzyme required to produce DNA out of the RNA chain of HIV in a critical step during its life cycle. In this way, these drugs keep the virus from reproducing.

SIDE EFFECTS

Abacavir: Its side effects may include severe hypotension; shortness of breath and cough; mouth ulcers, abdominal pain, diarrhea; joint pain; muscle pain or weak-ness; severe peeling of skin, tingling or burning of the skin; fever or chills; and severe allergic reactions.

Didanosine: Its side effects may include sore tongue or mouth, and severe diarrhea; jaundice; muscle or joint pain and tingling/numbness/pain and weakness

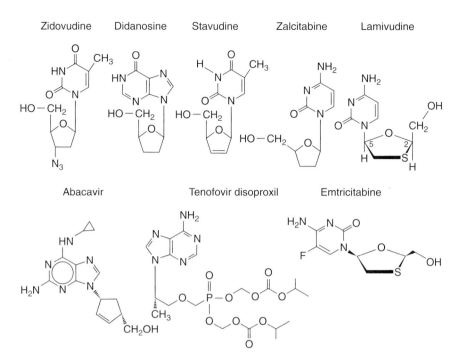

FIGURE 78-7   Molecular structures of nucleoside RT inhibitors.

in the limbs (peripheral neuropathy); pancreatitis; chills and fever; and headache and insomnia.

Emtricitabine: Its side effects may include change in the color of the skin (palms or soles of feet); tingling sensation; weakness of the limbs, and pain at joints and muscle.

Lamivudine: Its side effects may include muscle aches or weakness (mitochondrial toxicity) and tingling of the hands or feet (peripheral neuropathy); skin rash; fever and chills; and dizziness.

Stavudine: Its side effects may include hepatotoxicity; peripheral neuropathy such as numbness, tingling, burning or pain of the hands or feet; fatal lactic acidosis; sore throat; and itchy skin rashes.

Tenofovir: Its side effects may include muscle pain, numbness or tingling of the limbs, unusual tiredness, or weakness; and headache and dizziness.

Zidovudine: Its side effects may include shortness of breath; sore throat; liver damage with jaundice; dark urine; fever; muscle pain with unusual tiredness or weakness; bone marrow depression such as neutropenia and agranulocytosis; drowsiness and seizures; and allergic reactions such as skin rash and difficulty in breathing; and swelling of tissues.

DRUG INTERACTIONS

Abacavir

Abacavir and alcohol are both at least partially inactivated by alcohol dehydrogenase. Co-administration may decrease elimination of abacavir and increase its adverse effects.

Didanosine

See Box 78-1.

BOX 78-1

Basic Concepts of Didanosine Interactions

1. Most cases of pancreatitis caused by didanosine result from hypertriglyceridemia. When didanosine is co-administered with drugs that generate similar side effects, there is an increased risk of fatal pancreatitis. Those drugs include: **asparaginase** (an anticancer drug); **azathioprine** (an immunosuppressant); **estrogens** (*See* Ω-40 in Appendix A) (which can cause hypertriglyceridemia that can lead to pancreatitis in rare instances); **hydroxyurea** (an anticancer drug); **6-mercaptopurine** (a drug to treat acute lymphoblastic leukemia); **methyldopa** (an antihypertensive drug that may cause pancreatitis in rare instances); **metronidazole** (an antibiotic drug used against anaerobic bacteria that may cause pancreatitis in rare instances); **nitrofurantoin** (a urinary antiseptic that may cause pancreatitis in rare instances); **pentamidine** (a drug useful for leishmaniasis, including kala-azar and trypanosomiasis, that may cause pancreatitis in rare instances); **sulfonamide chemotherapeutics** (*See* Ω-70 in Appendix A); and **valproic acid** (an anticonvulsant that may cause pancreatitis in rare instances).

2. Didanosine is apt to cause peripheral neuropathy as manifested by tingling, numbness, or pain in the hands or feet. When co-administered with drugs that generate a similar neuropathy, greater incidence of neurologic disturbances may result. Those drugs include: **stavudine** (an anti-HIV drug that is prone to cause peripheral neuropathy); **zalcitabine** (an anti-HIV drug with a common

BOX 78-1 *(continued)*

side effect of peripheral neuropathy, which may be disabling); and **vinca alkaloids** (Fig. 78-8), especially vincristine.

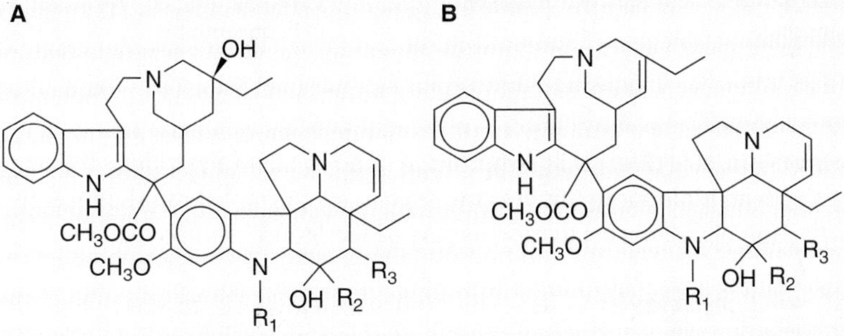

	R_1	R_2	R_3
Structure **A**			
Vinblastine	$-CH_3$	$-\overset{O}{\overset{\|}{C}}-OCH_3$	$-O-\overset{O}{\overset{\|}{C}}-CH_3$
Vincristine	$-CH$	$-\overset{O}{\overset{\|}{C}}-OCH_3$	$-O-\overset{O}{\overset{\|}{C}}-CH_3$
Vindesine	$-CH_3$	$-\overset{O}{\overset{\|}{C}}-NH_2$	$-OH$
Structure **B**			
Vinorelbine	$-CH_3$	$-\overset{O}{\overset{\|}{C}}-OCH_3$	$-O-\overset{O}{\overset{\|}{C}}-CH_3$

FIGURE 78-8 Molecular structures of vinca alkaloids. Reproduced, with permission, from Brunton LL, Lazo JS, and Parker KL. *Goodman and Gilman's The Pharmacological Basis of Therapeutics.* 11th ed. New York, NY: McGraw-Hill; 2006, p 1350.

Miscellaneous Interactions of Didanosine (DDS)

DDS ⟷ Allopurinol: Didanosine (Fig. 78-9) differs from other nucleoside analogues in that it has hypoxanthine, rather than any regular base, attached to the sugar ring. Thus, it yields hypoxanthine (Fig. 78-10) during its metabolism in the liver, which

FIGURE 78-9   Molecular structure of didanosine.

FIGURE 78-10   Molecular structure of hypoxanthine.

generates uric acid (Fig. 78-11) when acted upon by xanthine oxidase. If didanosine is taken with an inhibitor of this enzyme, such as allopurinol, it can significantly inhibit inactivation of didanosine to raise its plasma levels and incite its toxicity.

DDS ⬌ Ganciclovir: Didanosine and ganciclovir (Cytovene) (Fig. 78-12), a guanosine analogue, are frequently coadministered for treatment of HIV infection. Concurrent therapy raises plasma levels of didanosine not only to improve its therapeutic efficacy, but also to increase the potential for its toxicity. The mechanism responsible for increased didanosine concentrations may stem from competition of the two drugs for active secretion by the kidney tubules, but there are some who challenge this interpretation. To avoid this interaction, administer ganciclovir two hours before or one hour after didanosine.

DDS ⬌ Tenofovir: Combined administration of didanosine with tenofovir (Viread) (Fig. 78-13), an analog of adenosine (Fig. 78-14), raises plasma levels of didanosine to improve its therapeutic efficacy and enhance the potential for its toxicity. The mechanism responsible for increased didanosine concentrations may be the fact that tenofovir competes with didanosine for active secretion through the human organic anion transporter-1 (hOAT1) located at the basolateral membrane of the renal proximal tubules. Another possibility is that tenofovir inhibits the enzyme purine nucleoside phosphorylase (PNP), which is involved in degradation of didanosine. To avoid this interaction, administer tenofovir two hours before or one hour after didanosine.

Emtricitabine: This drug is poorly metabolized by the liver. Up to 80% of the administered dose is excreted in the urine unchanged, and its interaction with other drugs is not well documented.

Lamivudine (LVD)

LVD ⬌ Ribavirin: Both ribavirin and lamivudine can induce mitochondrial dysfunction (reduced respiratory chain enzyme activities) to cause clinical symptoms such as progressive muscle weakness at the lower limbs, acute respiratory failure,

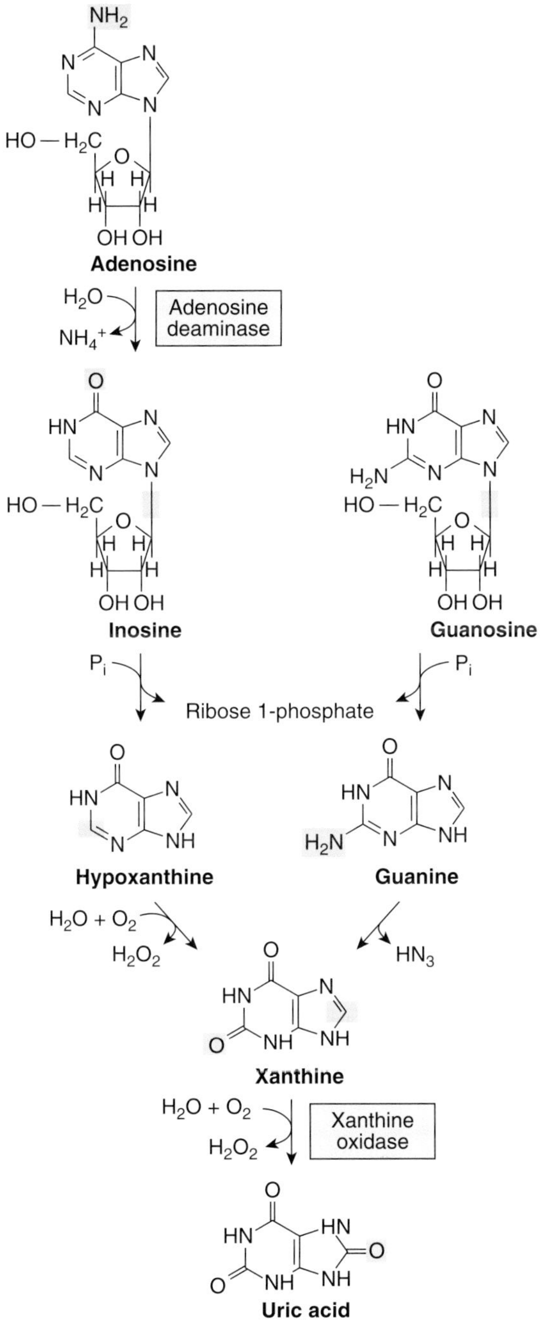

FIGURE 78-11 Xanthine oxidase site of action. Reproduced, with permission, from Murray RK, Bender DA, Botham KM, Kennelly PJ, Rodwell VW and Weil PA, eds. *Harper's Illustrated Biochemistry*. 28th ed. New York, NY: McGraw-Hill; 2009, p 299.

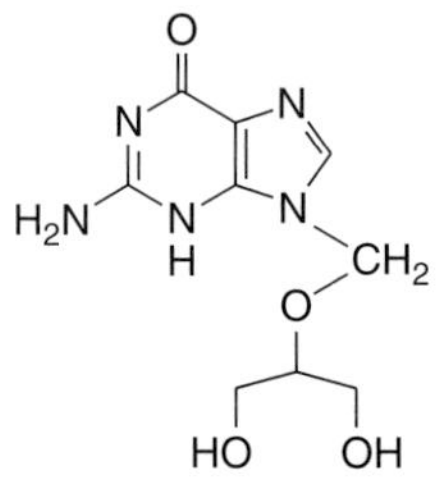

FIGURE 78-12   Molecular structure of ganciclovir.

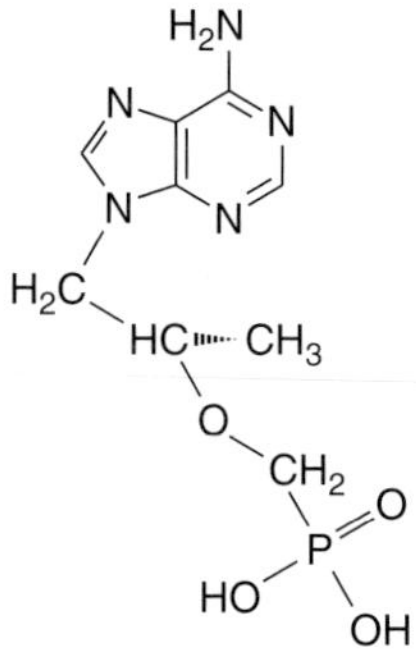

FIGURE 78-13   Molecular structure of tenofovir.

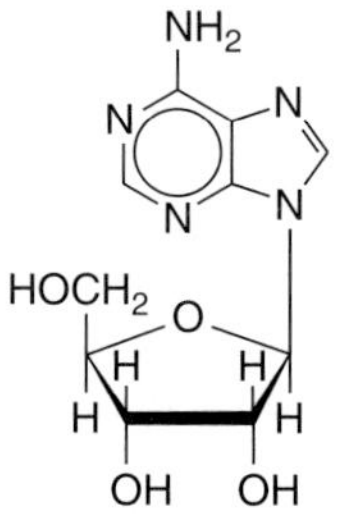

FIGURE 78-14   Molecular structure of adenosine.

and cardiac arrest that requires assisted ventilation. Concomitant use of ribavirin with lamivudine may result in increased risk of such adverse effects.

LVD ⟷ Trimethoprim/Sulfamethoxazole: As elimination of lamivudine depends more on renal excretion than its hepatic metabolism, if it is used in combination with trimethoprim/sulfamethoxazole, it may decrease renal clearance of lamivudine, increasing its serum concentrations and inciting its adverse effects.

LVD ⟷ Zalcitabine: To become an active agent, lamivudine (Fig. 78-15) has to be phosphorylated to its triphosphate form. When used in combination with zalcitabine, competition for phosphorylation may result, inhibiting activation of lamivudine and nullifying its antiretroviral effect. Therefore, it is prudent to avoid combination of the two.

Stavudine (STV)

See Box 78-2.

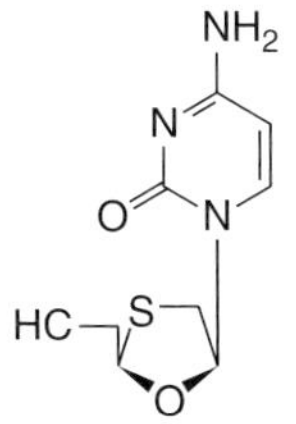

FIGURE 78-15 Molecular structure of lamivudine.

BOX 78-2

Basic Concepts of Stavudine Interactions

Stavudine is apt to cause side effects of peripheral neuropathy such as numbness, tingling, and burning or pain in the hands or feet. When co-administered with drugs that generate similar side effects, there may be an increased risk of neuropathy. Those drugs include: **carboplatin** (an anticancer drug whose high doses led to severe neuropathy in some patients); **didanosine** (an anti-HIV drug that causes peripheral neuropathy in about 15% of users); **isoniazid** (an antituberculotic drug); **paclitaxel** (an anticancer drug which is prone to produce neuropathy); **zalcitabine** (an anti-HIV drug proven to cause peripheral neuropathy); and **zidovudine** (an anti-HIV drug that can cause peripheral neuropathy with paresthesia and seizure).

Miscellaneous Interactions of Stavudine (STV)

STV ⟷ Hydroxyurea: Hydroxyurea has little or no anti-HIV activity by itself. However, by inhibition of cellular ribonucleoside reductase, it opposes the formation of deoxynucleoside triphosphate, with which stavudine (Fig. 78-16), a nucleoside analog, competes for binding to the enzyme revere transcriptase. Therefore, hydroxyurea enhances the anti-HIV effectiveness of stavudine (Zerit). Incidences of side effects of stavudine, such as fatal hepatic failure and severe neurotoxicity, were also increased when they were taken in combination.

STV ⟷ Ribavirin: Both stavudine and ribavirin can induce mitochondrial dysfunction (reduced respiratory chain enzyme activity), causing clinical symptoms such as progressive muscle weakness at the lower limbs, acute respiratory failure, and cardiac arrest that requires assisted ventilation. Concomitant use of stavudine with ribavirin may exacerbate such adverse effects.

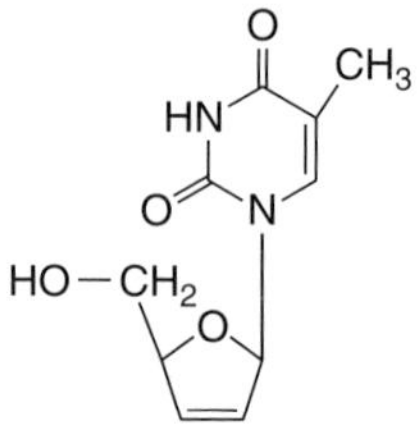

FIGURE 78-16   Molecular structure of stavudine.

Tenofovir (TFV)
Miscellaneous Interactions of Tenofovir (TFV)
TFV ⟷ CYP Isozymes: *See* Table 78-2.

TFV ⟷ Didanosine: Combined administration of tenofovir (Viread), an adenosine analog, with didanosine raises plasma levels of didanosine to improve its therapeutic efficacy and enhance its potential for toxicity. One possible mechanism responsible for the increase in didanosine concentrations is competition for active secretion through hOAT1, located at the basolateral membrane of the renal proximal tubules. Another possibility is that tenofovir inhibits the enzyme PNP, which is involved in the degradation of didanosine. Regardless, to avoid this interaction, administer tenofovir two hours before or one hour after didanosine.

TFV ⟷ Indinavir: Tenofovir is extensively excreted renally by means of glomerular filtration and active tubular secretion; whereas indinavir, another anti-HIV drug, is known to cause nephrolithiasis (kidney stone)-induced acute renal failure. Co-administration may result in increased serum levels of tenofovir.

BOX 78-3

Basic Concepts of Tenofovir Interactions

Tenofovir is not metabolized via any hepatic CYP enzyme but is eliminated via glomerular filtration and tubular secretion, mostly as unaltered drug. Hence, co-administration with a drug that reduces renal function or competes for tubular secretion may increase tenofovir's serum levels and incite its toxicity. Those drugs include: **adefovir** (a dug approved to treat chronic hepatitis-B that may compete with tenofovir for elimination through the kidney); **ganciclovir** (a drug that may compete with tenofovir for renal clearance); and **lopinavir/ritonavir** (a combined preparation shown to slow the renal clearance of tenofovir.)

TABLE 78-2 Tenofovir vs CYP Enzymes

Drug Name	1A2	2A6	2B6	2C8	2C9	2C18	2C19	2D6	2E1	3A4
Tenofovir	Inh									

Abbreviations: Sub, substrate of the enzyme; Inh, inhibits the enzyme; Ezi, induces the enzyme
Tenofovir is unusual in that it has a weak inhibitory effect on CYP1A2. Therefore, administration in combination with other drugs that require this enzyme for hepatic clearance may raise their blood levels and possibly incite their adverse effects.

Zidovudine

See Box 78-4.

Miscellaneous Interactions of Zidovudine (ZDV)

ZDV ⟷ Acetaminophen: The major metabolic pathway for both zidovudine and acetaminophen is by glucuronidation. Taken in combination, zidovudine appears to hinder elimination of acetaminophen by that process and let it be oxidized to generate its hepatotoxic free radical, called N-acetyl benzoquinoneimine. Caution is advised when the two are administered together.

BOX 78-4

Basic Concepts of Zidovudine Interactions

Zidovudine is apt to cause bone marrow depression as evidenced by neutropenia and agranulocytosis, and hence when it is co-administered with other drugs that also generate bone marrow suppression they may pull together toward life-threatening hematologic toxicities, requiring frequent monitoring of blood cell counts. Those drugs include **Azathioprine** [immunosuppressant, *See* miscellaneous interactions of Zidovudine]; **Chloramphenicol** [antibiotic]; **Dapsone** [this anti-leprosy drug may cause methemoglobinemia, and bone marrow suppression]; **doxorubicin** [anticancer drug that causes both cardiomyopathy and bone marrow depression]; **Etoposide** [anticancer drug]; **Fluorouracil** [anticancer drug]; **Ganciclovir** [a drug used to treat the symptoms of cytomegalovirus (CMV) infection of the eyes; Ganciclovir at concentrations of approximately 0.6 mg/L is known to be toxic to the human bone marrow]; **Interferon-Alfa** [Interferon-alfa may interfere with the growth of cancer cells and may be effective in leukemia, but it may cause bone marrow suppression]; **Methotrexate** [anticancer drug]; **Mitoxantrone** [anticancer drug]; **Topotecan** [anticancer drug]; and **Vinblastine** [anticancer drug]; and majority of classic **Anticancer Drugs** (*refer* to Ω-13 in the Appendix A).

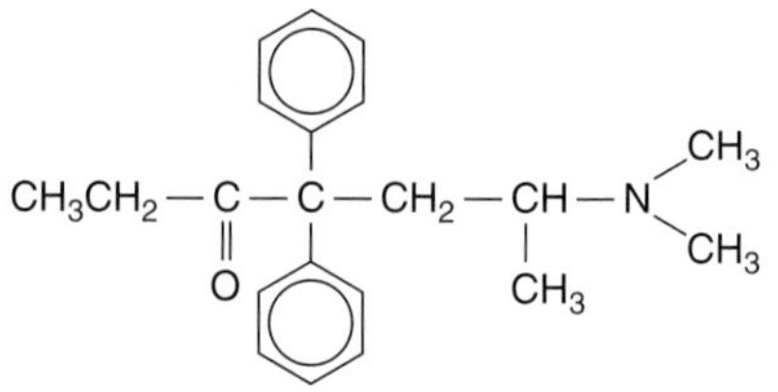

FIGURE 78-17   Molecular structure of methadone.

ZDV ⟷ Atovaquone: The major metabolic pathway for zidovudine is by glucuronidation, a process that atovaquone (Mepron), a drug with a broad-spectrum antiprotozoal activity, inhibits. Therefore, use of the two in conjunction can increase serum levels of zidovudine to incite its toxicity.

ZDV ⟷ Azathioprine: Zidovudine and mercaptopurine, to which azathioprine converts, have been associated with hematologic toxicities such as neutropenia and agranulocytosis. Therefore, concurrent use may amplify these hematologic toxicities.

ZDV ⟷ Methadone: Concurrent use of zidovudine and methadone (Fig. 78-17), a synthetic narcotic analgesic drug, can increase the blood levels of zidovudine (AZT) by about 40 % over the control value. The mechanism behind this observation remains obscure, even though methadone appears to interfere with the glucuronidation of zidovudine, its major metabolic pathway.

ZDV ⟷ Probenecid: Concomitant use of zidovudine with probenecid increases blood levels of zidovudine, prompting to generate its adverse effects. Probenecid, an acidic compound, appears to reduce excretion of zidovudine glucuronide, probably by competition for renal tubular secretion.

ZDV ⟷ Stavudine: Zidovudine may undercut the therapeutic efficacy of stavudine, probably by inhibiting the phosphorylation of stavudine, a process required for this drug's activation.

NON-NUCLEOSIDE RT INHIBITORS

Delavirdine, efavirenz, and nevirapine

MECHANISM OF ACTION

Unlike nucleoside RT inhibitors, these non-nucleoside reverse transcriptase (NNRT) inhibitors (Fig. 78-18) do not need phosphorylation before binding to

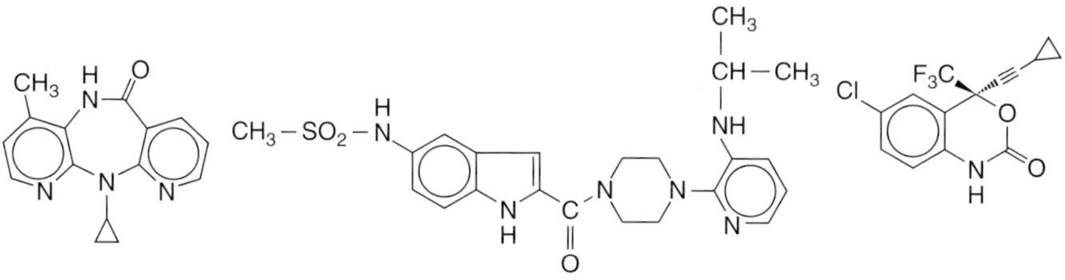

FIGURE 78-18 Molecular structures of delavirdine, efavirenz, and nevirapine.

and inhibiting the RT, for they can directly disrupt the catalytic site of the RT enzyme, and block activity of both the RNA-dependent and DNA-dependent DNA polymerases. Thus, there is no competition or cross-resistance between these two different classes of drugs.

SIDE EFFECTS

Delavirdine: Its side effects may include nausea, vomiting, and diarrhea; skin rash; fatigue, dizziness, and headache; and rarely, teratogenicity.

Efavirenz: Its side effects may include jaundice; redistribution of body fats (increased fat in the upper back and stomach areas, with decreased fat in the arms and legs); skin rash; dizziness, and rarely, teratogenicity.

Nevirapine: Its side effects may include liver damage (regular blood tests may be needed); muscle and/or joint aches; redistribution of body fats (increased fat in the upper back and stomach areas, with decreased fat in the arms and legs); tingling or numb hands or feet; pink eye (conjunctivitis); There is no known risk of teratogenicity with this drug.

DRUG INTERACTIONS
Delavirdine

See Box 78-5.

Miscellaneous Interactions of Delavirdine (DVD)

DVD ↔ CYP Isozymes: *See* Table 78-3.

BOX 78-5

Basic Concepts of Delavirdine Interactions

Delavirdine is poorly soluble at a pH greater than 3. Therefore, co-administration with drugs that increase the gastric pH can decrease absorption of delavirdine and undercut its antiretroviral effectiveness. Those drug include: **aluminum hydroxide; calcium carbonate; H2 blockers** (*See* Ω-45 in Appendix A); and **proton pump inhibitors** (*See* Ω-61 in Appendix A).

TABLE 78-3   NNRT Inhibitors vs CYP Enzymes

Drug Name	1A2	2A6	2B6	2C8	2C9	2C18	2C19	2D6	2E1	3A4
Delavirdine	Inh				Inh		Inh	Inh		Sub+ Inh
Efavirenz			Sub+ Inh		Inh		Inh	Sub		Sub
Nevirapine	Inh		Sub+ Ezi							Sub

1. Delavirdine is metabolized by the microsomal enzyme CYP3A4. Therefore, inhibition of this enzyme by other drugs may raise blood levels of delavirdine and possibly exacerbate its adverse effects. (*See* the left-hand column of Table-0 at the 'Introduction' for possible inhibitors of this enzyme.)
2. Delavirdine is an inhibitor of several microsomal cytochrome enzymes such as CYP1A2, 2C9, 2C19, 2D6 and 3A4. Therefore, co-administration with drugs that require these enzymes for hepatic clearance may raise their blood levels to incite their adverse effects. (*See* the middle column of Table-0 at the 'Introduction' for possible substrates of these enzymes.)
3. Efavirenz may inhibit hepatic enzymes CYP2B6, 2C9, and 2C19. Therefore, co-administration with drugs that require these enzymes for hepatic clearance may raise their blood levels to incite their adverse effects. (*See* the middle column of Table-0 at the 'Introduction' for possible substrates of these enzymes.)
4. Nevirapine inhibits hepatic enzyme CYP1A2. Therefore, co-administration with drugs that require this enzyme for hepatic clearance may raise their blood levels to possibly incite their adverse effects. (*See* the middle column of Table-0 at the 'Introduction' for possible substrates of this enzyme.)
5. Nevirapine is unusual in that it can induce CYP2B6. Therefore, co-administration with drugs requiring this enzyme for metabolic clearance may quicken their elimination, resulting in lowered blood levels and therapeutic insufficiency. (*See* the middle column of Table-0 at the 'Introduction' for possible substrates of this enzyme.)

DVD ⟷ Fosamprenavir: Fosamprenavir (Fig. 78-19) is an inactive prodrug that is rapidly and almost completely hydrolyzed by cellular phosphatases in the gut epithelium to amprenavir (Fig. 78-20), an active inhibitor of HIV protease. Delavirdine should not be coadministered with fosamprenavir, as it may impair the

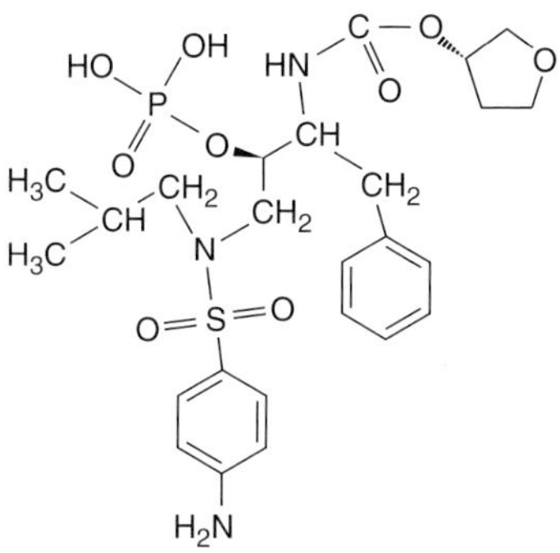

FIGURE 78-19 Molecular structure of fosamprenavir.

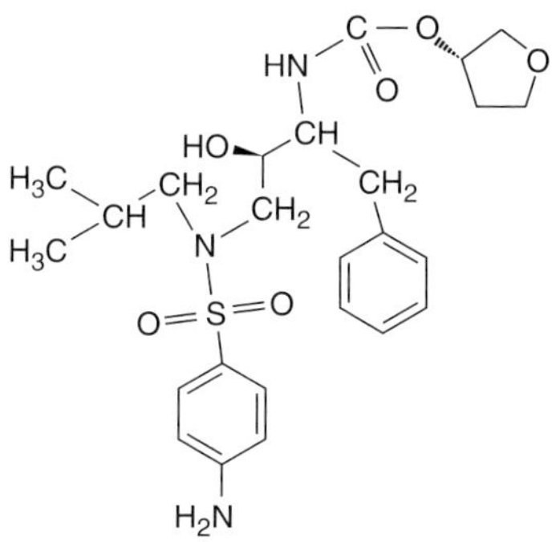

FIGURE 78-20 Molecular structure of amprenavir.

bioavailability of delavirdine by 60%, undercutting its virological response rate. The mechanism of interaction between the two is not well elucidated, but it is suspected that fosamprenavir, during its conversion to amprenavir in the gut, may hinder intestinal absorption of delavirdine.

Efavirenz

See Table 78-3.

Nevirapine

See Table 78-3.

PROTEASE INHIBITORS

Amprenavir, atazanavir, fosamprenavir, indinavir, lopinavir (which is usually used in combination with ritonavir), **nelfinavir, ritonavir, saquinavir,** and **tipranavir** (Fig. 78-21)

MECHANISM OF ACTION

For replication and maturation of HIV, the HIV enzyme proteases have to cut nonfunctional gag-pol polyproteins and gag polyproteins, both encoded by the HIV, into functional viral proteins. Protease inhibitors bind to the sites of polyproteins where the proteases normally work to cut, and by so doing prevent the enzyme from manufacturing the functional viral proteins required for viral replication and maturation.

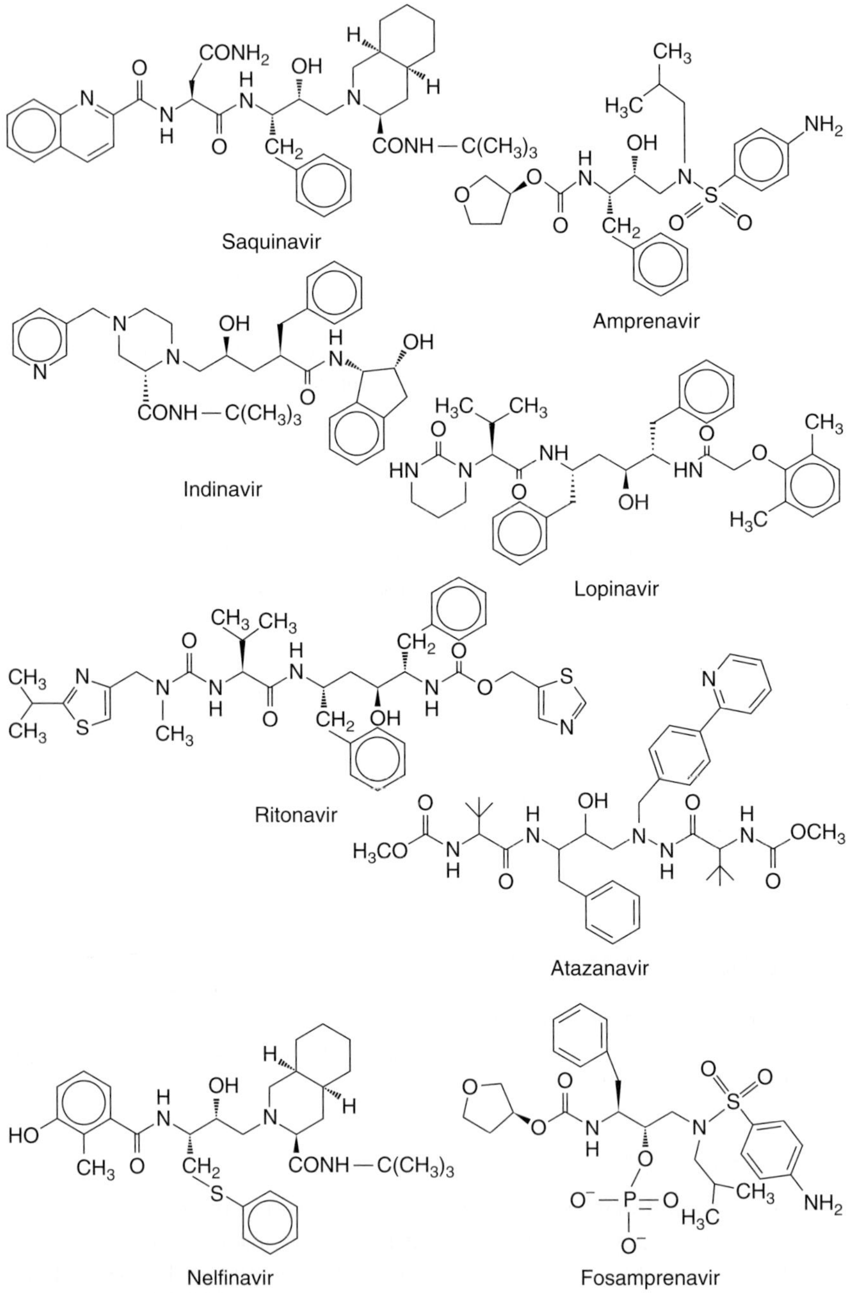

FIGURE 78-21   Molecular structures of protease inhibitors.

SIDE EFFECTS

Amprenavir: Its side effects may include nausea, vomiting, diarrhea, and stomach pain; unusual increase in urination or thirst; tingling or numbness; and rarely, skin rash.

Atazanavir: Its side effects may include unusual bleeding or bruising; jaundice; nausea, increased urination or thirst; fatigue; fever; and trouble sleeping and headache.

Fosamprenavir: Its side effects may include stomach and/or abdominal pain; skin rash; and fatigue and headache.

Indinavir: Its side effects may include cough; altered sense of taste, nausea, vomiting, stomach pain; weakness; blurred vision; and insomnia.

Lopinavir: (Kaletra [**Lopinavir + Ritonavir**]) The frequent side effects of this combined preparation include stomach pain, nausea, vomiting, and diarrhea; joint or muscle pain and weakness; skin rash; blurred vision; insomnia; and headache.

Nelfinavir: Its side effects may include stomach pain; increased urination or thirst; jaundice; blurred vision; fatigue; and dizziness.

Ritonavir: Its side effects may include altered taste, and stomach pain; numbness or tingling of mouth, hands or feet, muscle or joint pain, and weakness; blurred vision; and dizziness, drowsiness, and headache.

Saquinavir: Its side effects may include unusual bleeding or bruising; cough; persistent sore throat, stomach pain; jaundice; muscle or joint pain, loss of coordination, and severe weakness; skin rash; fever and chills; hearing or visual difficulty; and confusion and mental depression.

Tipranavir: Its side effects may include unusual bleeding (such as a nosebleed, blood in the urine or stool, and bleeding in the brain); cough; dark urine and clay-colored stools; jaundice and liver damage; blistering, peeling, or sunburn; fever or chills; blurred vision; and allergic reactions such as skin hives and difficulty in breathing.

DRUG INTERACTIONS

(*See* Appendix B-9: Interactions of Protease Inhibitors.) Lopinavir often comes in combination with ritonavir. The otherwise quick inactivation of lopinavir through

CYP3A4 can be thwarted by ritonavir, which is inhibitory to this enzyme. Hence, this interaction establishes increased anti-HIV activity of lopinavir. Also notable is that inducers of the enzyme, such as rifampin, may quicken inactivation of lopinavir and possibly result in lowered blood levels and insufficient therapeutic effectiveness of this drug. (*See* the right-hand column of Table-0 at the 'Introduction' for other possible inducers of the enzyme.)

ENFUVIRTIDE

This is a new class of polypeptide anti-HIV drug.

MECHANISM OF ACTION

At the start of the HIV invasion into host body cells, HIV has to bind to a cell receptor at the outside surface of a host CD4⁺ T-cell (a type of T-lymphocyte) via gp41-gp120 complex, a viral transmembrane protein, creating an entry pore to fuse with the host cell, before beginning HIV multiplication. Enfuvirtide binds to gp41 and prevents fusion between the host cell membrane and the viral membrane, to prevent uninfected host cells from becoming infected.

SIDE EFFECTS

Possible side effects of enfuvirtide include skin itchiness and swelling at the site of injection. Other side effects may include numbness in the feet or legs; fatigue; and dizziness and insomnia.

DRUG INTERACTIONS

This drug undergoes catabolism to its constituent amino acids, which subsequently recycle in the body. There has been no clinically important interaction reported.

79

Systemic Infections by Bacteria

Medications shown effective in the treatment of various bacterial infections include: (1) penicillin antibiotics such as **amoxicillin** (Amoxil, Trimox), Augmentin XR **(amoxicillin + potassium clavulanate),** and **penicillin-V;** (2) cephalosporin antibiotics such as **cefdinir** (Omnicef), **cefprozil** (Cefzil), **cefuroxime,** and **cephalexin.** (3) tetracycline antibiotics such as **doxycycline, minocycline,** and **tetracycline;** (4) fluoroquinolone antibiotics such as **ciprofloxacin, norfloxacin, ofloxacin,** and **pefloxacin;** (5) macrolide antibiotics such as **azithromycin** (Zithromax), **clarithromycin** (Biaxin), and **telithromycin** (Ketek); (6) **clindamycin;** (7) a combination of **sulfamethoxazole** with **trimethoprim** (Cotrimoxazole or Septrim); (8) **mupirocin** (Bactroban); (9) **nitrofurantoin;** and (10) **ethambutol, isoniazid,** or **rifampin** or a combination thereof.

PENICILLINS

Amoxicillin and **penicillin-V**

Augmentin XR represents amoxicillin plus potassium clavulanate. All penicillins are beta-lactam antibiotics (*See* Fig. 75-1), and were the first antibiotics discovered and found valuable in the treatment of staphylococcus infections and serious diseases such as syphilis. Many staphylococci became gradually resistant to penicillin, although they are still widely used in treatment of infections of most streptococci such as *Streptococcus pneumoniae,* and *Streptococcus pyogenes,* and by *Neisseria* such as *N. meningitidis.*

MECHANISM OF ACTION

See Chapter 12.

SIDE EFFECTS

See Chapter 12.

DRUG INTERACTIONS

See Appendix B-24: Interactions of Penicillins.

CEPHALOSPORINS

Cefdinir, cefprozil, cefuroxime, and **cephalexin** (Keflex)

All the cephalosporins have a broad-spectrum antibiotic effect (both Gram-positive and Gram-negative), especially against *Klebsiella,* where they are usually the drug of choice. However, some bacteria became resistant to this group of antibiotics, such as methicillin-resistant *Staphylococcus aureus* and *Streptococcus faecalis.*

MECHANISM OF ACTION

Their mechanism of action is identical to that of penicillin antibiotics. *See* Chapter 12.

SIDE EFFECTS

Possible side effects of cephalosporin antibiotics include bloody diarrhea, and stomach pain; nephrotoxicity (probably except ceftriaxone); headache, dizziness, and convulsions; and allergic reactions such as skin hives; difficulty in breathing; and swelling of the face, lips, tongue, or throat.

DRUG INTERACTIONS

See Appendix B-17: Interactions of Cephalosporins.

TETRACYCLINES

Doxycycline, minocycline, and **tetracycline**

Tetracyclines are broad-spectrum antibiotics effective against many gram-negative bacteria, and some Gram-positive bacteria such as streptococci (except *Streptococcus faecalis*). Tetracyclines are the drugs of choice for infections caused by *Brucella abortus, Shigella dysenteriae, Mycoplasma pneumoniae, Vibrio cholerae,* the *Chlamydia* species, and the *Rickettsia* species. However, they are not effective against *Bacteroides fragilis, Streptococcus faecalis, Pseudomonas aeruginosa,* and indole-positive Proteus such as *Proteus vulgaris,* nor against many staphylococci.

MECHANISM OF ACTION

See Chapter 17.

SIDE EFFECTS

See Chapter 17.

DRUG INTERACTIONS

See Appendix B-30: Interactions of Tetracyclines.

FLUOROQUINOLONE ANTIBIOTICS

Ciprofloxacin, norfloxacin, ofloxacin, and **pefloxacin**

Fluorinated quinolones are often used in the treatment of bone, joint, genital, gastrointestinal, and respiratory tract infections. Ciprofloxacin and ofloxacin were the most widely used because they had the greatest potency. Ciprofloxacin is active against many aerobic Gram-negative bacteria, and some Gram-positive bacteria such as staphylococci (though *Staphylococcus aureus* may be resistant) and some streptococci.

MECHANISM OF ACTION

They generate their antibacterial effect by inhibition of DNA gyrase, an essential bacterial enzyme that catalyzes the ATP-dependent introduction of negative supercoiling of double-stranded bacterial DNA, which is required for DNA replication.

SIDE EFFECTS

Possible side effects of fluorinated quinolones include diarrhea; jaundice (yellowing of the skin or eyes); seizures (convulsions); and allergic reactions such as skin hives and swelling of tissues.

DRUG INTERACTIONS

See Appendix B-28: Interactions of Quinolone Antibiotics.

MACROLIDE ANTIBIOTICS

Azithromycin, clarithromycin, and **telithromycin**

Macrolide antibiotics are often used to treat infections of the respiratory tract caused by susceptible bacteria, including staphylococci, streptococci, pneumococci, and enterococci. Their antibacterial spectrum extends to *Mycoplasma,* some *Rickettsia,* and some *Chlamydia,* for which penicillins do not work. Therefore, macrolides are a common substitute for patients with a penicillin allergy

MECHANISM OF ACTION

They bind to the 50s subunit of the bacterial 70s ribosome to inhibit bacterial protein synthesis. The binding blocks translocation of aminoacyl transfer ribonucleic acid (tRNA) from the A site to the P site. As the A site remains occupied, no new amino acid carried by another tRNA can attach to keep feeding on the growing end of the peptide chain.

SIDE EFFECTS

Azithromycin: Its possible side effects include uneven heartbeats; stomach pain, and bloody diarrhea; dizziness, tiredness, and headache; and rarely, allergic reactions such as skin hives.

Clarithromycin: Its possible side effects include irregular heartbeats; stomach upset, pseudomembranous colitis, and diarrhea (avoid using antidiarrheal agents or narcotic drugs, as these products may worsen symptoms); dark urine; jaundice; and headache. Upon prolonged use, oral or vaginal infections by fungi may result.

Telithromycin: This drug may cause strange taste in the mouth; dark urine; jaundice; visual disturbances (blurred vision, double vision, and difficulty in focusing); and dizziness. Rarely, this medication may cause a severe intestinal condition (pseudomembranous colitis) due to resistant bacteria.

DRUG INTERACTIONS

Azithromycin: *See* Appendix B-13: Interactions of Macrolide Antibiotics.

Clarithromycin: *See* Appendix B-13: Interactions of Macrolide Antibiotics.

Telithromycin: *See* Appendix B-13: Interactions of Macrolide Antibiotics.

CLINDAMYCIN

Clindamycin (Fig. 79-1) is used as a drug of choice in the treatment of infections either by Gram-negative anaerobic bacteria such as *Bacteroides fragilis* and *Fusobacterium varium* or by Gram-positive anaerobic bacteria such as *Propionibacterium acnes*. This drug has virtually no significant activity against most other Gram-negative bacteria.

MECHANISM OF ACTION

Clindamycin inhibits bacterial protein synthesis by binding to the 50S subunit of bacterial ribosome, probably inhibiting peptidyl transferase.

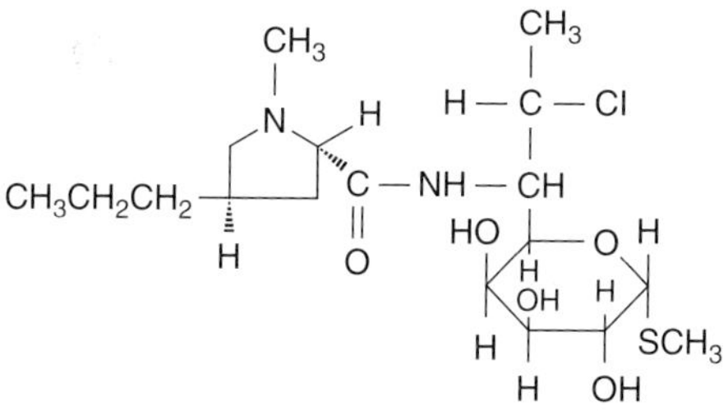

FIGURE 79-1 Molecular structure of clindamycin.

SIDE EFFECTS

Its possible side effect include upset stomach, mild persistent diarrhea, and blood and/or mucus in stool probably with pseudomembranous colitis; renal dysfunction; joint pain with swelling and loss of muscle tone; and jaundice; peeling, burning, or redness of the skin. Rarely, it may cause allergic reactions such as swelling of tissues. Upon prolonged use, it may cause oral or vaginal infections by fungi.

DRUG INTERACTIONS

See Box 79-1.

Miscellaneous Interactions of Clindamycin (CLM)

If applied topically there is no known interaction reported for clindamycin. But if taken orally or absorbed extensively from the skin, clindamycin may interact as in the following list.

CLM ⟷ Aminoglycoside Antibiotics: (*See* Ω-7 in Appendix A.) Most aminoglycoside antibiotics possess reversible nephrotoxicity, whereas clindamycin has no direct relationship to renal damage, but can induce renal dysfunctions such as oliguria and proteinuria. Rarely, combined use of clindamycin and an aminoglycoside antibiotic may cause acute renal failure. Careful monitoring of renal function is recommended.

CLM ⟷ Erythromycin: Both clindamycin and erythromycin appear to compete for the same ribosomal binding site to exert their antibacterial action. Thus, the bactericidal effect of clindamycin can be compromised by the bacteriostatic effect of erythromycin.

BOX 79-1

Basic Concepts of Clindamycin Interactions

If pseudomembranous colitis, which is characterized by abdominal pain, fever, and diarrhea that can induce dehydration, develops due to administration of clindamycin, do not use any drugs to correct the diarrhea, because it serves as a means of purging the toxin from the colon. Otherwise, it may make the intestinal condition worse. Those drugs to avoid in this circumstance include: **antidiarrheal drugs** (*See* Ω-17 in Appendix A) and **narcotic analgesics** (*See* Ω-52 in Appendix A).

CLM ⟷ Neuromuscular Blockers: (*See* Ω-53 in Appendix A.) Clindamycin is not a neuromuscular blocker, but it can cause muscle relaxation by a direct action on the muscle contractility. Its use in combination with authentic neuromuscular blockers has been shown to enhance the actions of such agents. Therefore, it should be used with caution in patients receiving a neuromuscular blocker.

SULFAMETHOXAZOLE PLUS TRIMETHOPRIM

This combination potentiates chemotherapeutic effectiveness and reduces development of drug-resistant bacteria. This preparation may be considered in the treatment of urinary tract infections by susceptible organisms such as *E. Coli*, *Klebsiella* species, *Enterobacter* species, *Proteus mirabilis*, and *Proteus vulgaris*; and in the treatment of *Pneumocystis Carinii* pneumonia.

MECHANISM OF ACTION

Sulfamethoxazole is a sulfonamide that works by interfering with incorporation of para-aminobenzoic acid (PABA) (Fig. 79-2) into dihydrofolate, the precursor from which tetrahydrofolate is formed (*See* Fig. 8-1). **Trimethoprim** (*See* Fig. 35-2),

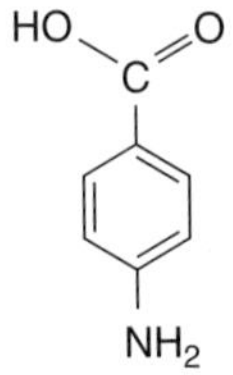

FIGURE 79-2   Molecular structure of PABA.

on the other hand, is a non-sulfonamide drug that works by inhibition of dihydro-folate reductase, the enzyme that catalyzes conversion of dihydrofolate to tetra-hydrofolate. As no tetrahydrofolate is formed by this two drug combination, the germs cannot synthesize thymine, an essential base required for the synthesis of bacterial DNA. Without DNA, there can be no proliferation of the bacteria.

SIDE EFFECTS

Sulfamethoxazole: This drug may cause diarrhea; headache, fatigue, and dizzi-ness; and allergic reactions such as skin hives; difficulty in breathing; and swelling of the face, lips, tongue, or throat.

Trimethoprim: This drug may cause irregular heartbeat; stomach upset, and diarrhea; decreased urination (nephrotoxicity); chills, fever, or sore throat; seizures; and allergic reactions such as skin hives and swelling of tissues.

DRUG INTERACTIONS

Sulfamethoxazole: *See* Chapter 35.

Trimethoprim: *See* Chapter 35.

MUPIROCIN

Mupirocin is bacteriostatic at low concentrations and bactericidal at high concen-trations. It is used topically to treat impetigo, furuncle, and other open wounds by Gram-positive germs including methicillin-resistant *Staphylococcus aureus* (MRSA), which is a significant cause of death in hospitalized patients.

MECHANISM OF ACTION

Mupirocin (Fig. 79-3) selectively but reversibly binds to bacterial isoleucyl-tRNA synthetase to prevent incorporation of isoleucine into bacterial proteins. The lack

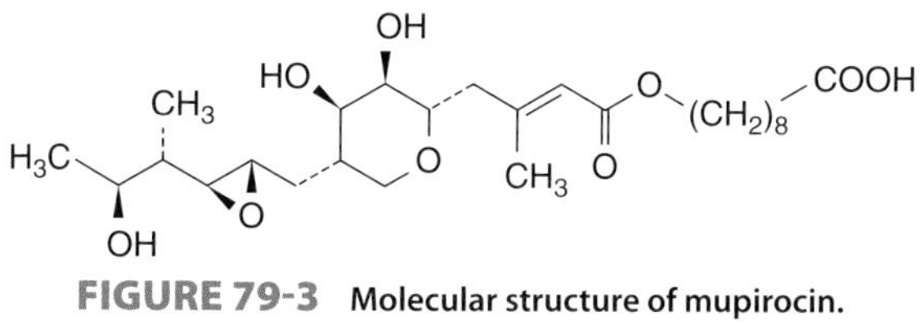

FIGURE 79-3   Molecular structure of mupirocin.

of one amino acid isoleucine inhibits synthesis of bacterial protein and bacterial RNA. Because of this unique mechanism of action, there is little likelihood that bacteria will become resistant to mupirocin.

SIDE EFFECTS
When applied topically it may cause blistering, itching, and irritation of the skin.

DRUG INTERACTIONS
It is not known whether other medications will interact with this medication applied topically.

NITROFURANTOIN
It has a broad spectrum antibacterial effect in acidic urine (pH below 6). It is usually used in treating urinary tract infections caused by *E. Coli*.

MECHANISM OF ACTION
Nitrofurantoin (Fig. 79-4) is reduced inside the bacterial cell by flavoproteins to many reactive intermediates that damage bacterial enzymes and DNA.

SIDE EFFECTS
Its side effects may include cough; stomach upset, nausea, and diarrhea; yellowish brown urine color (this is not a cause for concern and will disappear when the drug is terminated); muscle aches; tingling of the hands or feet; jaundice; fever and chills; and dizziness and headache.

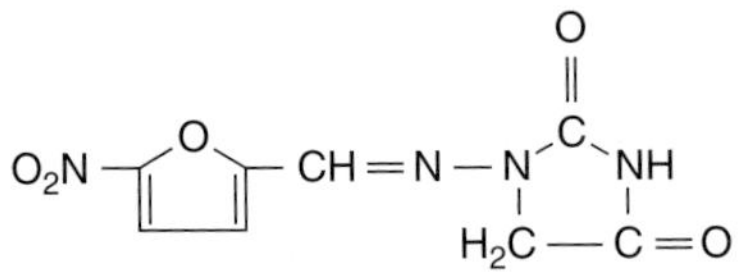

FIGURE 79-4   Molecular structure of nitrofurantoin.

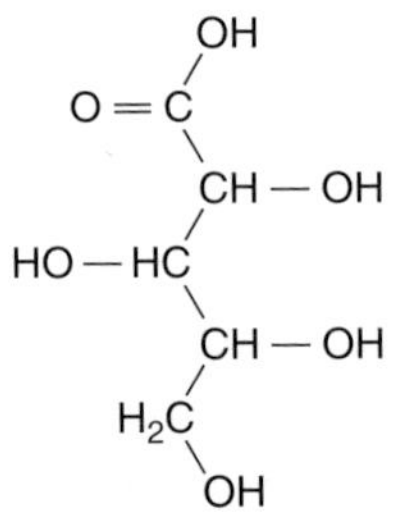

FIGURE 79-5   Molecular structure of arabinose.

DRUG INTERACTIONS

See Chapter 35.

ETHAMBUTOL, ISONIAZID, OR RIFAMPIN

Medications shown effective in the treatment of tuberculosis include: **ethambutol, isoniazid,** and **rifampin.** They are taken orally or by injection. Often two or more drugs are taken in combination to prevent development of bacterial resistance.

MECHANISM OF ACTION

Ethambutol: This drug usually has a bacteriostatic effect against *Mycobacterium tuberculosis.* It is used in combination with other antituberculotic agents, such as isoniazid and rifampicin. The unique cell wall of *Mycobacterium tuberculosis* consists of arabinogalactan, to which mycolic acid is attached. Mycolic acid attaches to the 5'-hydroxyl group of D-arabinose of arabinogalactan. Ethambutol (Fig. 79-6) appears to inhibit arabinosyl transferase, an enzyme that is involved in the production of arabinogalactan, and therefore appears to work by obstructing the formation of the bacterial cell wall.

Isoniazid: This drug has a tuberculocidal effect against actively growing *Mycobacterium tuberculosis.* However, isoniazid **(**Fig. 79-7) is a prodrug that must be activated by bacterial enzyme catalase and peroxidase to form an isonicotinic acyl anion, which then reacts with NADH to make an isonicotinic acyl-NADH complex that binds to the enoyl-acyl carrier protein reductase, thereby blocking the action of fatty acid synthase, and this binding prevents access of the natural substrates required for the synthesis of mycolic acid, an important component of the mycobacterial cell wall.

Rifampin: Rifampin binds to and inhibits DNA-directed RNA polymerase to oppose production of RNA of the tuberculotic bacteria.

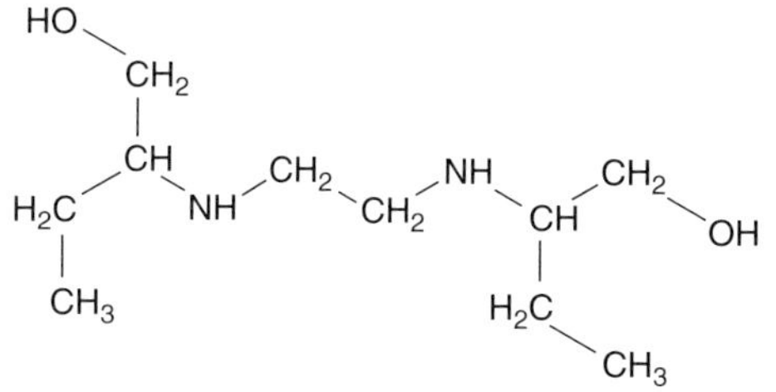

FIGURE 79-6 Molecular structure of ethambutol.

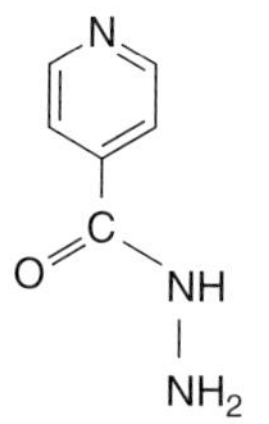

FIGURE 79-7 Molecular structure of isoniazid.

SIDE EFFECTS

Ethambutol: It may cause optic neuritis to impair visual acuity and loss of green color perception. Ethambutol is not recommended in children too young to monitor visual changes. It may also cause pain and swelling of joints; and headache and mental confusion. Unlike most other antituberculotic drugs, ethambutol it does not cause hepatotoxicity.

Isoniazid: Its side effects may include dyspnea; hemolytic anemia and thrombocytopenia; hepatitis; gynecomastia; peripheral neuropathy with pyridoxine deficiency; dizziness and seizure; and rarely, allergic reactions.

Rifampin: Its side effects may include heartburn, flatulence, epigastric distress, anorexia; jaundice (hepatotoxicity); ataxia, fatigue, and muscle pain; bone pain; thrombocytopenia; and skin rash (hives). Rifampin may turn urine dark yellow to orange-red, but this does not indicate medical emergency.

DRUG INTERACTIONS

Ethambutol: Its intestinal absorption is impaired by co-administration of aluminum hydroxide, an antacid; attapulgite (aluminum magnesium silicate), an antidiarrheal agent; or by co-administration of magaldrate (aluminum magnesium hydroxide hydrate), a drug used to treat peptic ulcers. Separate their administrations by a minimum of several hours.

Isoniazid: *See* Box 79-2.

Miscellaneous Interactions of Isoniazid (INZ)

INZ ⟷ Carbamazepine: Metabolic clearance of carbamazepine, an antiepileptic drug, via CYP3A4 is likely interrupted by concurrent administration of isoniazid, an inhibitor of the said enzyme. This results in elevated blood levels of carbamazepine, potentially inciting its adverse effects.

INZ ⟷ CYP Isozymes: *See* Table 79-1.

INZ ⟷ Dicumarol: Isoniazid used in combination with dicumarol tends to enhance the anticoagulant effects of dicumarol, increasing the incidence of bleeding. The mechanism behind this observation remains unclear.

INZ ⟷ Disulfiram: Disulfiram (Antabuse), a drug to treat chronic alcoholism, can generate peripheral neuropathies such as ataxia and muscular incoordination and, at high doses, psychotic reactions. Co-administration of isoniazid, an inhibitor of CYP3A4, with disulfiram, a substrate of CYP3A4, may lead to the

TABLE 80-1 Azole Antifungal Drugs vs CYP Enzymes

Drug Name	1A2	2A6	2B6	2C8	2C9	2C18	2C19	2D6	2E1	3A4
Fluconazole	Inh				Inh		Inh			Inh
Ketoconazole	Inh				Inh		Inh			Sub+ Inh
Voriconazole					Inh		Sub+ Inh			Sub+ Inh

1. Ketoconazole is processed through CYP3A4 for clearance, and inhibition of this enzyme by any other drug taken in combination may raise blood levels of ketoconazole and incite its adverse effects. (*See* the left-hand column of Table-0 at the 'Introduction' for possible inhibitors of the enzyme.)
2. Voriconazole, like the other azole antifungal drugs discussed, inhibits CYP2C9, 2C19 and 3A4. Therefore, co-administration with other drugs that require these enzymes for their metabolic clearance may result in their elevated blood levels, possibly exacerbating their adverse effects. (*See* the middle column of Table-0 at the 'Introduction' for possible substrates of these enzymes.)

CASPOFUNGIN OR MICAFUNGIN

These drugs are used by intravenous injection, and they exert excellent antifungal activity against a broad range of Candida species, including azole-resistant strain. Caspofungin is also used to treat invasive aspergillosis (Fig. 80-5) in patients resistant to other antifungal agents, such as amphotericin-B and itraconazole.

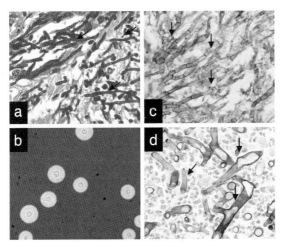

FIGURE 80-5 **Candida vs cryptococcus vs aspergillus.** Reproduced, with permission, from Chisholm-Burns MA, Wells BG, Schwinghammer TL, Malone PM, Kolesar JM, Rotschafer JC, and DiPiro JT, eds. *Pharmacotherapy: Principles & Practice.* New York, NY: McGraw-Hill; 2008, p 1219.

MECHANISM OF ACTION

The major essential components of fungal cell walls, not present in the mammalian cell wall, are 1,3-beta-D-glucan and mannan. These drugs inhibit 1,3-beta-D-glucan synthase, the enzyme essential for the synthesis of 1,3-beta-D-glucan, accounting for their fungicidal effect.

SIDE EFFECTS

Caspofungin: Its possible side effects include flushing of skin; abdominal pain, and diarrhea; liver damage (rare); numbness of the limbs and muscle ache; fever and chills; and headache.

Micafungin: This drug may cause acute renal failure; and may release histamine to cause side effects such as skin rash, itching, and vasodilation that leads to facial swelling. It may cause thrombophlebitis at the injection site.

DRUG INTERACTIONS

See Box 80-1.

BOX 80-1

Basic Concepts of Caspofungin Interactions

1. Caspofungin (Fig. 80-6), after intravenous injection, is spontaneously metabolized mainly by peptide hydrolysis and N-acetylation, letting only a minute amount (less than 2%) be eliminated unaltered in the urine. However, when

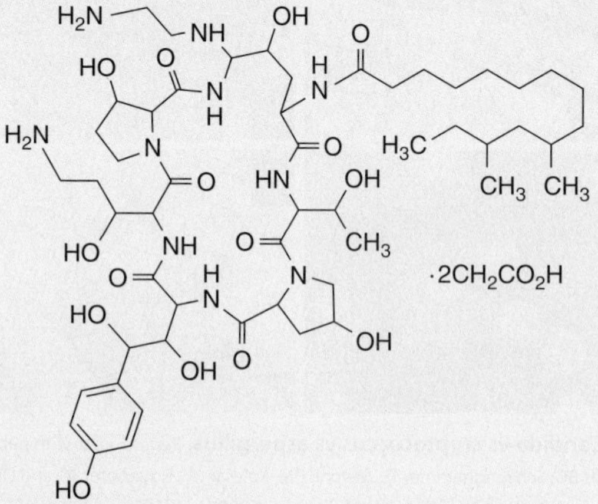

FIGURE 80-6 Molecular structure of caspofungin.

BOX 80-1 *(continued)*

caspofungin is taken with a drug that causes acute renal failure, clearance of caspofungin is decreased by 30% to 50%. An example includes: **cyclosporine** (an immunosuppressant).

2. Caspofungin is neither an inducer nor an inhibitor of hepatic microsomal CYP isozymes but is a substrate, though apparently a poor one. Therefore, co-administration with drugs known to induce CYP enzymes may quicken its hepatic clearance and lower its blood concentration and therapeutic value. Those drugs include: **dexamethasone** (a glucocorticoid); **phenytoin** (an anti-epileptic drug); and **rifampin** (an antibiotic).

Miscellaneous Interactions of Micafungin (MFG)

MFG ⟷ Itraconazole: Micafungin taken with itraconazole, another antifungal drug, may result in a slightly increased plasma concentration of itraconazole (about 10%), possibly providing an additive therapeutic effect against life-threatening, invasive aspergillosis.

MFG ⟷ Nifedipine: Micafungin used with nifedipine, a calcium channel blocker, results in a slightly increased plasma concentration of nifedipine (about 20%), to possibly exacerbate its adverse effects. The mechanism behind this observation remains uncharacterized.

MFG ⟷ Sirolimus: Micafungin used with sirolimus, an immunosuppressant, results in a slightly increased plasma concentration of sirolimus (about 22%), giving rise to greater incidence of adverse effects. The mechanism behind this observation remains unclear.

TERBINAFINE:

Topical cream or oral intake of terbinafine may be of help to treat jock itch, a tinea infection caused by several types of mold-like fungi called dermatophytes.
Terbinafine/ itraconazole combination exhibited a synergistic effect against the most of strains of Zygomycota, although lipid formulations of amphotericin-B are the treatments of choice for this life-threatening mold infections.

MECHANISM OF ACTION

Terbinafine (Fig. 80-7) inhibits the enzyme squalene epoxide involved in the synthesis of ergosterol, an essential component of the fungal cell membrane.

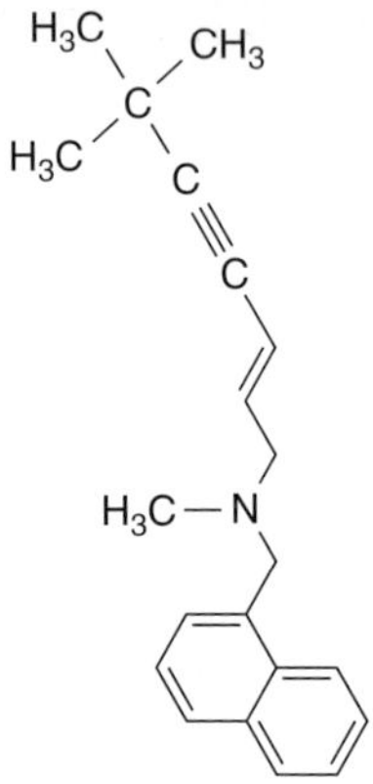

FIGURE 80-7   Molecular structure of terbinafine.

This leads to disrupted fungal membrane functions, causing death of the fungal cells.

SIDE EFFECTS

Side effects after topical application may include burning, redness or irritation for the first few days, and allergic reactions such as skin rash and itching; difficulty in breathing; and swelling of tissues.

DRUG INTERACTIONS

Terbinafine (TBF)

TABLE 80-2   Terbinafine vs CYP Enzymes

Drug Name	1A2	2A6	2B6	2C8	2C9	2C18	2C19	2D6	2E1	3A4
Terbinafine	Sub				Sub			Inh		Sub

1. Terbinafine is a strong inhibitor of CYP2D6. Therefore, co-administration with drugs that require this enzyme for hepatic clearance may raise their blood levels and possibly exacerbate their adverse effects. Examples include: desipramine and thioridazine. (*See* the middle column of Table-0 at the 'Introduction' for other possible substrates of this enzyme.)

2. Terbinafine is processed through CYP1A2, CYP2C9, and especially CYP3A4. Cimetidine inhibits all these enzymes to oppose inactivation of terbinafine, raising its blood levels and inciting its adverse effects. (*See* the left-hand column of Table-0 at the 'Introduction' for other possible inhibitors of these enzymes.) Rifampin induces all these enzymes to increase clearance of terbinafine, resulting in lowered blood levels and insufficient therapeutic effectiveness. (*See* the right-hand column of Table-0 at the 'Introduction' for other possible inducers of these enzymes.)

TBF ⟷ Cimetidine: Terbinafine is mainly cleared through CYP3A4. Its use in combination with Cimetidine, an inhibitor of CYP3A4, causes impaired metabolism of Terbinafine, raising its blood levels and inciting its adverse effects (*See* Table 80-2).

TBF ⟷ CYP Isozymes: *See* Table 80-2.

TBF ⟷ Tricyclic Antidepressants: (*See* Ω-76 in Appendix A.) By inhibition of CYP2D6, terbinafine opposes metabolic clearance of most, if not all, tricyclic antidepressants, including amitriptyline, desipramine, doxepin, and imipramine. This effect raises their blood levels to exacerbate their adverse effects. (*See* Table 80-2 and Table-0 at the 'Introduction'.)

CQN ⟷Cyclosporine: Metabolic clearance of cyclosporine heavily depends on CYP3A4, and clearance of chloroquine partially depends on this same enzyme. When used in combination they may compete for metabolic clearance, potentially resulting in impaired metabolism of cyclosporine, accounting for its elevated serum levels and greater incidences of adverse effects.

CQN ⟷ CYP Isozymes: *See* Table 81-1.

CQN ⟷ Digoxin: Digoxin is a substrate for the efflux P-glycoprotein (P-gp) transporter in the renal tubules. When digoxin is taken with another drug that inhibits

TABLE 81-1 Antimalarial Drugs vs CYP Enzymes

Drug Name	1A2	2A6	2B6	2C8	2C9	2C18	2C19	2D6	2E1	3A4
Chloroguanide							Sub			
Chloroquine				Sub				Inh		Sub
Halofantrine								Inh		Sub
Mefloquine										Sub
Primaquine	Inh									
Quinine								Inh		Sub+ Inh

Abbreviations: Sub, substrate of the enzyme; Inh, inhibits the enzyme; Ezi, induces the enzyme

1. Metabolic clearance of chloroguanide requires the presence of microsomal CYP2C19. Thus, inhibition of this enzyme by any drug taken in combination may raise blood levels of chloroguanide to possibly exacerbate its adverse effects. (*See* the left-hand column of Table-0 at the 'Introduction' for possible inhibitors of this enzyme.)
2. Chloroquine is metabolized mainly by CYP2C8 and, to a lesser extent, by CYP3A4. If chloroquine is co-administered with cimetidine, which is an inhibitor of both enzymes, the blood levels of chloroquine may rise to increase its potential for adverse effects.
3. Halofantrine, mefloquine , and quinine each require CYP3A4. Therefore, inhibition of this enzyme by any drug taken in combination may raise their blood levels and possibly exacerbate their adverse effects. (*See* the left-hand column of Table-0 at the 'Introduction' for possible inhibitors of this enzyme.)
4. Chloroquine, halofantrine, and quinine each have an inhibitory effect on CYP2D6. Therefore, administration in combination with drugs that require this enzyme for metabolic clearance may result in their elevated blood levels and incite their adverse effects. (*See* the middle column of Table-0 at the 'Introduction' for possible substrates of this enzyme.)
5. Only primaquine is an inhibitor of CYP1A2, and when used in combination with drugs that require this enzyme for clearance, it may elevate their blood levels and exacerbate their adverse effects. (*See* the middle column of Table-0 at the 'Introduction' for possible substrates of this enzyme.)
6. Only quinine is an inhibitor of CYP3A4, and when used in combination with other antimalarial drugs that require CYP3A4 for clearance, it may elevate their blood levels and incite their adverse effects. Such antimalarial drugs include: artemisinin, chloroquine, halofantrine, and mefloquine. (*See* the middle column of Table-0 at the 'Introduction' for other possible substrates of this enzyme.)

this efflux transporter, it will impair renal clearance of digoxin to elevate its serum concentrations and its cardiotoxic effects. Examples include: chloroquine.

MEFLOQUINE

Mefloquine (Fig. 81-3) is a 4-quinolinemethanol derivative, which acts as a blood schizonticidal agent active against all four species of malarial parasite (*P. falciparum, P. vivax, P. malariae,* and *P. ovale*), but is not active against their exoerythrocytic (hepatic) stages. Mefloquine is effective against malaria parasites resistant to chloroquine and other 4-aminoquinoline derivatives.

MECHANISM OF ACTION

Its exact mechanism of action is not fully characterized. Mefloquine, however, appears to inhibit hemozoin formation, and heme degradation. Further, mefloquine may form a toxic complex with free heme to damage the membranes of malarial parasites.

SIDE EFFECTS

Its side effects may include mild and rare prolongation of the Q-T interval at high doses; stomach upset, gastric pain, and diarrhea; hair loss; fever; ringing in the ears; and dizziness, headache, and lightheadedness.

DRUG INTERACTIONS

Mefloquine (MFQ)

MFQ ⟷ CYP Isozymes: *See* Table 81-1.

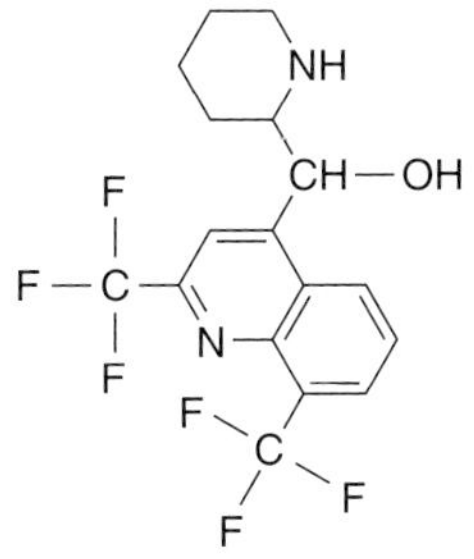

FIGURE 81-3 Molecular structure of mefloquine.

MFQ ↔ Halofantrine: The QT-elongation caused by halofantrine may be furthered by combined intake of mefloquine, which at regular doses has little such effect. Since both halofantrine and mefloquine are substrates of CYP3A4, the presence of mefloquine appears to deter, by competition, metabolic clearance of halofantrine; and the furthered Q-T elongation may cause life-threatening cardiac arrhythmias.

MFQ ↔ Metoclopramide: Metoclopramide quickens the speed of gastric emptying, and its concurrent administration with mefloquine may increase its absorption, raising blood levels of mefloquine and inciting its adverse effects.

MALARONE

Atovaquone + chloroguanide

MECHANISM OF ACTION

This combination product exerts a synergistic effects against development of the erythrocytic and exoerythrocytic stages of *Plasmodium* parasites, with little or no emergence of the resistance that occurs when atovaquone is used alone.

Atovaquone: Atovaquone (Fig. 81-4) closely resembles the chemical structure of CoQ-10 (ubiquinone) (*See* Fig. 54-3), and appears to selectively inhibit mitochondrial electron transport in sensitive parasites, such as Plasmodia and *Pneumocystis carinii*, inhibiting synthesis of ATP. However, this drug does not cause bone marrow depression, an important advantage in patients who have received bone marrow transplantation.

Chloroguanide: The prodrug chloroguanide (Proguanil) (Fig. 81-5) is converted primarily through CYP2C19 to cycloguanil (Fig. 81-6), its active metabolite, which inhibits the enzyme dihydrofolate reductase to interrupt the synthesis of thymine

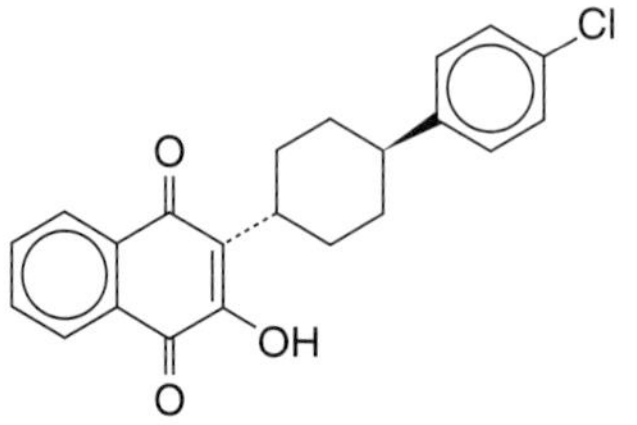

FIGURE 81-4   Molecular structure of atovaquone.

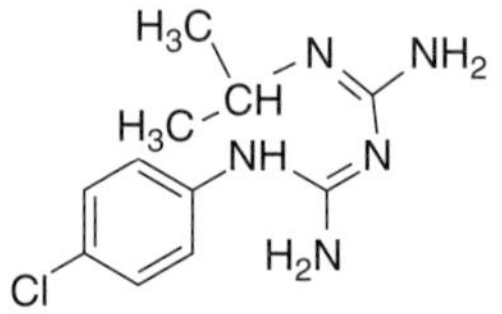

FIGURE 81-5   Molecular structure of chloroguanide.

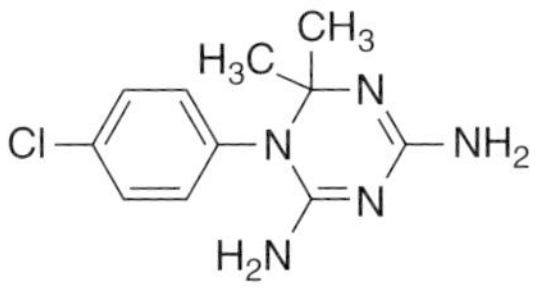

FIGURE 81-6   Molecular structure of cycloguanil.

required for the formation of deoxythymidylate, without which the synthesis of plasmodial DNA cannot be accomplished.

SIDE EFFECTS

This drug preparation appears to be extremely well tolerated with fewer side effects than other antimalarial medications. However, it may cause gastrointestinal upset and headache.

DRUG INTERACTIONS

Malarone (Atovaquone + Chloroguanide) (ACG)

ACG ⟷ CYP Isozymes: *See* Table 81-1.

ACG ⟷ Fat-Rich Foods: Foods rich in fat can enhance absorption of this medical preparation three-fold, yielding greater incidences of their adverse effects.

ACG ⟷ Rifampin: Co-administration of atovaquone with rifampicin or rifabutin was shown to reduce blood levels of atovaquone quite significantly. Therefore, induction of atovaquone's metabolism by those antibiotics is suspected but not yet confirmed.

ACG ⟷ Salicylates: (*See* Ω-64 in Appendix A.) In this preparation, atovaquone is extensively bound to blood proteins but can be displaced by other drugs that also bind extensively with higher affinity, such as salicylates. Therefore, such combination entails higher free drug concentrations of atovaquone with greater adverse effects.

ACG ⟷ Zidovudine: Atovaquone was shown to raise plasma concentrations of zidovudine by about 30%. It appears to decrease the rate of glucuronidation of zidovudine, its major metabolic pathway.

PRIMAQUINE

Primaquine (Fig. 81-7) is a derivative of 8-aminoquinoline. This drug destroys exoerythrocytic schizonts of all four *Plasmodium* species, especially of *P. vivax* and *P. ovale*. It is to be taken as a prophylactic for two weeks before entering and two

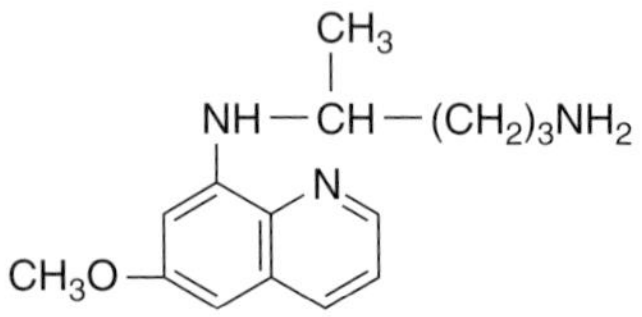

$$CH_3O - \underset{\displaystyle}{\text{quinoline ring}} - NH - \overset{\displaystyle CH_3}{\underset{\displaystyle}{CH}} - (CH_2)_3NH_2$$

FIGURE 81-7   Molecular structure of primaquine.

weeks after leaving an area where malaria is endemic. Since this drug has no red blood cell (RBC) schizonticidal effect, it is almost always used in combination with an RBC schizonticidal drug, such as chloroquine.

MECHANISM OF ACTION

The mechanism of action of primaquine is not well understood. It is speculated, however, that primaquine forms quinoline-quinone metabolites, which act as cellular oxidants. The plasmodial mitochondria exposed to primaquine become swollen and vacuolated, resulting in collapse of mitochondrial membrane potential, interfering with their electron transport in the parasites.

SIDE EFFECTS

Primaquine has a low incidence of adverse effects, except for drug-induced hemolytic anemia in patients with low levels of the enzyme glucose-6-phosphate dehydrogenase (urine turns brown or brown-black, but this does not usually indicate medical emergency). At high doses, primaquine may cause abdominal discomfort and granulocytopenia with increased susceptibility to bacterial infections.

DRUG INTERACTIONS

No clinically important interactions have been reported, but it appears to inhibit CYP1A2. (*See* Table 81-1.)

HALOFANTRINE

Halofantrine is used in the treatment of chloroquine-resistant and multi-drug resistant *P. falciparum* malaria. This drug has an RBC schizonticidal effect, but has no effect against the exoerythrocytic form of the parasites.

MECHANISM OF ACTION

The precise mechanism of action is not understood, but it is postulated that halofantrine (Fig. 81-8) interferes with the process whereby toxic heme is neutralized

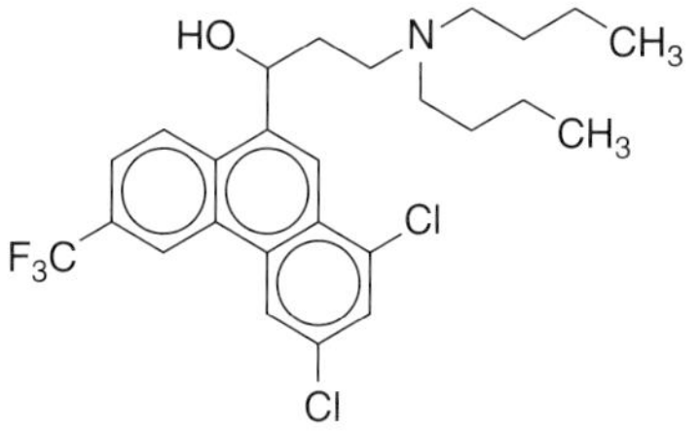

FIGURE 81-8   Molecular structure of halofantrine.

by plasmodium. The toxic metabolite accumulates to break open the internal cell membranes of the parasites, resulting in their death.

SIDE EFFECTS

Possible side effects include elongation of the Q-T interval on electrocardiogram; cough; diarrhea, stomach pain, and loss of appetite; muscle pain; tremors; and dizziness and headache.

DRUG INTERACTIONS

See Box 81-2.

Miscellaneous Interactions of Halofantrine (HFT)

HFT ⟷ CYP Isozymes: *See* Table 81-1.

HFT ⟷ Diuretics: (*See* Ω-49 and Ω-73 in Appendix A.) Co-administration of halofantrine, a QT-prolonging drug, with a drug that causes hypokalemia, such as a loop or thiazide diuretic, may predispose the patient to torsade de pointes.

HFT ⟷ Gastric Antacids: Concurrent administration of halofantrine and a gastric antacid, such as magnesium carbonate or aluminum hydroxide, diminishes intestinal absorption of halofantrine.

HFT ⟷ Mefloquine: Halofantrine induces a dose-related prolongation of the Q-T interval and this effect may be enhanced by prior intake of mefloquine, which at regular doses has little such effect. Since both halofantrine and mefloquine are substrates of CYP3A4, it appears that the presence of mefloquine deters, by competition, metabolic clearance of halofantrine; and the furthered Q-T elongation may bring about torsade de pointes.

BOX 81-2

Basic Concepts of Halofantrine Interactions

Halofantrine is apt to prolong the Q-T interval, and when co-administered with drugs that also tend to elongate the Q-T interval, the life-threatening arrhythmia of torsade de pointes may result. Those drugs include: **chloroquine** (an antimalarial and amebicidal drug); **chlorpromazine** (an antipsychotic drug); **disopyramide** (an antiarrhythmic agent); **droperidol** (a tranquilizer used to alleviate nausea and vomiting); **haloperidol** (an antipsychotic drug); **pimozide** (Fig. 81-9) (an atypical antipsychotic drug); and **sotalol** (a beta blocker).

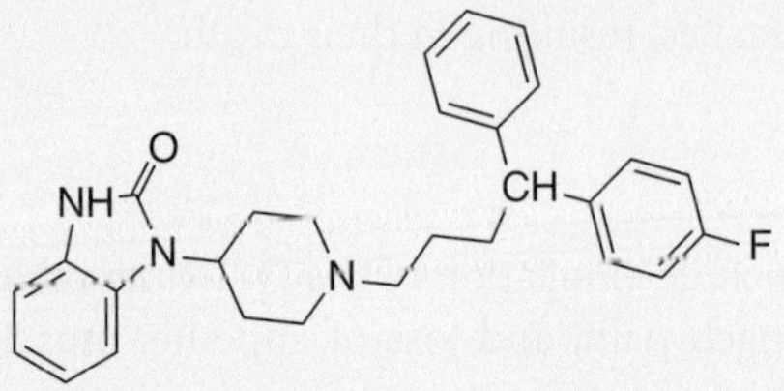

FIGURE 81-9   Molecular structure of pimozide.

HFT ⟷ Methadone: Methadone inhibits cardiac potassium channels to elongate the Q-T interval, and concurrent use with halofantrine, which also elongates the Q-T interval, may lead to torsade de pointes.

QUININE

Quinine, until 1959, was the drug of choice for treatment of acute attack of malaria, and still is a drug of choice for treating malaria caused by chloroquine-resistant *Plasmodium falciparum,* where it is used in combination with pyrimethamine or a sulfonamide such as sulfadiazine or sulfadoxine. Quinine is a schizonticidal drug, which is less effective and more toxic than chloroquine.

MECHANISM OF ACTION

The mechanism of action of quinine is not fully resolved, but it is thought that this drug may interfere with polymerization of toxic heme to inert crystalline hemozoin by the parasites. The toxic free heme then accumulates in the parasites, leading to their death.

SIDE EFFECTS

Side effects of quinine may include cardiac arrhythmia (with Q-T elongation); nausea, and diarrhea; dark colored urine with mild renal impairment; jaundice;

BOX 81-3

Basic Concepts of Quinine Interactions

1. Quinine is apt to prolong the Q-T interval as a side effect, and when co-administered with drugs that generate similar side effects, Torsade de Pointes may result. Those drugs include: **chloroquine** (an antimalarial and amebicidal drug); **chlorpromazine** (an antipsychotic drug); **disopyramide** (an antiarrhythmic agent); **droperidol** (a tranquilizer used to alleviate nausea and vomiting); **halofantrine** (an antimalarial drug); **haloperidol** (an antipsychotic drug); **pimozide** (an atypical antipsychotic drug); and **sotalol** (a beta blocker).

2. Quinine may depress the hepatic enzymes that synthesize the vitamin K-dependent blood clotting factors, and when co-administered with drugs that tend to cause bleeding, prolonged hemorrhage may result. Those drugs include: **dicumarol** (an oral anticoagulant) and **warfarin** (an oral anticoagulant).

---

muscle weakness; hearing or visual disturbances; headache, dizziness, and confusion; and allergic reactions such as skin hives; difficulty in breathing; and swelling of the face, lips, tongue, or throat.

DRUG INTERACTIONS

See Box 81-3.

Miscellaneous Interactions of Quinine (QNN)

QNN ⟷ Amantadine: Quinine may increase serum levels and the risk of toxicity of amantadine. The organic cation transport mechanisms for amantadine in the distal renal tubules appear to be inhibited by quinine.

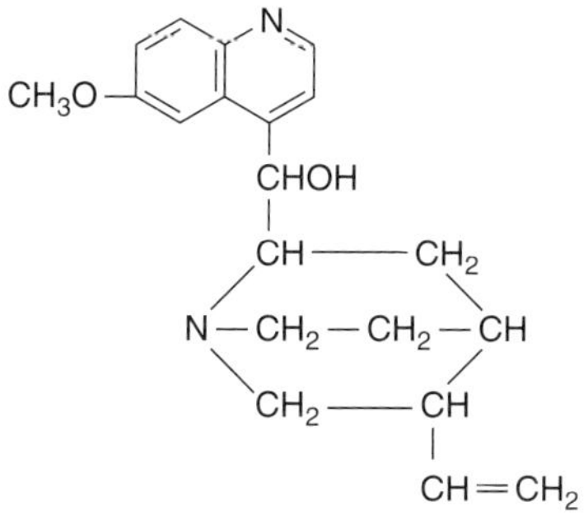

FIGURE 81-10   Molecular structure of quinine.

QNN ⟷ Baking Soda: Quinine (Fig. 81-10) is a basic drug, and alkaline pH of urine caused by administration of an alkalinizing agent such as baking soda can shift to greater amounts of the nonionized form of quinine, which is readily diffused back from tubular fluid into circulation, raising its serum concentrations and inching up its toxicities.

QNN ⟷ CYP Isozymes: *See* Table 81-1.

QNN ⟷ Digoxin: Quinine may raise serum concentrations of digoxin, leading to increased incidences of cardiac arrhythmia by digoxin. It was shown that quinine reduces digoxin excretions by inhibiting the P-gp (Fig. 81-11) transporter in the renal tubules.

QNN ⟷ Diuretics: (*See* Ω-49 and Ω-73 in Appendix A.) Co-administration of quinine, a Q-T elongating drug, with drugs that cause hypokalemia, such as loop or thiazide diuretics, may predispose patients to torsade de pointes.

QNN ⟷ Succinylcholine: Quinine has its own skeletal muscle relaxant effect, and when used in combination with a neuromuscular blocker such as succinyl-choline, life-threatening paralysis of respiratory muscle may ensue.

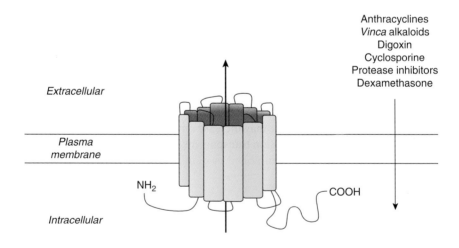

P-glycoprotein

FIGURE 81-11   **P-glycoprotein transporter.** Reproduced, with permission, from DiPiro JT, Talbert RL, Yee GC, Matzke GR, Wells BG, and Posey LM, eds. *Pharmacotherapy: A Pathologic Approach.* 6th ed. New York, NY: McGraw-Hill; 2005, p 1730.

Dysentery

82

Dysentery refers to intestinal inflammation characterized by abdominal pain, and frequent, intense diarrhea with bloody, mucus-laden feces. Dysentery is commonly caused either by the bacteria *Shigella dysenteriae* or by the protozoa *Entamoeba histolytica*.

Medications shown effective in the treatment of dysentery include: (1) **metronidazole** (Flagyl); (2) **iodoquinol** (Diquinol and others); (3) **paromomycin** (Humatin); and (4) **diloxanide** (Furamide).

METRONIDAZOLE

This drug is usually given for 10 days, either by mouth or directly into the veins (intravenously injected).

MECHANISM OF ACTION

The $-NO_2$ group of metronidazole (*See* Fig. 22-4) is reduced to $-NH_2$ by nitrate reductase, which works in conjunction with ferredoxin, an iron-sulfur protein that functions as an electron carrier in the anaerobic parasites by undergoing reversible Fe(ll)-Fe(lll) transitions. This reduction process generates a superoxide radical, which in turn reacts with DNA to destroy the phosphodiester bondage of the DNA. Therefore, metronidazole inhibits synthesis of protozoal nucleic acid to kill amoebas residing in the wall of the intestine, blood, and abscess of the liver. Resistance to this drug is by altered nitrate reductase.

SIDE EFFECTS

Possible side effects of metronidazole include nausea, loss of appetite, and metallic taste; numbness or tingling of extremities (peripheral neuropathy); seizures; headaches; and rarely, skin rash. At high doses, metronidazole can cause serious Stevens-Johnson syndrome or toxic epidermal necrolysis. Metronidazole may turn urine brown-black, but this does not usually indicate medical emergency.

DRUG INTERACTIONS

Metronidazole (MNZ)

MNZ ⟷ Alcohol: Alcoholic beverages should be avoided for at least 24 hours after taking metronidazole. The combination can generate disulfiram-like reactions, such as tachycardia, nausea, vomiting, abdominal cramps, and flushing. Do not give metronidazole to patients who have taken disulfiram within the previous two weeks, otherwise acute psychosis or confusion may result.

MNZ ⟷ Carbamazepine: Metronidazole may increase the serum levels of carbamazepine and its risk of toxicity. One possible mechanism of this interaction is that carbamazepine is a substrate of CYP3A4, and metronidazole has an inhibitory effect on this enzyme.

MNZ ⟷ Cholestyramine: Administering metronidazole with bile-sequestrants such as cholestyramine may impair its intestinal absorption.

MNZ ⟷ Cyclosporine: Since metronidazole is an inhibitor of the enzyme CYP3A4, co-administration with cyclosporine, which requires this enzyme for clearance, may raise blood levels of cyclosporine, exacerbating its toxic effects.

MNZ ⟷ CYP Isozymes: *See* Table 82-1.

MNZ ⟷ Lithium: Metronidazole inhibits renal excretion of lithium. Therefore, plasma levels of lithium may be elevated with increase risk of toxicity.

TABLE 82-1 Metronidazole vs CYP Isozymes

Drug Name	1A2	2A6	2B6	2C8	2C9	2C18	2C19	2D6	2E1	3A4
Metronidazole					Inh + Sub					Inh

1. Hepatic inactivation of metronidazole requires the presence of microsomal CYP2C9. Therefore, inhibition of this enzyme by any drug taken in combination may raise blood levels of metronidazole to exacerbate its adverse effects. Those strong inhibitors of CYP 2C9 include: fluconazole. (*See* the left-hand column of Table-0 at the 'Introduction' for other possible inhibitors of this enzyme.) Induction of this enzyme by carbamazepine and phenobarbital taken together may lower blood levels of metronidazole to therapeutic insufficiency. (*See* the right-hand column of Table-0 at the 'Introduction' for other possible inducers of this enzyme.)

2. Metronidazole functions as an inhibitor of the hepatic enzymes CYP2C9 and CYP3A4. Co-administration with drugs that require these enzymes for hepatic clearance may cause elevation of their blood levels and increased incidence of adverse effects. (*See* the middle column of Table-0 at the 'Introduction' for possible substrates of these enzymes.)

MNZ ↔ Zalcitabine: Metronidazole and zalcitabine both cause numbness or tingling of extremities (peripheral neuropathy). Concomitant use may lead to an enhanced risk of disabling peripheral neuropathies.

IODOQUINOL

Since iodoquinol is poorly absorbed from the gastrointestinal tract, it reaches high concentrations in the intestinal lumen.

MECHANISM OF ACTION

Iodoquinol produces its amebicidal effect at the site of amebal infections, but its precise mechanism of action is poorly understood. It is postulated that it may inhibit ATPase, the enzyme involved in energy metabolism of amoebas.

SIDE EFFECTS

Side effects of iodoquinol may include abdominal cramps, diarrhea, and rectal irritation or itching; numbness or tingling of arms or legs; thyroid enlargement owing to its iodine content; optic neuritis and atrophy with vision changes, especially in children after long-term use; seizures; vertigo; and allergic reactions such as skin rash and itching; difficulty in breathing; and swelling of tissues.

DRUG INTERACTIONS

As iodoquinol in its molecule (Fig. 82-1) contains high concentrations (64%) of organically bound iodine, it is recommended to carefully observe responses to thyroid medications taken together, such as levothyroxine and methimazole.

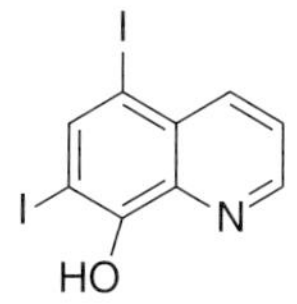

FIGURE 82-1 Molecular structure of iodoquinol.

PAROMOMYCIN

Paromomycin is considered a luminal amebicidal agent, since it acts principally in the intestinal lumen.

MECHANISM OF ACTION

The precise mechanism of action of paromomycin remains elusive but it is speculated that it inhibits synthesis of protozoal proteins.

SIDE EFFECTS

Its side effects may include diarrhea; rarely, neuromuscular blockade; decreased hearing or ringing in the ears; dizziness; and allergic reactions such as skin rash and itching; and difficulty in breathing.

DRUG INTERACTIONS

See Box 82-1.

Miscellaneous Interactions of Paromomycin (PMN)

PMN ⟷ Digoxin: Paromomycin appears to reduce the rate and extent of digoxin absorption. Concurrent administration with digoxin may decrease digoxin's bioavailability by 30-82% to undercut its therapeutic effectiveness.

BOX 82-1

Basic Concepts of Paromomycin Interactions

1. Paromomycin, like other aminoglycosides, has a potential to cause neuromuscular blocking effects. When co-administered with drugs that generate similar effects, respiratory paralysis may result. Those neuromuscular blocking drugs include: **capreomycin** (an antituberculotic agent with a neuromuscular depressant effect); **polymyxin-B** (an antibiotic with a neuromuscular depressant effect); and **vecuronium** (an authentic neuromuscular blocker).

2. Paromomycin tends to cause ototoxicity as a side effect, and when co-administered with drugs that also generate ototoxicity, a greater incidence of this adverse effect may result. Those drugs include: **cisplatin** (an anticancer drug with a high incidence of ototoxicity) and **ethacrynic acid** (a loop diuretic with a higher incidence of ototoxicity than other loop diuretics).

DILOXANIDE

This drug kills amoebas in the intestinal lumen, and not in extraintestinal tissue. Since it generates few serious side effects, this drug may best be used in the treatment of asymptomatic intestinal amebiasis.

MECHANISM OF ACTION

Its mechanism of action is yet to be clearly elucidated. It is presumed to inhibit protein synthesis in amoebas.

SIDE EFFECTS

Side effects of diloxanide may include stomach pain, nausea, loss of appetite, flatulence, and diarrhea; and skin rash.

DRUG INTERACTIONS

There is no clinically important interaction reported.

83

Helminthiasis

Helminthiasis refers to infestations of intestinal or extra-intestinal tissues by parasitic worms. Most of these worms or parasites enter the human body either by the mouth or through the skin. Helminths include nematodes, cestodes, trematodes, and filaria. Their energy for survival is provided by anaerobic glycolysis (breakdown of glucose under oxygen-free condition).

Medications shown effective in the treatment of helminthiasis include: (1) **mebendazole** (Vermox); (2) **albendazole;** (3) **pyrantel pamoate;** (4) **thiabendazole** (Mintezol); (5) **niclosamide;** (6) **praziquantel;** (7) **diethylcarbamazine;** and (8) **ivermectin.**

MEBENDAZOLE

Mebendazole (Fig. 83-1) is a broad-spectrum nematocidal agent. It is a drug of choice in infestation by intestinal nematodes, including whipworm (*Trichuris trichiura*), common roundworm (*Ascaris lumbricoides*), pinworm (*Enterobius vermicularis*), and hookworm (*Necator americanus).* Mebendazole may also become a drug of choice in infections by pork worm (*Trichinella spiralis*).

MECHANISM OF ACTION

Mebendazole binds to tubulin to inhibit its polymerization into microtubules. The loss of cytoplasmic microtubules impairs uptake of glucose by the larval and adult stages of the susceptible parasites, resulting in decreased production

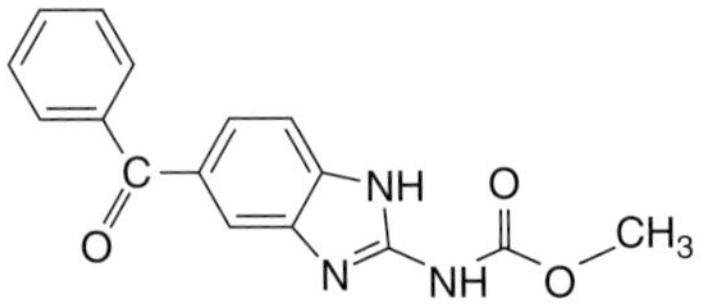

FIGURE 83-1 Molecular structure of mebendazole.

of adenosine triphosphate (ATP), with consequent energy depletions, immobilization, and eventual death of the parasites.

SIDE EFFECTS

Possible side effects of mebendazole (Vermox) include abdominal pain, diarrhea, nausea, alopecia (loss of hair at high doses); unusual muscle weakness; and skin rash and itching.

DRUG INTERACTIONS

Mebendazole (MBZ)

MBZ ⟷ Cimetidine: Blood levels of mebendazole may increase if taken with food; cimetidine, an H2 antagonist; or with an inhibitor of several CYP enzymes including CYP3A4, to foster greater incidence of adverse effects. However, hepatic clearances of mebendazole by CYP enzymes in humans are not clearly elucidated.

MBZ ⟷ Insulin: Mebendazole has been reported to increase secretions of insulin to decrease plasma glucose concentrations in type-1 and type-2 diabetic patients. This action may result in a reduced requirement for insulin during treatment with mebendazole.

MBZ ⟷ Metronidazole: High doses of metronidazole alone rarely cause Stevens-Johnson Syndrome (SJS) or toxic epidermal necrolysis (TEN), but those incidences are reportedly higher when used in combination with mebendazole. The mechanism of this serious interaction remains uncharacterized.

MBZ ⟷ Phenytoin: If mebendazole is taken with phenytoin, an antiepileptic drug and an inducer of CYP3A4 and a few other CYP enzymes, the latter quickens metabolic clearance of mebendazole to lower its blood levels. However, hepatic clearances of mebendazole by specific CYP enzymes in humans are not clearly understood.

ALBENDAZOLE

Albendazole is a broad-spectrum nematocidal agent. It is effective against intestinal nematodes, including whipworm (*Trichuris trichiura*), common roundworm (*Ascaris lumbricoides*), pinworm (*Enterobius vermicularis*), and hookworm (*Necator americanus*). Albendazole is also effective against tapeworms (pork tapeworm, beef tapeworm, dwarf tapeworm, and dog tapeworm [causing Hydatid disease]), and it appears that albendazole is more active than mebendazole against threadworm (*Strongyloides stercoralis*) and pork worm (*Trichinella spiralis*).

MECHANISM OF ACTION

Albendazole damages microtubules and thereby inhibits cellular glucose uptake, similar to mebendazole.

SIDE EFFECTS

Side effects of albendazole may include leukopenia (reversible reduction of white blood cells) and thrombocytopenia; abdominal pain, nausea, and vomiting; acute renal failure; alopecia (loss of hair); and allergic reactions such as skin rash.

DRUG INTERACTIONS

Albendazole (ABZ)

ABZ ⟷ Cimetidine: Albendazole (Fig. 83-2) is metabolically cleared through CYP3A4, and so inhibition of this enzyme by cimetidine is known to increase serum levels of albendazole. *See* Table 83-1.

ABZ ⟷ CYP Isozymes: *See* Table 83-1.

ABZ ⟷ Fatty Meal: Serum levels of albendazole may be increased if taken with a fatty meal (increases oral bioavailability by four to five times) to exacerbate its adverse effects.

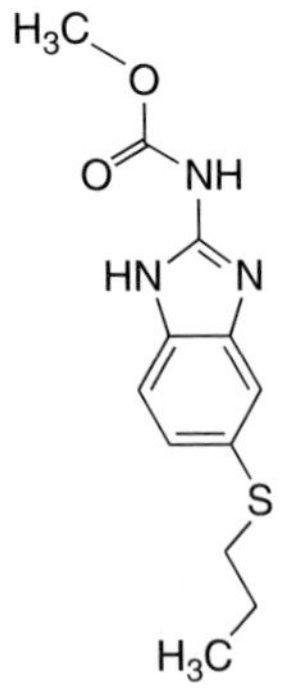

FIGURE 83-2   Molecular structure of albendazole.

TABLE 83-1 Anthelmintics vs CYP Enzymes

Drug Name	1A2	2A6	2B6	2C8	2C9	2C18	2C19	2D6	2E1	3A4
Albendazole										Sub
Praziquantel										Sub
Thiabendazole	Inh									

1. Many anthelmintic drugs either do not interact with CYP isozymes, or their natures of interaction are not as clearly elucidated as the drugs shown in this table. They include diethylcarbamazine, ivermectin, mebendazole, niclosamide, and pyrantel pamoate .

2. Both albendazole and praziquantel are metabolically cleared through CYP3A4, and so inhibition of this enzyme by drugs taken together may raise their blood levels to potentially exacerbate their adverse effects. (*See* the left-hand column of Table-0 at the 'Introduction' for possible inhibitors of this enzyme).

3. Both albendazole and dexamethasone, a glucocorticoid, require the enzyme CYP3A4 for clearance. Thus, concurrent administration may cause competition for the same enzyme to possibly result in elevated blood levels of albendazole that might exacerbate its adverse effects. Anticonvulsants such as carbamazepine, phenytoin, and phenobarbital (all inducers of CYP3A4) appear to enhance the metabolic clearance of albendazole to result in reduced serum levels of albendazole. (*See* the right-hand column of Table-0 at the 'Introduction' for other possible inducers of this enzyme.)

4. Thiabendazole is unusual in that it inhibits CYP1A2, and so co-administration with drugs that require this enzyme for metabolic clearance may result in elevated blood levels of those unmetabolized drugs to incite their adverse effects. Theophylline, for instance, heavily depends on this enzyme for its clearance, and co-administration with thiabendazole may elevate serum levels of theophylline and exacerbate its adverse effects, including severe nausea and vomiting. (*See* the middle column of Table-0 at the 'Introduction' for other possible substrates of this enzyme.)

PYRANTEL PAMOATE

This is a drug of choice in infestations by intestinal nematodes such as common roundworm, pinworm, and hookworm, but not against whipworm, which is resistant to this drug.

MECHANISM OF ACTION

Pyrantel (Fig. 83-3) inhibits the enzyme cholinesterase in the myoneural system of the worms, and produces spastic paralysis of their muscles. The paralyzed

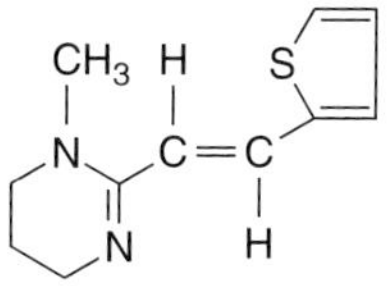

FIGURE 83-3 Molecular structure of pyrantel.

nematodes are unable to hold on to the intestinal mucosa of the host and are slowly expelled.

SIDE EFFECTS

Side effects of pyrantel pamoate may include nausea, vomiting, anorexia, abdominal cramps, and diarrhea; and skeletal muscle weakness.

DRUG INTERACTIONS

Pyrantel Pamoate (PPT)

PPT ⟷ Piperazine: If pyrantel pamoate is used in combination with piperazine, another drug useful against common roundworm, the anthelmintic efficacy of pyrantel pamoate may be lost because depolarization of the parasitic membrane caused by pyrantel pamoate is counteracted by hyperpolarization of the parasitic membrane caused by piperazine.

THIABENDAZOLE

Thiabendazole (Fig. 83-4) is a drug of choice against threadworm (*Strongyloides stercoralis*) and cutaneous larva migrans (*Ancylostoma braziliense*).

MECHANISM OF ACTION

Thiabendazole inhibits fumarate reductase, a helminth-specific enzyme that is essential for generation of ATP in the parasites. Thiabendazole also binds to tubulin to interfere with the microtubular function of the sensitive helminths.

SIDE EFFECTS

Side effects of thiabendazole may include angioedema; leucopenia and hyperglycemia; drying of mucous membranes; abdominal pain, and diarrhea; hematuria and crystalluria; cholestasis and jaundice; muscle numbness or incoordination; xanthopsia (yellowish vision) and blurred vision; tinnitus (ringing in the ear); Stevens-Johnson syndrome (a skin disorder); and delirium, dizziness, hallucination, and seizure.

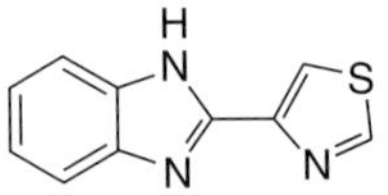

FIGURE 83-4   Molecular structure of thiabendazole.

DRUG INTERACTIONS

See Table 83-1.

NICLOSAMIDE:

Niclosamide is a drug of choice in infections by tapeworms (*Taenia* species), except by dwarf tapeworm (*Hymenolepis nana*), for which praziquantel is the drug of choice.

MECHANISM OF ACTION

Niclosamide inhibits cellular uptake of glucose, and inhibits phosphorylation of ADP, which is required to generate ATP in the anaerobic tapeworms. Each tapeworm has a scolex (head and neck part), proglottids (body segments), and ova. The ova of pork tapeworm (*Taenia solium*), unlike those of beef tapeworm (*Taenia saginata*), can hatch inside the human intestine to develop infective larvae that later causes cysticercosis. Niclosamide can damage the scolex and proglottids but not the ova. Therefore, to eradicate the ova of pork tapeworm and thereby to prevent eventual cysticercosis, a saline purge with sodium sulfate or magnesium sulfate two hours after administration of niclosamide is recommended. In fact, for eradication of pork tapeworm, praziquantel or albendazole is more effective than niclosamide.

SIDE EFFECTS

Possible side effects of niclosamide include abdominal cramps, loss of appetite, and diarrhea; itching at the rectal area; lightheadedness and dizziness. There is no contra-indication for the use of niclosamide in both small children and pregnant women.

DRUG INTERACTIONS

Ethanol taken in combination can dissolve and increase intestinal absorption of niclosamide, inciting its adverse effects. Alcohol intake should be restricted during treatment with niclosamide.

PRAZIQUANTEL

Praziquantel is a drug of choice against dwarf tapeworm (*Hymenolepis nana)* and fish tapeworm (*Diphyllobothrium latum*). Praziquantel is also highly active against all forms of blood flukes (*Schistoma* species), liver flukes (*Opisthorchis* species), and lung flukes *(Paragonimus westermanii).*

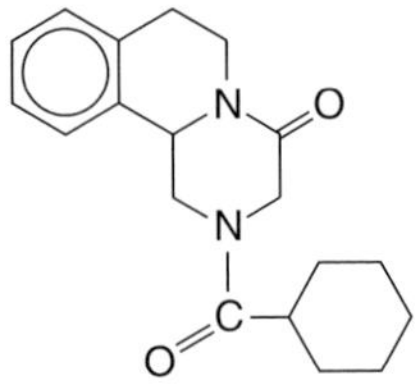

FIGURE 83-5   Molecular structure of praziquantel.

MECHANISM OF ACTION

Praziquantel (Fig. 83-5) works by changing membrane permeability so as to allow massive influx of calcium ions into parasite tissues, to bring about excessive muscle contractions, followed by spastic paralysis of those parasites.

SIDE EFFECTS

Possible side effects of praziquantel include diaphoresis (copious sweating); abdominal pain, loss of appetite, nausea, vomiting, and diarrhea; skin rash and urticaria with itching; fever; and drowsiness and dizziness.

DRUG INTERACTIONS

See Table 83-1.

DIETHYLCARBAMAZINE

Diethylcarbamazine is active against the microfilariae of *Wuchereria bancrofti, Loa loa,* and of *Onchocerca volvulus,* but adult forms of *Onchocerca volvulus* are resistant.

MECHANISM OF ACTION

Diethylcarbamazine appears to promote phagocytosis of the parasites by fixed macrophages of the reticuloendothelial system. Although adult filarial worms may not respond as quickly, they too may eventually be eradicated by this drug.

SIDE EFFECTS

Side effects of diethylcarbamazine may include painful and tender glands in neck, armpits, or groin; joint pain; unusual tiredness or weakness; fever; tunnel vision, and night blindness; and Mazzotti reactions with intense and long-lasting itching and swelling of the face, especially of the eyes.

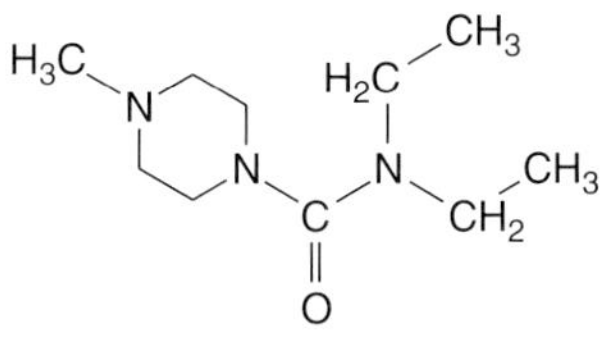

FIGURE 83-6   Molecular structure of diethylcarbamazine.

DRUG INTERACTIONS

Diethylcarbamazine (Fig. 83-6) is a basic drug and if the urine is made alkaline by taking an alkalinizing agent such as sodium bicarbonate or sodium lactate, diethylcarbamazine turns increasingly into its nonionized form, which has greater lipid-solubility and is more readily back-diffused through the renal tubules. This effect raises the serum levels of diethylcarbamazine and exacerbates its adverse effects.

IVERMECTIN

This is a drug of choice for infections by *Onchocerca volvulus* that causes "river blindness." Ivermectin is also active against threadworm (*Strongyloides stercoralis*). Furthermore, ivermectin is active against intestinal nematodes such as common round worm, pinworm, whipworm, and to a lesser degree, hookworm. It is not effective against tapeworm or *Schistosoma*. A single dose of ivermectin is taken orally on an empty stomach, and may require a follow up doses after three months. This drug is not recommended in pregnant or lactating women or in children under five years old.

MECHANISM OF ACTION

Ivermectin (Fig. 83-7) appears to work at the parasites' gamma-aminobutyric acid (GABA) receptors to increase the influx of chloride ions, leading to hyperpolarization and paralysis of the parasites' muscles. Ivermectin was shown not to kill adult *Onchocerca*, but it blocks the release of microfilariae from the adult female parasites.

SIDE EFFECTS

Side effects of ivermectin may include hypotension and transient tachycardia; anemia, eosinophilia, and leucopenia; peripheral and facial edema; abdominal pain; myalgia, tremor, and muscle weakness; arthralgia; hyperthermia; Stevens-Johnson Syndrome; and dizziness and headache.

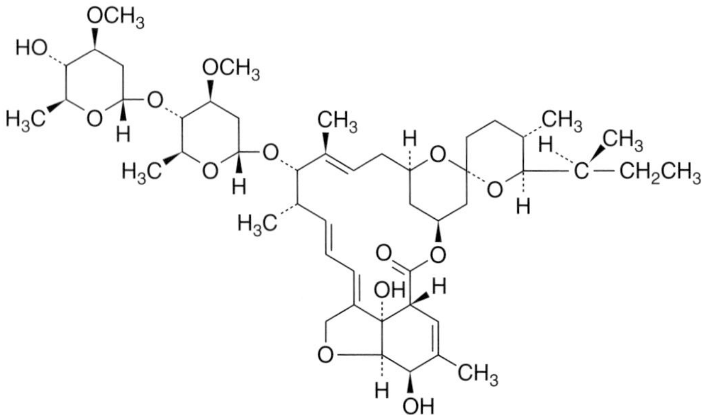

FIGURE 83-7   Molecular structure of ivermectin.

DRUG INTERACTIONS

As ivermectin is usually given as a one-time dose, or because its dosing interval is as long as 12 months, its interactions with other drugs are thought to be uncommon, but the following interactions cannot be excluded.

Ivermectin (IVM)

IVM ⟷ Alcohol: The absorption of ivermectin is significantly affected by the presence of alcohol. Co-administration of alcohol and ivermectin significantly increases serum levels of ivermectin to generate such side effects as weakness, confusion, and lack of coordination. Although the side effects are not significantly alarming, it would be prudent to avoid alcohol while on ivermectin therapy.

IVM ⟷ Cyclosporine: If ivermectin is co-administered with cyclosporine, it may cause elevated ivermectin concentrations in the brain, producing such neurotoxicities as ataxia, tremors, mydriasis, and vomiting. Cyclosporine appears to interrupt the functions of the P-glycoprotein transporter at the blood-brain barrier, which effluxes ivermectin, allowing more ivermectin to enter into the brain.

IVM ⟷ High-Fat Meal: Bioavailability of ivermectin will be increased two to three fold when administered following a high fat meal.

IVM ⟷ Ketoconazole: Ivermectin is a substrate of multidrug-resistance (MDR) P-glycoprotein but ketoconazole is an inhibitor of such transporter. Therefore, ketoconazole, when used in combination, may increase the intestinal absorption of ivermectin, raising its serum concentration and arousing its adverse effects.

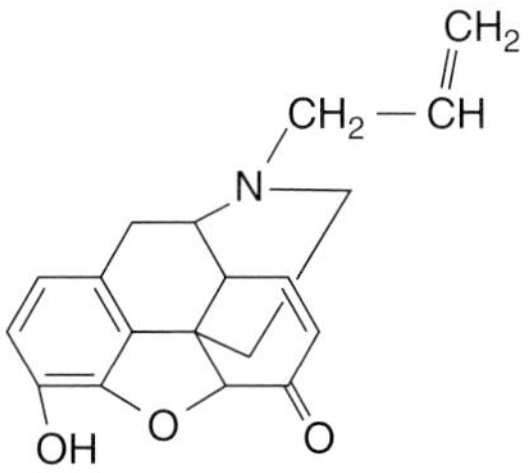

FIGURE 84-3   Molecular structure of naloxone.

constipation, all mediated through activation of the mu receptors. Naloxone also competes at other opioid receptors, such as kappa and sigma receptors.

SIDE EFFECTS

Side effects of naloxone may include tachycardia and increased blood pressure; pulmonary edema; nausea and vomiting; and seizure.

DRUG INTERACTIONS

Naloxone can decrease therapeutic efficacy of narcotic analgesics used in combination, and even can precipitate acute withdrawal reactions in patients physically dependent on narcotic drugs.

N-ACETYLCYSTEINE

To minimize or reverse necrotic damage of the liver caused by acetaminophen, it is recommend to take 0.1 gram per kilogram of body weight of N-acetylcysteine within 12 hours of overdose with acetaminophen. Signs of liver damage may include nausea, vomiting, and abdominal pain, with elevated blood levels of liver enzymes, such as aspartate aminotransferase (AST) and alanine aminotransferase (ALT), all released from the damaged liver cells.

MECHANISM OF ACTION

Acetaminophen at recommended therapeutic doses is inactivated mainly by glucuronidation (50%) and sulfate conjugation (30%); and only about 5% of the drug undergoes microsomal oxidation (mainly by CYP2E1, and to a lesser extent by CYP1A2) to form N-acetyl-p-benzoquinoneimine (NAPQI), a hepatotoxic metabolite. With higher doses of acetaminophen, portions of the oxidation pathway become enlarged, generating a greater amount of toxic metabolites that act as free radical oxidizing agents. Elimination of this toxic metabolite depends on

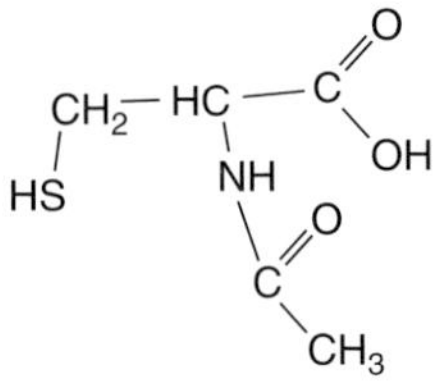

FIGURE 84-4   Molecular structure of N-acetylcysteine.

conjugation with the -SH group of the reduced form of glutathione (chemically, r-glutamylcysteinylglycine). When the drug doses are too excessive, the toxic metabolite formed can quickly exhaust the reduced form of glutathione available, and the non-conjugated toxic metabolite snatches electrons away from liver tissue, leading to necrotic damage. N-acetylcysteine (Fig 84-4) works by donating its -SH group to help regenerate the reduced form of glutathione, which can bolster the body's natural detoxification mechanism.

SIDE EFFECTS

Side effects of N-acetylcysteine may include skin rash, urticaria, and itching.

DRUG INTERACTIONS

Activated charcoal can adsorb N-acetylcysteine to decrease its bioavailability and therapeutic effectiveness. It is not known whether other medications will interact with this medication.

SODIUM POLYSTYRENE SULFONATE

To treat hyperkalemia, which causes fatal arrhythmia by blockade of cardiac A-V conduction, oral intake of 15-40 grams of sodium polystyrene sulfonate, one to four times a day, may help reduce the blood potassium.

MECHANISM OF ACTION

Sodium polystyrene sulfonate is a potassium-binding ion-exchange resin that removes potassium and other cationic electrolytes from the blood stream, in exchange for sodium ions partially released from the drug.

SIDE EFFECTS

Side effects may include irregular pulse; hypokalemia and hypocalcemia; sodium retention; gastric irritation, loss of appetite, stomach pain, and diarrhea or constipation; muscle cramps; and dizziness.

DRUG INTERACTIONS

No clinically significant interactions have been documented.

HYDROXOCOBALAMIN, AMYL NITRITE, OR SODIUM NITRITE

For the treatment of cyanide poisoning, the following treatments are recommended: (1) hydroxocobalamin (5 g IV infused over 15 minutes); and (2) amyl nitrite, sodium nitrite, and sodium thiosulfate (a 0.3 ml of amyl nitrite inhaled for up to 30 seconds and then 300 mg of sodium nitrite i.v. injected, followed by 12.5 g sodium thiosulfate I.V over 10 minutes, as one of dosing plans recommended for initial treatment).

MECHANISM OF ACTION

Cyanide is toxic because it is bound to and inactivates cytochrome oxidase, an enzyme essential for mitochondrial respiration. Hydroxocobalamin takes up cyanide into its own molecule, to remove its availability, freeing the cytochrome oxidase. The nitrites (both amyl nitrite and sodium nitrite) oxidize normal hemoglobin to methemoglobin, which because of its high affinity for binding to cyanide can pull away the toxic cyanide from the enzyme cytochrome oxidase. Thiosulfate reacts with the cyanide thus released, to form relatively nontoxic thiocyanate (-SCN), which is excreted in the urine.

SIDE EFFECTS

Hydroxocobalamin: It may cause peripheral vascular thrombosis; diarrhea; and allergic reactions such as skin rash and itching.

Amyl Nitrite or **Sodium Nitrite:** They may cause bluish-colored skin; tiredness; and seizure; and allergic reactions such as difficulty in breathing; and skin rash and itching.

Sodium Thiosulfate: sodium thiosulfate may cause nausea and vomiting; muscle cramps; blurred vision; ringing in the ears; and hallucinations.

DRUG INTERACTIONS

Hydroxocobalamin: It is not known whether other medications will interact with this medication.

Amyl Nitrite or **Sodium Nitrite** or **sodium thiosulfate:** *See* Box 84-2.

Sodium Thiosulfate: Interactions of injected sodium thiosulfate with other drugs is not well documented.

BOX 84-2

Basic Concepts of Amyl Nitrite or Sodium Nitrite Interactions

Both **amyl nitrite** and **sodium nitrite** rapidly generate vasodilation, and when co-administered with drugs that also generate vasodilation, a precipitous fall of blood pressure may result. Those drugs include: **sildenafil** (Viagra); **tadalafil** (Cialis); and **vardenafil** (Levitra*).*

Miscellaneous Interactions of Amyl Nitrite or Sodium Nitrite (ASN)

ASN ⟷ Ethanol: Amyl nitrite and sodium nitrite are sources of nitric oxide, which causes rapid vasodilation through formation of C-GMP, to lower blood pressure, flush facial skin, and increase heart rate. As alcohol also causes vasodilation through its oxidation product acetaldehyde, taking amyl nitrite or sodium nitrite shortly after drinking alcohol may worsen side effects of the nitrites, to cause severe hypotension and cardiovascular collapse.

ATROPINE

To treat poisoning by nerve gas such as sarin, or by warfare agents such as soman (Fig. 84-7) and tabun (Fig. 84-8), or by insecticides such as parathion (*See* Fig. 84-1), it is recommend to take atropine (*See* Fig. 25-2), to be used in conjunction with pralidoxime or obidoxime. At low doses of the above organophosphate poisons, the muscarinic effects of acetylcholine predominate. Thus, atropine, a nonspecific muscarinic antagonist, may be administered first: 1 to 2 mg of atropine sulfate can be administered intravenously every ten minutes until reversal of cholinergic symptoms, such as salivation and miosis, is achieved.

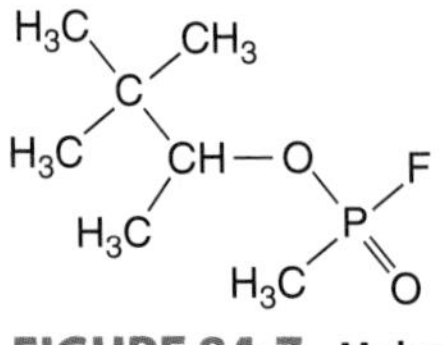

FIGURE 84-7 Molecular structure of soman.

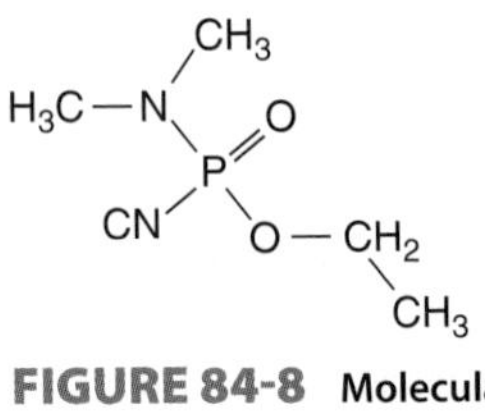

FIGURE 84-8 Molecular structure of tabun.

MECHANISM OF ACTION

The aforementioned toxic agents work by irreversible inhibition of cholinesterase, the enzyme that inactivates acetylcholine. If the above agents inhibit this enzyme, excessive amounts of acetylcholine will be accumulated at the wide-spread muscarinic receptors to interact with and generate cholinergic crisis. Atropine competitively binds to the muscarinic receptors, to minimize or even completely reverse the muscarinic cholinergic symptoms.

SIDE EFFECTS

Side effects of atropine may include cardiac arrhythmia (tachycardia); flushing and hypotension; dyspnea, laryngospasm, and pulmonary edema; bloating, xerostomia (dry mouth), delayed gastric emptying, constipation; skeletal muscle weakness and ataxia; angle-closure glaucoma, blurred vision, cycloplegia, dry eyes, and mydriasis; skin rash and urticaria; and disorientation, fever, and hallucinations.

DRUG INTERACTIONS

See Appendix B-15: Interactions of Belladonna Alkaloids.

OBIDOXIME OR PRALIDOXIME

While muscarinic cholinergic symptoms, such as excessive salivation and miosis, can be reversed by injection of atropine, the nicotinic toxicity of acetylcholine, such as paralysis of respiratory muscles, cannot be reversed by atropine, as it has only blocking effects on the muscarinic receptors and not on the nicotinic receptors. To reverse paralysis of respiratory muscles mediated through activation of the nicotinic receptors, artificial respiration, taken in conjunction with prompt injections of pralidoxime or obidoxime, is helpful. Suggested dosing plans in adults include pralidoxime (1–2 g intravenously over 15-30 minute period, and after about an hour, a second dose of 1-2 g will be indicated if muscle weakness persists); and obidoxime (a single dose of 250 mg IV followed by continuous infusion of 750 mg/24 hour).

MECHANISM OF ACTION

Both pralidoxime (Fig. 84-9) and obidoxime (Fig. 84-10) each have a negatively charged group in their molecules, which has affinity toward and interacts with the positively charged phosphorus of the above organophosphate poisons, so as to extract the poison away from the enzyme cholinesterase and set it free. The now liberated enzyme cholinesterase destroys acetylcholine existing in excess, alleviating cholinergic crisis.

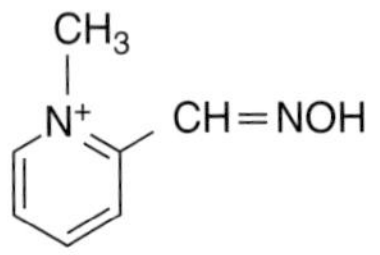

CH₃
|
N⁺   CH=NOH

FIGURE 84-9   Molecular structure of pralidoxime.

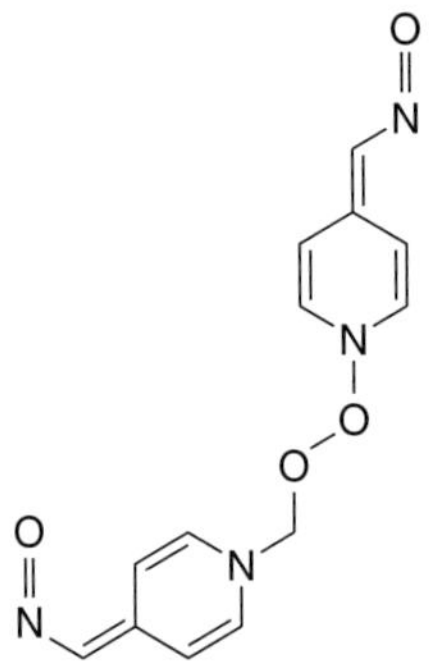

FIGURE 84-10   Molecular structure of obidoxime.

SIDE EFFECTS

Obidoxime: Side effects of obidoxime include pain at the site of injection; paresthesias (abnormal sensations) of the face muscles, such as heat and tension, mainly in the lips and cheeks as the most peculiar side effect; and xerostomia (dryness of the mouth).

Pralidoxime: Side effects of pralidoxime include rapid heartbeat; hyperventilation (over breathing); spasm of the larynx; liver damage; muscle rigidity and weakness; kidney damage; blurred or double vision; and skin rash.

DRUG INTERACTIONS

Obidoxime: It is unknown if other medications will interact with this one.

Pralidoxime (PDX)

PDX ⟷ Morphine: Acetylcholine is an important neurotransmitter involved in regulations of tone and contractility of skeletal muscle, smooth muscle, and cardiac muscle. The principal action of pralidoxime is limited to reactivation of the enzyme cholinesterase outside of the CNS, since the drug cannot enter the brain. The cholinesterase thus freed by pralidoxime can now destroy acetylcholine. On the other hand, morphine opposes the release of existing acetylcholine from the cholinergic nerve terminals. Therefore, if the two are taken together, the deficiency of acetylcholine would become too great to sustain normal cholinergic function, possibly culminating in wide-spread neurologic disturbances.

PDX ⟷ Succinylcholine: Succinylcholine (Fig. 84-11) binds to nicotinic receptors to cause initial depolarization (or stimulation of skeletal muscle), but its continuous occupation of the receptors causes depolarizing neuromuscular blockade

PENICILLAMINE

To remove copper, oral intake of penicillamine (Cuprimine, Depen), 20-30 mg/kg daily, given in 4 equally divided doses, may be of help.

MECHANISM OF ACTION

Penicillamine chelates copper to make a metal complex which is harmlessly removed by the kidneys.

SIDE EFFECTS

Side effects of penicillamine include abdominal pain, diarrhea; blood in the urine, and rarely, depressed kidney function; muscle weakness; poor wound healing; bone marrow depression; jaundice; increased wrinkling of the skin; double vision; ringing in the ears; and allergic reactions such as skin rash and itching; difficulty in breathing; and swelling of tissues.

DRUG INTERACTIONS

See Box 84-3.

Miscellaneous Interactions of Penicillamine (PLM)

PLM ⟷ Chloroquine and Other Antimalarial Drugs: Penicillamine is metabolized in the body and is excreted in the urine and feces. Blood levels of penicillamine may rise to cause hematologic and dermatologic adverse effects when it is taken with chloroquine (Aralen) or other chemically related antimalarial drugs, such as quinine (Quinamm), mefloquine (Lariam), hydroxychloroquine (Plaquenil), and primaquine; and even with chemically unrelated pyrimethamine (Daraprim). The mechanism behind these observations has not been established.

PLM ⟷ Digoxin: Penicillamine appears to decrease absorption of digoxin and decrease blood levels of digoxin to undercut its therapeutic effectiveness.

PLM ⟷ Gold Preparations: Like penicillamine, gold preparations can depress the bone marrow and impair kidney function. Such gold preparations include: auranofin (Ridaura), aurothioglucose (Solganal), and gold sodium thiomalate (Myochrysine, Aurolate). When any of these gold preparations is used in combination with penicillamine it may cause dangerous additive toxicities.

PLM ⟷ Indomethacin: Combined use of penicillamine with indomethacin in patients with rheumatoid arthritis caused a significant increase in blood levels and toxicity of penicillamine, but the exact mechanism behind this observation remains unclear.

BOX 84-3

Basic Concepts of Penicillamine Interactions

1. Penicillamine is well absorbed from the GI tract and can chelate many poly-valent cations, such as aluminum, calcium, copper, iron, magnesium, and zinc to increase their urinary excretions. Those drugs that oppose the intestinal absorption of penicillamine to undercut its therapeutic effectiveness include: **gastric antacids** (*See* Ω-11 in Appendix A) (probably because gastric antac-ids raise gastric pH, which tends to oxidize penicillamine (Fig. 84-15) to its dis-ulfide form that is not well absorbed from the GI tract); **ferrous sulfate;** and **sucralfate** (an oral medication useful for treatment of gastrointestinal ulcers).

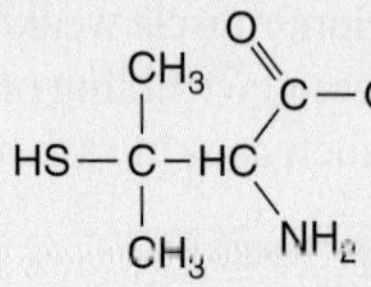

FIGURE 84-15   Molecular structure of penicillamine.

2. Penicillamine may cause bone marrow depression as is evidenced by throm-bocytopenia and leucopenia. When it is co-administered with drugs that generate similar side effects, there is a greater incidence of hematologic toxicity. Those drugs include: **amphotericin-B** (an antifungal drug that has rare incidence of bone marrow depression, causing easy bruising or bleed-ing and anemia); **azathioprine** (an anticancer drug); and **thioguanine** (an anticancer drug).

PLM ⟷ Levodopa: Penicillamine depletes pyridoxine (vitamin B-6), which is a coenzyme for dopa decarboxylase, the enzyme required for the conversion of levodopa to dopamine. Hence, penicillamine tends to oppose the formation of dopamine from levodopa and tends to raise blood levels and adverse effects of levodopa.

PLM ⟷ Probenecid: Though penicillamine interacts with insoluble cystine to make it a soluble penicillamine-cysteine-mixed disulfide, to reduce the urinary concentration of cystine (cystinuria being prone to produce urolithiasis), admin-istration of penicillamine together with probenecid is contraindicated in patients affected by cystinuria, for probenecid blocks renal excretions of the soluble mixed disulfide, undermining the therapeutic benefit of penicillamine in such patients.

APPENDIXES

Major Drugs in Therapeutic Classifications

Ω-1   **ACE inhibitors** include: benazepril, captopril, enalapril, fosinopril, lisino-pril, moexipril, quinapril, and ramipril.

Ω-2   **Adrenergic beta-2 agonists** include: albuterol (Ventolin, Proventil), metaproterenol (Alupent), pirbuterol (Maxair), and terbutaline.

Ω-3   **Aldosterone antagonists** include: canrenone, eplerenone, and spirono-lactone.

Ω-4   **Alpha-2 activators** include: clonidine, guanfacine, and methyldopa (Al-domet).

Ω-5   **Alpha agonists** include: methoxamine, norepinephrine, oxymetazoline, and phenylephrine.

Ω-6   **Alpha blockers** include: alfuzosin (UroXatral), doxazosin (Cardura), tamsulosin (Flomax), and terazosin (Hytrin).

Ω-7   **Aminoglycoside antibiotics** include: amikacin, gentamicin, kanamycin, neomycin, netilmicin, paromomycin, streptomycin, and tobramycin.

Ω-8   **Anabolic steroids** include: ethylestrenol, fluoxymesterone, methyltestos-terone, nandrolone, oxandrolone, oxymetholone, and stanozolol.

Ω-9   **Anesthetics agents** include: desflurane, enflurane, halothane, isoflurane, nitrous oxide, and sevoflurane.

Ω-10   **Angiotensin receptor blockers** include: irbesartan, losartan, olmesartan, telmisartan, and valsartan.

Ω-11   **Antacids** include: aluminum hydroxide (AlternaGEL, Amphojel), aluminum carbonate (Basaljel), aluminum hydroxide with magnesium hydroxide (Maalox, Mylanta), bismuth subsalicylate (Pepto-Bismol), calcium carbonate (Rolaids, Titralac, Tums), magnesium hydroxide (Phillips' Milk of Magnesia), and sodium bicarbonate (Bicarbonate of soda, Alka-Seltzer).

Ω-12   **Antiarrhythmic drugs** include: adenosine, amiodarone, atenolol, digoxin, diltiazem, disopyramide, dofetilide, esmolol, flecainide, ibutilide, lidocaine, metoprolol, mexiletine, moricizine, procainamide, propafenone, propranolol, quinidine, timolol, tocainide, and verapamil. Among the above, class-Ia antiarrhythmic drugs include: disopyramide, procainamide, quinidine; class-Ib drugs include: lidocaine, mexiletine, and tocainide; class-Ic drugs include: flecainide, moricizine, and propafenone; class-ll antiarrhythmic drugs include: atenolol, esmolol, metoprolol, propranolol, and timolol; class-lll drugs include: amiodarone, dofetilide, and ibutilide; class-IV drugs include: diltiazem, and verapamil; and miscellaneous antiarrhythmic drugs include: adenosine and digoxin.

Ω-13   **Anticancer drugs** often used include: actinomycin, altretamine, amsacrine, bleomycin, busulfan, capecitabine, carboplatin, carmustine, cisplatin, cyclophosphamide, cytarabine, dacarbazine, dactinomycin, daunorubicin, docetaxel, doxorubicin, epirubicin, estramustine, etoposide, fludarabine, 5-fluorouracil, gemcitabine, hydroxyurea, idarubicin, ifosfamide, irinotecan, mechlorethamine, melphalan, mercaptopurine, methotrexate, mitoxantrone, paclitaxel, procarbazine, thioguanine, thiotepa, topotecan, vinblastine, vindesine, and vinorelbine.

Ω-14   **Anticholinergic agents** include: ipratropium (Atrovent), oxitropium (Oxivent), scopolamine, and tiotropium (Spiriva).

Ω-15   **Anticholinesterase agents** include: demecarium, echothiophate, isoflurophate, neostigmine, and physostigmine.

Ω-16   **Anticoagulants** often used include: acenocoumarol (Nicoumalone), heparin (various heparins exist), and warfarin.

Ω-17   **Antidiarrheal drugs** include: attapulgite (found in Kaopectate), bismuth subsalicylate (Pepto-Bismol); diphenoxylate, and loperamide.

Ω-18   **Antiglaucoma drugs** most frequently used include: Beta blockers such as betaxolol, carteolol, levobunolol, metipranolol, and timolol; Carbonic anhydrase inhibitors such as acetazolamide, brinzolamide, dorzolamide, and methazolamide; relatively selective Alpha-Agonists such as apraclonidine, and brimonidine; Cholinergic drugs such as carbachol, and pilocarpine; and Prostaglandin preparations such as latanoprost; and further, epinephrine is also effective in lowering intraocular pressure for glaucoma.

Ω-19   **Antihistamines** include: acrivastine, azelastine (Astelin, Astepro), brompheniramine, cetirizine, chlorpheniramine (Chlor-Trimeton), clemastine (Tavist), cyproheptadine (Periactin), desloratadine (Clarinex), diphenhydramine (Benadryl), fexofenadine (Allegra), hydroxyzine (Atarax), levocetirizine (Xyzal), loratadine, olopatadine (Patanase), and promethazine (Phenergan).

Ω-20   **Antihypertensive drugs** include the following groups: (1) ACE inhibitors; (2) alpha-1 blockers; (3) alpha-2 activators; (4) angiotensin-receptor blockers; (5) beta blockers; (6) calcium-channel blockers; and (7) diuretic drugs. *See* appropriate rows in this Appendix A for members of each group.

Ω-21   **Antithyroid drugs** include: carbimazole, methimazole, potassium perchlorate, and propylthiouracil.

Ω-22   **Antiplatelet drugs** include: abciximab (ReoPro), aspirin, clopidogrel (Plavix), dipyridamole (Persantine), eptifibatide (Integrilin), ticlopidine (Ticlid*),* and tirofiban (Aggrastat).

Ω-23   **Azole antifungal drugs** include: clotrimazole, fluconazole, itraconazole, ketoconazole, miconazole, and voriconazole.

Ω-24   **Barbiturates** include: amobarbital, butalbital, mephobarbital (Mebaral), methohexital (Brevital), pentobarbital, phenobarbital, secobarbital, thiamylal (Surital), and thiopental (Pentothal).

Ω-25   **Belladonna alkaloids include:** atropine and scopolamine.

Ω-26   **Benzodiazepine antianxiety drugs** include: alprazolam (Xanax), bromazepam (Lexotan), chlordiazepoxide, clorazepate (Tranxene), diazepam, halazepam (Paxipam), lorazepam (Ativan), nitrazepam (Mogadon), oxazepam (Serax), and prazepam (Centrax).

Ω-27   **Beta blockers:** (1) Beta-1-selective (or cardio-selective) blockers include: acebutolol, atenolol, betaxolol, bisoprolol, esmolol, and metoprolol; and (2) Non-cardioselective beta blockers include: carteolol, levobunolol, metipranolol, nadolol, penbutolol, pindolol, propranolol, sotalol, and timolol.

Ω-28   **Bile acid sequestrants** include: cholestyramine (Questran, Questran, Prevalite, Locholest), colesevelam (WelChol), and colestipol (Colestid),

Ω-29   **Bone marrow depressants:** Many anticancer drugs suppress bone marrow, and they include: busulfan, carboplatin, carmustine, chlorambucil, cisplatin, cladribine, cyclophosphamide, cytarabine, dactinomycin, doxorubicin, fluorouracil, ifosfamide, lomustine, mechlorethamine, mercaptopurine, methotrexate, mitomycin, plicamycin, procarbazine, thioguanine, and vinblastine.

Ω-30   **Bronchodilators** include: albuterol (Ventolin, Proventil), metaproterenol (Alupent), pirbuterol (Maxair), and terbutaline.

Ω-31   **Calcium-channel blockers** include: amlodipine (Norvasc), aranidipine (Sapresta), barnidipine, felodipine (Plendil), nicardipine (Cardene), nifedipine (Procardia, Adalat), nimodipine (Nimotop), nisoldipine (Baymycard, Sular, Syscor), nitrendipine (Nitrepin, Baylotensin), and verapamil.

Ω-32   **Cephalosporin antibiotic drugs** include: cefaclor, cefamandole, cefdinir, cefotetan, cefoxitin , cefpodoxime, cefprozil, ceftibuten, ceftriaxone, cefuroxime, and cephalexin.

Ω-33   **Cholesterol-lowering drugs** include: Bile-acid sequestrants such as cholestyramine, and colestipol; niacin (nicotinic acid); Inhibitors of cholesterol absorption such as ezetimibe; and Statins such as fluvastatin, lovastatin, mevastatin, pitavastatin, pravastatin, rosuvastatin, and simvastatin.

Ω-34   **Cholinomimetic drugs:** Direct-acting cholinomimetic drugs include: carbachol, bethanechol, cevimeline, and pilocarpine; and Indirect-acting cholinomimetic drugs (by reversible inhibition of cholinesterase, the enzyme that destroy acetylcholine) include: donepezil, edrophonium, neostigmine, physostigmine, pyridostigmine, rivastigmine, and tacrine.

Ω-35   **Contraceptives (oral.)** commonly in use include the following combinations: (1) ethinyl estradiol + desogestrel (Apri, Kariva); (2) ethinyl estradiol + drospirenone (Yasmin 28); (3) ethinyl estradiol + etonogestrel (NuvaRing); (4) ethinyl estradiol + levonorgestrel (Aviane, Trivora-28); (5) ethinyl estradiol + norelgestromin (Ortho Evra); (6) ethinyl estradiol + norethindrone (Estrostep Fe, Necon 1/35); (7) ethinyl estradiol + norgestimate (Ortho Tri-Cycle, Sprintec, Trinessa, Tri-Sprintec); and (8) ethinyl estradiol + norgestrel (Low-Ogestrel).

Ω-36   **COX-2 inhibitors** include: celecoxib, rofecoxib (Bextra, Celebrex, Vioxx), and valdecoxib.

Ω-37   **Dopamine agonists** include: apomorphine (APO-go), bromocriptine (Parlodel), cabergoline (Cabaser, Dostinex), pergolide (Celance), pramipexole (Mirapex), and ropinirole (Requip).

Ω-38   **Erectile dysfunction drugs** include: sildenafil (Viagra), tadalafil (Cialis), and vardenafil (Levitra).

Ω-39   **Ergot alkaloids** include: dihydroergocornine, dihydroergocristine, dihydroergocryptine, dihydroergotamine, ergonovine, and ergotamine.

Ω-40   **Estrogens** include: conjugated equine estrogens (Premarin); esterified estrogens (Estratab, Menest); estradiol; estradiol valerate (Estrace); estropipate; ethinyl estradiol; and synthetic conjugated estrogen (Cenestin, Enjuvia).

Ω-41   **Ganglionic blockers** include: mecamylamine and trimethaphan.

Ω-42   **Glucocorticoids** include: beclomethasone, betamethasone, budesonide, clobetasol, cortisol, dexamethasone, flunisolide, fluorometholone, fluticasone, hydrocortisone, methylprednisolone, mometasone, prednisolone, prednisone, and triamcinolone.

Ω-43   **Hemorrhagic drugs** include: cefamandole, cefoperazone, cefotetan, dextrothyroxine (Choloxin); and NSAIDs such as aspirin and phenylbutazone.

Ω-44   **Hepatotoxic drugs** include: acetaminophen, aflatoxins, arsenic, carbon tetrachloride, isoniazid, phenylbutazone, and zidovudine.

Ω-45   **H2 blockers** include: cimetidine (Tagamet), famotidine (Pepcid), nizatidine (Axid), and ranitidine (Zantac).

BTB ↔ Bronchodilators: (*See* Ω-30 in Appendix A.) As bronchodilation is mediated through activation of beta-adrenergic receptors in the bronchial tree, beta blockers can counteract the efficacy of bronchodilators.

BTB ↔ Calcium-Channel Blockers: (*See* Ω-31 in Appendix A.) Both parties have a negative inotropic and chronotropic effect on the heart, and when taken in combination, they may lead to additive or supra-additive effects such as depressed myocardial contractility and slowed atrioventricular conduction speed, possibly resulting in hypotension that can bring about vertigo or syncope.

BTB ↔ Cholinomimetic Drugs: (*See* Ω-34 in Appendix A.) Concurrent intake of a cholinergic drug, having potential to slow cardiac conduction speed, with a beta-adrenergic blocker may cause excessive slowing of impulse conduction at the A-V node.

BTB ↔ Digoxin: Both parties slow the A-V conduction speed and lower the heart rate. When taken together, they may lead to the third-degree AV block, also known as complete heart block.

BTB ↔ Epinephrine: Simultaneous use of epinephrine (Adrenaline) and a non-selective beta blocker can result in a potentially life-threatening hypertensive crisis. This is because the beta blocker cancels out the beta agonistic effect (vasodilation) of epinephrine without affecting its alpha agonistic effect (vasoconstriction), allowing the unmasked alpha effect to cause tremendous vasoconstriction to shoot up the blood pressure.

BTB ↔ Ergot Alkaloids: (*See* Ω-39 in Appendix A.) Both parties favor vasoconstrictions, and co-administration may lead to peripheral ischemia, causing cold extremities and even peripheral gangrene.

BTB ↔ Flecainide: Both parties have a similar effect on the A-V conduction speed, and when used in combination, they may bring in bradycardia, fall of blood pressure, and even atrioventricular blockade.

BTB ↔ Insulin: Concurrent administration of insulin with a beta-adrenergic blocker masks signs of hypoglycemia caused by insulin, since many signs of sympathetic activation triggered by hypoglycemia can be removed by the beta blocker.

BTB ↔ Methyldopa: Patients taking methyldopa and a beta blocker in combination may rarely experience paradoxical hypertensive responses to epinephrine released by excessive physiologic stresses, probably because the beta blocker cancels out the beta agonistic effects of epinephrine (vasodilation) without affecting its alpha agonistic effect (vasoconstriction), permitting the unmasked alpha effects to contribute to the rise of the pressure.

BTB ↔ NSAIDs: (*See* Ω-54 in Appendix A.) The hypotensive effect of beta blockers can be impaired by combined use with an NSAID, as NSAIDs can inhibit the renal excretions of sodium to raise the extracellular fluid (ECF) volume.

BTB ↔ Propantheline: The negative chronotropic (heart rate-slowing) effect of propranolol or other beta blockers may be counteracted by combined use with propantheline, an anticholinergic drug that tends to increase the heart rate.

ADDITIONAL INDIVIDUAL INTERACTIONS: BETA BLOCKERS

Labetalol (LBT) metoprolol (MTP), propranolol (PRP), and sotalol (STL)

LBT ↔ Alpha blockers: (*See* Ω-6 in Appendix A.) Labetalol is unusual in that it has both alpha and beta blocking effects. When the alpha receptors that mediate vasoconstriction are blocked by both labetalol and a pure alpha blocker used in combination, excessive fall of blood pressure may result. In fact, a severe fall of blood pressure is more likely with labetalol than with other pure beta blockers.

MTP ↔ Antithyroid Drugs: Clearance of metoprolol is increased in hyperthyroidism. Therefore, antithyroid drugs such as methimazole and propylthiouracil may reduce clearance of metoprolol to increase its serum concentrations and adverse effects, including excessive fall of blood pressure and lowered heart rate. For this reason, a reduced dose of metoprolol should be considered in such patients.

PRP ↔ Haloperidol: Propranolol may raise blood levels and adverse effects of haloperidol when used in combination. One possible mechanism of this interaction is that haloperidol is at least partially cleared through CYP1A2 and propranolol is inhibitory to this enzyme.

PRP ↔ Lidocaine: Propranolol, unlike most other beta blockers, reduces hepatic blood flow and thereby diminishes hepatic clearance of lidocaine to elevate its blood levels and adverse effects.

PRP ↔ Oral Hypoglycemic Agents: (*See* Ω-55 in Appendix A.) Propranolol delays beta-2-mediated glycogenolysis to slow recovery from hypoglycemia caused by insulin or by oral hypoglycemic agents.

STL ↔ Moxifloxacin: When sotalol and moxifloxacin, both of which tend to cause elongation of the Q-T interval, are taken in combination, a life-threatening ventricular arrhythmia called torsade de pointes may result.

STL ⬌ Succinylcholine: Sotalol prolongs action potential duration, and may prolong muscle relaxation caused by succinylcholine when used in combination.

STL ⬌ Ziprasidone: When these two drugs, both of which tend to cause elongation of the Q-T interval, are taken in combination, they may lead to a life-threatening ventricular arrhythmia.

Beta blockers vs CYP Isozymes

Drug Name	1A2	2A6	2B6	2C8	2C9	2C18	2C19	2D6	2E1	3A4
Bisoprolol								Sub		
Carvedilol								Sub		
Labetalol								Sub + Inh		
Metoprolol								Sub		
Pindolol								Sub		
Propranolol	Sub + Inh				Sub	Sub		Sub	Sub	Sub

1. Acebutolol, atenolol, esmolol, nadolol, and sotalol (all not shown here) either do not interact with cytochrome P450 (CYP) isozymes, or their natures of interaction are not as clearly elucidated as other drugs shown above.

2. Blood concentrations of all the above beta blockers, with possible exception for propranolol, may rise in the presence of any inhibitor of CYP2D6, such as bupropion, fluoxetine, paroxetine, and quinidine. (See left-hand column of Table-0 at the 'Introduction' for other possible inhibitors.)

3. Propranolol has an inhibitory effect on CYP1A2. Co-administration with other drugs that require this enzyme for metabolic clearance may result in elevated blood levels to exacerbate their adverse effects. Examples include: theophylline. (For other possible substrates, See the middle column of Table-0 at the 'Introduction'.)

4. Labetalol is unusual in that it inhibits CYP2D6. Co-administration with drugs that require this enzyme for metabolic clearance may result in elevated blood levels of those unmetabolized drugs to exacerbate their adverse effects. Examples include: imipramine. (For other possible substrates of this enzyme, See the middle column of Table-0 at the 'Introduction'.)

APPENDIX B-2: INTERACTIONS OF ALPHA BLOCKERS

COMMON THEME INTERACTIONS: ALPHA BLOCKERS (ABK)

Alfuzosin, doxazosin, tamsulosin, and terazosin

ABK ↔ Alcohol: Alpha blockers may potentiate the risk of alcohol-induced hypotension, especially in patients who experience flushing during drinking alcohol (those are individuals who are deficient in aldehyde dehydrogenase).

ABK ↔ Blood Pressure Lowering Agents: When an alpha blocker that removes vasoconstriction is taken in conjunction with any other drug that lowers blood pressure, it may lead to an excessive fall in pressure to cause syncope, especially in patients with acute myocardial infarction. Those drugs include: **ACE inhibitors** (*See* Ω-1 in Appendix A), **anesthetic agents** (*See* Ω-9 in Appendix A.), **beta blockers** (*See* Ω-27 in Appendix A), **calcium-channel blockers** (*See* Ω-31 in Appendix A), **ED Drugs** (*See* Ω-38 in Appendix A), **ganglionic blockers** (*See* Ω-41 in Appendix A), **nitroglycerin,** and **vasodilators** (*See* Ω-78 in Appendix A).

ABK ↔ NSAIDs: (*See* Ω-54 in Appendix A.) Non-steroidal anti-inflammatory drugs (NSAIDs) tend to retain sodium and water, and may cause mild elevation in blood pressure. Therefore, they may mitigate the antihypertensive effect of alpha blockers.

Alpha Blockers vs CYP Isozymes

Drug Name	1A2	2A6	2B6	2C8	2C9	2C18	2C19	2D6	2E1	3A4
Alfuzosin										Sub
Doxazosin										Sub
Tamsulosin										Sub

1. All of the alpha blockers depend on the microsomal enzyme CYP3A4 for their elimination. Therefore, inhibition of this enzyme by other drugs taken in combination may impair their metabolism, raising their blood levels and inciting their adverse effects. (*See* the left-hand column of Table-0 at the 'Introduction' for inhibitors of this enzyme.)

2. Terazosin, unlike the above three, is not metabolically processed via hepatic CYP isozymes.

can further the loss of potassium. The resultant hypokalemia may increase the tendency toward cardiac arrhythmia, especially in people taking digoxin (Lanoxin).

TZD ⟷ Lithium: Both hydrochlorothiazide and trichlormethiazide reduce renal clearance of lithium to raise its blood levels and risk of toxicity, such as tremor, and cerebellar ataxia.

TZD ⟷NSAIDs (*See* Ω-54 in Appendix A.) NSAIDs tend to retain sodium and water to counteract the therapeutic efficacy of thiazides in lowering blood pressure.

TZD ⟷ Oral Hypoglycemic Agents (*See* Ω-55 in Appendix A.) Both hydrochlorothiazide and trichlormethiazide can raise blood levels of glucose to impair therapeutic efficiency of oral hypoglycemic agents.

TZD ⟷ Probenecid: Probenecid competes with both hydrochlorothiazide and trichlormethiazide for renal tubular secretions to interfere with their elimination, resulting in elevated blood levels and adverse effects of the thiazide diuretics.

TZD ⟷ Q-T Elongators: Some drugs tend to elongate the QT-interval and this tendency is facilitated by hypokalemia caused by thiazide diuretics. When used in combination, they may pull together toward the life-threatening ventricular arrhythmia of torsade de pointes.

TZD ⟷ (Sennosides): Chronic use of sennosides or hydroxyanthracene glycosides derived from senna leaves, may cause a significant loss of fluid and such electrolytes as sodium and potassium, to further the hypokalemia caused by a thiazide diuretic, and to thereby generate many adverse effects on the heart and the skeletal muscles.

TZD ⟷ Topiramate: Topiramate, an anticonvulsant useful in treating epilepsy and migraine headaches, has a rare tendency to produce hypokalemia. When used in combination with a thiazide diuretic, it may further the loss of serum potassium to invite cardiac arrhythmia.

TZD ⟷ Trimethoprim: Trimethoprim, an inhibitor of renal cationic secretion, can decrease the renal tubular secretions of thiazide diuretics to raise their blood levels and adverse effects.

APPENDIX B-5: INTERACTIONS OF LOOP DIURETICS

COMMON THEME INTERACTIONS: LOOP DIURETICS (LOP)

Bumetanide, ethacrynic acid, and furosemide

Parentheses below indicate an herb.

LOP ⟷ ACE Inhibitors: (*See* Ω-1 in Appendix A.) Loop diuretics shrink ECF volume and thereby potentiate the hypotensive effect of ACE blockers, possibly resulting in an excessive fall of blood pressure.

LOP ⟷ Arginine: Severe hypokalemia caused by a loop diuretic can be counteracted by L-arginine, which raises blood levels of potassium probably by attenuating the secretions of aldosterone from the adrenal cortex.

LOP ⟷ Aminoglycoside Antibiotics: (*See* Ω-7 in Appendix A.) Both loop diuretics (especially ethacrynic acid) and aminoglycoside antibiotics have a tendency to cause ototoxicity, and when used in combination they may pull together toward an additive risk of that toxicity.

LOP ⟷ Aspirin: Aspirin tends to retain sodium and water, and may undercut the blood pressure-lowering effect of loop diuretics.

LOP ⟷ Bile Acid Sequestrants: (*See* Ω-28 in Appendix A.) Cholesterol-lowering anionic exchange resins, such as cholestyramine and colestipol, bind loop diuretics such as bumetanide, ethacrynic acid, and furosemide to reduce their intestinal absorption, and thereby to undercut their therapeutic efficiencies.

LOP ⟷ Chlorthalidone: Both loop diuretics and chlorthalidone can lower blood levels of potassium and magnesium. When used in combination, they may lead to an additional loss of such minerals, to incite cardiac arrhythmia.

LOP ⟷ COX-2 Inhibitors: (*See* Ω-36 in Appendix A.) COX-2 inhibitors, such as celecoxib and rofecoxib (which was withdrawn from the market in the United States in 2004 due to risks of myocardial infarction), tend to retain sodium and water to raise ECF volume. Co-administration of a COX-2 inhibitor with a loop diuretic may undercut the diuretic and antihypertensive efficacies of the loop.

LOP ⟷ Digoxin: Loop diuretics cause loss of blood potassium, leading to hypokalemia, which promotes the arrhythmogenic tendency of digoxin.

VPM ⟷ Dantrolene: Hyperkalemia has been reported following co-administration of dantrolene and verapamil. Hyperkalemia tends to foster myocardial depression, cardiac arrest, and heart block.

VPM ⟷ Digoxin: Verapamil can inhibit digoxin transporter protein to inhibit its urinary excretion with consequent rise of digoxin in circulation. Verapamil may also displace digoxin from its tissue binding sites. The increased blood levels of digoxin may prompt complete heart block.

VPM ⟷ Pramipexole: Verapamil may reduce clearance of pramipexole and stoke its adverse effects. The mechanism behind this interaction is not fully elucidated, but verapamil appears to inhibit P-gp-mediated efflux of pramipexole.

VPM ⟷ Vincristine: Verapamil can inhibit P-gp, a membrane-bound protein that mediates an energy-dependent (ATP hydrolysis) efflux of exogenous substances. When used in combination, verapamil can block efflux of vincristine, a substrate of the transporter, to increase its blood levels and toxicities.

Calcium-Channel Blockers vs CYP Isozymes

Drug Name	1A2	2A6	2B6	2C8	2C9	2C18	2C19	2D6	2E1	3A4
Amlodipine	Inh			Sub	Inh			Inh		Sub Inh
Diltiazem	Inh									Sub Inh
Isradipine										Sub
Nifedipine	Inh									Sub
Nitrendipine										Sub
Verapamil	Sub Inh			Sub Inh	Sub					Sub Inh

1. Amlodipine, diltiazem, and verapamil inhibit the CYP3A4 isoenzyme to cause a reduction in metabolic clearance of CYP3A4 substrates such as amiodarone, atorvastatin, buspirone, cyclosporine, and imipramine to raise their blood concentrations and adverse effects. (See the middle column of Table-0 at the 'Introduction' for other possible substrates of this enzyme.)

2. All the above calcium-channel blockers are processed at least partially through CYP3A4 for clearance. Therefore, inhibition of this enzyme by any other drug taken in combination may raise blood levels of these drugs and possibly exacerbate their adverse effects, with possible exceptions of verapamil and amlodipine, which are both processed by other CYP enzymes as well. (See the left-hand column of Table-0 at the 'Introduction' for inhibitors of this enzyme.)

3. All of the above calcium-channel blockers, except for isradipine and nitrendipine, inhibit CYP1A2. Therefore, administration of any of them in combination with drugs that require this enzyme for metabolic clearance may result in elevated blood levels, possibly inciting their adverse effects. (See the middle column of Table-0 at the 'Introduction' for substrates of the enzyme.)

APPENDIX B-8: INTERACTIONS OF ALPHA AGONISTS

COMMON THEME INTERACTIONS: ALPHA AGONISTS (OPP)

Oxymetazoline, phenylephrine, or **pseudoephedrine**
Oxymetazoline is used as a nasal spray. Phenylephrine is used by injection. Pseudoephedrine is administered orally.

OPP ⟷ Anesthetics: Some anesthetic agents, such as enflurane and halothane, but not desflurane and isoflurane, can sensitize myocardium, potentially causing a cardiac arrhythmia when combined with an alpha agonist.

OPP ⟷Beta Blockers: (*See* Ω-27 in Appendix A.) Vasoconstriction caused by the above drugs may be potentiated by combined use with a beta blocker.

OPP ⟷ Digoxin: Oxymetazoline or pseudoephedrine may somewhat enhance the cardiac arrhythmia caused by a digitalis glycoside, such as digoxin.

OPP ⟷ Ergot alkaloids: (*See* Ω-39 in Appendix A.) The risk for vasoconstriction leading to cerebral ischemia or ischemia of the extremities is increased by concurrent use of an alpha agonist and an ergot alkaloid.

OPP ⟷ MAO Inhibitors: (*See* Ω-51 in Appendix A.) All of the above alpha agonists need the enzyme monoamine oxidase (MAO) for their inactivation in the liver. Therefore, if any of them is used in combination with an MAO inhibitor, hypertensive crisis may ensue.

OPP ⟷ Midodrine: The use of any of the above alpha-agonists may enhance the pressor effects of midodrine, a medication useful to treat postural hypotension, and may cause alarming hypertensive responses.

OPP ⟷ Sodium Bicarbonate: If urine is made alkaline in pH, such as by administration of sodium bicarbonate, the urinary excretions of pseudoephedrine, a strongly basic drug, will be decreased, elevating its blood levels to sustain longer-lasting therapeutic and adverse effects.

APPENDIX B-9: INTERACTIONS OF PROTEASE INHIBITORS

COMMON THEME INTERACTIONS: PROTEASE INHIBITORS (PRI)

Amprenavir, atazanavir, fosamprenavir, indinavir, lopinavir, nelfinavir, rito-navir, saquinavir, and **tipranavir;** where fosamprenavir (Lexiva, Telzir) is a phosphate ester prodrug of amprenavir.

PRI ⟷ Didanosine: Gastrointestinal absorption of amprenavir, atazanavir, or fosamprenavir tends to be reduced by combination with didanosine, since it is buffered with calcium carbonate and magnesium hydroxide to prevent its gastric degradation. To avoid this, take the above drugs two hours before or one hour after didanosine.

PRI ⟷ Gastric pH Raisers: Elevated gastric pH may reduce absorption of amprenavir, atazanavir, fosamprenavir , and tipranavir. Those pH-raisers include: **gastric antacids** (*See* Ω-11 in Appendix Box-A); **H2 blockers** (*See* Ω-45 in Appendix A); and **proton-pump inhibitors** (*See* Ω-61 in Appendix A). To avoid this problem, separate administration by at least two hours.

PRI ⟷ High-Fat Meal: A high-fat meal substantially increases gastrointestinal absorption of saquinavir, lopinavir, nelfinavir, and tipranavir, but reduces absorption of amprenavir and indinavir.

ADDITIONAL INDIVIDUAL INTERACTIONS

Atazanavir (ATZ), fosamprenavir (FSP), indinavir (IDV), and **lopinavir (LPV),** where fosamprenavir (*See* Fig. 78-19) is a prodrug of amprenavir (*See* Fig. 78-20)

ATZ ⟷ Tenofovir: Tenofovir (*See* Fig. 78-13), an analog of adenosine 5'-monophosphate, is not a protease inhibitor, as it inhibits HIV replication by interfering with viral RNA-dependent DNA polymerase. Tenofovir is not metabolized via a hepatic CYP enzyme but is eliminated mainly by tubular secretions largely as unaltered drug. Co-administration with atazanavir results in elevated tenofovir levels, supposedly because some efflux transporter of tenofovir is inhibited by atazanavir, causing its accumulation in the renal proximal tubular cells, leading to nephrotoxicity. An additional possibility raised is that tenofovir may lead to loss of virological response and possible resistance to atazanavir.

APPENDIX B-10: INTERACTIONS OF ANTIHISTAMINES, FIRST-GENERATION

COMMON THEME INTERACTIONS: ANTIHISTAMINES (AHT-1)

Brompheniramine, chlorpheniramine, cyproheptadine, clemastine, dimenhydrinate, diphenhydramine, doxylamine, hydroxyzine, meclizine, promethazine, pyrilamine, and triprolidine

AHT-1 ⬌ Agents Causing Drowsiness: All of the above first-generation antihistamines have drowsiness as a side effect. Because of possible additive CNS depressions such as extreme drowsiness and dizziness, avoid taking any of the above with an agent that also causes CNS depression. Those drugs include: **alcohol, alpha-2 activators** (*See* Ω-4 in Appendix A), **benzodiazepine antianxiety drugs** (*See* Ω-26 in Appendix A), **narcotic analgesics** (*See* Ω-52 in Appendix A), **sedative/hypnotic drugs** (*See* Ω-65 in Appendix A), and **tricyclic antidepressants** (*See* Ω-76 in Appendix A).

AHT-1 ⬌Anticholinergic Agents: (*See* Ω-14 in Appendix A.) All of the above first-generation antihistamines have a potential anticholinergic action, and combined use with an authentic anticholinergic agent can bring about severe anticholinergic adverse effects such as mydriasis, diplopia, tachycardia, pyrexia, loss of coordination, and urinary retention.

AHT-1 ⬌ Azelastine: Concurrent use of any of the above first generation antihistamines with azelastine, a second generation antihistamine having some sedations, especially at high doses, can further the sedating effect of the first antihistamine.

AHT-1 ⬌ MAO Inhibitors: (*See* Ω-51 in Appendix A.) Prolonged and intensified anticholinergic effects of the above first-generation antihistamines may ensue if any of them is taken with an MAO inhibitor. Two weeks separation between the two is recommended.

AHT-1 ⬌ Sodium Nitroprusside: All of the above first-generation antihistamines have a tendency to lower blood pressure. To avoid severe fall of blood pressure, avoid taking any of them in conjunction with sodium nitroprusside, a rapid-acting vasodilator.

AHT-1 ⬌ Tramadol: If tramadol is taken with a first-generation antihistamine, such as diphenhydramine or doxylamine, an alarming CNS depression may ensue, causing severe respiratory depression.

ADDITIONAL INDIVIDUAL INTERACTIONS

Cyproheptadine (CPH) and **promethazine (PRM)**

CPH ⟷ Fluoxetine: Cyproheptadine is unusual in that it is not only an antagonist at histamine receptors but also at serotonin receptors. When it is taken with fluoxetine, an antidepressant that works by blocking reuptake of serotonin, its therapeutic power may be nullified.

PRM ⟷ Epinephrine: Hypotension associated with overdoses of promethazine should not be treated with epinephrine because promethazine has an alpha-adrenergic blocking side effect that can unmask the beta agonistic effect (vasodilation) of epinephrine to reverse its vasopressor effect at high doses (so-called epinephrine reversal), leading to serious fall of blood pressure.

PRM ⟷ MAO Inhibitors: (*See* Ω-51 in Appendix A.) Don't take promethazine in conjunction with any drug that inhibits MAO because it will increase the incidence of extrapyramidal side effects of promethazine.

Antihistamines vs CYP Isozymes

Drug Name	1A2	2A6	2B6	2C8	2C9	2C18	2C19	2D6	2E1	3A4
Brompheniramine								Inh		
Chlorpheniramine								Sub + Inh		Sub
Clemastine								Inh		
Diphenhydramine							Sub	Sub + Inh		
Hydroxyzine								Inh		
Promethazine								Sub		

Abbreviations: Sub, substrate of the enzyme; Inh, inhibits the enzyme; Ezi, induces the enzyme

1. Cyproheptadine, doxylamine, meclizine, pyrilamine, and triprolidine (not shown), either do not interact with CYP isozymes, or their natures of interaction are not as clearly elucidated as other drugs shown above.

2. All of the above antihistamines except promethazine inhibit the enzyme CYP2D6. Administration in combination with drugs that require this enzyme for metabolic clearance may result in their elevated blood levels to exacerbate their adverse effects. (*See* the middle column of Table-0 at the 'Introduction' for possible substrates of this enzyme.)

3. As promethazine requires CYP2D6 for its metabolic clearance, inhibition of this enzyme by any other drug taken in combination may raise blood levels of promethazine to possibly exacerbate its adverse effects. (*See* the left-hand column of Table-0 at the 'Introduction' for possible inhibitors of the enzyme.)

APPENDIX B-11: INTERACTIONS OF ANTIHISTAMINES, SECOND-GENERATION

COMMON THEME INTERACTIONS: ANTIHISTAMINES, SECOND-GENERATION (AHT-2)

Azelastine, cetirizine, fexofenadine, desloratadine, and **loratadine**

AHT-2 ←→ Alcohol: Second-generation antihistamines have little or no sedation, but because of a possible additive effect avoid taking ethanol concomitantly, especially with azelastine.

ADDITIONAL INDIVIDUAL INTERACTIONS

Azelastine (AZT), cetirizine (CTZ), and **fexofenadine (FXF)**

AZT ←→ Antihistamines (*See* Ω-19 in Appendix A) Concurrent use of azelastine with any first-generation antihistamines, such as triprolidine, may generate additive anticholinergic and sedative effects.

CTZ ←→ Theophylline: Theophylline caused some decrease in the clearance of cetirizine, but no such evidence exists for azelastine, desloratadine, loratadine, or fexofenadine.

FXF ←→ Antacids: (*See* Ω-11 in Appendix A.) Gastric antacids, such as aluminum hydroxide and magnesium hydroxide, may inhibit intestinal absorption of fexofenadine but does not significantly inhibit azelastine, cetirizine, or loratadine.

Antihistamines, Second-Generation vs CYP Isozymes

Drug Name	1A2	2A6	2B6	2C8	2C9	2C18	2C19	2D6	2E1	3A4
Azelastine								Sub		Sub
Desloratadine										Sub
Fexofenadine										Sub
Loratadine							Inh	Sub		Sub

Abbreviations: Sub, substrate of the enzyme; Inh, inhibits the enzyme; Ezi, induces the enzyme

1. Cetirizine (not shown) either does not interact with CYP isozymes, or its nature of interaction is not as clearly elucidated as other drugs shown above

2. Since desloratadine and fexofenadine require CYP3A4 for clearance, inhibition of this enzyme by any other drug taken in combination may raise their blood levels to possibly exacerbate their adverse effects. (*See* the left-hand column of Table-0 at the 'Introduction' for possible inhibitors of this enzyme).

APPENDIX B-12: INTERACTIONS OF ATYPICAL ANTIPSYCHOTIC DRUGS

COMMON THEME INTERACTIONS: ATYPICAL ANTIPSYCHOTIC DRUGS (APS)

Aripiprazole, clozapine, olanzapine, quetiapine, risperidone, and sertindole

APS ↔ Alcohol: Do not use any of the above drugs in combination with alcohol or other CNS depressants, as it could lead to severe neuronal depression. Those drugs include: benzodiazepines, carbamazepine, and tricyclic antidepressants.

APS ↔ Anticholinergic Agents: (*See* Ω-14 in Appendix A.) Among the above drugs, clozapine, olanzapine, and risperidone have a significant anticholinergic effect, and if taken in combination with an authentic anticholinergic agent, a potentiated anticholinergic symptoms may be generated. Note that quetiapine has minimal anticholinergic effect, and aripiprazole has little or no anticholinergic effect.

APS ↔ Antihypertensive Drugs: (*See* Ω-20 in Appendix A.) Antihypertensive drugs may cause excessive fall of blood pressure when used in combination with atypical antipsychotics.

APS ↔ Bone Marrow Depressants: (*See* Ω-29 in Appendix A.) Do not use clozapine, olanzapine, or risperidone in combination with a drug known to depress bone marrow, to avoid the risk of severe myelosuppression.

ADDITIONAL INDIVIDUAL INTERACTIONS: ATYPICAL ANTIPSYCHOTIC DRUGS

Clozapine (CLZ) and olanzapine (OZP)

CLZ ↔ Lithium: Co-administration of clozapine with lithium may generate neuroleptic malignant syndrome, which will consist of neurologic emergency in most cases with symptoms such as tremors, involuntary muscle movements, confusion, and seizure. The mechanism behind this observation remains unclear.

CLZ ↔ Risperidone: Risperidone may increase the blood levels and adverse effects of clozapine used in combination. One possible mechanism of this interaction is that clozapine is at least partially cleared through CYP2D6, an enzyme inhibited by risperidone.

OZP ↔ Alpha-2 Activators: (*See* Ω-4 in Appendix A.) Since olanzapine itself has a potential for causing hypotension, its co-administration with an alpha-2 activator may possibly bring about a severe fall of blood pressure.

OZP ⟷ Dopamine Agonists: (*See* Ω-37 in the Box-A at Appendix A.) Olanzapine is an antagonist at both serotonin receptors and dopamine receptors. When used in combination with a dopamine receptor agonist useful in the treatment of Parkinson disease, it may reverse the therapeutic actions of the latter.

OZP ⟷ Epinephrine: As olanzapine has a moderate alpha-adrenergic blocking effect, it may unmask the vasodilating beta-agonistic effect of epinephrine to result in serious fall of blood pressure.

OZP ⟷ Terazosin: Because olanzapine may lower blood pressure, its co-administration with terazosin, an alpha blocker, may result in excessive hypotension.

Atypical Antipsychotics vs CYP Isozymes

Drug Name	1A2	2A6	2B6	2C8	2C9	2C18	2C19	2D6	2E1	3A4
Aripiprazole							Sub	Sub		Sub
Clozapine	Sub + Inh						Sub	Sub + Inh		Sub
Olanzapine	Sub + Inh						Sub	Sub		
Quetiapine								Sub		Sub
Risperidone								Sub + Inh		Sub
Sertindole								Sub + Inh		Sub + Inh

Abbreviations: Sub, substrate of the enzyme; Inh, inhibits the enzyme; Ezi, induces the enzyme

1. Estrogens in oral contraceptives are partially metabolized by CYP3A4, the same enzyme that is at least partially involved in clearance of all of the above drugs except olanzapine. When taken together, they may compete with each other for the same enzyme for metabolic clearance, resulting in increased plasma concentrations and adverse effects of those above drugs.

2. Both clozapine and olanzapine have an inhibitory effect on CYP1A2 and therefore, administration of either in combination with drugs that require this enzyme for metabolic clearance may result in their elevated blood levels to possibly exacerbate their adverse effects. (*See* the middle column of Table-0 at the 'Introduction' for possible substrates of the enzyme.)

3. Clozapine, risperidone, and sertindole have an inhibitory effect on CYP2D6. Thus, co-administration with drugs that require this enzyme for metabolic clearance may result in their elevated blood levels, inciting their adverse effects. (*See* the middle column of Table-0 at the 'Introduction' for possible substrates of the enzyme.)

4. Sertindole exerts an inhibitory effect on both CYP2D6 and CYP3A4 (unique here). Therefore, administration in combination with drugs that require these enzymes for metabolic clearance may result in their elevated blood levels to exacerbate their adverse effects. (*See* the middle column of Table-0 at the 'Introduction' for possible substrates of these enzymes.)

APPENDIX B-13: INTERACTIONS OF MACROLIDE ANTIBIOTICS

COMMON THEME INTERACTIONS: MACROLIDE ANTIBIOTICS (MAB)

Azithromycin, clarithromycin, erythromycin, and **telithromycin**

MAB ⟷ Chloramphenicol: Any of the above macrolide antibiotics may compete with chloramphenicol for binding to the same 50S subunit of bacterial ribosomes, antagonizing the antibacterial effect of chloramphenicol. Thus, it is advised to separate their times of administration.

MAB ⟷ Clindamycin: Any of the above macrolide antibiotics may compete with clindamycin for binding to the same 50S subunit of bacterial ribosomes, antagonizing the antibacterial effect of clindamycin. Thus, it is prudent to avoid administering these drugs in combination.

MAB ⟷ Lincomycin: Any of the above macrolide antibiotics may compete with lincomycin for binding to the same 50S subunit of bacterial ribosomes, antagonizing the antibacterial effect of lincomycin. Therefore, it is advised to separate their times of administration.

ADDITIONAL INDIVIDUAL INTERACTIONS

Azithromycin (AZM) and **erythromycin (ERM)**

AZM ⟷ Antacids: (*See* Ω-11 in Appendix A.) Antacids containing aluminum or magnesium decrease peak azithromycin blood levels, to undermine its therapeutic efficiency.

AZM ⟷ Digoxin: Co-administration of azithromycin with digoxin may increase digoxin levels and its toxicities. It may be due to azithromycin-induced inhibition of P-gp proteins that promote efflux of digoxin in the intestine and kidney.

AZM ⟷ Doxorubicin: It appears that azithromycin inhibits binding of doxorubicin to the efflux P-gp so as to elevate its blood levels and overcome resistance of tumor cells to doxorubicin.

AZM ⟷ Nelfinavir: Co-administration of azithromycin with nelfinavir results in elevated serum levels of azithromycin to exacerbate its adverse effects. Since azithromycin does not interact with CYP isozymes, inhibition of P-gp by nelfinavir is thought responsible for this observation.

AZM ⟷ Tetracycline Antibiotics: (*See* Ω-72 in Appendix A.) The bactericidal effect of azithromycin can be diminished by combined use with tetracyclines, bacteriostatic drugs.

ERM ⟷ Colchicine: Erythromycin used in combination may increase the serum levels and the risk of toxicity of colchicine. One possible mechanism of this interaction is that colchicine is cleared through CYP3A4, and this enzyme is inhibited by erythromycin.

ERM ⟷Pimozide: Erythromycin used in combination may raise blood levels and cardiotoxicity of pimozide as evidenced by prolongation of the Q-T interval. One possible mechanism of this interaction is that pimozide is mainly cleared through CYP3A4, and erythromycin is inhibitory to this enzyme.

ERM ⟷ Thiazide Diuretics (*See* Ω-73 in Appendix A.) Erythromycin tends to elongate the Q-T interval, and when used in combination with thiazide diuretics that cause hypokalemia, it may predispose patients to torsade de pointes, a life-threatening ventricular arrhythmia.

Macrolide Antibiotics vs CYP Isozymes

Drug Name	1A2	2A6	2B6	2C8	2C9	2C18	2C19	2D6	2E1	3A4
Azithromycin										Inh
Clarithromycin	Inh									Sub + Inh
Erythromycin	Sub + Inh									Sub + Inh
Telithromycin										Sub + Inh

Abbreviations: Sub, substrate of the enzyme; Inh, inhibits the enzyme; Ezi, induces the enzyme

1. Clarithromycin and telithromycin requires CYP3A4 for metabolic clearance. Thus, inhibition of this enzyme by drugs taken in combination can raise blood levels of these two drugs to possibly exacerbate their adverse effects. (*See* the left-hand column of Table-0 at the 'Introduction' for possible inhibitors of the enzyme.)

2. All above drugs exert an inhibitory effect on CYP3A4 and hence administration in combination with other drugs that require this enzyme for metabolic clearance may result in elevated blood levels to incite their adverse effects. (*See* the middle column of Table-0 at the 'Introduction' for possible substrates of the enzyme).

3. Clarithromycin and erythromycin exert an inhibitory effect on CYP1A2. Therefore, administration of either in combination with drugs that require this enzyme for metabolic clearance may result in elevated blood levels and incite their adverse effects. (*See* the middle column of Table-0 at the 'Introduction' for possible substrates of the enzyme.)

APPENDIX B-17: INTERACTIONS OF CEPHALOSPORINS

COMMON THEME INTERACTIONS: CEPHALOSPORINS (CPS)

Cefaclor, cefamandole, cefdinir, cefotetan, cefoxitin, cefpodoxime, cefprozil, ceftibuten, ceftriaxone, cefuroxime, and cephalexin

CPS ⟷ Aminoglycoside Antibiotics: (*See* Ω-7 in Appendix A.) All of the above cephalosporins, except for cefamandole and cefoxitin, have a potential for nephrotoxicity. The risk of nephrotoxicity tends to be increased by combined use with any aminoglycoside antibiotics, such as gentamicin and tobramycin.

CPS ⟷ Antacids: (*See* Ω-11 in Appendix A.) Gastric antacids, such as aluminum hydroxide and magnesium hydroxide, may decrease intestinal absorption of cefuroxime, cefdinir, cefpodoxime, cephalexin, and, to a lesser degree, cefaclor. The bioavailability of cefprozil, unlike all others above, was not affected when was administered five minutes following an antacid.

CPS ⟷ Contraceptives (Oral) (*See* Ω-35 in Appendix A.) In common with other antibiotics, all the above cephalosporins tend to oppose intestinal reabsorption of estrogens to result in reduced effectiveness of the estrogens contained in oral contraceptive pills.

CPS ⟷ Loop Diuretics: (*See* Ω-49 in Appendix A.) All of the above cephalosporins, except for cefamandole and cefoxitin, have a potential for nephrotoxicity. Risk of nephrotoxicity is increased by combined use with a loop diuretic, such as ethacrynic acid or furosemide. The mechanism behind this observation remains unclear.

CPS ⟷ Methotrexate: Renal excretion of methotrexate, an anticancer drug, is impaired by combined use with an organic acid such as the above cephalosporins antibiotics.

CPS ⟷ Penicillins: (*See* Ω-56 in Appendix A.) Patients known to be allergic to penicillins should avoid taking cefuroxime or cephalexin, since some patients may have allergic reactions (potentially even anaphylaxis) to these cephalosporins.

CPS ⟷ Probenecid: Renal excretions of cefamandole, cefdinir, cefotetan, cefprozil, ceftibuten, and cefuroxime are known to be impaired by combined use with probenecid, to result in elevated plasma concentrations and increased adverse effects of them. However, probenecid delayed, but did not diminish, renal excretion of cefoxitin.

ADDITIONAL INDIVIDUAL INTERACTIONS: CEPHALOSPORINS

Cefamandole, cefoperazone, cefotetan, cefoxitin, and **ceftriaxone (CFO);** and **Cephalexin (CFL)**

CFO ⟷ Anticoagulants: (*See* Ω-16 in Appendix A.) Concurrent use of cefamandole with heparin, dalteparin, enoxaparin, warfarin, or any other anticoagulant may increase the risk of bleeding.

CFO ⟷ Thrombolytic Agents: (*See* Ω74 in Appendix A.) Concurrent use of cefamandole with any thrombolytic agent may increase the risk of excessive bleeding.

CFL ⟷ Metformin: If cephalexin is coadministered with metformin, an oral antidiabetic drug, the former decreases renal clearance of the latter to increase blood levels and adverse effects of metformin.

APPENDIX B-18: INTERACTIONS OF GASTRIC ANTACIDS

COMMON THEME INTERACTIONS: GASTRIC ANTACIDS (ACC)

Aluminum hydroxide and calcium carbonate

ACC ⟷ Digoxin: Aluminum hydroxide or calcium carbonate taken in combination with digoxin may decrease intestinal absorption of digoxin. However, if blood levels of calcium are elevated by calcium carbonate, the likelihood of cardiac arrhythmia caused by digoxin may increase.

ACC ⟷ Drugs Requiring Acidic pH For Absorption: Both aluminum hydroxide and calcium carbonate can neutralize acidity of stomach fluid to decrease intestinal absorption of many drugs. Those drugs that require acidic pH for their best absorption include: **allopurinol** (an antigout drug); **atazanavir** (an anti-HIV drug whose solubility decreases as gastric pH increases); **cyanocobalamin (vitamin B-12); delavirdine** (an anti-HIV drug whose solubility decreases as gastric pH increases above 3); **diazepam; gefitinib** (a lung cancer drug whose absorption decreases if gastric pH rises above 5); **glucocorticoids** (*See* Ω-42 in Appendix A); **isoniazid** (an antituberculotic drug); **iron salts; itraconazole** (an antifungal drug whose absorption requires gastric acidity); **ketoconazole** (an antifungal drug whose absorption requires gastric acidity); **penicillamine** (a metal chelator); **phenothiazine antipsychotic drugs** (*See* Ω-58 in Appendix A); **phenytoin** (an antiepileptic drug); **protease inhibitors** (*See* Ω-59 in Appendix A) such as amprenavir, atazanavir, fosamprenavir, and tipranavir; **quinolone antibiotics** such as ciprofloxacin, levofloxacin, norfloxacin, and ofloxacin; and **tetracyclines** such as doxycycline , minocycline, and tetracycline.

ADDITIONAL INDIVIDUAL INTERACTIONS:

Aluminum hydroxide (AHD) and calcium carbonate (CBN)

AHD ⟷ Sodium Polystyrene Sulfonate: If sodium polystyrene sulfonate is administered with a cation-donating antacid such as aluminum hydroxide, it engenders systemic alkalosis that may bring about seizures.

CBN ⟷ Alendronate: Calcium is known to interfere with the absorption of alendronate, a drug approved to treat osteoporosis.

CBN ⟷ Aminoglycoside Antibiotic (*See* Ω-7 in Appendix A.) Being a cationic drug, calcium carbonate can dilute the intracellular negative charge of bacteria, the driving force for an aminoglycoside antibiotic to enter the cell, thereby diminishing its antibacterial effect.

CBN ⟷ Cholesterol-Lowering Resins: Normal calcium absorption from the intestine is impaired by combined use with a cholesterol-lowering resin such as cholestyramine or colestipol.

CBN ⟷ Estrogens: (*See* Ω-40 in Appendix A.) In the treatment of osteoporosis, taking calcium with estrogens may improve mineralization of the bones, leading to increased bone density.

CBN ⟷ Thiazide Diuretics: (*See* Ω-73 in Appendix A.) Thiazide diuretics, such as hydrochlorothiazide, promote reabsorption of calcium in the kidney to raise its blood levels. When used in combination, calcium carbonate may quicken the rise of calcium levels caused by the diuretics.

APPENDIX B-19: INTERACTIONS OF MAGNESIUM SALTS

COMMON THEME INTERACTIONS: MAGNESIUM SALTS (MHC)

Magnesium hydroxide and **magnesium citrate**

MHC ⟷ Aminoglycoside Antibiotics: (*See* Ω-7 in Appendix A.) Being a cationic drug, magnesium salts can dilute the intracellular negative charge of bacteria, the driving force for aminoglycoside antibiotics to enter the bacterial cell, and thus can diminish their antibacterial effect. Besides, magnesium salts can cause neuromuscular blockade to potentiate the neuromuscular blocking side effect of aminoglycoside antibiotics.

MHC ⟷ Antibiotics: (*See* Ω-62 in Appendix A for quinolone antibiotics, and Ω-72 for tetracycline antibiotics.) Magnesium tends to impair intestinal absorption of both quinolone antibiotics such as ciprofloxacin and moxifloxacin; and tetracycline antibiotics such as doxycycline, minocycline, and tetracycline. Therefore, magnesium should be taken two to four hours before or after taking these medications, to prevent interference with their absorptions.

MHC ⟷ Calcium-Channel Blockers: (*See* Ω-31 in Appendix A.) Co-administration of a magnesium salt with a calcium-channel blocker such as verapamil may prove unwise, as it may increase unpleasant side effects of the calcium-channel blocker such as dizziness, nausea, and fluid retention.

MHC ⟷ Digoxin: Magnesium hydroxide taken with digoxin can undercut the effectiveness of the digitalis, because elevated serum levels of magnesium counteract calcium ions required for the improved cardiac contractility by digoxin.

MHC ⟷ Diuretics: (*See* Ω-49 in Appendix A for loop diuretics and Ω-73 for thiazide diuretics.) The diuretics tend to deplete magnesium ions, and symptoms of magnesium deficiency include: muscle tremors or twitching, fatigue, irritability, and insomnia. Therefore, it is suggested to prescribe a powerful diuretic together with a supplementary dose of magnesium.

MHC ⟷ Iron Salts: Magnesium hydroxide may neutralize acidity of the stomach to decrease intestinal absorption of iron salts.

MHC ⟷ Ketoconazole: Absorption of ketoconazole, an antifungal drug, requires normal acidic pH of the stomach, and when acidity is diluted by magnesium hydroxide, the absorption of ketoconazole is destined to decrease.

MHC ↔ Neuromuscular Blockers: (*See* Ω-53 in Appendix A.) Magnesium can cause neuromuscular blockade and can potentiate effects of authentic neuromuscular blockers to lead to respiratory paralysis.

MHC ↔ Nitrofurantoin: Magnesium salts decrease both the rate and extent of intestinal absorption of nitrofurantoin (Macrodantin, Furadantin, others), an antibiotic agent.

MHC ↔Oral Hypoglycemic Agents: (*See* Ω-55 in Appendix A.) Magnesium has been shown to increase the rate and extent of absorption of oral antidiabetic drugs such as glipizide and glyburide, increasing their blood levels and promoting their hypoglycemic effect. Furthermore, magnesium appears to enhance tissue sensitivity to insulin.

MHC ↔ Sodium Polystyrene Sulfonate: If sodium polystyrene sulfonate is administered with a cation-donating antacid, such as magnesium hydroxide, it engenders systemic alkalosis that may bring about seizures.

MHC ↔ Terbutaline: Magnesium co-administered with terbutaline, a bronchodilator for asthma patients, can greatly increase the risk of pulmonary edema, heart palpitations, and nervousness, all caused by the latter.

MHC ↔ Tiludronate: Magnesium tends to impair intestinal absorption of tiludronate, a drug used for the treatment of osteoporosis. However, magnesium is known to have a less significant effect on the intestinal absorption of alendronate, another drug used for treatment of osteoporosis.

APPENDIX B-20: INTERACTIONS OF GLUCOCORTICOIDS

COMMON THEME INTERACTIONS: GLUCOCORTICOIDS (GCC)

Beclomethasone, budesonide, clobetasol, dexamethasone, flunisolide, fluorometholone, fluticasone, methylprednisolone, mometasone, prednisolone, prednisone, and triamcinolone

Prednisone is rapidly and almost entirely converted to its active metabolite, prednisolone, in the liver through a non-CYP-mediated pathway.

GCC ⟷ Aluminum Hydroxide: Aluminum hydroxide may neutralize acidity of the stomach to decrease intestinal absorption of glucocorticoids.

GCC ⟷ Amphotericin-B: The above corticosteroids tend to cause depletion of potassium. Therefore, co-administration with amphotericin-B, a potassium-depleting antifungal agent, can lead to excessive hypokalemia.

GCC ⟷ Anticholinesterase Agents: (*See* Ω-15 in Appendix A.) A corticosteroid such as prednisolone may interact with nicotinic receptors at neuromuscular junctions, to diminish effectiveness of anticholinesterase agents, such as neostigmine and pyridostigmine, in the treatment of myasthenia gravis, allowing a profound muscular weakness to continue.

GCC ⟷ Aspirin: Aspirin taken in combination with a glucocorticoid can increase the risk of gastrointestinal bleeding.

GCC ⟷ Calcium Carbonate: Calcium carbonate may neutralize acidity of the stomach to decrease intestinal absorption of glucocorticosteroids.

GCC ⟷ Cyclosporine: If cyclosporine, an immunosuppressant, is used in combination with another immunosuppressant, additive suppression may occur. Such drugs include: glucocorticosteroids.

GCC ⟷ Diuretics: (*See* Ω-49 and Ω-73 in Appendix A.) The above glucocorticoids tend to cause depletion of potassium, and co-administration with a potassium-depleting diuretic, such as furosemide or hydrochlorothiazide, can lead to excessive hypokalemia.

GCC ⟷ Interleukin-2 (IL-2): Glucocorticoids may decrease the antitumor efficacy of IL-2 due to their inhibitory effect on the immune system.

GCC ⟷ NSAIDs: (*See* Ω-54 in Appendix A.) When taken with an NSAID, such as aspirin, ibuprofen or naproxen, all the above corticosteroids can increase the risk of gastrointestinal bleeding.

GCC ⟷ Oral Hypoglycemic Agents: (*See* Ω-55 in Appendix A.) The glucocorticoids mentioned above increase concentrations of blood glucose, undercutting the therapeutic effectiveness of antidiabetic drugs.

Glucocorticoids vs CYP Isozymes

Drug Name	1A2	2A6	2B6	2C8	2C9	2C18	2C19	2D6	2E1	3A4
Beclomethasone										Sub
Budesonide										Sub
Clobetasol										Sub
Dexamethasone		Ezi		Ezi				Ezi		Sub
Flunisolide										Sub
Fluticasone										Sub
Methylprednisolone										Sub
Mometasone										Sub
Prednisolone										Sub
Prednisone							Ezi			Sub
Triamcinolone										Sub

Abbreviations: Sub, substrate of the enzyme; Inh, inhibits the enzyme; Ezi, induces the enzyme

1. Fluorometholone (not shown), unlike all of the others above, is either not processed through any CYP enzymes or its relationship with CYP is not fully elucidated.
2. Metabolic clearance of all of the above glucocorticoids requires the presence of microsomal CYP3A4. Therefore, inhibition of this enzyme by any other drug taken in combination, such as an azole antifungal drug, may raise blood levels of the above drugs to possibly exacerbate their adverse effects. (*See* the left-hand column of Table-0 at the 'Introduction' for other possible inhibitors of this enzyme.)
3. Dexamethasone and albendazole both require the enzyme CYP3A4 for their clearance. Thus, concurrent administration may cause competition for the same enzyme for clearance, possibly resulting in elevated blood levels of unmetabolized albendazole that might incite its adverse effects.
4. Note that dexamethasone induces more than one CYP enzyme, quickening metabolic clearance of the drugs that depend on these enzymes.
5. Only prednisone induces CYP2C19. Therefore, co-administration with drugs requiring this enzyme for metabolic clearance may quicken their elimination, resulting in lowered blood levels and therapeutic effectiveness. (*See* the middle column of Table-0 at the 'Introduction' for possible substrates of this enzyme.)

APPENDIX B-21: INTERACTIONS OF H2 BLOCKERS

COMMON THEME INTERACTIONS: H2 BLOCKERS (H2B)

Cimetidine, famotidine, nizatidine, and ranitidine

Parentheses below indicate an herb.

H2B ⟷ Drugs Requiring Acidic pH For Absorption: H2 blockers suppress normal secretions of acid by parietal cells to dilute acidity of the stomach fluid, thereby decreasing the intestinal absorption of many drugs. Those drugs include: **allopurinol** (an antigout drug); **atazanavir** (an anti-HIV drug whose solubility decreases as gastric pH increases); **cyanocobalamin (vitamin B-12); delavirdine** (an anti-HIV drug whose solubility decreases as gastric pH increases above 3); **diazepam; gefitinib** (a drug used for lung cancer, whose absorption decreases if the gastric pH rises above 5); **glucocorticoids** (*See* Ω-42 in Appendix A); **isoniazid** (an antituberculotic drug); i**ron salts; itraconazole** (an antifungal drug whose absorption requires gastric acidity); **ketoconazole** (an antifungal drug whose absorption requires gastric acidity); **penicillamine** (a metal chelator); **phenothiazine antipsychotic drugs** (*See* Ω-58 in Appendix A); **phenytoin** (an antiepileptic drug); **protease inhibitors** (*See* Ω-59 in Appendix A) such as amprenavir and atazanavir; **quinolone antibiotics** such as ciprofloxacin, levofloxacin, norfloxacin, and ofloxacin; and **tetracyclines** such as doxycycline, minocycline, and tetracycline.

H2B ⟷ (Turmeric): If turmeric (*See* Fig. 54-5) is taken orally, it increases the production of stomach acid to counteract effectiveness of such H2 receptor blockers as cimetidine (Tagamet), famotidine (Pepcid), nizatidine (Axid), and ranitidine (Zantac).

ADDITIONAL INDIVIDUAL INTERACTIONS
Cimetidine (CMT)

CMT ⟷ Carmustine: Co-administration of cimetidine and carmustine enhances the bone marrow depressant effect of carmustine. The mechanism of this interaction is unclear.

CMT ⟷ Lomustine: Co-administration of cimetidine and lomustine enhances the bone marrow depressant effects of lomustine. The mechanism of this interaction is unclear.

CMT ⟷ Gabapentin: Gabapentin is not highly metabolized by the microsomal CYP enzymes. Thus, inhibitors of CYP have little effect on its metabolic clearance. However, cimetidine was shown to reduce renal clearance of gabapentin to elevate its serum levels and adverse effects.

CMT ⟷ Pramipexole: Cimetidine may inhibit the renal excretion of pramipexole, leading to increased plasma levels and adverse effects.

H2 Blockers vs CYP Isozymes

Drug Name	1A2	2A6	2B6	2C8	2C9	2C18	2C19	2D6	2E1	3A4
Cimetidine	Inh			Inh	Inh	Inh	Inh	Inh	Inh	Inh
Famotidine	Inh									
Ranitidine	Inh							Inh		Inh

1. Nizatidine (not shown) either does not interact with CYP isozymes, or its natures of interaction are not as clearly elucidated as other drugs shown above.
2. As cimetidine inhibits so many CYP enzymes, its co-administration with drugs that require those enzymes may interrupt their metabolic clearance, leading to increased blood levels and adverse effects. Examples include: procainamide, lidocaine, verapamil, and warfarin. (See the middle column of Table-0 at the 'Introduction' for other possible substrates of these enzymes.)
3. Famotidine exerts an inhibitory effect on CYP1A2 only, and administration in combination with drugs that require this enzyme for metabolic clearance may result in elevated blood levels to stir up their adverse effects. (See the middle column of Table-0 at the 'Introduction' for possible substrates of this enzyme.)
4. Ranitidine was shown to increase the serum levels of procainamide (a substrate of CYP2D6) and increase the risk of its adverse effects.

PPX ⟷ Cimetidine: Pramipexole is not highly metabolized by microsomal CYP enzymes, but is mainly eliminated via renal tubular secretion. Cimetidine, a known inhibitor of renal tubular secretion, may compete with pramipexole for renal clearance, elevating its blood levels and increasing the incidence of adverse effects.

PPX ⟷ Diltiazem: When used in combination, diltiazem, which is eliminated via cationic renal secretion, may compete with pramipexole for renal clearance, to elevate its blood levels and increase its adverse effects.

PPX ⟷ Quinidine: Quinidine, which is eliminated via cationic renal secretion, can elevate blood levels and adverse effects of pramipexole, probably by interrupting its renal clearance.

PPX ⟷ Ranitidine: Pramipexole is not highly metabolized by microsomal CYP enzymes, as its main route of its elimination is via renal tubular secretion. Ranitidine may compete with pramipexole for renal clearance, elevating its blood levels and increasing its therapeutic and adverse effects.

PPX ⟷ Triamterene: Triamterene taken in combination can compete for renal clearance of pramipexole, to elevate its blood levels and stir up its adverse effects.

RPL ⟷ Levodopa: Ropinirole, when used in combination, may increase the blood levels of levodopa to foster its adverse effect of dyskinesia. The exact mechanism behind this observation is not yet clearly defined.

Dopamine Agonists vs CYP Isozymes

Drug Name	1A2	2A6	2B6	2C8	2C9	2C18	2C19	2D6	2E1	3A4
Bromocriptine	Inh									Inh Sub
Ropinirole	Inh Sub							Inh		

Abbreviations: Sub, substrate of the enzyme; Inh, inhibits the enzyme; Ezi, induces the enzyme

1. Pramipexole (not shown), unlike the other two above, is not highly metabolized by microsomal CYP enzymes.
2. Metabolic clearance of bromocriptine requires the presence of microsomal CYP3A4. Therefore, inhibition of this enzyme by any other drug taken in combination may raise blood levels of bromocriptine to possibly exacerbate its adverse effects. (*See* the left-hand column of Table-0 at the 'Introduction' for possible inhibitors of the enzyme.)
3. Hepatic inactivation of ropinirole requires the presence of microsomal CYP1A2. Therefore, inhibition of this enzyme by any other drug taken in combination may raise blood levels of ropinirole to possibly incite its adverse effects. (*See* the left-hand column of Table-0 at the 'Introduction' for possible inhibitors of the enzyme.)

APPENDIX B-24: INTERACTIONS OF PENICILLINS

COMMON THEME INTERACTIONS: PENICILLINS (PCN)

Amoxicillin, ampicillin, dicloxacillin, and **penicillin V**

PCN ⟷ Allopurinol: Concurrent administration of amoxicillin, ampicillin, or penicillin V with allopurinol substantially increases the incidence of skin rash as compared to patients receiving one of the antibiotics alone. It is not known whether this potentiation of rash is due to allopurinol itself or due to hyperuricemia caused by the above antibiotics in these patients.

PCN ⟷ Antacids: (*See* Ω-11 in Appendix A.) Gastric antacids such as aluminum hydroxide and magnesium hydroxide may decrease intestinal absorption of the above penicillins.

PCN ⟷ Contraceptives (Oral): (*See* Ω-35 in Appendix A.) Amoxicillin, ampicillin, and penicillin V, in common with other broad-spectrum antibiotics, may reduce intestinal reabsorption of estrogens of contraceptive pills, with consequent reduction of their serum concentrations and a possibly failed contraception.

PCN ⟷Epinephrine: One of the best ways to counter a penicillin allergy is injection of 0.2 ml of 0.1% epinephrine by subcutaneous (SC) or intravenous (IV) route, and repeat if no response is obtained in a few minutes. Inhalation of epinephrine is also an option.

PCN ⟷ Methotrexate: Renal excretion of methotrexate is impaired by combined use with an organic acid such as a penicillin.

PCN ⟷ Probenecid: If used in combination, probenecid decreases renal excretions of amoxicillin, ampicillin, and penicillin V, to elevate their blood levels and increase their therapeutic and adverse effects.

PCN ⟷ Proton-Pump Inhibitors: (*See* Ω-61 in Appendix A.) Proton-pump inhibitors block gastric acid pump to raise the gastric pH and thereby enhance absorption of acid-labile antibiotics such as ampicillin, nafcillin, and penicillin, promoting their therapeutic and adverse effects.

PCN ⟷ Tetracycline Antibiotics: (*See* Ω-72 in Appendix A.) A bacteriostatic antibiotic such as tetracycline may antagonize the bactericidal effect of the above penicillins. Therefore, it is prudent to avoid such combination.

APPENDIX B-25: INTERACTIONS OF PHENOTHIAZINE ANTIPSYCHOTIC DRUGS

COMMON THEME INTERACTIONS: PHENOTHIAZINES (PTZ)

Chlorpromazine and **prochlorperazine**

Parentheses below indicate an herb.

PTZ ⟷ Alcohol: Both chlorpromazine and prochlorperazine may enhance CNS depression caused by any sedative agent, including alcohol. Alcohol can also increase the incidence of extrapyramidal adverse effects of both chlorpromazine and prochlorperazine.

PTZ ⟷ Alpha-2 Activators: (*See* Ω-4 in Appendix A.) Both chlorpromazine and prochlorperazine have a hypotensive side effect, and when taken in combination with an alpha-2 activator, it may cause an alarming fall of blood pressure.

PTZ ⟷ Amphetamine or Dextroamphetamine: Dopamine released by amphetamine or dextroamphetamine cannot work on its receptors in the presence of a dopamine-receptor blocker, such as chlorpromazine or prochlorperazine, accounting for insufficient CNS effects of amphetamine and dextroamphetamine.

PTZ ⟷ Antacids: (*See* Ω-11 in Appendix A.) Gastric antacids, such as aluminum hydroxide and calcium carbonate, may neutralize acidity of the stomach to decrease intestinal absorption of phenothiazine antipsychotic drugs.

PTZ ⟷ Anticholinergic Agents: (*See* Ω-14 in the Appendix A.) Both chlorpromazine and prochlorperazine have some anticholinergic side effects. Co-administration of either with other drugs that possess similar effects may generate additive anticholinergic signs such as tachycardia, blurred vision, and, confusion. They should not be used in combination, especially in patients with a narrow-angle glaucoma, where they, by increasing the intraocular pressure, can make it worse.

PTZ ⟷Cevimeline: Concurrent intake of cevimeline, a muscarinic agonist, with chlorpromazine or prochlorperazine, each of which has some antimuscarinic side effects, may offset the therapeutic efficacy of cevimeline.

PTZ ⟷ Dofetilide: Co-administration of prochlorperazine or chlorpromazine with dofetilide (Tikosyn), an antiarrhythmic drug, increases the risk of paradoxical cardiac arrhythmia with elongated Q-T interval.

PTZ ↔ Dopamine Agonist: (*See* Ω-37 in Appendix A.) The clinical effectiveness of such dopamine agonists as bromocriptine and pramipexole may be counteracted by combined use with a dopamine antagonist, such as chlorpromazine or prochlorperazine.

PTZ ↔ Epinephrine: The blood pressure-elevating effect of epinephrine at high doses may be reverted to a blood pressure-lowering effect (so-called epinephrine reversal), if epinephrine is used in combination with a drug that blocks alpha-adrenergic receptors. Those drugs having an alpha blocking effect include: phenothiazines antipsychotic drugs such as chlorpromazine (Thorazine), fluphenazine (*Duraclon*), mesoridazine (Serentil), and perphenazine (Etrafon).

PTZ ↔ (Evening Primrose) Co-administration of prochlorperazine or chlorpromazine with this herb can result in seizures (convulsions). The mechanism behind this observation is yet to be explored.

PTZ ↔ Lithium: Lithium lowers plasma concentrations of chlorpromazine probably by increasing its gut metabolism, while chlorpromazine lowers plasma concentrations of lithium probably by increasing its uptake into RBC, and increasing its renal excretions. When used together they may generate erratic neuronal responses such as confusion, delirium, seizure and disorientation.

PTZ ↔ Loperamide: The tendency toward CNS depression by loperamide, a drug used to treat diarrhea, may possibly be enhanced by combined intake of any phenothiazine antipsychotic drug.

PTZ ↔ MAO Inhibitors: (*See* Ω-51 in Appendix A.) Co-administration of prochlorperazine or chlorpromazine with an MAO inhibitor, such as procarbazine, may result in increased risk of extrapyramidal side effects.

PTZ ↔ Narcotic Analgesics: (*See* Ω-52 in Appendix A.) If any narcotic drug is taken with chlorpromazine or prochlorperazine, it may cause increased risk of respiratory depression, hypotension, and profound sedations that impair driving skills.

PTZ ↔ Piracetam: Piracetam is a drug used to enhance cognition and memory, and may increase the risk of hyperkinesia caused by such antipsychotic drug as chlorpromazine and prochlorperazine when used in combination. The mechanism for this observation is yet to be explored.

PTZ ↔ Sedatives/Hypnotics: (*See* Ω-65 in Appendix A.) Co-administration of a sedative, such as eszopiclone or zaleplon, with a phenothiazine may potentiate CNS depression, causing serious drowsiness and respiratory depression.

PTZ ↔ Tramadol: Inherent side effects of tramadol (Ultram), an analgesic drug, include convulsions, and the risk of this side effect increases when used in combination with prochlorperazine or chlorpromazine. One possibility is that tramadol is at least partially cleared through CYP2D6 and prochlorperazine requires this enzyme for its clearance (generating substrate competition), and this enzyme is inhibited by chlorpromazine.

PTZ ⟷ Tretinoin: Tretinoin topical can interact with a number of drugs to make skin more sensitive to sunlight. They include: phenothiazine antipsychotic drugs such as chlorpromazine (Thorazine), fluphenazine (Permitil, Prolixin), perphenazine (Trilafon), prochlorperazine (Compazine), and promethazine (Phenergan, Promethegan).

PTZ ⟷ Zotepine: Co-administration of prochlorperazine or chlorpromazine with zotepine (Nipolept), an atypical antipsychotic drug, may increase the risk of convulsions. The mechanism behind this observation remains unclear.

ADDITIONAL INDIVIDUAL INTERACTIONS
Chlorpromazine (CPZ) and **prochlorperazine (PCP)**

CPZ ⟷ Diazoxide: Chlorpromazine appears to increase the release of epinephrine from the adrenal medulla, which in turn causes breakdown of glycogen to raise blood glucose levels. Diazoxide, an antihypertensive agent, on the other hand, inhibits the release of insulin from the pancreas to raise blood glucose. When used in combination, they may set the serum glucose level excessively high, requiring increased doses of antidiabetic drugs.

CPZ ⟷ Diuretics (*See* Ω-49 and Ω-73 in Appendix A.) Chlorpromazine tends to elongate the Q-T interval, and when taken together with a thiazide or loop diuretic that induces hypokalemia, it is likely to aggravate the cardiac arrhythmia toward torsade de pointes.

CPZ ⟷ Drugs That Elongate the Q-T Intervals: Chlorpromazine itself tends to elongate the Q-T interval on EKG, and when taken in combination with other drugs that also cause the elongation, it may increase the effect, possibly leading to the life-threatening ventricular arrhythmia of torsade de pointes. Those Q-T elongating drugs include: **amiodarone, bepridil** (a drug for the treatment of chronic stable angina), **clarithromycin, disopyramide, dofetilide** (an antiarrhythmic drug), **domperidone** (a drug used to increase contractility of the stomach and bowel), **erythromycin, halofantrine** (a drug used to treat malaria), **ibutilide** (an antiarrhythmic drug), **pimozide** (an antipsychotic drug), **quinidine,** and **thioridazine** (an antipsychotic drug).

PCP ⟷ Deferoxamine: Combined use of prochlorperazine with deferoxamine (also known as **d**esferrioxamine) may cause transient loss of consciousness lasting up to 72 hours. The neurotoxicity of deferoxamine to ocular tissue may also be enhanced by concurrent use with prochlorperazine.

PCP ⟷ Dofetilide: Prochlorperazine may increase the serum levels of dofetilide probably by inhibiting its active renal transport. The elevated serum levels of dofetilide may bring about paradoxical elongation of the Q-T interval and even the life-threatening torsade de pointes.

PCP ⟷ Irinotecan: When irinotecan, an anticancer drug, was used in combination with prochlorperazine, there was increased incidence of akathisia (a syndrome characterized by inability to sit still) caused by prochlorperazine. The mechanism behind this observation remains unclear.

Phenothiazines vs CYP Isozymes

Drug Name	1A2	2A6	2B6	2C8	2C9	2C18	2C19	2D6	2E1	3A4
Chlorpromazine	Sub				Sub			Sub + Inh		
Prochlorperazine								Sub		

Abbreviations: Sub, substrate of the enzyme; Inh, inhibits the enzyme; Ezi, induces the enzyme

1. Chlorpromazine inhibits CYP2D6. Therefore, co-administration with drugs that require this enzyme for metabolic clearance may result in elevated blood levels and increased adverse effects. (*See* the middle column of Table-0 at the 'Introduction' for possible substrates of the enzyme).

2. Prochlorperazine requires CYP2D6 for its clearance and thus, inhibition of this enzyme by any drug taken in combination may raise blood levels of prochlorperazine to possibly exacerbate its adverse effects. (*See* the left-hand column of Table-0 at the 'Introduction' for possible inhibitors of the enzyme.)

APPENDIX B-26: INTERACTIONS OF PROGESTERONE OR PROGESTOGENS

COMMON THEME INTERACTIONS: PROGESTOGENS (PRG)

Note that progestogens in oral contraceptives may increase the risk of thromboembolic disorders. Their use is usually contraindicated in those with thromboembolism.

PRG ⟷ Azole Antifungal Drugs: (*See* Ω-23 in Appendix A.) The therapeutic effectiveness of progestogens in oral contraceptives may sometimes be undercut by co-administration with azole antifungals, such as fluconazole, itraconazole, and ketoconazole. The mechanism behind this observation remains obscure.

PRG ⟷ Carbamazepine: Carbamazepine, an inducer of CYPA4, increases the metabolic clearance of progestogens, a substrate of CYPA4, with consequent risk of failed contraception, menstrual irregularities, and breakthrough bleeding.

PRG ⟷ Mycophenolate Mofetil: Mycophenolate mofetil can reduce the effectiveness of norethindrone, a progestogen, causing contraceptive failure. Mycophenolate did not affect average serum levels of FSH, LH, and progesterone. The mechanism behind this observation remains unclear.

PRG ⟷ Oral Hypoglycemic Agents: (*See* Ω-55 in Appendix A.) High doses of progestogen increases the risk of hyperglycemia and glucose intolerance in patients with diabetes. Therefore, progestogens can undermine the therapeutic effectiveness of antidiabetic drugs such as glimepiride, glipizide, and tolbutamide.

PRG ⟷ Tetracycline Antibiotics: (*See* Ω-72 in Appendix A.) Tetracyclines may decrease gastrointestinal flora, which may decrease the enterohepatic recycling of contraceptive steroids, undermining the contraceptive effectiveness of progestogens.

Progestogens vs CYP Isozymes

Drug Name	1A2	2A6	2B6	2C8	2C9	2C18	2C19	2D6	2E1	3A4
Drospirenone	Inh									
Medroxyprogesterone										Sub
Norethindrone							Ezi			Sub

Abbreviations: Sub, substrate of the enzyme; Inh, inhibits the enzyme; Ezi, induces the enzyme

1. Except for drospirenone, the above progestogens requires CYP3A4 for metabolic clearance and when used in combination with other substrates of CYP3A4, such as cyclosporine and doxorubicin, they compete for the same enzyme for clearance, resulting in elevated blood levels of unmetabolized cyclosporine and doxorubicin that might incite their adverse effects, such as hepatotoxicity with cyclosporine, and bone marrow depression with doxorubicin. (See the middle column of Table-0 at the 'Introduction' for other possible substrates of this enzyme.) Aminoglutethimide, phenobarbital, rifampin, and (St. John's wort) are known inducers of CYP3A4 and therefore, co-administration with medroxyprogesterone or norethindrone may quicken their elimination to result in lowered blood levels and failed contraceptive effectiveness. (See the right-hand column of Table-0 at the 'Introduction' for other possible inducers of the enzyme.)

2. Only drospirenone inhibits CYP1A2. Therefore, its administration in combination with drugs that require this enzyme for metabolic clearance may result in elevated blood levels to stir up their adverse effects. (See the middle column of Table-0 at the 'Introduction' for possible substrates of this enzyme.)

3. Norethindrone, unlike other progestogens in oral contraceptive pills, can induce CYP2C19 and thus, co-administration with other drugs that are metabolized through this enzyme may result in lowered blood levels and insufficient therapeutic effectiveness. (See the middle column of Table-0 at the 'Introduction' for possible substrates of the enzyme.)

APPENDIX B-27: INTERACTIONS OF PROTON-PUMP INHIBITORS

COMMON THEME INTERACTIONS: PROTON-PUMP INHIBITORS (PPI)

Esomeprazole, lansoprazole, omeprazole, pantoprazole, and **rabeprazole**

Parentheses below indicate an herb.

PPI ⟷ Digoxin: Esomeprazole, lansoprazole, omeprazole, pantoprazole, and rabeprazole were shown to slightly increase the absorption of digoxin, raising its blood levels and promoting its tendency toward cardiac arrhythmia.

PPI ⟷ Drugs Requiring Acidic pH For Absorption: Proton-pump inhibitors can reduce the acidity of stomach fluid, decreasing the intestinal absorption of many drugs. Those drugs include: **allopurinol** (an antigout drug); **atazanavir** (an anti-HIV drug whose solubility decreases as gastric pH increases); **cyanocobalamin (vitamin B-12); delavirdine** (an anti-HIV drug whose solubility decreases as gastric pH increases above 3); **diazepam; erlotinib** (a drug to treat metastatic non-small cell lung cancer, whose solubility is reduced in pH greater than 5); **gefitinib** (a drug used for lung cancer, whose absorption decreases if the gastric pH rises above 5); **glucocorticoids** (*See* Ω-42 in Appendix A); **indinavir** (an anti-HIV drug); **isoniazid** (an antituberculotic drug); **iron salts; itraconazole** (an antifungal drug whose absorption requires gastric acidity); **ketoconazole** (an antifungal drug); **penicillamine** (a metal chelator); **phenothiazine antipsychotic drugs** (*See* Ω-58 in Appendix A); **phenytoin** (an antiepileptic drug); **protease inhibitors** such as amprenavir, atazanavir, fosamprenavir, and tipranavir; **quinolone antibiotics** such as ciprofloxacin, levofloxacin, norfloxacin, and ofloxacin; and **tetracyclines** such as doxycycline, minocycline, and tetracycline.

PPI ⟷ Penicillins: (*See* Ω-56 in Appendix A.) All of the above drugs block gastric acid pump to raise gastric pH, and thereby enhance absorption of acid-labile medications such as ampicillin, nafcillin, and penicillin, increasing their blood concentrations and potential for adverse effects.

PPI ⟷ (Turmeric): Turmeric (*See* Fig. 54-5) taken by mouth may increase the production of stomach acid, to counteract the effectiveness of the above proton-pump inhibitors.

Proton-Pump Inhibitors vs CYP Isozymes

Drug Name	1A2	2A6	2B6	2C8	2C9	2C18	2C19	2D6	2E1	3A4
Esomeprazole							Inh			
Lansoprazole	Ezi						Sub + Inh	Inh		Sub
Omeprazole	Inh + Ezi			Inh	Inh + Sub		Inh + Sub			Inh + Sub
Pantoprazole							Inh + Sub			
Rabeprazole							Inh + Sub			

Abbreviations: Sub, substrate of the enzyme; Inh, inhibits the enzyme; Ezi, induces the enzyme

1. All proton-pump inhibitors inhibit CYP2C19, although inhibition by rabeprazole is known to be milder than by others. Therefore, their administration in combination with drugs that require this enzyme for metabolic clearance may result in elevated blood levels to exacerbate their adverse effects. (See the middle column of Table-0 at the 'Introduction' for possible substrates of the enzyme.)

2. Pantoprazole and rabeprazole both require CYP2C19 for their metabolic clearance. Therefore, inhibition of this enzyme by any other drug taken in combination may raise their blood levels to incite their adverse effects. (See the left-hand column of Table-0 at the 'Introduction' for possible inhibitors of the enzyme.)

APPENDIX B-28: INTERACTIONS OF QUINOLONE ANTIBIOTICS

COMMON THEME INTERACTIONS: QUINOLONE ANTIBIOTICS (QAB)

Ciprofloxacin, moxifloxacin (Avelox), norfloxacin, ofloxacin, and pefloxacin

QAB ⟷ Antacids: (*See* Ω-11 in Appendix A.) Intestinal absorption of the above antibiotics can be inhibited by concurrent use of gastric antacids, such as aluminum hydroxide, calcium carbonate, and magnesium hydroxide.

QAB ⟷ Antiarrhythmic Drugs: (*See* Ω-12 in Appendix A.) By acting on the intracardiac potassium channels, quinolone antibiotics such as ciprofloxacin, norfloxacin, ofloxacin, pefloxacin, and especially sparfloxacin, may prolong the Q-T interval. When any one of them is taken in combination with another arrhythmogenic drug that tends to prolong the Q-T interval, it may lead to torsade de pointes, a life-threatening ventricular arrhythmia. Those Q-T elongating drugs include: a**miodarone, amitriptyline, disopyramide, procainamide,** and **quinidine.**

QAB ⟷ Cyclosporine: Quinolone antibiotics, such as ciprofloxacin, norfloxacin, ofloxacin, and pefloxacin, may cause acute tubular necrosis or interstitial nephritis. When used in combination with cyclosporine, an immunosuppressant highly toxic to the kidney, they may generate a synergistic nephrotoxicity.

QAB ⟷ Digoxin: Any of the above drugs may raise serum levels of digoxin by mechanisms yet to be defined.

QAB ⟷ Exenatide: Exenatide taken concurrently with a quinolone antibiotic, such as ciprofloxacin, levofloxacin, or ofloxacin, can decrease intestinal absorption of the quinolone, lowering its blood levels and decreasing its antibiotic effects. To avoid this interaction, administer any one of these oral antibiotics one hour before injection of exenatide.

QAB ⟷ Iron Salts: Intestinal absorption of ciprofloxacin and pefloxacin can be inhibited by concurrent use of iron salts.

QAB ⟷ Magnesium Hydroxide: Magnesium tends to impair intestinal absorption of quinolone antibiotics such as ciprofloxacin and moxifloxacin. Therefore, magnesium should be taken two to four hours before or after taking any of the above medications to avoid interference.

QAB ⟷ Mitoxantrone: Concurrent oral intake of mitoxantrone may decrease absorption of quinolone antibiotics, undermining their antibiotic effect.

QAB ⟷ NSAIDs: (*See* Ω-54 in Appendix A.) Ciprofloxacin, norfloxacin, ofloxacin, and pefloxacin are known to cause CNS stimulation as evidenced by tremors, restlessness, and convulsions. These neurologic adverse effects may be aggravated when taken in combination with an NSAID, such as aspirin or naproxen. This may be due to a synergistic inhibitory effect of quinolones and NSAIDs on the binding of GABA (an inhibitory neurotransmitter) to its receptors in the CNS.

QAB ⟷ Probenecid: When used in combination, probenecid decreases renal excretion of ciprofloxacin, norfloxacin, ofloxacin, and probably pefloxacin as well.

QAB ⟷ Sucralfate: Intestinal absorption of ciprofloxacin can be inhibited by concurrent use of sucralfate.

QAB ⟷ Theophylline: Quinolone antibiotics, such as ciprofloxacin, clinafloxacin, enoxacin, grepafloxacin, norfloxacin, ofloxacin, and pefloxacin, can decrease metabolic clearance of theophylline to raise its serum levels and incite its adverse reactions on the cardiovascular system and the CNS. A possible mechanism for this interaction is that theophylline is a strong substrate of CYP1A2 and the above quinolones are inhibitory to this enzyme.

QAB ⟷ Tretinoin: Tretinoin topical can interact with the following drugs to make skin more sensitive to sunlight. They include: quinolone antibiotics such as ciprofloxacin (Cipro), lomefloxacin (Maxaquin), ofloxacin (Floxin), and sparfloxacin (Zagam).

QAB ⟷ Zinc Salts: Zinc sulfate can bind to ciprofloxacin, and greatly reduces intestinal absorption of ciprofloxacin as much as by 20%. Hence, it is unwise to take the two in combination.

PXT ⟷ Nefazodone: Nefazodone may increase blood levels and the incidence of serotonin syndrome caused by paroxetine. One possible mechanism of this interaction is that paroxetine is at least partially cleared through CYP2D6 and CYP3A4, and nefazodone is inhibitory to these enzymes.

PXT ⟷ Risperidone: Paroxetine may increase blood levels and adverse effects of risperidone. One possible mechanism of this interaction is that both drugs are at least partially cleared through CYP2D6 and CYP3A4, and they may compete for clearance by these same enzymes, resulting in accumulation of unmetabolized risperidone.

SRT ⟷ Levothyroxine: Sertraline was shown to decrease the effect of levothyroxine taken by hypothyroid patients, elevating blood levels of TSH. The mechanism of interaction between the two drugs is not well established.

APPENDIX B-30: INTERACTIONS OF TETRACYCLINES

COMMON THEME INTERACTIONS: TETRACYCLINES (TCS)

Chlortetracycline, doxycycline, minocycline, and tetracycline

TCS ⟷ Acitretin: Because both acitretin and a tetracycline can cause increased intracranial pressure, their concurrent use is contraindicated.

TCS ⟷Antacids: (*See* Ω-11 in Appendix A.) Gastric antacids, such as aluminum hydroxide, calcium carbonate, and magnesium hydroxide, neutralize the acidity of stomach fluid to decrease intestinal absorption of tetracycline antibiotics.

TCS ⟷Attapulgite: Attapulgite, an antidiarrheal agent, may decrease gastrointestinal absorption and bioavailability of tetracyclines, undercutting their antibacterial effect.

TCS ⟷ Azithromycin: The bactericidal effect of azithromycin may be diminished by combined use with a tetracycline, a bacteriostatic drug.

TCS ⟷ Bismuth Subsalicylate: Bismuth subsalicylate can oppose the intestinal absorptions of tetracyclines, reducing their blood levels and lowering therapeutic efficiency.

TCS ⟷ Cyanocobalamin (Vitamin B-12.) Like all vitamin B complex members, cyanocobalamin impairs intestinal absorption of tetracyclines to undercut their effectiveness. Therefore, a few hours separation between the two is recommended.

TCS ⟷ Dicumarol: By chelation of calcium ions required for blood clotting, and decimation of intestinal flora required to manufacture vitamin K, all the above tetracyclines can enhance the therapeutic and adverse effects of oral anticoagulants, such as dicumarol and warfarin, including excessive bleeding.

TCS ⟷ Digoxin: Co-administration of any of the above tetracyclines with digoxin may raise serum levels of digoxin, increasing its tendency toward cardiac arrhythmia.

TCS ⟷ Ergot Alkaloids: (*See* Ω-39 in Appendix A.) An ergot alkaloid, such as ergometrine (used for migraine headache), is apt to cause arterial vasoconstriction by activation of both alpha-adrenergic and serotonin receptors, as well as by inhibition of the release of endothelial-derived relaxation factor. A group of side effects called "ergotism" include not only vasoconstriction that can cause gangrene of the limbs, but also abdominal cramps, and even seizures. Data suggests that tetracyclines taken in combination may increase the plasma concentrations and toxicities of ergot alkaloids, but the precise mechanism behind this observation is yet to be fully characterized.

TCS ⟷ Ethinyl Estradiol: Tetracyclines can reduce the enterohepatic recycling of ethinyl estradiol contained in oral contraceptive pills and may thereby diminish the effectiveness of this estrogen, possibly resulting in contraceptive failure.

TCS ⟷ Isotretinoin: Administration of isotretinoin should be avoided shortly before, during, or shortly after taking chlortetracycline, doxycycline, minocycline, or tetracycline, since it would increase the chance of pseudotumor cerebri.

TCS ⟷ Lithium: Rarely, tetracyclines may decrease clearance of lithium to increase its serum levels and risk of toxicity.

TCS ⟷ Magnesium: Some antibiotics chelate magnesium to form a complex which cannot be effectively absorbed through the gastrointestinal tract. Those tetracycline antibiotics include: demeclocycline (Declomycin), doxycycline (Vibramycin, Monodox, Doxy, and others), minocycline (Minocin, Dynacin, and others), oxytetracycline (Terramycin, and others), and tetracycline (Sumycin, Achromycin V, and others).

TCS ⟷ Methotrexate: Tetracyclines, when taken in combination, can increase serum levels of methotrexate, portending toxicities such as bone marrow depression. This interaction may be based on the ability of tetracyclines to displace methotrexate from its protein-binding sites.

TCS ⟷ Methoxyflurane: Concurrent use of chlortetracycline or tetracycline with methoxyflurane, a general anesthetic agent, has reportedly caused fatal renal failure.

TCS ⟷ Penicillins: (*See* Ω-56 in Appendix A.) The bacteriostatic effect of a tetracycline antibiotic may undermine the bactericidal effect of penicillin. Therefore, it is prudent not to use them in combination.

TCS ⟷ Tretinoin: Tretinoin topical can interact with the following drugs to make skin more sensitive to sunlight. They include: tetracycline antibiotics such as demeclocycline (Declomycin), doxycycline (Doryx, Vibramycin), and minocycline (Minocin).

TCS ⟷ Warfarin: As all the above tetracyclines chelate calcium ions required for blood clotting, and kill the intestinal flora that manufactures vitamin K, these antibiotics can enhance the oral anticoagulants effect of warfarin.

ADDITIONAL INDIVIDUAL INTERACTIONS
Tetracycline (TTC)

TTC ⟷ Atovaquone: Tetracycline, when used in combination, can reduce the blood levels and effectiveness of atovaquone, a drug useful in the treatment of malaria and *Pneumocystis carinii* pneumonia. The mechanism of interaction behind this observation is not fully clarified.

Tetracyclines vs CYP Isozymes

Drug Name	1A2	2A6	2B6	2C8	2C9	2C18	2C19	2D6	2E1	3A4
Doxycycline										Sub+ Inh

Abbreviations: Sub, substrate of the enzyme; Inh, inhibits the enzyme; Ezi, induces the enzyme

1. Chlortetracycline, minocycline, and tetracycline (not shown), either do not interact with CYP isozymes, or their natures of interaction are not as clearly elucidated as doxycycline.
2. Doxycycline requires CYP3A4 for its inactivation. Therefore, inhibition of this enzyme by any other drug taken in combination may raise blood levels of doxycycline to possibly exacerbate its adverse effects. (*See* the left-hand column of Table-0 at the 'Introduction' for possible inhibitors of this enzyme.) Its metabolism may be accelerated by drugs that induce microsomal CYP3A4 enzymes to result in insufficient therapeutic effectiveness. Those CYP3A4 inducers include: carbamazepine, phenobarbital, phenytoin, and rifampin. (*See* the right-hand column of Table-0 at the 'Introduction' for other possible inducers of this enzyme.)
3. Doxycycline exerts an inhibitory effect on CYP3A4. Therefore, its administration in combination with drugs that require this enzyme for metabolic clearance may result in elevated blood levels to exacerbate their adverse effects. (*See* the middle column of Table-0 at the 'Introduction' for possible substrates of this enzyme.)

OPA ⟷ ED Drugs: (*See* Ω-38 in Appendix A.) Because of a possible precipitous fall of blood pressure, use of sildenafil, tadalafil, or vardenafil in conjunction with an opioid analgesic, such as codeine or morphine, is contraindicated.

OPA ⟷ Flumazenil: Flumazenil, a benzodiazepine antagonist, can decrease the effect of narcotic analgesics and may even precipitate acute withdrawal reactions in physically dependent patients.

OPA ⟷ MAO Inhibitors: (*See* Ω-51 in Appendix A.) None of the above drugs require the enzyme MAO for metabolic clearance, but this enzyme is essential for inactivations of histamine, serotonin, and catecholamines, all released by the above drugs. Therefore, use of fentanyl, morphine, or meperidine within 14 days of receiving an MAO inhibitor, such as isocarboxazid (Marplan) or tranylcypromine, may beget potentially fatal reactions, including hypotension, tachycardia, hyperpyrexia, and life-threatening respiratory depression.

OPA ⟷ Metoclopramide: The effects of metoclopramide on gastrointestinal motility are antagonized by any of the above narcotic analgesics as well as by an authentic anticholinergic agent.

OPA ⟷ Narcotic Antagonists: Narcotic antagonists such as naloxone can reverse various effects of narcotic agonists, including analgesia, miosis, constipation, and respiratory depression. In fact, in an emergency situation where overdose of an opioid caused fatal respiratory depression, timely use of the antagonist may prove life-saving.

OPA ⟷ Pralidoxime: While morphine or other opiates limit availability of acetylcholine by inhibiting its release from cholinergic neurons, pralidoxime destroys available acetylcholine by reactivation of enzyme acetylcholinesterase. If the two are taken in combination, neurologic toxicity owing to lack of the cholinergic transmitter may result, which include disruption of cognitions, and chemical denervation of the skeletal muscle, causing weakness or paralysis of the muscles.

ADDITIONAL INDIVIDUAL INTERACTIONS

Fentanyl (FTN), methadone (MTD), morphine (MRP), and **oxycodone (OXC)**

FTN ⟷ Amiodarone: Amiodarone taken in combination with fentanyl may increase the adverse cardiovascular effects of the latter, including hypotension, bradycardia, and reduced cardiac output. One possible mechanism for this observation is that fentanyl is a strong substrate of CYP3A4, whereas amiodarone has an inhibitory effect on this enzyme.

MTD ⟷ Cocaine: Methadone inhibits cardiac potassium channels, causing elongation of the Q-T interval. Concurrent use of methadone with cocaine, a drug that also elongates the Q-T interval, is contraindicated, as it might cause the life-threatening arrhythmia of torsade de pointes.

MTD ⟷ Diuretics: (*See* Ω-49 and Ω-73 in Appendix A.) As methadone elongates the Q-T interval, its co-administration with a diuretic that depletes potassium may lead to the life-threatening arrhythmia of torsade de pointes.

Opioid Analgesics vs CYP Isozymes

Drug Name	1A2	2A6	2B6	2C8	2C9	2C18	2C19	2D6	2E1	3A4
Codeine								Sub		Sub
Fentanyl								Sub		Sub
Hydrocodone								Sub		Sub
Meperidine								Sub		
Methadone			Sub		Sub		Sub	Inh		Sub
Morphine								Sub		
Oxycodone								Sub		Sub

1. Codeine Is regarded as an inactive prodrug that must be O-demethylated at position 3 by the enzyme CYP2D6 to morphine, which is its active form. Therefore, co-administration of codeine with an inhibitor of CYP2D6 can make codeine an ineffective or insufficiently active drug. For instance, if cimetidine, an inhibitor of many CYP enzymes including CYP2D6, is taken in combination, the therapeutic effectiveness of codeine may be compromised.

2. Hydrocodone is also an inactive prodrug that must be o-demethylated mainly by CYP2D6 to hydromorphone, its active metabolite, which is then processed by CYP3A4 to its inactive norhydrocodone. Thus, medications that inhibit the enzyme CYP2D6, such as paroxetine and ritonavir, would likely the decrease analgesic effect of hydrocodone. (*See* the left-hand column of Table-0 at the 'Introduction' for other possible inhibitors of this enzyme.)

3. Methadone is unusual in that it has an inhibitory effect on CYP2D6. Thus, its administration in combination with drugs that require this enzyme for metabolic clearance may result in elevated blood levels to stir up their adverse effects. In addition, methadone, by inhibition of CYP2D6, which is required for the activation of codeine, may decrease the analgesic effect of codeine. (*See* the middle column of Table-0 at the 'Introduction' for possible substrates of the enzyme.)

4. Opiate withdrawal syndrome was generated by combined use of methadone, a CYP2B6 substrate, with nevirapine, an inducer of CYP2B. Nevirapine may increase the metabolism of methadone to decrease its blood concentration and therapeutic efficiency

5. Since all the above narcotics except methadone are at least partially processed by CYP2D6, their combination with fluvoxamine or sertraline, both antidepressants and substrates of CYP2D6, may cause substrate competition and could elevate blood levels of fluvoxamine or sertraline to possibly exacerbate adverse effects including serotonin syndrome.

6. A small amount of morphine appears N-demethylated by CYP2D6 to form normorphine, whose analgesic efficacy is far lower than morphine (about 5 to 10%). Morphine is mainly inactivated by glucuronidation at position 3. Thus, CYP2D6 plays only a minor role and its inhibition leads to little clinical consequence.

MTD ⟷ Foscarnet: Foscarnet, a drug useful in the treatment of cytomegalovirus infections, can generate such adverse effects as renal tubular acidosis and Q-T elongation. Its co-administration with methadone, which also elongates the Q-T, may further the elongation, possibly leading to the life-threatening ventricular arrhythmia of torsade de pointes.

MTD ⟷ Sotalol: Co-administration of methadone and sotalol, both tending to elongate the Q-T interval, may bring about the rare but life-threatening ventricular arrhythmia of torsade de pointes.

MTD ⟷ Zidovudine: Co-administration of methadone with zidovudine may cause increased blood levels of zidovudine to amplify its adverse effects including influenza-like symptoms. One possible mechanism for this observation is that both methadone and its inactive metabolite N-demethyl methadone formed by CYP 3A4 are known to oppose inactivation of zidovudine via glucuronidation.

MRP ⟷ Gabapentin: Morphine may compete with gabapentin for clearance by glucuronidation, raising the blood levels of gabapentin and exacerbating its adverse effects.

OXC ⟷ Carisoprodol: Co-administration of carisoprodol, a centrally acting skeletal muscle relaxant, with oxycodone, a narcotic pain-killer, may make the CNS depressant effect of oxycodone worse, resulting in life-threatening respiratory depression and unconsciousness, requiring medical intervention. It is known that carisoprodol is metabolized to meprobamate, which is a Class IV controlled substance with significant potential for abuse and dependency, and has such CNS-depressant effects as hypotension; respiratory depression; and coma. Since there is no evidence that they interact at pharmacokinetic level interfering with each other's metabolism, it is thought they rather interact at pharmacodynamic level to generate dangerous additive CNS depressant effects.

Actinomycin, (*see* dactinomycin)
Activated charcoal, 143, 295, 569
  drug interactions with
    ipecac, 145
    minerals, 145
    oral medications, 145
    mechanism of action, 145
    side effects, 145
Actonel (*see* risedronate)
Actos (*see* pioglitazone)
Acyclovir
  drug interactions
    aminoglycoside antibiotics, 503
    CYP isozymes, 503–504
    mycophenolate mofetil, 503
    NSAIDs, 503
    probenecid, 504
    mechanism of action, 502
    molecular structure, 503
    side effects, 503
Adder all XR (*see* amphetamine
    dextroamphetamine)
Addison disease
  medications for
    cortisone + hydrocortisone, 362–363
    fludrocortisone, 362–365
Adenocard (*see* adenosine)
Adenosine
  mechanism of action, 43
  molecular structure, 514
  side effects, 43
ADHD. *see* Attention deficit hyperactivity
    disorder
Adoxa, (*see* doxycycline)
Adrenal gland, 366
Adrenergic alpha blockers
  drug interactions, 188
  mechanism of action, 188
  members of, 188
  side effects, 188
Adrenergic beta-2 agonists, 364
  drug interactions, 117–119
  mechanism of action, 117
  members of, 117
  side effects, 117
Adrenocorticotropic hormone (ACTH), 366
Adriamycin (*see* doxorubicin)
Adrucil (*see* fluorouracil)
Advil (*see* ibuprofen)

Aethoxysclerol (*see* polidocanol)
Afinitor (*see* everolimus)
Afrin (*see* oxymetazoline)
Akatinol (*see* memantine)
Alanine aminotransferase (ALT), 573
Alanine, molecular structure, 355
Albalon (*see* naphazoline)
Albendazole, 560–561
  drug interactions with
    cimetidine, 562
    CYP isozymes, 562–563
    fatty meal, 562
    mechanism of action, 562
    molecular structure, 562
    side effects, 562
Albuterol aerosol, 116
  drug interactions, 117–119
  mechanism of action, 117
  side effects, 117
Albuterol ipratropium
  drug interactions with
    anticholinergic agents, 118
    beta blockers, 118
    digoxin, 118
    MAO inhibitors, 119
    sympathomimetic drugs, 119
    tricyclic antidepressants, 119
  mechanism of action, 117
  side effects, 117
Albuterol
  drug interactions with
    beta blockers, 118
    fludrocortisone, 118
    MAO inhibitors, 118
    sympathomimetic drugs, 118
  mechanism of action, 117
  side effects, 117
Albuterol nebulizer solution, 116
  drug interactions, 117–119
  mechanism of action, 117
  side effects, 117
Alcohol, 402, 411
Aldactone (*see* spironolactone)
Aldara (*see* imiquimod)
Aldosterone antagonists
  drug interactions with, 24
    CYP isozymes, 25
    digoxin, 25
    ibuprofen, 25

indomethacin, 25
licorice, 25
naproxen, 25
mechanism of action, 23
side effects, 24
Alefacept
drug interactions with
anakinra, 252
cyclophosphamide, 252
mechanism of action, 251
side effects, 251–252
Alendronate, 411
drug interactions with
aminoglycosides, 210
antacids, 210
aspirin, 210
CYP isozymes, 210–211
estrogens, 211
NSAIDs, 211
mechanism of action, 209
molecular structures, 211
side effects, 210
Aleve (*see* naproxen)
Alfuzosin, 180
drug interactions, 188, 206
mechanism of action, 188, 206
side effects, 188, 206
Algesia
medications for
acetaminophen, 395–399
ergotamine, 396, 404–407, 427
NSAIDs, 395, 399–400
opioid analgesics, 395, 400–401
topiramate, 396, 407
tramadol, 395, 401–403
triptans, 395, 403–404
Allegra (*see* fexofenadine)
Allergic reaction, 425
medications for
antihistamines, first-generation,
426, 431
epinephrine, 426–428
glucocorticoids, 426, 430–431
leukotriene receptor blockers, 426
mast cell stabilizers, 426, 432
Allopurinol
drug interactions with, 222
captopril, 197
chlorpropamide, 198

cyclophosphamide, 198
penicillins, 198
pentostatin, 198
porfirmer, 198
mechanism of action,
196–197, 221
molecular structures, 197
side effects, 197, 222
Almotriptan, 395
drug interactions, 404
mechanism of action, 403–404
molecular structure of, 404
side effects, 404
Aloprim (*see* allopurinol)
Alosetron
drug interactions with
CYP isozymes, 160
mechanism of action, 159
molecular structure of, 160
side effects, 159
Alpha$_2$ activators, 351, 353
Alpha agonists, 406, 427
Alpha blockers, 18, 427
drug interactions, 206
mechanism of action, 206
members of, 206
side effects, 206
Alpha$_1$ blockers, 1
drug interactions, 4
mechanism of action, 3
members of, 3
side effects, 3–4
Alpha$_2$ blockers
drug interactions with, 5–6
beta blockers, 5
insulin, 5
prazosin, 5
tricyclic antidepressants, 6
verapamil, 6
mechanism of action, 4
members of, 4
side effects, 4
Alpha lipoic acid, 351, 353, 356
Alprazolam
drug interactions, 258
mechanism of action, 257
side effects, 257–258
ALT (alanine aminotransferase), 573
Altace (*see* ramipril)

Alteplase
  drug interactions, 60
  mechanism of action, 60
  side effects, 60
Altretamine
  drug interactions with
    chloramphenicol, 491
    CYP enzymes and, 491
    live vaccines, 491
    MAO inhibitors, 491
    pyridoxine, 492
    zidovudine, 492
  mechanism of action, 490
  molecular structure, 491
  side effects, 490
Aluminum acetate, 244
  drug interactions, 245
  mechanism of action, 245
  side effects, 245
Aluminum hydroxide, 146, 166, 535
  drug interactions, 147
  mechanism of action, 146
  side effects, 147
Alzheimer disease
  medications for
    anticholinesterase agents, 301–304
      donepezil, 301
      galantamine, 301
      memantine, 302, 304–305
      rivastigmine, 301–302
      tacrine, 302
Amantadine, 164, 193, 305, 326
  drug interactions with, 507
    alcohol, 329
    chasteberry, 329
    influenza virus vaccine, 330
    levodopa, 330
    quinidine, 330
    risperidone, 330
    triamterene, 330
  mechanism of action, 328, 507
  molecular structure of, 507
  side effects, 329, 507
Amaryl, (glimepiride), 353
Ambien, (see zolpidem)
Amerge, (see naratriptan)
American Heart Association
  hypertension, defined by, 1
Amevive (alefacept)

Amiloride, 15, 184
  molecular structure, 40
Aminoglycoside antibiotics, 229, 463
  drug interactions with, 101–102
    anticholinesterase agents, 102
    cationic drugs, 102
    clindamycin, 102
    loop diuretics, 103
    topotecan, 103
  mechanism of action, 101
  members of, 101
  side effects, 101
4-Aminoquinoline, molecular
    structure, 544
Amiodarone, 158, 171
  drug interactions with, 34
    cholestyramine, 33
    CYP isozymes, 35
    digoxin, 35–36
    echinacea, 36
  mechanism of action, 32
  molecular structure, 35
  side effects, 32–33
Amitiza, (lubiprostone)
Amitriptyline, 263, 267
  drug interactions, 268, 288
  mechanism of action, 268, 288
  members, 287
  molecular structures, 287
  side effects, 268, 288
Amlexanox
  drug interactions, 128
  mechanism of action, 127
  side effects, 127
Amlodipine, 1, 318
  drug interactions, 10
  mechanism of action, 10
  side effects, 10
Ammonium chloride, 273
Amoxicillin, 95, 146, 199, 525
  drug interactions, 96, 153, 199, 526
  mechanism of action, 95–96, 152, 199, 525
  side effects, 96, 152, 199, 525
Amoxil, (see amoxicillin)
Amphetamine, 114
  drug interactions, 439
  mechanism of action, 439
  molecular structure, 27
  side effects, 439

Amphetamine dextroamphetamine, 269
    drug interactions with
        CYP isozymes, 272, 273
        dextromethorphan, 272
        digoxin, 272
        MAO inhibitor, 273
    mechanism of action, 272
    side effects, 272
Amphotericin, 102, 364
Amphotericin-B, 588
Ampicillin, 95, 199
    drug interactions, 96, 199
    mechanism of action, 95–96, 199
    side effects, 96, 199
Amprenavir
    mechanism of action, 521
    molecular structure of, 521–522
    side effects, 523
Amyl nitrite, 180, 569, 580
    drug interactions, 579–580
    mechanism of action, 579
    side effects, 579
Anabolic steroids
    drug interactions with, 213
        CYP isozymes, 214
        insulin, 214
    mechanism of action, 213
    members of, 213
    side effects, 213
Anaprox (see naproxen)
Anastrozole
    drug interactions with
        CYP isozymes, 480
    mechanism of action, 479
    molecular structure, 478
    side effects, 480
Anbesol (see benzocaine)
Anemia
    medications for
        antithymocyte globulin, 65
        cyanocobalamin, 65
        cyclosporine, 65
        darbepoetin alfa, 65
        epoetin alfa, 65
        ferrous fumarate, 65–66
        ferrous sulfate, 65–66
        folic acid, 65
        granulocyte colony-stimulating factor (GCSF), 65

        granulocyte macrophage colony-stimulating factor (GM-CSF), 65
        immunosuppressive agents, 65
Anesthetic agents, 18
Angina pectoris
    medications for
        beta blockers, 45, 47
        calcium-channel blockers, 45, 47
        vasodilators, 45–46
Angiotensin-converting enzyme (ACE), 21
    inhibitors, 1, 184, 290, 411
        drug interactions, 9, 20, 22
        mechanism of action, 6, 9, 20–21
        molecular structures of, 7–8
        side effects, 9, 20–22
Angiotensin-receptor blockers (ARBs), 1, 290
    drug interactions, 10, 22
    mechanism of action, 9, 22
    members of, 9
    side effects, 9–10, 22
Anisoyl group, molecular structure, 48
Anistreplase
    drug interactions, 60
    mechanism of action, 60
    side effects, 60
Antiarrhythmic drugs
    drug interactions with
        caffeine, 44
        theophylline, 44
    mechanism of action, 43
    members of, 43
    side effects, 43
Antibiotics
    drug interactions, 153
    mechanism of action, 152
    members of, 151
    side effects, 152–153
Anticholinergic medications
    agents, 107, 164, 193
        drug interactions, 164, 167, 192
        mechanism of action, 163, 166, 191–192
        members of, 163, 166
        side effects, 163–164, 166–167, 192
    drug interactions with, 327
        digoxin, 328
        galantamine, 328
        tacrine, 328
    mechanism of action, 327
    side effects, 327

Anticholinesterase agents (ACAs)
  drug interactions with
    cholinomimetic drugs, 302
    CYP isozymes, 303–304
    haloperidol, 30304
    levodopa, 304
    neostigmine, 229–230
    pyridostigmine, 229–230
    succinylcholine, 304
  mechanism of action, 228–229, 302
  members of, 228, 302
  side effects, 229, 302
Anticoagulants, 149, 183, 293, 410
Antidiarrheal drugs, 530
Antidiuretic hormone (ADH), 360
Antihistamines, 164, 402
  drug interactions, 339, 415, 431
    first- and second-generation, 93–94
  mechanism of action, 93, 339, 415, 431
  members of, 93, 339, 415
  side effects, 339, 415, 431
    first and second generation, 93
Antihistaminic antianxiety drugs (*see*
    hydroxyzine)
Antihistaminic antiemetics
  drug interactions, 335
  mechanism of action, 334
  side effects, 334–335
Antiplatelet drugs, 183, 293
Antipsychotic drugs, 427
Antithymocyte globulin
  drug interactions, 70
  mechanism of action, 69–70
  side effects, 70
Antivert (*see* meclizine)
Antizol (*see* fomepizole)
Anturane (*see* sulfinpyrazone)
Anu-Med (*see* phenylephrine)
Anusol-HC (hydrocortisone ointment), 176
Aphthasol (*see* amlexanox)
Aphthous ulcer
  medications for
    amlexanox, 127–128
    dexamethasone, 127, 129–130
    sulfonated phenol topical solution,
      127–128
    tetracycline, 127–129
    triamcinolone, 127, 129–130

Apri (ethinyl estradiol + desogestrel), 417
Arabinose, molecular structure, 532
Aralene (*see* chloroquine)
ARBs (*see* angiotensin receptor blockers)
L-Arginine, 181
  drug interactions with, 183
    lysine, 184
    NSAIDs, 184
  mechanism of action, 182
  molecular structure of, 182
  side effects, 182
Aricept (*see* donepezil)
Arimidex (*see* anastrozole)
Aripiprazole
  drug interactions, 299
  mechanism of action, 299
  molecular structure, 298
  side effects, 299
Armour thyroid, 372
  drug interactions, 375
  mechanism of action, 374
  side effects, 374
Aromasin (*see* exemestane)
Aromatase inhibitors
  drug interactions with, 481
    CYP enzymes, 480
  mechanism of action, 479–480
  members of, 478
  side effects, 480
Artane (*see* trihexyphenidyl)
Arthritis, 217
Ascorbic acid, 419
Asparaginase, 510
Aspartate aminotransferase, 573
Aspartic acid, molecular structure, 315
Aspirin, 131–132, 202, 224, 226, 395, 408,
    465, 478
  drug interactions with, 135, 400, 409
    cyclosporine, 411
    lithium, 411
    potassium citrate, 412
    sulfinpyrazone, 412
    trimethoprim, 412
  mechanism of action, 133, 399, 409
  molecular structure of, 409
  side effects, 133, 400, 409
AST (aspartate aminotransferase) 573
Astelin (*see* azelastine)

Asthma
    dyphylline, 119–120
    medications for
        adrenergic beta 2 agonists, 116–119
        glucocorticoids, 116, 120–121
        montelukast, 116–117
        xanthine derivative, 116
Atacand (*see* candesartan)
Atazanavir
    mechanism of action, 521
    molecular structures of, 522
    side effects, 523
Atenolol, 1
    drug interactions with, 3
    mechanism of action, 2
    side effects, 2–3
Ativan (*see* lorazepam)
Atomoxetine, 269
    drug interactions with
        albuterol, 271
        CYP isozymes, 271
        epinephrine, 272
        MAO inhibitors, 272
    mechanism of action, 271
    molecular structure, 269
    side effects, 271
Atorvastatin, 318
    drug interactions, 80
    mechanism of action, 78, 80
    molecular structures, 79
    side effects, 80
Atovaquone, 518
    drug interactions with
        CYP isozymes, 549
        fat-rich foods, 549
        rifampin, 549
        salicylates, 549
        zidovudine, 549
    mechanism of action, 548
    molecular structure, 548
    side effects, 549
Atovaquone + chloroguanide, 549
    drug interactions with
        CYP isozymes, 549
        fat-rich foods, 549
        rifampin, 549
        salicylates, 549
        zidovudine, 549

    mechanism of action, 548–549
    members, 548
    side effects, 549
Atretol (*see* carbamazepine)
Atropine, 124, 569, 580
    drug interactions, 581
    mechanism of action, 581
    molecular structures of, 163
    side effects, 581
Attention deficit hyperactivity disorder
        (ADHD)
    medications for
        Adderall XR, 272–273
        atomoxetine, 271–272
        methylphenidate, 269–271
Atypical antipsychotic drugs
    drug interactions, 299
    mechanism of action, 299
    members of, 299
    side effects, 299
Avalide (irbesartan +
        hydrochlorothiazide)
Avandia (rosiglitazone), 350
Avapro (irbesartan
Aviane (ethinyl estradiol
        levonorgestrel), 417
Avodart (*see* dutasteride; tamsulosin)
Axert (*see* almotriptan)
Axura (*see* memantine)
Azathioprine, 102, 197, 202, 228, 230, 463,
        465, 510, 588
    drug interactions with
        allopurinol, 231–232
        cyclosporine, 232
        live vaccines, 232
        methotrexate, 232
        NSAIDs, 232
        olsalazine, 232
        trimethoprim-sulfamethoxazole,
            232–233
        and zidovudine, 233
    mechanism of action, 231
    molecular structure, 231
Azelaic acid
    drug interactions, 244
    mechanism of action, 244
    molecular structure of, 244
    side effects, 244

Azelastine, 90, 426, 431
  drug interactions, first- and second-
    generation, 93–94
  mechanism of action, 93
  side effects, first- and second-
    generation, 93
Azelex, (cream/gel azelaic acid), 243
Azilect (*see* rasagiline)
Azithromycin, 95, 388, 525, 527
  drug interactions, 101, 390, 528
  mechanism of action, 98, 100, 390, 528
  molecular structures, 99
  side effects, 98, 390, 528
Azole antifungal drugs
  drug interactions, 538–539
  mechanism of action, 537
  members of, 537
  relation with CYP enzymes, 539
  side effects, 538
Azulfidine (*see* sulfasalazine)

B
Baclofen (BCF), 104, 234, 353, 356
  drug interactions with, 105, 236
    alcohol, 105
    ibuprofen, 106
    morphine, 106
    oral hypoglycemic agents, 106
    tricyclic antidepressants, 106
  mechanism of action, 105, 236
  molecular structure, 105
  side effects, 105, 236
Bacteria, systemic infections
  medications for
    cephalosporins, 526
    clindamycin, 528–530
    ethambutol, 533–536
    fluoroquinolone antibiotics, 527
    isoniazid, 533–536
    macrolide antibiotics, 527–528
    mupirocin, 531–532
    nitrofurantoin, 532–533
    penicillins, 525–526
    rifampin, 533–536
    sulfamethoxazole plus trimethoprim,
      530–531
    tetracyclines, 526–527
Bactrim, see sulfamethoxazole +
  trimethoprim

Bactroban (*see* mupirocin)
Barbiturates, 402
Bayotensin, see nitrendipine
Beclomethasone, 89, 426, 430
  drug interactions, 90
  mechanism of action, 90
  side effects, 90
Beconase (*see* beclomethasone)
Bed-wetting
  medications for
    anticholinergic agents, 191
    dicyclomine, 191–192
    hyoscyamine, 191
    oxybutynin, 191
    tolterodine, 191
Benadryl (*see* diphenhydramine)
Benazepril, 1
  drug interactions, 9, 20
  mechanism of action, 6, 9, 20
  molecular structure of, 7
  side effects, 9, 20
Benemid (*see* probenecid)
Benicar (*see* olmesartan)
Benign prostatic hyperplasia (BPH), 188
  medications for
    adrenergic alpha blockers, 188
    alfuzosin, 188
    5-alpha reductase inhibitors, 188–190
    doxazosin, 188
    dutasteride, 188
    finasteride, 188
    tamsulosin, 188
    terazosin, 188
Bentyl (*see* dicyclomine)
Benylin-DM (*see* dextromethorphan)
Benzocaine, 131, 176
  drug interactions, 132, 176
  mechanism of action, 131–132, 176
  molecular structure of, 131
  side effects, 132, 176
Benzodent, see benzocaine
Benzodiazepine (BDZ)
  antianxiety drugs, 402
  drug interactions with, 258, 323
  mechanism of action, 257, 322
  members of, 257
  molecular structures, 258
  receptors, 259
  sedatives

drug interactions, 416
  mechanism of action, 416
  members of, 415
  side effects, 416
  side effects, 257–258, 323
Benzonatate, 110
  drug interactions, 115
  mechanism of action, 115
  side effects, 115
Benztropine
  drug interactions, 328
  mechanism of action, 327
  side effects, 327
Bepridil, 158
Beta-adrenergic blockers, 351, 353
  drug interactions, 23
  mechanism of action, 22
  side effects, 22–23
Beta blockers, 1, 18
  drug interactions, 3, 43, 47
  mechanism of action, 2, 42, 47
  members of, 1–2, 42, 47
  side effects, 2–3, 43, 47
Betahistine
  drug interactions, 335
  mechanism of action, 335
  molecular structure, 335
  side effects, 335
Betapace (see sotalol)
Bethanechol, 41, 154, 193, 206
  drug interactions
    ganglionic blockers with, 155
  mechanism of action, 155
  molecular structure of, 155
  side effects, 155
Biaxin (see clarithromycin)
BiCNU (see carmustine)
Bifemelane
  drug interactions, 307
  mechanism of action, 306
  molecular structure, 306
  side effects, 307
Bisacodyl, 168
  drug interactions with
    antacids, 170
    digoxin, 170
    milk with, 170
  mechanism of action, 170
  side effects, 170

Bismuth subsalicylate, 146, 173–174, 226
  drug interactions with
    aspirin, 149
    oral hypoglycemic agents, 149
    tetracycline antibiotics, 149
  mechanism of action, 148–149
  side effects, 149
Bisoprolol, 1
  drug interactions, 3, 23, 47
  mechanism of action, 2, 22
  side effects, 2–3, 22–23
Bitter gourd, 353, 356
Black cohosh, 351, 353
Bleomycin
  drug interactions, 456
  mechanism of action, 455
  side effects, 456
Bonine (see meclizine)
Boniva (see ibandronate)
BPH (see Benign prostatic
    hyperplasia)
Brain cancer
  medications for
    carmustine, 450
    lomustine, 450
    nitrosourea derivatives, 450–451
    procarbazine, 450
    temozolomide, 450
Breast cancer
  medications for
    anastrozole, 478
    aromatase inhibitors, 478–480
    capecitabine, 478–482
    docetaxel, 480, 482
    epirubicin, 478, 483
    exemestane, 478
    goserelin, 478, 483
    letrozole, 478
    paclitaxel, 478, 482
    selective estrogen receptor modulators,
      478, 483–486
    tamoxifen, 478
    toremifene, 478
    trastuzumab, 478, 486–487
Breast engorgement
  medications for
    azithromycin, 388, 390
    bromocriptine, 388–389
    cabergoline, 388–389

Brevibloc (*see* esmolol)
Brinzolamide, 321
Brodspec (*see* tetracycline)
Bromocriptine, 107, 380, 388
    drug interactions with, 330, 389
        alcohol, 382
        chasteberry, 383
        CYP isozymes, 383
        isometheptene, 383
        sage, 383
    mechanism of action, 330, 382, 389
    side effects, 330, 382, 389
Brompheniramine, 89, 426, 431
    drug interactions, first- and second-
        generation, 93–94
    mechanism of action, 93
    side effects, first- and second-generation, 93
Bronchitis, 95
    ciprofloxacin, 98
    medications
        aminoglycoside antibiotics, 95,
          101–103
        cephalosporin antibiotics, 95–97
        fluoroquinolone antibiotic, 95
        macrolide antibiotics, 95, 98–101
        penicillins, 95–96
Budesonide, 89, 116, 426, 430
    drug interactions, 90, 121
    mechanism of action, 90, 120–121
    side effects, 90, 121
Bulk cathartics
    drug interactions, 169
    mechanism of action, 169
    members of, 168
    side effects, 169
Bumetanide, 1
    drug interactions, 23, 64
    mechanism of action, 23, 64
    molecular structure of, 11
    side effects, 23, 64
Bumex (*see* bumetanide)
Bupropion, 281
    drug interactions with, 268, 275, 438
        alcohol, 286
        CYP isozymes, 286–287
        guanfacine, 286
        MAO inhibitors, 286
        nicotine, 286
    mechanism of action, 268, 275, 286, 438
    molecular structure, 263
    side effects, 268, 275, 286, 438
Buspirone, 257, 259, 309
    drug interactions with
        CYP enzymes, 261
        CYP isozymes, 260
        diltiazem, 260
        MAO inhibitors, 260–261
        verapamil, 261
    mechanism of action, 260
    molecular structure, 260
    side effects, 260
Busulfan
    drug interactions with
        acetaminophen, 473
        chloramphenicol, 473
        cyclophosphamide, 473
        CYP isozymes, 473
        live vaccines, 474
        6-thioguanine, 474
    mechanism of action, 472
    molecular structure, 472
    side effects, 473
Busulfex (*see* busulfan)
Butalbital + acetaminophen + caffeine, 396
    drug interactions with, 396
        acetylcysteine, 397
        alcohol, 397
        caffeine, 397
        CYP isozymes, 397
        echinacea, 397
        MAO inhibitors, 397
        metyrapone, 397
        quinolone antibiotics, 398
        theophylline, 398
        zidovudine, 398
    mechanism of action, 396
    side effects, 396

C

Cabergoline, 388
    drug interactions with
        haloperidol, 388
        macrolides, 388
        metoclopramide, 389
        phenothiazine antipsychotic
          drugs, 389

mechanism of action, 388
side effects, 388
Caduet (*see* amlodipine)
Cafergot (*see* ergotamine)
Caffeine, 114
    molecular structure of, 398
Calan (*see* verapamil)
Calcitonin-salmon
    drug interactions, 213
    mechanism of action, 212
    side effects, 212
Calcium carbonate, 146, 535
    drug interactions, 147, 216
    mechanism of action, 146, 215
    side effects, 147, 215–216
Calcium-channel blockers, 1, 40, 180
    drug interactions, 10, 42, 47
    mechanism of action, 10, 41, 47
    members of, 41, 47
    side effects, 10, 42, 47
Calcium disodium edetate, 569
    drug interactions, 585
    mechanism of action, 584
    molecular structure, 585
    side effects, 584
Camptosar (*see* irinotecan)
Cancer
    characteristics, 440
    treatments
        chemotherapy, 440
        radiation, 440
        surgery, 440
    types of, 440
Cancidas (*see* caspofungin)
Candesartan, 1
    drug interactions, 10
    mechanism of action, 9
    side effects, 9–10
Candida vs *Cryptococcus* vs
        Aspergillus, 539
Canrenone, 184
Capecitabine
    drug interactions with
        chloramphenicol, 481
        CYP isozymes, 481–482
        leucovorin, 481
        live vaccines, 481
        zidovudine, 481

mechanism of action, 480
    molecular structure, 481
    side effects, 481
Capoten (*see* captopril)
Capreomycin, 558
Captopril, 1
    drug interactions, 9, 20
    mechanism of action, 6, 9, 20
    molecular structure of, 7
    side effects, 9, 20
Carafate (*see* sucralfate)
Carbamazepine, 294, 315
    drug interactions with, 316
        alcohol, 294
        clozapine, 295
        CYP isozymes, 295
        lithium, 296
        MAO inhibitors, 296
        valerian, 296
        valproic acid, 296
        vasopressin, 296
    mechanism of action, 294, 316
    molecular structure, 265
    side effects, 294, 316
Carbex (*see* selegiline)
Carbonic anhydrase inhibitors, 411
Carboplatin, 443
    drug interactions, 490, 492
    mechanism of action, 489, 492
    molecular structure, 492
    side effects, 489, 492
Cardiac arrhythmia
    medications for
        adenosine, 32
        adrenergic beta blockers, 32, 42–43
        antiarrhythmic drugs, 32, 44
        calcium-channel blockers, 32, 34, 41–46
        cibenzoline, 32
        diltiazem, 32
        esmolol, 32
        lidocaine, 32
        procainamide, 32
        propranolol, 32
        quinidine, 32
        sodium-channel blockers, 32, 36–41
        sotalol, 32
        tocainide, 32
        verapamil, 32

Cardizem (*see* diltiazem)
Cardura (*see* doxazosin)
Carisoprodol, 234
    drug interactions with
        alcohol, 234–235
        CYP isozymes, 235
        magnesium hydroxide, 235
        monoamine oxidase (MAO), 235
        opioids, 236
    mechanism of action, 234
    molecular structure of, 236
    side effects, 234
Carmustine
    drug interactions with
        chloramphenicol, 451
        CYP isozymes, 451
        live vaccines, 451
    mechanism of action, 450
    molecular structures, 450
    side effects, 451
Carmustine and lomustine
    drug interactions with
        chloramphenicol, 451
        CYP isozymes, 451
        live vaccines, 451
Carpal tunnel syndrome
    medications for
        cortisone, 239–240
        hydrocortisone, 239–240
        nonsteroidal antiinflammatory drugs
            (NSAIDs), 239, 241–242
Cartia (*see* diltiazem)
Cartia XT (*see* diltiazem)
Carvedilol, 1
    drug interactions, 3, 23
    mechanism of action, 2, 22
    molecular structure, 2
    side effects, 2–3, 22–23
Caspofungin, 537, 539
    drug interactions, 540–541
    mechanism of action, 540
    molecular structure of, 540
    side effects, 540
Cefaclor, 95
    drug interactions, 96
    mechanism of action, 96
    molecular structures, 97
    side effects, 96

Cefamandole, molecular structures, 51
Cefdinir, 95, 525
    drug interactions, 96, 526
    mechanism of action, 96, 526
    molecular structures, 97
    side effects, 96, 526
Cefpodoxime, 95
    drug interactions, 96
    mechanism of action, 96
    molecular structures, 97
    side effects, 96
Cefprozil, 95, 525
    drug interactions, 96, 526
    mechanism of action, 96, 526
    molecular structures, 97
    side effects, 96, 526
Cefuroxime, 95, 388, 525
    drug interactions, 96, 390, 526
    mechanism of action, 96, 390, 526
    molecular structures, 97
    side effects, 96, 390, 526
Cefzil (*see* cefprozil)
Celebrex (*see* celecoxib)
Celecoxib
    drug interactions, 219
    mechanism of action, 219
    side effects, 219
Centrally-acting skeletal muscle relaxants
    and CYP enzymes, 235
    drug interactions, 234–236
    mechanism of action, 234
    members of, 234
    side effects, 234
Centrax (*see* prazepam)
Cephalexin, 95, 388, 525
    drug interactions, 96, 390, 526
    mechanism of action, 96, 390, 526
    molecular structures, 97
    side effects, 96, 390, 526
Cephalosporin antibiotics, 224, 419
    drug interactions, 96, 390
    mechanism of action, 96, 390
    members of, 96
    molecular structures, 97
    side effects, 96, 390
Cephalosporins
    members of
        drug interactions, 526

mechanism of action, 526
side effects, 526
molecular structures, 51
Cervical cancer
medications for
cisplatin, 487, 489
fluorouracil, 487, 489
ifosfamide, 487–489
Cetirizine, 90, 426, 431
drug interactions, first- and second-
generation, 93–94
mechanism of action, 93
side effects, first- and second-
generation, 93
Cevimeline, 156
drug interactions with
beta blockers, 124
bethanechol, 124
CYP isozymes, 124
tolazoline, 125
mechanism of action, 123
side effects, 123
Chamomile
cut and dried flowers, 410
partial feature of, 410
Chasteberry
cut and dried form of, 108
partial feature of, 108
Chemical poisoning, 569
antidotes
activated charcoal, 570
amyl nitrite, 579–580
atropine, 580–581
calcium disodium edetate, 584–585
deferoxamine, 585–586
dimercaprol, 583–584
epinephrine, 572
flumazenil, 577–578
fomepizole, 576–577
glucagon, 571
hydroxocobalamin, 579–580
ipecac syrup, 570–571
Mesna, 575
N-acetylcysteine, 573–574
naloxone, 572–573
obidoxime, 580–583
oxygen therapy, 578–579
penicillamine, 587–588
pralidoxime, 580–583

sodium nitrite, 579–580
sodium polystyrene sulfonate,
574–575
methanol and ethanol, metabolic
pathway, 576
Chloral hydrate, 402
Chloramphenicol, 442–443, 446, 478
Chloraseptic, 131
Chlorhexidine gluconate
drug interactions, 137
mechanism of action, 136
molecular structure of, 136
side effects, 136
Chloroguanide
drug interactions with
CYP isozymes, 549
fat-rich foods, 549
rifampin, 549
salicylates, 549
zidovudine, 549
mechanism of action, 548
molecular structure, 548
side effects, 549
Chloroquine, 158, 552, 554
drug interactions with
alcohol, 545
cyclosporine, 546
CYP isozymes, 546
digoxin, 546–547
mechanism of action, 544–545
molecular structure, 544
side effects, 545
8-Chlorotheophylline
molecular structure of, 139
Chlorpheniramine, 89, 110, 318, 426, 431
drug interactions, first- and second-
generation, 93–94
mechanism of action, 93
side effects first- and second-
generation, 93
Chlorpheniramine + hydrocodone
drug interactions, 111
side effects, 110
Chlorpromazine, 104, 273, 382, 552–553
drug interactions, 105, 300
mechanism of action, 104, 300
molecular structure, 104
side effects, 105, 300
Chlorpropamide, 201

Chlorthalidone, 1, 158, 171
  drug interactions with
    digoxin, 11
    lithium, 11
    NSAIDs, 12
    toremifene, 12
  mechanism of action, 10
  molecular structure, 2
  side effects, 11
Chlor-Trimeton (see chlorpheniramine)
Cholestyramine, 159, 169
  drug interactions with
    ezetimibe, 161
    gotu kola, 161
    vitamins, 161
  mechanism of action, 160
  side effects, 160
Choriocarcinoma
  medications for
    cisplatin, 494, 498
    cyclophosphamide, 494, 498
    dactinomycin, 494–496
    etoposide, 494, 496
    methotrexate, 494
    vincristine, 494, 496–498
Chronic fatigue syndrome
  medications
    bupropion, 275
    modafinil, 274–275
    selegiline, 276–277
Cialis (see tadalafil)
Cibalith-S (see lithium carbonate)
Cibenzoline
  drug interactions with
    caffeine, 44
    theophylline, 44
  mechanism of action, 43
  side effects, 43
Cimetidine, 146, 166
  drug interactions, 147
  mechanism of action, 147
  side effects, 147
Cipralan (see cibenzoline)
Cipro (see ciprofloxacin)
Ciprofloxacin, 95, 173, 359
  drug interactions, 98, 175, 200, 527
  mechanism of action, 98, 175, 200, 527
  side effects, 98, 175, 200, 527
Cis-diaminedichloroplatinum, 461

Cisplatin, 102, 443, 461, 469, 489, 498, 558
  drug interactions with, 463, 490, 492
    aldesleukin, 462
    live vaccination, 462
    loop diuretics, 462
    vinorelbine, 463
    zalcitabine, 463
  mechanism of action, 461–462,
    489, 492
  molecular structure, 462
  side effects, 462, 489, 492
Citalopram
  drug interactions, 283
  mechanism of action, 282
  members, 282
  molecular structure, 282
  side effects, 282
Citrucel (see methylcellulose)
Clarinex (see desloratadine)
Clarithromycin, 95, 146, 318, 525, 527
  drug interactions, 101, 153, 528
  mechanism of action, 98, 100, 152, 528
  molecular structures, 99
  side effects, 98, 153, 528
Claritin (see loratadine)
Clemastine, 89, 426, 431
  drug interactions, first- and second-
    generation, 93–94
  mechanism of action, 93
  side effects first- and second-
    generation, 93
Clindamycin, 229, 525
  drug interactions with
    aminoglycoside antibiotics, 529
    erythromycin, 529
    neuromuscular blockers, 530
  mechanism of action, 528
  molecular structure, 529
  side effects, 529
Clobetasol
  drug interactions, 250
  mechanism of action, 250
  molecular structure, 246
  side effects, 250
  and triamcinolone, 246
Clofibrate, 212, 224
  molecular structure, 225
Clomiphene, 376
  drug interactions, 379

mechanism of action, 378–379
side effects, 379
Clonazepam
    drug interactions, 258, 323
    mechanism of action, 257, 322
    side effects, 257–258, 323
Clonidine, 1
    drug interaction with
        bupropion, 6
        cyclosporine, 6
        entacapone, 6
        lithium, 6
    mechanism of action, 4
    molecular structure of, 4
    side effects, 4
Clopidogrel, 410
    and CYP enzymes, 59
    drug interactions with, 58
        abciximab, 58
        aspirin, 58
        NSAIDs, 59
        omeprazole, 59
        valproic acid, 59
        warfarin, 59
    mechanism of action, 58
    molecular structure, 58
    side effects, 58
Clozapine, 193
    drug interactions, 296, 299
    mechanism of action, 296, 299
    molecular structure, 296, 299
    side effects, 296, 299
Clozaril (see clozapine)
Codeine, 110, 395
    drug interactions, 112–113, 401
    mechanism of action, 111–112, 401
    molecular structure, 112
    side effects, 112–113, 401
Cogentin (see benztropine)
Cognex (see tacrine)
Colace (see docusate sodium)
Colchicine
    and CYP enzymes, 223
    drug interactions, 223
    mechanism of action, 222
    molecular structure, 222
    side effects, 222
Colestipol, 169
Combivent (see albuterol + ipratropium)

Compazine (see prochlorperazine)
Concerta (see methylphenidate)
Condylomata
    medications for
        fluorouracil, 185–187
        imiquimod, 185–186
        podofilox gel, 185–186
Condylox (see podofilox gel)
Congestive heart failure
    medications for
        aldosterone-receptor blockers, 21
        angiotensin-converting enzyme
            (ACE), 21
        angiotensin-receptor blockers, 21
        bisoprolol, 21
        captopril, 21
        carvedilol, 21
        digoxin, 21
        enalapril, 21
        eplerenone, 21
        furosemide, 21
        lisinopril, 21
        losartan, 21
        metoprolol, 21
        spironolactone, 21
        valsartan, 21
Constipation
    medications
        bisacodyl, 168, 170
        bulk cathartics, 168–169
        docusate sodium, 168–170
        lubiprostone, 168
        magnesium citrate, 168, 172
        polyethylene glycol, 168, 172
        sennosides, 168, 170–171
CoQ10, molecular structure, 311
Cordarone (see amiodarone)
Coreg (see carvedilol)
Corgard (see nadolol)
Cortef (see cortisone + hydrocortisone)
Cortifoam (hydrocortisone ointment)
Cortisone
    drug interactions, 239
        anticholinesterase agents, 240
        CYP isozymes, 240
        diuretics, 240
        licorice, 240
        cut and dried root, 241
        leaves in nature, 241

Cortisone (*Cont'd.*)
    oral hypoglycemic agents, 241
    mechanism of action, 239
    side effects, 239
Cortisone + hydrocortisone
    adrenocorticotropic hormone
        (ACTH), 362
    drug interactions, 363
    mechanism of action, 362
    side effects, 362
Cotrimoxazole (*see* sulfamethoxazole +
    trimethoprim)
Coumadin (*see* warfarin)
Coumarin derivatives, molecular
    structures, 52
Covera (*see* verapamil)
Cozaar (*see* losartan)
Cream aluminum acetate, 243
Cream/gel azelaic acid, 243
Crestor (*see* rosuvastatin)
Cromolyn sodium, 89, 426
    drug interactions, 91, 432
    histamine, molecular structure, 91
    leukotrienes, molecular structure, 91
    mechanism of action, 90–91, 432
    molecular structure, 91
    side effects, 91, 432
Cuprimine (*see* penicillamine)
Cushing disease
    medications for
        ketoconazole, 366–367
        metirapone, 366–368
        methimazde or propylthiovracil
            (MPT), 366–368
Cyanocobalamin
    drug interactions with, 68–69
        alcohol, 69
        chloramphenicol, 69
        gastric antacids, 69
        H-2 blockers, 69
        neomycin, 69
        proton-pump inhibitors, 69
        tetracycline, 69
    mechanism of action, 67
    molecular structure, 68
    side effects, 68
Cyanokit (*see* hydroxocobalamin)
Cyclobenzaprine, 234

drug interactions with
    alcohol, 234–235
    CYP isozymes, 235
    magnesium hydroxide, 235
    monoamine oxidase (MAO), 235
    opioids, 236
mechanism of action, 234
molecular structure, 265
side effects, 234
Cycloguanil, molecular structure, 549
Cyclophosphamide, 34, 102, 487
    drug interactions, 461, 498
    mechanism of action, 460, 498
    side effects, 461, 498
Cyclosporine, 102, 107, 202, 228, 230,
        497, 541
    drug interactions with
        acetazolamide, 70
        caspofungin, 70
        ciprofloxacin, 74
        colchicine, 72
        CYP isozymes, 73
        digoxin, 72
        doxorubicin, 72
        fibrate drugs, 73
        hydroxychloroquine, 73
        ivermectin, 73
        levofloxacin, 74
        live vaccines, 73
        metoclopramide, 74
        metronidazole, 74
        moxifloxacin, 74
        nephrotoxic, 74
        nifedipine, 74
        norfloxacin, 74
        pefloxacin, 74
        rabeprazole, 74
    mechanism of action, 69–70, 231
    molecular structure, 70
    side effects, 70
Cycrin (*see* medroxyprogesterone)
Cyproheptadine, 89
    drug interactions, 92
    mechanism of action, 91–92
    molecular structure, 92
    side effects, 92
Cystitis/urethritis
    medications for

amoxicillin, 199
ampicillin, 199
ciprofloxacin, 199
nitrofurantoin, 199, 203–204
norfloxacin, 199
ofloxacin, 199
penicillins, 199
phenazopyridine, 199, 204–205
quinolone antibiotics, 199–200
sulfamethoxazole + trimethoprim,
    199–203
sulfa preparation, 199
urinary antiseptics, 199
urinary tract analgesics, 199
Cytomel (liothyronine), 372
Cytotec (*see* misoprostol)
Cytovene (*see* ganciclovir)
Cytoxan (*see* cyclophosphamide)

D

Dacarbazine
    drug interactions, 456
    mechanism of action, 455
    molecular structure, 456
    side effects, 456
Dactinomycin
    drug interactions with
        chloramphenicol, 495
        live vaccine, 496
        vinblastine, 496
        zidovudine, 496
    mechanism of action, 495
    molecular structure, 495
    side effects, 495
Danazol, 380
    drug interactions with
        anisindione, 381
        CYP isozymes, 381
        oral contraceptives, 381
    mechanism of action, 380–381
    molecular structure of, 380
    side effects, 381
Dandelion, 351, 353
Danocrine (*see* danazol)
Dapsone, molecular structure, 203
Darbepoetin alfa
    drug interactions, 74
    mechanism of action, 74

side effects, 74
Daunorubicin, 487
DDP (cis-diaminedichloroplatinum), 161
DDS (*see* didanosine)
Debacterol (*see* sulfonated phenol topical
    solution)
Decadron (*see* dexamethasone)
Deferoxamine, 569
    drug interactions with, 585
        aluminum, 586
        prochlorperazine, 586
        vitamin C, 586
    mechanism of action, 585
    molecular structure, 586
    side effects, 585
Delavirdine
    drug interactions with
        CYP isozymes, 519–520
        fosamprenavir, 520
    mechanism of action, 518–519
    molecular structure of, 519
    side effects, 519
Denileukin
    drug interactions, 460
    mechanism of action, 459
    side effects, 459–460
Depakene (*see* divalproex)
Depakote (*see* divalproex)
Depen (*see* penicillamine)
Deponit (*see* nitroglycerin)
N-desethylamiodarone, molecular
    structure, 35
Desipramine, 263, 267
    drug interactions, 268, 288
    mechanism of action, 268, 288
    members, 287
    molecular structures, 287
    side effects, 268, 288
Desloratadine, 90
    drug interactions, first- and second-
        generation, 93–94
    mechanism of action, 93
    side effects, first- and second-
        generation, 93
Desmopressin
    drug interactions, 360
    mechanism of action, 360
    side effects, 360

Desogestrel, 380
Detrol (*see* tolterodine)
Dexamethasone, 127, 426, 430, 541
   drug interactions, 130
   mechanism of action, 129–130
   molecular structure, 129
   side effects, 130
Dextroamphetamine
   drug interactions, 439
   mechanism of action, 439
   side effects, 439
Dextromethorphan, 110, 305, 437
   drug interactions with, 112
      alcohol, 114
      CYP isozymes, 114
      MAO inhibitors, 114
   mechanism of action, 113
   side effects, 113
Dextrostat (*see* dextroamphetamine)
DiaBeta (*see* glyburide)
Diabetes insipidus
   medications for
      desmopressin, 360
      hydrochlorothiazide, 360–161
      vasopressin, 360
Diabetes mellitus
   medications for
      exenatide, 349
      glimepiride, 349
      glipizide, 349
      glyburide, 349
      insulin, 349–352
      metformin, 349, 355–356
      pioglitazone, 349
      PPAR-gamma, 349, 356–358
      rosiglitazone, 349
      second-generation sulfonylureas, 349,
         352–353
Dialose (*see* docusate sodium)
Diamox (*see* acetazolamide)
Diarrhea
   medications for
      bismuth subsalicylate, 173–174
      opiate agonist, 173–174
      quinolone antibiotics, 173, 175
Diazepam, 107, 293, 318, 413
   drug interactions, 258, 416
   mechanism of action, 257, 416

side effects, 257–258, 416
Dibucaine, 176
   drug interactions, 176
   mechanism of action, 176
   side effects, 176
Diclofenac
   drug interactions, 219
   mechanism of action, 219
   side effects, 219
Dicumarol, 102, 213, 215, 364, 370, 553
Dicyclomine, 159, 166, 326
   drug interactions with, 167, 192
      alcohol, 164
      antiarrhythmic drugs, 164
      antiglaucoma drugs, 164
      lavender, 164
      levodopa, 165
      narcotic analgesics, 165
      phenothiazine antipsychotic drugs, 165
   mechanism of action, 163, 166, 191–192
   side effects, 163–164, 166, 192
Didanosine, 197, 497
   drug interactions with, 510–511
      allopurinol, 512–513
      emtricitabine, 512
      ganciclovir, 512
      tenofovir, 512
   mechanism of action, 508
   molecular structure of, 512
   side effects, 508
Diethylcarbamazine, 560
   drug interactions, 567
   mechanism of action, 566
   molecular structure, 567
   side effects, 566
Diflunisal, molecular structure, 225
Digitalis glycoside
   drug interactions, 26–28
   mechanism of action, 26
   side effects, 26
Digitek (*see* digoxin)
Digitoxin, molecular structure, 25
Digitoxose, molecular structure, 25
Digoxin, 44, 169
   drug interactions with, 26–27
      albuterol, 28
      brimonidine, 28
      fluoxetine, 28

ginseng, 28–29
hawthorn, 29
levalbuterol, 28
magnesium, 29
midodrine, 29
neomycin, 29
NSAIDs, 29
penicillamine, 30
phenytoin, 30
procarbazine, 30
propafenone, 30
quinolone antibiotics, 30
spironolactone, 31
SSRI members, 31
sulfamethoxazole-trimethoprim, 31
sulfasalazine, 31
telmisartan, 31
thyroid drugs, 31
trazodone, 31
mechanism of action, 26
side effects, 26
Dihydroergotamine, 437
Dihydrotestosterone, molecular
structure, 189
Dilacor (*see* diltiazem)
Dilantin (*see* phenytoin)
Dilor (*see* dyphylline)
Diloxanide, 555
drug interactions, 559
mechanism of action, 559
side effects, 559
Diltia (*see* diltiazem)
Diltiazem, 1
drug interactions, 10, 42
mechanism of action, 10, 42
molecular structure, 42
side effects, 10, 42
Dimenhydrinate, 139
drug interactions, 142, 339
mechanism of action, 141, 339
molecular structure of, 141
side effects, 142, 339
Dimercaprol, 569
drug interactions, 584
mechanism of action, 583
molecular structure, 584
side effects, 584
Dinagen (*see* piracetam)

Diovan (*see* valsartan)
Diphenhydramine, 89, 413, 426, 431
drug interactions, 339, 415
first- and second-generation, 93–94
mechanism of action, 93, 339, 415
molecular structure of, 139
side effects, 339, 415
first- and second-generation, 93
Diphenoxylate
drug interactions with
alcohol, 174
barbiturates, 174
MAO inhibitors, 174
quinidine, 174
mechanism of action, 173–174
molecular structure of, 173
side effects, 174
Diphosphonates
drug interactions, 210
mechanism of action, 209
members of, 209
side effects, 210
Dipyridamole, 44
Diquinol (*see* iodoquinol)
Disopyramide, 34, 158, 552–553
Ditropan (*see* oxybutynin)
Diuretics, 1, 40, 290, 411
bumetanide, 13
drug interactions, 11–12, 15–16,
23, 195
ethacrynic acid, 13
furosemide, 13
hydrochlorothiazide, 13
mechanism of action, 10, 14, 23, 195
members of, 10, 13, 195
potassium chloride, 13
side effects, 11, 23, 14–15, 195
spironolactone, 13
triamterene, 13
Divalproex
drug interactions, 314
mechanism of action, 313
molecular structure, 313
side effects, 314
Docetaxel
drug interactions, 444, 482
mechanism of action, 444, 482
side effects, 444, 482

Docusate sodium, 168
    drug interactions, 170
    mechanism of action, 169
    side effects, 170
Dofetilide, 171, 202
Domeboro (see cream aluminum
        acetate), 243
Domperidone
    drug interactions
        CYP isozymes with, 157–158
    mechanism of action, 157
    side effects, 157
Donepezil
    drug interactions, 302–304
    mechanism of action, 302
    molecular structure, 301
    side effects, 302
Dihydrophenylacetic acid (DOPAC),
        molecular structure, 332
Dopamine agonists, 107, 452
    drug interactions, 330
    mechanism of action, 330
    members of, 330
    side effects, 330
Dopar (see levodopa)
Doryx (see doxycycline)
Dostinex (see cabergoline)
Doxazosin, 1, 180
    drug interactions, 4, 188, 206
    mechanism of action, 3, 206
    members of, 3
    molecular structure, 3
    side effects, 3–4, 188, 206
Doxepin, 263, 267
    drug interactions, 268, 288
    mechanism of action, 268, 288
    members, 287
    molecular structures, 287
    side effects, 268, 288
Doxil (see doxorubicin)
Doxorubicin (DXR), 454, 469, 487, 490, 493
    drug interactions with, 461
        azithromycin, 456–457
        cyclosporine, 457
        CYP isozymes, 457
        digoxin, 457
        live vaccines, 457
        trastuzumab, 457
    mechanism of action, 454–455, 460
    molecular structures, 455
    side effects, 455–456, 461
Doxorubicin + bleomycin + vinblastine +
        dacarbazine (ABVD)
    drug interactions, 456–459
    mechanism of action, 454–455
    members of, 454
    side effects, 455–456
Doxycycline, 136
    drug interactions with, 527
        tetracyclines, 137–138
    mechanism of action, 137, 526
    side effects, 137, 527
Doxylamine, 89, 413, 426, 431
    drug interactions, 415
        first- and second generation,
            93–94
    mechanism of action, 93, 415
    side effects, 415
        first- and second-generation, 93
Dramamine (see dimenhydrinate)
Droperidol, 427, 552–553
Drospirenone, 380
Drugs
    for peptic ulcers, 154, 156
    therapeutic group interactions
        ACE inhibitors, 602–603
        alpha agonists, 614
        alpha blockers, 600–601
        angiotensin-receptor blockers (ARB),
            609–610
        antifungal drugs, 625–626
        antihistamines, first-generation,
            618–619
        second-generation, 620
        atypical antipsychotic drugs, 621–622
        benzodiazepines, 629–630
        beta blockers, 596–599
        calcium-channel blockers, 611–613
        cephalosporins, 631–632
        dopamine agonists, 646–647
        gastric antacids, 633–634
        glucocorticoids, 637–638
        H2 blockers, 639–640
        loop diuretics, 606–608
        macrolide antibiotics, 623–624
        magnesium salts, 635–636

NSAIDs, 641–645
   opioid analgesics, 670–673
   penicillins, 648
   phenothiazines, 649–652
   progestogens, 653–654
   protease inhibitors, 615–617
   proton-pump inhibitors, 655–656
   quinolone antibiotics, 657–659
   SSRIs, 661–663
   tetracyclines, 664–666
   thiazide diuretics, 604–605
   tricyclic antidepressants, 667–669
Dulcolax (*see* bisacodyl)
Duloxetine
   drug interactions with
      alcohol, 279
      CYP isozymes, 279
      MAO inhibitors, 279
      propafenone, 279
      venlafaxine vs CYP enzymes, 280
   mechanism of action, 278
   molecular structure, 278
   side effects, 279
Duragesic (*see* fentanyl)
Dutasteride
   drug interactions, 198, 207
   mechanism of action, 198, 207
   molecular structure, 198
   side effects, 198, 207
Duvoid (*see* bethanechol)
Dyclonine, 131
   drug interactions, 132
   mechanism of action, 131–132
   molecular structure of, 131
   side effects, 132
Dynacin (minocycline)
Dynacirc (isradipine)
Dyphylline, 116
   drug interactions, 120
   mechanism of action, 120
   molecular structure of, 119
   side effects, 120
Dysentery
   medications for
      diloxanide, 559
      iodoquinol, 557
      metronidazole, 555–557
      paromomycin, 557

Dyspepsia
   medications for
      domperidone, 157–158
      metoclopramide, 157–158

E
Ebixa (*see* memantine)
Econopred (*see* prednisolone)
Eczema
   medications for
      glucocorticoid, 250
      immunosuppressants, 246–250
Edecrin (*see* ethacrynic acid)
Edema
   treatment for
      angiotensin-converting enzyme (ACE)
         inhibitors, 13
      benazepril, 13
      bumetanide, 13
      captopril, 13
      diuretics, 13–17
      enalapril, 13
      ethacrynic acid, 13
      furosemide, 13
      hydrochlorothiazide, 13
      lisinopril, 13
      nitroglycerin, 13
      ramipril, 13
      sodium nitroprusside, 13
      vasodilators, 13, 17–19
Efalizumab, 251
   drug interactions with
      anakinra, 252
      cyclophosphamide, 252
   mechanism of action, 251
   side effects, 252
Efavirenz
   drug interactions with, 520
   mechanism of action, 518–519
   molecular structure of, 519
   side effects, 519
Efudex (*see* fluorouracil)
Elavil (*see* amitriptyline)
Eldepryl (*see* selegiline)
Elidel (*see* pimecrolimus cream)
Ellence (*see* epirubicin)
Emadine (*see* emedastine)
Emcyt (*see* estramustine)

Emedastine, 426
    drug interactions, 432
    mechanism of action, 432
    side effects, 432
Emtricitabine
    mechanism of action, 509
    molecular structure of, 509
    side effects, 509
Enalapril, 1
    drug interactions, 9, 20
    mechanism of action, 6, 9, 20
    molecular structure of, 7
    side effects, 9, 20
Enbrel (see etanercept)
Enfuvirtide
    drug interactions, 524
    mechanism of action, 524
    side effects, 524
Ephedrine, 277, 406
Epilepsy
    medications for
        benzodiazepines, 313, 322–323
        carbamazepine, 313
        clonazepam, 313
        divalproex, 313–314
        gabapentin, 313, 315
        lamotrigine, 313
        levetiracetam, 313, 315
        lorazepam, 313
        oxcarbazepine, 313
        phenobarbital, 313
        phenytoin, 313
        pregabalin, 313, 315
        sodium-channel blockers, 313,
            315–316
Epinephrine, 406, 569
    drug interactions with, 426, 572
        anesthetic agents, 427
        beta blockers, 428
        digoxin, 428
        guanethidine, 428
        levothyroxine, 428
        MAO inhibitor, 428
    mechanism of action, 426, 572
    molecular structure, 27
    side effects, 426, 572
EpiPen (see epinephrine)
Epirubicin, 487

    drug interactions, 483
    mechanism of action, 483
    side effects, 483
Eplerenone
    CYP enzymes and, 25
    mechanism of action, 23
    molecular structure, 24
    side effects, 24
Epoetin alfa
    drug interactions, 74
    mechanism of action, 74
    side effects, 74
Eprosartan, 1
    drug interactions, 10
    mechanism of action, 9
    side effects, 9–10
Eptifibatide, 410
    drug interactions, 60
    mechanism of action, 59
    side effects, 60
Erectile dysfunction (ED), 18–19
    medications for
        phosphodiesterase inhibitors,
            179–181
        pycnogenol, 179, 181–183
        relation with CYP enzymes, 181
ERG. (see Ergoloid mesylates)
Ergoloid mesylates
    drug interactions with
        beta blockers with, 309
        CYP isozymes with, 309–310
        MAO Inhibitors with, 309
    mechanism of action, 308
    side effects, 308
Ergomar (see ergotamine)
Ergosterol, molecular structure of, 538
Ergot alkaloids, molecular structures, 331
Ergotamine, 396, 404–407, 427
    drug interactions with
        amyl nitrite, 405
        beta blockers, 406
        CYP isozymes, 406–407
        dopamine, 406
    mechanism of action, 404
    side effects, 405
Erythromycin, 95, 318
    drug interactions, 101
    mechanism of action, 98, 100

molecular structures, 99
side effects, 98–100
Escitalopram
  drug interactions, 283
  mechanism of action, 282
  members, 282
  side effects, 282
Esidrix (*see* hydrochlorothiazide)
Eskalith (*see* lithium carbonate)
Esmolol
  drug interactions, 43
  mechanism of action, 42
  molecular structure, 42
  side effects, 43
Esomeprazole, 146
  drug interactions, 148
  mechanism of action, 147
  side effects, 148
Estazolam, 413
  drug interactions, 416
  mechanism of action, 416
  side effects, 416
Estradiol
  drug interactions with
    anticoagulants, 385
    black cohosh, 385
    cholesterol-lowering drugs, 385
    CYP isozymes, 385
    insulin, 385
    licorice, 386
    NSAIDs, 386
    vasodilators, 386
  mechanism of action, 384
  molecular structure of, 384
  side effects, 385
Estramustine
  drug interactions, 501
  mechanism of action, 501
  molecular structure, 501
  side effects, 501
Estrogen + progestogen, 417
  drug interactions, 421
  mechanism of action, 418
  members of, 417
  side effects, 419
Estrogens, 510
Estrostep Fe (ethinyl estradiol +
    norethindrone), 417

Eszopiclone
  drug interactions, 414
  mechanism of action, 413–414
  molecular structure of, 413
  side effects, 414
Etanercept, 251
  drug interactions with
    anakinra, 252
    cyclophosphamide, 252
  mechanism of action, 251
  side effects, 252
Ethacrynic acid, 1, 558
  drug interactions, 12, 23
  mechanism of action, 10, 23
  molecular structure of, 11
  side effects, 11, 23
Ethambutol, 525
  drug interactions, 534
  mechanism of action, 533
  side effects, 534
Ethanolamine oleate
  drug interactions, 77
  mechanism of action, 77
  side effects, 77
Ethinyl estradiol, 417
  drug interactions with
    anticoagulants, 419–420
    black cohosh, 420
    chasteberry, 420
    cholesterol-lowering drugs, 420
    CYP isozymes, 420
    dantrolene, 420
    didanosine, 420
    insulin, 420
    licorice, 420
    NSAIDs, 420
    ropinirole, 420–421
    thyroid preparations, 421
    vasodilators, 421
  mechanism of action, 418
  relation with CYP enzymes, 421
  side effects, 418
Ethinyl estradiol + desogestrel, 417
Ethinyl estradiol + drospirenone, 417
Ethinyl estradiol + etonogestrel, 417
Ethinyl estradiol + norelgestromin, 417
Ethinyl estradiol + norethindrone, 417
Ethinyl estradiol + norgestimate, 417

Ethinyl estradiol + norgestrel, 417
Etodolac
    drug interactions, 219
    mechanism of action, 219
    side effects, 219
Etonogestrel, 380
    molecular structure of, 418
Etopophos (*see* etoposide)
Etoposide, 441, 496, 499
    drug interactions with
        cyclosporine, 441
        CYP isozymes, 442
        live vaccines, 442
        warfarin, 442
    mechanism of action, 441
    molecular structures, 441
    side effects, 441
Etretinate, molecular structure, 253
Everolimus
    CYP enzymes, 468
    drug interactions, 467
    mammalian target of rapamycin
        (mTOR), 467
    mechanism of action, 467
    side effects, 467
Evista (*see* raloxifene)
Evra (ethinyl estradiol +
        norelgestromin)
Exelon (*see* rivastigmine)
Exemestane
    CYP enzymes and, 480
    drug interactions, 480
    mechanism of action, 479
    molecular structure, 478
    side effects, 480
Exenatide
    drug interactions, 358–359
    mechanism of action, 358
    side effects, 358
Ex-lax (*see* sennosides)
Extina (*see* ketoconazole)
Ezetimibe
    interactions, 83
        cyclosporine with, 83
        saturated fat, 84
    mechanism of action, 82
    molecular structure, 83
    side effects, 83

F
Famotidine, 146, 166
    drug interactions, 147
    mechanism of action, 147
    side effects, 147
Fareston (*see* toremifene)
Femara (*see* letrozole)
Fenofibrate
    drug interactions with
        bile acid sequestrants, 85
        bitter gourd, 85
        cyclosporine, 85
        ezetimibe, 86
        gotu kola, 86
        repaglinide, 86
    mechanism of action, 84
    molecular structure, 84
    side effects, 84–85
Fenofibric acid, molecular structure, 84
Fentanyl
    drug interactions, 401
    mechanism of action, 401
    molecular structure, 34
    side effects, 401
Fenugreek, 351, 353, 356
Ferrous sulfate or ferrous fumarate
    drug interactions with, 65
        ciprofloxacin, 66
        demeclocycline, 66
        doxycycline, 66
        levofloxacin, 66
        lomefloxacin, 66
        minocycline, 66
        norfloxacin, 66
        ofloxacin, 66
        tetracycline, 66
    mechanism of action, 65
    side effects, 65
Fexofenadine, 90, 426, 431
    drug interactions, first- and second-
        generation, 93–94
        pseudoephedrine with, 94
    mechanism of action, 93
    side effects, first- and second-generation, 93
Fibrates
    drug interactions, 85
    mechanism of action, 84
    side effects, 84

Finasteride
  drug interactions, 198, 207
    CYP isozymes with, 198
  mechanism of action, 198, 207
  molecular structure, 198
  side effects, 198, 207
First-generation antihistamines
  drug interactions, 431
  mechanism of action, 431
  members of, 431
  side effects, 431
Flagyl (*see* metronidazole)
Flatulence
  medications for
    activated charcoal, 143, 145
    rifaximin, 143–144
    simethicone, 143–144
Flexeril (*see* cyclobenzaprine)
Flomax (*see* tamsulosin)
Flonase (*see* fluticasone)
Flovent HFA (*see* fluticasone)
Floxin (*see* ofloxacin)
Fluconazole, 537
  drug interactions, 538–539
  mechanism of action, 537
  molecular structure of, 537
  side effects, 538
Fludara (*see* fludarabine)
Fludarabine
  drug interactions, 475
  mechanism of action, 474
  molecular structure, 474
  side effects, 474–475
Fludrocortisone, 362
  drug interactions with, 363
    antihypertensive drugs, 364
    CYP isozymes, 364
    digoxin, 365
    insulin, 365
    live vaccines, 365
    midodrine, 365
    NSAIDs, 365
    oral hypoglycemic agents, 365
  mechanism of action, 363
  molecular structure of, 363
  side effects, 363
Flumadine (*see* rimantadine)
Flumazenil, 569

  drug interactions, 578
  mechanism of action, 577
  molecular structure, 577
  side effects, 578
Flunisolide, 426, 430
Fluorometholone, 426, 430
Fluor-Op (*see* fluorometholone)
Fluoroplex (*see* fluorouracil)
Fluoroplex (*see* fluorouracil)
Fluoroquinolone antibiotics, 525
  drug interactions, 527
  mechanism of action, 527
  members, 527
  side effects, 527
Fluoroquinolones
  basic structure, 448
  molecular structure, 448
Fluorouracil, 489
  drug interactions with, 187
    bone marrow depressants, 470
    CYP isozymes, 471
    hydroxyurea, 470
    live vaccines, 470–471
    zidovudine, 471
  mechanism of action, 186, 469
  molecular structure, 187
  side effects, 187, 470
Fluoxetine, 92, 277
  drug interactions, 264, 283
  mechanism of action, 263–264, 282
  members, 282
  molecular structure, 282
  side effects, 264, 282
Flutamide
  CYP enzymes and, 500
  drug interactions, 500
  mechanism of action, 500
  molecular structure, 500
  side effects, 500
Fluticasone, 89, 116, 426, 430
  drug interactions, 90, 121
  mechanism of action, 90, 120–121
  side effects, 90, 121
Fluvastatin
  drug interactions with
    cholestyramine, 80
    digoxin, 81
    exenatide, 81

Fluvastatin (cont'd.)
  mechanism of action, 80
  molecular structures, 79
  side effects, 80
Folic acid
  drug interactions with, 66
    cholestyramine, 67
    colestipol, 67
    phenytoin, 67
    pyrimethamine, 67
    sulfasalazine, 67
  mechanism of action, 66
  molecular structures, 66
  side effects, 66
Follicle-stimulating hormone (FSH), 376
  drug interactions, 377
  mechanism of action, 377
  side effects, 377
Fomepizole, 569, 576
  drug interactions, 577
  mechanism of action, 577
  side effects, 577
Fosamax (see alendronate)
Fosamprenavir, 520
  mechanism of action, 521
  molecular structure of, 521–522
  side effects, 523
Fosinopril, 1
  drug interactions, 9
  mechanism of action, 6, 9
  molecular structure of, 7
  side effects, 9
Four-drug combination
  drug interactions, 461
  mechanism of action, 460–461
  members of, 460
  molecular structure, 460
  side effects, 461
Fungi infections
  for medications
    azole antifungal drugs, 537–539
    caspofungin, 537, 539–541
    micafungin, 537, 539–541
    terbinafine, 537, 541–543
Furamide (see diloxanide)
Furosemide, 1, 158
  drug interactions, 23, 64
  mechanism of action, 23, 64
  molecular structure of, 11
  side effects, 23, 64

G
Gabapentin
  drug interactions with
    antacids, 315
    cimetidine, 315
    morphine, 315
  mechanism of action, 314
  molecular structure and BABA, 314
Gabarone (see gabapentin)
Gamma-aminobutyric acid (GABA)
  derivative
    drug interactions, 307
    mechanism of action, 306
    side effects, 307
  molecular structure, 292
Gamma-aminobutyric acid (GABA)
    activators, 413
  drug interactions with
    alcohol, 414
    aminoglutethimide, 414
    CYP isozymes, 414–415
    flumazenil, 414
    imipramine, 414
    thioridazine, 414
  mechanism of action, 413–414
  members of, 413
  side effects, 414
Ganciclovir, 512
  molecular structure, 514
Garlic, 352–353, 356
Gastric antacids, 167
  drug interactions, 147
  mechanism of action, 146
  side effects, 147
Gastroesophageal reflux disease
    (GERD)
  medications for
    bethanechol, 154–156
    drugs for peptic ulcers, 154, 156
    metoclopramide, 154
GCSF (see granulocyte colony-stimulating
    factor)
Gemcitabine
  drug interactions, 445
  mechanism of action, 444
  molecular structure, 445
  side effects, 444
Gemfibrozil
  drug interactions, 85
  mechanism of action, 84

molecular structure, 84
side effects, 84
Gemtuzumab ozogamicin
  drug interactions, 475
  mechanism of action, 475
  side effects, 475
Gemzar (*see* gemcitabine)
Gentamicin, 95
  bacitracin, 102
  drug interactions, 101–102
  mechanism of action, 101
  polymyxin B, 102
  side effects, 101
Gerimal (*see* Ergoloid mesylates)
Gingivitis
  chlorhexidine gluconate, 136–137
  doxycycline, 137–138
  hydrogen peroxide, 138
  medications for
    gel, 136
    mouthwash, 136
  minocycline, 137–138
Ginkgo biloba, 410
Ginseng, 352–353
Glimepiride, 353
Glipizide, 353
Glucagon, 569
  drug interactions with
    beta blockers, 571
    warfarin, 571
  mechanism of action, 571
  side effects, 571
Glucocorticoids, 228, 352–353, 356, 410
  drug interactions, 90, 121, 177, 250,
    430–431
  mechanism of action, 90, 120–121, 176,
    218, 250, 430
  members of, 90, 120, 218, 250, 430
  prednisone
    drug interactions, 230
    mechanism of action, 230
    side effects, 230
  side effects, 90, 121, 177, 218, 250, 430
(*see also* clobetasol, and triamcinolone)
Glucophage (*see* metformin),
Glucosamine + chondroitin sulfate
  drug interactions, 214–215
    aspirin with, 215
  mechanism of action, 214
  side effects, 214

Glucotrol (glipizide), 353
Glutamic acid, molecular structure, 314
Glyburide, 318, 353
Glycolax (*see* polyethylene glycol)
Glycoprotein llb/llla receptor
    antagonists
  drug interactions, 60
  mechanism of action, 59
  side effects, 60
Glycopyrrolate, 146
  drug interactions, 151
  mechanism of action, 151
  side effects, 151
Glynase (*see* glyburide)
GM-CSF (*see* granulocyte macrophage
    colony-stimulating factor), 65
Gonadotropin-releasing hormone
    analogues, 376
  drug interactions, 378
  mechanism of action, 378
  side effects, 378
Goserelin
  drug interactions, 500
  mechanism of action, 499
  side effects, 499
Gotu kola, 352–353, 356
Gout
  medications for
    allopurinol, 221–222
    colchicine, 222–223
    ibuprofen, 221, 227
    indomethacin, 221, 227
    naproxen, 221, 227
    NSAIDs, 221, 227
    probenecid, 221
    sulfinpyrazone, 221
    uricosuric agents, 221, 223–226
Granulocyte colony-stimulating factor
    (GCSF), 65
Granulocyte-macrophage colony-
    stimulating factor (GM-CSF), 65
  drug interactions, 75
  mechanism of action, 75
  side effects, 75
Gravol (*see* dimenhydrinate)
Guanethidine, 351, 353
Guanfacine, 1
  mechanism of action, 4
  molecular structure of, 4
  side effects, 4

H

Halcion (*see* triazolam)
Haldol (*see* haloperidol)
Halfan (primaquine; halofantrine)
Halofantrine, 553
    drug interactions with
        CYP isozymes, 551
        diuretics, 551
        gastric antacid, 551
        mefloquine, 551
        methadone, 552
    mechanism of action, 550–551
    molecular structure, 551
    side effects, 551
Haloperidol, 273, 382, 427, 552–553
    molecular structure of, 389
Hawthorn berries, 30, 410
Helicobacter pylori, 157
Helminthiasis
    medications for
        albendazole, 561–563
        diethylcarbamazine, 566–567
        ivermectin, 567–568
        mebendazole, 560–561
        niclosamide, 565
        praziquantel, 565–566
        pyrantel pamoate 563–564
        thiabendazole, 564–565
Hemorrhage
    medications for
        bumetanide, 61
        furosemide, 61
        oxymetazoline, 61–62
        phenylephrine, 61–62
        vasopressin, 61–63
Hemorrhoids
    therapies for
        glucocorticoids, 176–177
        local anesthetic, 176
        phenylephrine, 176–177
Heparin
    drug interactions with
        cephalosporins, 49
        chamomile, 51
        dextran, 49
        fludrocortisone, 51
        valproic acid, 51
    Low-molecular-weight heparin (LMWH)
        interactions

        antiplatelet drugs, 50
        argatroban, 50
        human antithrombin III, 50
        nonsteroidal anti-inflammatory
            drugs, 51
        salicylates, 51
        thrombolytic agents, 50
    mechanism of action, 49
    side effects, 49
Hepatotoxic drugs, 535
Herceptin (*see* trastuzumab)
Herpes infections
    herpes simplex virus (HSV) type-1 and
        type-2, 502
    medications for
        acyclovir or valacyclovir, 502–504
        penciclovir or famciclovir, 504–505
Hexalen (*see* altretamine)
Hiccup
    medications for
        baclofen, 104–106
        metoclopramide, 104, 1107–109
        phenothiazines, 104–105
High blood pressure (*see* hypertension)
Histamine
    drug interactions, 91
    mechanism of action, 90–91
    molecular structure, 91
    side effects, 91
HIV infections, 507
    drug interactions with, 510–514
    medication
        enfuvirtide, 524
        nucleoside reverse transcriptase (RT)
            inhibitors, 508–518
        non-nucleoside RT inhibitors,
            518–521
        protease inhibitors, 521–524
HMG CoA reductase, site of action, 80
Hodgkin lymphoma
    medications for
        adriamycin, bleomycin, vinblastinev,
            and dacarbazine ABVD, 454–459
        doxorubicin, 454
        etoposide, 454, 459–460
H2 blockers, 167, 535
    drug interactions, 147
    mechanism of action, 147
    side effects, 147

Humalog (insulin lispro), 350
Human chorionic gonadotropin
    (hCG), 376
  drug interactions, 378
  mechanism of action, 377
  side effects, 377
Human insulin injection, 350
Human insulin isophane, 350
Human menopausal gonadotropin, 376
  drug interactions, 377
  luteinizing hormone (LH), 376
  mechanism of action, 376
  side effects, 376
Humatin (*see* paromomycin)
Humulin N (human insulin isophane), 350
Humulin 70/30 (human insulin
    isophane), 350
Hycamtin (*see* topotecan)
Hycoclear (*see* hydrocodone)
Hydergine see Ergoloid mesylates
Hydrochlorothiazide, 13
  drug interactions, 15, 195, 361
  mechanism of action, 14, 361
  members of, 195
  molecular structure, 2
  side effects, 14–15, 195, 361
Hydrocodone, 110, 395
  drug interactions, 111, 401
  mechanism of action, 110, 401
  members of, 110
  molecular structure, 111
  side effects, 110, 401
Hydrocortisone
  drug interactions with, 177, 239
    anticholinesterase agents, 240
    CYP isozymes, 240
    diuretics, 240
    licorice, 240
    cut and dried root, 241
    leaves in nature, 241
    oral hypoglycemic agents, 241
  mechanism of action, 176, 239
  side effects, 177, 239
Hydrocortisone ointment, 176
Hydrogen peroxide, 131, 136
  drug interactions, 132, 138
  mechanism of action, 132, 138
  side effects, 132, 138
Hydromorphone, molecular structure, 111

Hydroxocobalamin, 569
  drug interactions, 579–580
  mechanism of action, 579
  side effects, 579
Hydroxychloroquine
  drug interactions with
    acetaminophen, 218
    CYP isozymes, 218
    digoxin, 218
    penicillamine, 218
    sotalol, 218
  mechanism of action, 217
  side effects, 217
Hydroxyurea, 510
Hydroxyzine, 89, 257, 426, 431
  drug interactions, 262, 392
    first and second generation, 93–94
  mechanism of action, 93, 261, 391
  side effects, 262, 391
    first- and second-generation, 93
Hyoscyamine, 159, 166
  drug interactions, 164, 167, 192
  mechanism of action, 163, 166, 191–192
  side effects, 164, 166, 192
Hypercortisolism (*see* Cushing disease)
Hyperemesis gravidarum
  medications for
    hydroxyzine, 391–392
    metoclopramide, 391–392
    ondansetron, 391
    promethazine, 391–393
Hyperlipidemia
  medications for
    atorvastatin, 78
    ezetimibe, 78
    fenofibrate, 78
    fluvastatin, 78
    gemfibrozil, 78
    lovastatin, 78
    niacin, 78
    pravastatin, 78
    rosuvastatin, 78
    simvastatin, 78
Hypertension
  medications for
    ACE inhibitors, 1, 6–9
    alpha-1 blockers, 1, 3–4
    alpha-2 activators, 1, 4–6
    angiotensin-receptor blockers, 1, 9–10

Hypertension (*Cont'd.*)
  beta blockers, 1
  calcium channel blockers, 1, 10
  diuretics, 1, 10–12
Hyperthyroidism
  medications for
    propranolol, 369, 371
    sodium iodine, 369, 371
    thioamides, 369–370
Hypoadrenocortisolism (*see* Addison disease)
Hypogonadism
  medications for
    clomiphene, 376, 378–379
    follicle-stimulating hormone (FSH), 376–377
    gonadotropin-releasing hormone analogues, 376, 378
    human chorionic gonadotropin (hCG), 376–378
    human menopausal gonadotropin (hMG), 376–377
Hypothyroidism
  medications for
    armour thyroid, 372, 374–375
    synthetic thyroid hormones, 372
    thyrotropin alfa, 372, 375
Hypoxanthine, molecular structure, 512
Hytrin (*see* terazosin)
Hyzaar (*see* losartan)

I

Ibandronate, 411
  drug interactions with
    aminoglycosides, 210
    antacids, 210
    aspirin, 210
    CYP enzymes, 210–211
    estrogens, 211
    NSAIDs, 211
  molecular structures, 211
Ibuprofen, 212, 395, 408
  drug interactions, 219, 227, 242, 400, 412
  mechanism of action, 219, 227, 241, 399, 412
  molecular structure, 242
  side effects, 219, 227, 242, 400, 412
Ibutilide, 158

Idamycin (*see* idarubicin)
Idarubicin
  drug interactions, 476
  mechanism of action, 475–476
  side effects, 476
Idebenone
  drug interactions, 310
  mechanism of action, 310
  molecular structure, 311
  side effects, 310
Ifex (*see* ifosfamide)
Ifosfamide, 102, 499
  drug interactions with
    aminoglycosides antibiotics, 488
    bone marrow depressants, 488
    CYP isozymes, 488
    live vaccines, 488–489
    warfarin, 489
  mechanism of action, 488
  molecular structure, 487
  side effects, 488
Imdur (*see* isosorbide mononitrate)
Imipramine, 263, 267
  drug interactions, 268, 288
  mechanism of action, 268, 288
  members, 287
  molecular structures, 287
  side effects, 268, 288
Imiquimod, 471
  drug interactions, 186, 472
  mechanism of action, 186, 472
  molecular structure, 186
  side effects, 186, 472
Imitrex (*see* sumatriptan)
Immunosuppressants, 228
  drug interactions with, 231–233, 248
    alcohol, 249
    azole antifungals, 249
    clotrimazole, 249
    CYP isozymes, 249
    danazol, 249
    live vaccines, 249
    NSAIDs, 249–250
  mechanism of action, 231, 246–247
  members of, 230, 246
  side effects, 231, 247–248
Immunosuppressive agents
  drug interactions

mechanism of action, 69–70
side effects
Imodium (*see* loperamide)
Imuran (*see* azathioprine)
Indapamide, 38
Inderal (*see* propranolol)
Indinavir, 318
   mechanism of action, 521
   molecular structures of, 522
   side effects, 523
Indocin (*see* indomethacin)
Indomethacin, 212
   drug interactions, 219, 227
   mechanism of action, 219, 227
   side effects, 219, 227
Infertility
   medications for
     clomiphene, 376, 378–379
     follicle-stimulating hormone (FSH),
       376–377
     gonadotropin-releasing hormone
       analogues, 376, 378
     human chorionic gonadotropin (hCG),
       376–378
     human menopausal gonadotropin
       (hMG), 376–377
Infliximab, 251
   drug interactions with
     anakinra, 252
     cyclophosphamide, 252
   mechanism of action, 251
   side effects, 252
Influenza
   medications for
     oseltamivir, 506–507
     rimantadine, 507
   viruses types A, B and C, 505
Inhibitors of 5-alpha reductase
   drug interactions, 189, 207
     CYP isozymes and, 190
   mechanism of action, 189, 207
   members of, 189, 207
   side effects, 189, 207
Ionamin (*see* phentermine)
Insomnia
   medications for
     benzodiazepine (BDZ) sedatives, 413,
       415–416

gama-amino butyric acid (GABA)
     activators, 413–415
   sedating antihistamines,
     413, 415
Inspra (*see* eplerenone)
Insulin, 215
   drug interactions, 350–352
     alcohol with, 350
   mechanism of action, 350
   side effects, 350
Insulin aspart, 350
Insulin glargine, 350
Insulin lispro, 350
Intestinal cramps
   medications for
     anticholinergic agents, 166–167
     gastric antacids, 166–167
     H2 blockers, 166–167
Iodoquinol, 555
   drug interactions, 557
   mechanism of action, 557
   molecular structure, 557
   side effects, 557
Ipecac syrup, 569
Ipratropium, molecular structure, 119
Irbesartan, 1
   drug interactions, 10
   mechanism of action, 9
   side effects, 9–10
Irbesartan + hydrochlorothiazide, 1
Irinotecan
   drug interactions with
     chloramphenicol, 493
     CYP isozymes, 494
     live vaccines, 494
     zidovudine, 494
   mechanism of action, 493
   molecular structures, 443
   side effects, 493
Irritable bowel syndrome (IBS)
   medications for
     alosetron, 159–160
     anticholinergic agents, 159,
       163–165
     cholestyramine, 159–161
     loperamide, 159, 161–163
     tegaserod, 159, 165
Ismo (*see* isosorbide mononitrate)

Isoniazid, 525
    drug interactions with
        carbamazepine, 534
        CYP isozymes, 534
        dicumarol, 534
        disulfiram, 534–535
        meperidine, 535
        phenytoin, 535
    mechanism of action, 533
    molecular structure, 533
    side effects, 534
Isoproterenol, 427
Isoptin (*see* verapamil)
Isosorbide dinitrate, molecular
        structure, 180
Isosorbide mononitrate
    drug interactions with, 45
        ACE inhibitors, 46
        alpha blockers, 46
        anesthetic agents, 46
        beta blockers, 46
        erectile dysfunction drugs, 46
        ganglionic blockers, 46
        nitroglycerin, 46
    mechanism of action, 45
    side effects, 45
Isradipine, 1
    drug interactions, 10
    mechanism of action, 10
    side effects, 10
Ivermectin, 560
    drug interactions with
        alcohol, 568
        cyclosporine, 568
        high fat meal, 568
        ketoconazole, 568
    mechanism of action, 567
    molecular structure, 568
    side effects, 567

K

Kaletra (*see* lopinavir + ritonavir)
Kaolin, 545
Kariva (ethinyl estradiol +
        desogestrel), 417
Kayexalate (*see* sodium polystyrene
        sulfonate)
Keflex (*see* cephalexin)

Ketamine, 305
Ketek (*see* telithromycin)
Ketoconazole, 366, 537
    drug interactions, 367, 538–539
    mechanism of action, 367, 537
    molecular structure of, 537
    side effects, 367, 538
Ketoprofen
    drug interactions, 242
    mechanism of action, 241
    molecular structure, 242
    side effects, 242
Ketorolac, 224
    molecular structure, 225
Kidney cancer
    medications for
        everolimus, 467
        sorafenib tosylate, 467–468
        sunitinib malate, 467–469
Klonopin (*see* clonazepam)
Kuric (*see* ketoconazole)

L

Labetalol, 1, 18
    interactions with drug, 3
    mechanism of action, 2
    molecular structure of, 2
    side effects, 2–3
Lamictal (*see* lamotrigine)
Lamisil (*see* terbinafine)
Lamivudine
    drug interaction with
        ribavirin, 512
        trimethoprim-sulfamethoxazole, 514
        zalcitabine, 514
    mechanism of action, 509
    molecular structure of, 509, 515
    side effects, 509
Lamotrigine
    drug interactions, 316
    mechanism of action, 316
    side effects, 316
Lanosterol, molecular structure, 367
Lanoxin (*see* digoxin)
Lansoprazole
    drug interactions, 148
    mechanism of action, 147
    side effects, 148

Lantus, (insulin glargine), 350
Lariam (*see* mefloquine)
Larodopa (*see* levodopa)
Laryngitis, 95
  ciprofloxacin, 98
  medications for
    aminoglycoside antibiotics, 95,
      102–103
    cephalosporin antibiotics, 95–97
    fluoroquinolone antibiotics, 95
    macrolide antibiotics, 95, 98–101
    penicillins, 95–96
Lasix (*see* furosemide)
Lavender, cut and dried
    flower, 165
Leflunomide, 465
Lepirudin
  drug interactions, 52
  mechanism of action, 51–52
  side effects, 52
Letrozole
  CYP enzymes and, 480
  drug interactions, 480
  mechanism of action, 479
  molecular structure, 479
  side effects, 480
Leukemia
  medications for
    busulfan, 472–474
    fludarabine, 472, 474–475
    gemtuzumab ozogamicin, 472,
      474–475
    idarubicin, 472, 475
    mitoxantrone, 472, 476–477
    teniposide, 472, 477–478
Leukotrienes
  drug interactions, 91
  mechanism of action, 90–91
  molecular structure, 91
  side effects, 91
Leuprolide, 378
  drug interactions, 500
  mechanism of action, 499
  side effects, 499
Levalbuterol, 116
  drug interactions with
    beta blockers, 118
    fludrocortisone, 118

    MAO inhibitors, 118
    sympathomimetic drugs, 118
  mechanism of action, 117
Levaquin (*see* levofloxacin), 359
Levitra (*see* vardenafil)
Levodopa, 107
  drug interactions with
    antipsychotic drugs, 325
    chasteberry, 325
    ethaverine, 326
    halothane, 326
    iron salts, 327
    MAO inhibitors, 327
    metoclopramide, 327
    pyridoxine, 327
    tacrine with, 327
  mechanism of action, 325
  molecular structure, 324–325
  side effects, 325
Levofloxacin, 359
Levonorgestrel, 380, 417
Levorotary isomer (*see* hyoscyamine)
Levothroid (levothyroxine), 372
Levothyroxine, 372
Levothyroxine
  drug interactions with, 372
    alpha lipoic acid, 373
    amiodarone, 373
    barbiturates, 373
    carbamazepine, 373
    digoxin, 373
    estrogens, 374
    ketamine, 374
    ritonavir, 374
    sertraline, 374
  mechanism of action, 372
  side effects, 372
Levoxyl (levothyroxine), 372
Lidocaine, 131
  drug interactions with, 132, 220
    acetazolamide, 37
    antiarrhythmic drugs, 37
    CYP isozymes, 37–38
  mechanism of action, 36, 131–132, 220
  molecular structure, 36
  side effects, 37, 132, 220
Lidoderm (*see* lidocaine)
Linolenic acid, molecular structure, 57

Lioresal (*see* baclofen)
Liothyronine, 372
  drug interactions with, 372
    alpha lipoic acid, 373
    amiodarone, 373
    barbiturates, 373
    carbamazepine, 373
    digoxin, 373
    estrogens, 374
    ketamine, 374
    ritonavir, 374
    sertraline, 374
  mechanism of action, 372
  side eff ects, 372
Liotrix, 372
Lisinopril, 1
  drug interactions, 9, 20
  mechanism of action, 6, 9, 20–21
  molecular structure of, 7
  side effects, 9, 20
Lithane, see lithium carbonate
Lithium, 169
Lithium carbonate
  drug interactions with
    calcium channel blockers, 290
    carbamazepine, 290
    COX-2 inhibitors, 290
    doxycycline, 290
    haloperidol, 290
    methyldopa, 291
    metronidazole, 291
    NSAIDs, 291
    phenothiazine antipsychotic drugs, 291
    sodium bicarbonate, 291
  mechanism of action, 289
  side effects, 289
Lithobid (*see* lithium carbonate)
Liver cancer
  medications for
    cisplatin, 461–463
    doxorubicin, 461, 467
    methotrexate, 461, 463–467
LMWH (low-molecular-weight heparin), 48
Local anesthetics
  drug interactions, 132, 176
  mechanism of action, 131–132, 176
  members of, 131, 176
  side effects, 132, 176
Lodine (*see* etodolac)

Lomustine
  CYP enzymes and, 450
  drug interactions with
    chloramphenicol, 451
    CYP isozymes, 451
    live vaccines, 451
  mechanism of action, 450
  molecular structures, 450
  side effects, 450
Loop diuretics, 10, 13, 34, 38, 171, 364
  drug interactions, 15, 64
  mechanism of action, 14, 64
  side effects, 15, 64
Loperamide (LPM), 159, 173
  drug interactions with, 163, 174
    bile acid sequestrants, 162
    CYP isozymes, 162
    phenothiazines antipsychotic
      drugs, 162
    tricyclic antidepressants, 162
  mechanism of action, 161–162, 173–174
  molecular structure of, 173
  side effects, 162, 174
Lopinavir
  mechanism of action, 521
  molecular structures of, 522
  side effects, 523
Lopinavir + ritonavir, 523
Lopressor (*see* metoprolol)
Loratadine, 426, 431
Lorazepam, 413
  drug interactions, 258, 323, 416
  mechanism of action, 257, 322, 416
  side effects, 257–258, 323, 416
Lortab (*see* hydrocodone)
Losartan, 1, 318
  drug interactions, 10, 22
  mechanism of action, 9, 22
  side effects, 9–10, 22
Lotrel (*see* amlodipine)
Lotronex (*see* alosetron)
Lovastatin, 359
  drug interactions, 80
  mechanism of action, 79–80
  molecular structures, 79
  side effects, 80
Low-molecular-weight heparin
    (LMWH), 48
  interactions

antiplatelet drugs, 50
    argatroban, 50
    human antithrombin-III, 50
    non-steroidal anti-inflammatory
        drugs, 51
    salicylates, 51
    thrombolytic agents, 50
mechanism of action, 49
side effects, 49
Low-Ogestrel (ethinyl estradiol +
    norgestrel), 417
Lubiprostone
    drug interactions, 168
    mechanism of action, 168
    side effects, 168
Lufyllin (*see* dyphylline)
Lunesta (*see* eszopiclone)
Lung cancer
    medications for
        docetaxel, 440
        etoposide, 440
        gemcitabine, 440
        paclitaxel, 440
        porfirmer, 440
        topotecan, 440
        vinorelbine, 440
Lupron (leuprolide)
Lustral (*see* sertraline)

M

Macrobid (*see* nitrofurantoin)
Macrolide antibiotics
    drug interactions, 101, 528
    mechanism of action, 98, 100, 528
    members of, 98, 527
    molecular structures, 99–100
    side effects, 98–101, 528
Magnesium, 352–353
Magnesium citrate, 168, 234
    drug interactions, 172, 238
    mechanism of actions, 172, 238
    side effects, 172, 238
Magnesium hydroxide, 146
    drug interactions, 147
    mechanism of action, 146
    side effects, 147
Magnesium trisilicate, 545
Malaria
    antimalarial drugs and CYP enzymes, 546

medications
    chloroquine, 544–547
    halofantrine, 550–551
    malarone, 548–549
    mefloquine 547–548
    primaquine, 549–550
    quinine, 552–554
parasites
    Plasmodiam falciparum, 547
    P. malariae, 547
    P. ovale, 547
    P. vivax, 547
P-glycoprotein transporter, 554
Malarone (*see atovaquone + chloroguanide*)
Mania
    medications for
        carbamazepine, 289, 294–296
        clozapine, 289, 297
        divalproex, 289, 291–294
        lithium carbonate, 289–291
MAO (monoamine oxidase) inhibitors
    drug interactions with, 264–265
        alcohol, 266
        antihistamine, 267
        atomoxetine, 267
        buspirone, 267
        chlorpropamide, 267
        CYP isozymes, 267
        ginseng, 267
    mechanism of action, 264
    members of, 264
    side effects, 264
MAO-B inhibitors
    drug interactions, 332
    mechanism of action, 332
    members of, 332
    serotonin oxidation, 333
    side effects, 332
MAP kinases (mitogen-activated protein
    kinases), 590
Maprotiline, molecular structure, 266
Mast cell stabilizers
    drug interactions, 432
    mechanism of action, 432
        degranulation by allergen
            sensitization, 433
    members of, 432
    side effects, 432
Matulane (*see* procarbazine)

Maxalt (*see* rizatriptan)
Maxidex (*see* dexamethasone)
Mebendazole
    drug interactions with
        cimetidine, 561
        insulin, 561
        metronidazole, 561
        phenytoin, 561
    mechanism of action, 560–561
    molecular structure, 560
    side effects, 561
Mechlorethamine, molecular structure, 498
Meclizine, 89, 139
    drug interactions, 142, 339
        first- and second-generation, 93–94
    mechanism of action, 93, 141, 339
    side effects, 142, 339
        first- and second-generation, 93
Medipren (*see* ibuprofen)
Medrol (*see* methylprednisolone)
Medroxyprogesterone, 417, 421
    drug interactions with, 387
        azole antifungal drugs, 537–539
        CYP isozymes, 421–422
        oral hypoglycemic agents, 422–423
    mechanism of action, 386, 422
    molecular structure of, 422
    side effects, 387, 422
Mefloquine, 107, 554
    drug interactions with
        CYP isozymes, 547
        halofantrine, 548
        metoclopramide, 548
    mechanism of action, 547
    molecular structure, 547
    side effects, 547
Meloxicam
    drug interactions, 219
    mechanism of action, 219
    side effects, 219
Memantine, 302, 304–305
    drug interactions
        CYP enzymes inhibitors with, 305
    mechanism of action, 304
    molecular structure, 305
    side effects, 305
Memory impairment
    medications for
        bifemelane, 306

ergoloid mesylates, 306, 308–310
gamma-an botynic acid (GABA),
    306–307
idebenone, 306, 310–311
oxiracetam, 306
piracetam, 306–308
piribedil, 306, 308
vinpocetine, 306, 311–312
Menopause
    medications for
        estradiol, 384–386
        paroxetine, 384, 387
        prempro, 384, 386–387
Menstrual dysfunction
    medications for
        bromocriptine, 380, 382–383
        danazol, 380–381
        progestogens, 380, 383
Mental depression
    medications
        bupropion, 286–287
        duloxetine, 278–279
        mirtazapine, 285–286
        selective serotonin reuptake
            inhibitors, 282–283
        trazodone, 283–285
        tricyclic antidepressants,
            287–288
        venlafaxine, 280–282
Meperidine, 437
    molecular structure, 266
Mepron, see atovaquone
mercaptopurine, 197, 510
    molecular structure of, 231
Meridia (*see* sibutramine)
Meropenem, 224
    molecular structure, 225
Mesna, 569
    drug interactions, 575
    mechanism of action, 575
    side effects, 575
Mesnex (*see* mesna)
Mestinon (*see* pyridostigmine)
Metamucil (*see* psyllium)
Metaxalone, 234
    drug interactions with
        alcohol, 234–235
        CYP isozymes, 235
        magnesium hydroxide, 235

monoamine oxidase (MAO), 235
    opioids, 236
mechanism of action, 234
side effects, 234
Metformin
    drug interactions with
        alcohol, 355
        cephalexin, 355
        CYP isozymes with, 355
        metformin, 356
        nifedipine, 356
    mechanism of action, 355
    side effects, 355
Methadone, 319, 395
    drug interactions, 401
    mechanism of action, 401
    molecular structure of, 518
    side effects, 401
Methadose (see methadone)
Methenamine mandelate, 273
Methimazole
    drug interactions, 370
    mechanism of action, 369
    molecular structure of, 369
    relation with CYP enzymes, 370
    side effects, 369–370
Methimazole
    drug interactions with
        CYP isozymes, 370
        digoxin, 370
        phenothiazine antipsychotic drugs, 370
    mechanism of action, 369
    side effects, 369–370
Methocarbamol, 234
    drug interactions with
        alcohol, 234–235
        CYP isozymes, 235
        magnesium hydroxide, 235
        monoamine oxidase (MAO), 235
        opioids, 236
    mechanism of action, 234
    side effects, 234
Methotrexate, 34, 201–202, 224, 411, 463,
        465, 478, 494
    drug interactions with
        aldesleukin, 464
        amiodarone, 464
        cisplatin, 465
        CYP substrate, 465

digoxin, 466
doxycycline, 466
echinacea, 466
live vaccines, 466
NSAIDs, 466
procarbazine, 466
teniposide, 466
theophylline, 466
zidovudine, 466
    mechanism of action, 463
    side effects, 463–464
    and tetrahydrofolate, 464
Methylcellulose, 168
    drug interactions, 169
    mechanism of action, 169
    side effects, 169
Methyldopa, 1, 510
    mechanism of action, 4
    molecular structure of, 4
    side effects, 4
Methylphenidate, 269
    drug interactions with
        alcohol, 270
        CYP isozymes, 270
        MAO inhibitors, 270–271
        phenytoin, 271
        vasopressors, 271
    mechanism of action, 269–270
    molecular structure, 269
    side effects, 270
Methylprednisolone, 116
    drug interactions, 121
    mechanism of action, 120–121
    side effects, 121
Metoclopramide, 104, 157–158,
        382, 391
    drug interactions with, 141, 154, 392
        alcohol, 108
        cabergoline, 108
        chasteberry, 108
        cyclosporine, 108
        CYP isozymes, 108–109
        digoxin, 108
        MAO inhibitors, 108
        selective serotonin reuptake inhibitors
            (SSRIs), 109
        succinylcholine, 109
    mechanism of action, 107, 140, 154, 392
    side effects, 107, 141, 154, 392

Metoprolol, 1
  drug interactions with, 3, 23, 47
  mechanism of action, 2, 22
  side effects, 2–3, 22–23
MetroCream (*see* metronidazole)
MetroGel (*see* metronidazole)
Metronidazole, 146, 243, 510, 555
  drug interactions with, 153, 244
    alcoholic, 556
    carbamazepine, 556
    cholestyramine, 556
    cyclosporine, 556
    CYP isozymes, 556–557
    lithium, 556
    zalcitabine, 557
  mechanism of action, 152, 243, 555
  molecular structure of, 152
  side effects, 153, 243, 555
Metyrapone, 366
  drug interactions with
    acetaminophen, 368
    phenytoin, 368
  mechanism of action, 367
  molecular structure of, 368
  side effects, 368
MFQ (*see* mefloquine)
Miacalcin (*see* calcitonin-salmon)
Micafungin, 537, 539
  drug interactions with, 540
    itraconazole, 541
    nifedipine, 541
    sirolimus, 541
  mechanism of action, 540
  side effects, 540
Micardis (telmisartan)
Micronase (*see* glyburide)
Midazolam
  drug interactions, 258
  mechanism of action, 257
  side effects, 257–258
Midodrine, 427
Mifepristone, 417
  drug interactions with
    carbamazepine, 423
    erythromycin, 424
  mechanism of action, 423
  molecular structure of, 423
  side effects, 423

Minitran (*see* nitroglycerin)
Minocin (*see* minocycline)
Minocycline, 136
  drug interactions, 527
    with tetracyclines, 137–138
  mechanism of action, 137, 526
  side effects, 137, 527
Mintezol (*see* thiabendazole)
Mirapex (*see* pramipexole)
Mirtazapine
  drug interactions with
    alcohol, 285
    alpha-2 activators, 285
    CYP isozymes, 285
    diazepam, 286
    MAO inhibitors, 286
  mechanism of action, 285
  molecular structure, 285
  side effects, 285
Misoprostol, 146
  drug interactions, 151
  mechanism of action, 150–151
  molecular structure of, 150
  side effects, 151
Mitogen-activated protein (MAP)
    kinases, 90
Mitoxantrone (MXT)
  drug interactions with
    aldesleukin, 476
    chloramphenicol, 476
    CYP isozymes, 477
    live vaccines, 477
    zidovudine, 477
  mechanism of action, 476
  side effects, 476
Mobic (*see* meloxicam)
Modafinil
  drug interactions with
    CYP isozymes, 274
    MAO inhibitors, 275
    phenobarbital, 275
  mechanism of action, 274
  selegiline
    and CYP enzymes, 275
  side effects, 274
Moexipril, 1
  drug interactions, 9
  mechanism of action, 6, 9

molecular structure of, 8
side effects, 9
Mometasone, 116, 426, 430
   drug interactions, 121
   mechanism of action, 120–121
   side effects, 121
Montelukast, 116, 426
   drug interactions with, 116–117, 429–430
      CYP isozymes, 117
   mechanism of action, 116, 428–429
   molecular structure of, 428
   side effects, 116, 429
Morphine, 395
   drug interactions, 401
   mechanism of action, 401
   molecular structure, 113
   side effects, 401
Motion sickness
   medications for
      antihistamines, 338
      dimenhydrinate, 338
      diphenhydramine, 338
      meclizine, 338
      promethazine, 338
      scopolamine, 338
Motrin (*see* ibuprofen)
Moxifloxacin, 34
Mupirocin, 525
   drug interactions, 532
   mechanism of action, 531–532
   methicillin-resistant *Staphylococcus
      aureus* (MRSA), 531
   molecular structure, 531
   side effects, 532
Muscle spasticity
   medication for
      baclofen, 236
      centrally-acting skeletal muscle
         relaxants, 234–236
      magnesium citrate, 238
      tizanidine, 236–238
Myasthenia gravis
   medications for
      anticholinesterase agents, 228–230
      glucocorticoids, 228, 230
      immunosuppressants, 228, 230–233
Mycamine (*see* micafungin)
Mycophenolate mofetil, 224–225, 411

molecular structure, 319
Myleran (*see* busulfan)
Mylicon (*see* simethicone)
Mylotarg (*see* gemtuzumab ozogamicin)
Myocalm (*see* piracetam)
Myocardial infarction
   medications for
      abciximab, 48
      alteplase, 48
      anistreplase, 48
      clopidogrel, 48, 58–59
      eptifibatide, 48
      glycoprotein llb/llla receptor
         antagonists, 48, 59–60
      reteplase, 48
      streptokinase, 48
      thrombolytic agents, 48
      urokinase, 48

N
Nabumetone
   drug interactions, 219
   mechanism of action, 219
   side effects, 219
Nadolol, 1
   drug interactions, 3, 47
   mechanism of action, 2, 47
   side effects, 2–3, 47
Nafarelin, 378
Naloxone, 569
   drug interactions, 573
   mechanism of action, 572–573
   molecular structure, 573
   side effects, 573
Namenda (*see* memantine)
Naphazoline, 426
   drug interactions with
      MAO inhibitors, 434
      sympathomimetic drug, 434
   mechanism of action, 432
   molecular structure of, 434
   side effects, 433–434
Naprosyn (*see* naproxen)
Naproxen, 212, 319, 395
   drug interactions, 219, 227, 242, 400
   mechanism of action, 219, 227, 241, 399
   molecular structure, 242
   side effects, 219, 227, 242, 400

Naratriptan, 395
    drug interactions, 404
    mechanism of action, 403–404
    molecular structure of, 404
    side effects, 404
Narcan (*see* naloxone)
Narcotic analgesics, 107, 530
Nardil (*see* phenelzine)
Nasacort (*see* triamcinolone)
Nasacort AQ (*see* triamcinolone)
NasalCrom (*see* cromolyn sodium)
Nasarel (*see* flunisolide)
Nasonex (*see* mometasone)
Nausea
    dimenhydrinate, 141–142
    meclizine, 141–142
    medications for
        antihistamines, 139
        metoclopramide, 139–141
        ondansetron, 139–140
        promethazine, 141–142
Navelbine (*see* vinorelbine)
Nebracetam (*see* piracetam)
Necon 1/35 (*see* ethinyl estradiol +
        norethindrone)
Nefazodone, 309, 437
Nelfinavir
    mechanism of action, 521
    molecular structures of, 522
    side effects, 523
Neostigmine, 41
    drug interactions with
        anticholinesterase agents, 229–230
        beta blockers, 229
        glucocorticoids, 230
        lithium, 230
    mechanism of action, 228–229
    molecular structure, 228
    side effects, 229
Neosynephrine (*see* phenylephrine)
Nephrolithiasis
    medications for
        allopurinol, 195–198
        diuretic agents, 195–196
        hydrochlorothiazide, 195
        potassium citrate, 195–196
        trichlormethiazide, 195
Neurontin (*see* gabapentin)

Nevirapine
    drug interactions with, 520
    mechanism of action, 518–519
    molecular structure of, 519
    side effects, 519
Nexavar (*see* sorafenib tosylate)
Nexium (*see* esomeprazole)
Niacin
    drug interactions, 86–87
        aspirin, 87
        colestipol, 87
        gotu kola, 87
        repaglinide, 87
        statin drugs, 88
    mechanism of action, 86
    side effects, 86
Niaspan (*see* niacin)
Niclosamide, 560
    drug interactions with ethanol, 565
    mechanism of action, 565
    side effects, 565
Nicotinic acid
    drug interactions, 86
    mechanism of action, 86
    molecular structure, 86
    side effects, 86
Nifedipine, 1, 497
    drug interactions, 10
    mechanism of action, 10
    side effects, 10
Nitrendipine, 1
    drug interactions, 10
    mechanism of action, 10
    side effects, 10
Nitro-Bid (*see* nitroglycerin)
Nitro-Dur (*see* nitroglycerin)
Nitrofurantoin, 510, 525
    drug interactions with, 533
        antacids, 204
        anticholinergic agents, 204
        didanosine, 204
        phenytoin, 204
        zalcitabine, 204
    mechanism of action, 203, 532
    molecular structure, 532
    side effects, 203, 532
Nitroglycerin, 180
    drug interactions with

N-acetylcysteine, 18–19
  alcohol, 19
  alteplase, 19
  aspirin, 19
  L-carnitine, 19
  L-cysteine, 19
  diuretics, 19
  heparin, 19
  neuromuscular blockers, 19
  vitamin C, 19
  mechanism of actions, 17
  molecular structure, 17
  side effects, 17–18
Nitroglycerin mononitrate
  drug interactions with
    alteplase, 46
    L-carnitine, 46
    heparin, 46
    isosorbide, 46
    neuromuscular blockers, 46
Nitroglycerin sublingual
  drug interactions, 45
  mechanism of action, 45
  side eff ects, 45
Nitrol (*see* nitroglycerin)
Nitrolingual (*see* nitroglycerin)
Nitropress (*see* sodium nitroprusside)
Nitroquick (*see* nitroglycerin; nitroglycerin
    sublingual)
S-nitrosothiol, molecular structure, 17
Nitrosourea derivatives
  CYP enzymes and, 450
  drug interactions, 451
  mechanism of action, 450
  members of, 450
  side effects, 450
Nitrostat (*see* nitroglycerin; nitroglycerin
    sublingual)
Nizatidine, 146, 166
  drug interactions, 147
  mechanism of action, 147
  side effects, 147
Nizoral (*see* ketoconazole)
NMDA (*see* *N*-methyl D-aspartate)
N-methyl-*D*-aspartic acid (NMDA),
    113, 302
  molecular structure, 114
Non-Hodgkin lymphoma
  medications for
    cyclophosphamide, 459
    denileukin, 459–560
    doxorubicin, 459
    four-drug combination, 459–561
    prednisone, 459
    vincristine, 459
Non-nucleoside RT inhibitors
  drug interactions, 519–521
  mechanism of action, 518
  side effects, 519
Nonsteroidal antiinflammatory drugs
    (NSAIDs), 59, 217, 221, 227, 353,
    395, 410, 465
  drug interactions, 219, 227, 242, 400
  mechanism of action, 219, 227,
    241, 399
  members of, 219, 241, 399
  side effects, 219, 227, 242, 400
Nootropil (*see* piracetam)
Norco (*see* hydrocodone)
Norelgestromin, 380
Norepinephrine, 277, 452
  molecular structure, 265
Norethindrone, 380
  molecular structure, 318
Norfloxacin, 173
  drug interactions, 175, 200, 527
  mechanism of action, 175, 200, 527
  side effects, 175, 200, 527
Norgestimate, 380
  molecular structure of, 418
Norgestrel, 380
  molecular structure of, 418
Norhydrocodone
  molecular structure, 111
Normodyne (*see* labetalol)
Noroxin (*see* norfloxacin)
Norpramin (*see* desipramine)
Nortriptyline, 263, 267
  drug interactions, 268, 288
  mechanism of action, 268, 288
  members of, 287
  molecular structures, 287
  side effects, 268, 288
Norvasc (*see* amlodipine)
Novantrone (*see* mitoxantrone)
NovoLog (insulin aspart)

NSAIDS (*see* nonsteroidal antiinflammatory drugs)
Nucleoside reverse transcriptase (RT) inhibitors
  drug interactions, 510–518
  mechanism of action, 508
  members of, 508
  molecular structures of, 509
  side effects, 508–510
Numzident (*see* benzocaine)
Nupercainal (*see* dibucaine)
Nuprin (*see* ibuprofen)
NuvaRing (ethinyl estradiol + etonogestrel), 417

O

Obesity
  medications for
    amphetamine, 435
    bupropion, 435, 438
    dextroamphetamine, 435
    orlistat, 435–436
    phentermine, 435–436
    sibutramine, 435, 437–438
Obidoxime, 569
  drug interactions with
    morphine, 582
    succinylcholine, 582–583
    theophylline, 583
  mechanism of action, 581
  molecular structure, 582
  side effects, 582
Odontalgia
  acetaminophen, 132–135
  aspirin, 132–135
  local anesthetics, 131–132
  medications for
    hydrogen peroxide, 131–132
    lozenges or dental creams, 131
    oral analgesic drugs, 131
Ofloxacin, 173, 359
  drug interactions, 175, 200, 527
  mechanism of action, 175, 200, 527
  side effects, 175, 200, 527
Olanzapine, 427
  drug interactions, 299
  mechanism of action, 299
  molecular structure, 298

  side effects, 299
Olmesartan, 1
Olopatadine, 426
  drug interactions, 432
  mechanism of action, 432
  side effects, 432
Omega-3 fatty acids, 410
Omeprazole, 146, 465
  drug interactions, 148
  mechanism of action, 147
  side effects, 148
Omnicef (*see* cefdinir; cefuroxime; cephalexin)
Omnipen (*see* ampicillin)
Oncovin (*see* vincristine)
Ondansetron, 139, 391
  drug interactions, 140
  mechanism of action, 139–140
  members of, 139
  relation with CYP isozymes, 140
  side effects, 140
Ontak (*see* denileukin)
Opiate agonists
  drug interactions, 174
  mechanism of action, 173–174
  members of, 173
  side effects, 174
Opioid analgesics, 395
  drug interactions, 401
  mechanism of action, 401
  members of, 400
  side effects, 401
Oracea (*see* doxycycline)
Oral anticoagulants
  drug interactions, 52
  mechanism of action, 52
  side effects, 52
Oral hypoglycemic agents, 215
Orlistat
  drug interactions, 436
  mechanism of action, 436
  side effects, 436
Ortho, Evra (*see* ethinyl estradiol + norelgestromin), 417
Ortho Tri-Cyclen (*see* ethinyl estradiol + norgestimate), 417
Oseltamivir
  drug interactions, 506–507

mechanism of action, 506
molecular structure of, 506
side effects, 506
Osteoarthrosis
  medications for
    celecoxib, 217
    diclofenac, 217
    etodolac, 217
    glucocorticoids, 217–220
    hydroxychloroquine, 217–218
    ibuprofen, 217
    indomethacin, 217
    lidocaine, 217
    meloxicam, 217
    nabumetone, 217
    naproxen, 217
    nonsteroidal anti-inflammatory drugs
      (NSAIDs), 217
    piroxicam, 217
    prednisolone, 217
    prednisone, 217
    tenoxicam, 217
Osteoporosis
  medications for
    alendronate, 209
    anabolic steroids, 209, 213–214
    calcitonin-salmon, 209, 211–212
    calcium carbonate + vitamin D, 209,
      215–216
    diphosphonates, 209–211
    glucosamine + chondroitin sulfate, 209,
      214–215
    ibandronate, 209
    oxandrolone, 209
    raloxifene, 209, 211–212
    risedronate, 209
    selective estrogen-receptor
      modulators, 209
    testosterone, 209
Ovarian cancer
  medications for
    altretamine, 490–492
    carboplatin, 490, 492
    cisplatin, 490
    doxorubicin liposomal, 490, 493
    irinotecan, 490, 493–494
    paclitaxel, 490, 493
    topotecan, 490, 494

Ovidrel. see Human chorionic gonadotropin
    (hCG)
Oxandrolone
  drug interactions, 213
    CYP enzymes, 214
  mechanism of action, 213
  molecular structure, 213
  side effects, 213
Oxcarbazepine
  drug interactions with
    activated charcoal, 317
    CYP isozymes, 317
    MAO inhibitors, 318
  mechanism of action, 316
  molecular structure, 316
  side effects, 316
Oxybutynin, 326
  drug interactions with, 192
    CYP isozymes, 194
    digoxin, 192
    levodopa, 192
  mechanism of action, 191–192
  molecular structure, 191
  side effects, 192
Oxycodone, 395
  drug interactions, 401
  mechanism of action, 401
  molecular structure of, 400
  side effects, 401
OxyContin (see oxycodone)
Oxygen therapy, 569
  drug interactions, 579
  mechanism of action, 578
  side effects, 578
Oxymetazoline
  drug interactions, 62
  mechanism of action, 61
  molecular structure, 61
  side effects, 61
Oxymorphone, molecular
    structure, 400
Oxytocin
  drug interactions with, 63
    sage with, 63
    vasopressors with, 64
  mechanism of action, 63
  molecular structure, 63
  side effects, 63

P

Pacerone (see amiodarone)
Paclitaxel, 445, 463, 482, 490, 493
    drug interactions with, 446
        cisplatin, 447
        CYP isozymes, 447
        live vaccines, 447
        stavudine, 447
        trastuzumab, 447
    mechanism of action, 445
    molecular structures, 446
    side effects, 446
Pamelor (see nortriptyline)
Pancuronium, 102
Panmycin (see tetracycline)
Pantoprazole, 146
    drug interactions, 148
Para-aminobenzoic acid (PABA)
    molecular structure, 530–531
Paraplatin (see carboplatin)
Parathion, molecular structure, 569
Parkinson disease
    medications for
        amantadine, 324
        anticholinergic, 324, 327–328
        benztropine, 324
        bromocriptine, 324
        dopamine agonists, 324, 330–331
        dopamine releasers, 324
        levodopa, 324–327
        MAO-B inhibitors, 324, 332–333
        pramipexole, 324
        rasagiline, 324
        ropinirole, 324
        selegiline, 324
        trihexyphenidyl, 324
Parlodel (see bromocriptine)
Parnate (see tranylcypromine)
Paromomycin, 555
    drug interactions with
        digoxin, 558
    mechanism of action, 558
    side effects, 558
Paroxetine, 281
    drug interactions, 264, 283, 387
    mechanism of action, 263–264, 282, 387
    members, 282
    molecular structure, 282
    side effects, 264, 282, 387
Patanol (see olopatadine)

Paxil (see paroxetine)
Pefloxacin
    drug interactions, 527
    mechanism of action, 527
    side effects, 527
Penciclovir or famciclovir
    drug interactions
        digoxin, 505
        probenecid, 505
        theophylline, 505
    mechanism of action, 505
    molecular structure, 504
    side effects, 505
Penicillin, 225, 419, 465, 525
    drug interactions, 199, 526
    mechanism of action, 199, 525
    members of, 199, 525
    molecular structures of, 425
    side effects, 199, 525
Penicillin antibiotics
    drug interactions, 96
    mechanism of action, 95–96
    members of, 95
    side effects, 96
Penicillin V
    drug interactions, 96
    mechanism of action, 95–96
    side effects, 96
Penicillamine, 225, 569
    drug interactions with
        chloroquine and antimalarial
            drugs, 587
        digoxin, 587
        gold preparations, 587
        indomethacin, 587
        levodopa, 588
        molecular structure, 588
        probenecid, 588
    mechanism of action, 587
    side effects, 587
Peptic ulcers
    Helicobacter pylori (H. pylori), 146
    medications for
        antibiotics, 146, 151–153
        anticholinergic, 146
        bismuth subsalicylate, 146,
            148–149
        gastric antacids, 146–147
        H-2 blockers, 146–147
        misoprostol, 146, 150–151

proton-pump inhibitors, 146–148
   sucralfate, 146, 150
misoprostol, 150–151
   proton-pump inhibitors, 147–148
   sucralfate, 150
Pepto-Bismol (*see* bismuth subsalicylate)
Pergolide, 326
Pergonal (*see* Human menopausal)
   gonadotropin
Periactin, see cyproheptadine
Peroxisome proliferator-activated receptor-
   gamma (PPAR-gamma), 349,
   356–358
Phenazopyridine
   drug interactions, 205
   mechanism of action, 204
   side effects, 205
Phenelzine, 263
   drug interactions with, 264–265
      alcohol, 266
      antihistamine, 267
      atomoxetine, 267
      buspirone, 267
      chlorpropamide, 267
      CYP isozymes, 267
      ginseng, 267
   molecular structure, 106
Phenergan (*see* promethazine)
Phenobarbital, 225
   drug interactions with
      alcohol, 320
      CYP enzymes, 320–321
      narcotic analgesics, 320
      probenecid, 320
   mechanism of action, 319
   molecular structure, 321
   side effects, 320
Phenothiazine antipsychotic drugs, 107, 124,
   193, 402, 326, 427
   drug interactions, 105, 300
   mechanism of action, 104, 300
   members of, 105, 300
   side effects, 105, 300
Phenoxybenzamine, 427
Phentermine
   drug interactions with
      CYP isozymes, 436
      MAO inhibitors, 436
   mechanism of action, 435
   side effects, 435

Phentolamine, 427
Phenylbutazone, 465
Phenylephrine, 176
   drug interactions, 62
   mechanism of action, 61
   molecular structure, 62
   side effects, 61
Phenylephrine suppository
   drug interactions with
      antihypertensive drugs, 177
      MAO inhibitors, 177
      tricyclic antidepressants, 177
   mechanism of action, 177
   side effects, 177
Phenytoin, 293, 315, 541
   drug interactions with
      CYP isozymes, 318
      sucralfate, 318
      thyroid preparation, 319
   mechanism of action, 316
   side effects, 316
Phosphodiesterase inhibitors
   drug interactions, 180–181
   mechanism of action,
      179–180
   members of, 179
   side effects, 180
Photofrin (*see* porfimer)
Pilocarpine, 123, 193
   drug interactions with
      anticholinergic agents, 125
      beta blockers, 125
      cholinomimetic drugs, 125
      CYP isozymes, 125
   mechanism of action, 125
   side effects, 125
Pimecrolimus cream
   drug interactions with, 248
      alcohol, 249
      azole antifungal drugs, 249
      clotrimazole, 249
      CYP isozymes, 249
      danazol, 249
      live vaccines, 249
      NSAIDs, 249–250
   mechanism of action, 246–247
   molecular structure, 247
   side effects, 247
Pimozide, 382, 552–553
   molecular structure, 552

Pindolol, 1
  drug interactions, 3, 47
  mechanism of action, 2, 47
  side effects, 2–3, 47
Pioglitazone
  drug interactions with
    CYP isozymes, 357
    gemfibrozil, 357
    propranolol, 357
    salicylates, 357
  mechanism of action, 357
  molecular structure, 349
  side effects, 357
Piracetam
  drug interactions with, 336
    alcohol, 307
    amphetamine, 307
    anticoagulant, 307
    chlorpromazine, 307
    thyroid preparations, 307–308
  mechanism of action, 307, 336
  molecular structure, 336
  side effects, 307, 336
Piribedil
  drug interactions, 308
  mechanism of action, 308
  side effects, 308
Piroxicam, 219
  drug interactions, 219
  mechanism of action, 219
  side effects, 219
Plaquenil (see hydroxychloroquine)
Platinol (see cisplatin)
Plavix (see clopidogrel)
Podofilox gel
  drug interactions, 185
  mechanism of action, 185
  side effects, 185
Polidocanol
  drug interactions, 76
  mechanism of action, 76
  side effects, 76
Polycillin (see ampicillin)
Polyethylene glycol, 168
  drug interactions, 172
  mechanism of action, 172
  side effects, 172
Polymyxin-B, 558

Porfirmer
  drug interactions, 448
  mechanism of action, 447
  side effects, 448
Potassium chloride, 40
  drug interactions, 15–16
  side effects, 15
Potassium citrate
  drug interactions with
    amiloride, 196
    antihypertensive drugs, 196
    canrenone, 196
    digoxin, 196
    quinidine, 196
    salicylates, 196
    spironolactone, 196
    triamterene, 196
  mechanism of action, 196
  side effects, 196
Potassium clavulanate, 146
PPAR-gamma (see peroxisome
      proliferator-activated receptor-
      gamma)
PPAR-gamma activators
  drug interactions, 357
  mechanism of action, 356
  members of, 356
  side effects, 356
Pralidoxime
  drug interactions with
    morphine, 582
    succinylcholine, 582–583
    theophylline, 583
  mechanism of action, 581
  molecular structure, 582
  side effects, 582
Pramipexole, 326
  drug interactions, 330
  mechanism of action, 330
  molecular structure, 331
  side effects, 330
Pramoxine, 176
  drug interactions, 176
  mechanism of action, 176
  side effects, 176
Pravastatin
  drug interactions, 80
  mechanism of action, 78, 80

molecular structures, 79
side effects, 80
Prazepam, 257
   drug interactions, 258
   mechanism of action, 257
   side effects, 257–258
Praziquantel, 560, 565
   drug interactions, 563, 566
   mechanism of action, 566
   molecular structure, 566
   side effects, 566
Pred Forte (*see* prednisolone)
Prednisolone, 116, 426, 430
   drug interactions, 121
   mechanism of action, 120–121, 218
   members of, 218
   molecular structure, 219
   side effects, 121, 218
Prednisone, 116, 228, 426, 430
   drug interactions, 121, 230, 461
   mechanism of action, 120–121, 218,
      230, 460
   members of, 218
   molecular structure, 219
   side effects, 121, 218, 230, 461
Pregnancy
   medications for
      estrogen + progestogen, 417–421
      medroxyprogesterone, 417, 421–423
      mifepristone, 417, 423–424
Pregnyl [(*see* human chorionic gonadotropin
      (hCG)]
Preparation H (*see* phenylephrine)
Prevacid (lansoprazole), 146
Prilosec (*see* omeprazole)
Primaquine, 549
   drug interactions, 550
   halofantrine, 554
   mechanism of action, 550
   molecular structure, 550
   side effects, 550
Principen (*see* ampicillin)
Prinivil (*see* lisinopril)
Probalan (*see* probenecid)
Probenecid, 149, 202, 411, 465
   drug interactions with
      acyclovir, 224
      CYP isozymes, 226

famciclovir, 224
      ganciclovir, 224
      hydroxyurea, 226
      nitrofurantoin, 226
      valacyclovir, 224
      zalcitabine, 226
      zidovudine, 226
   mechanism of action, 223
   molecular structure, 223
   side effects, 223
Procainamide, 156, 202
   drug interactions with
      antiarrhythmic drugs, 38
      CYP isozymes, 39
      trimethoprim, 39
   mechanism of action, 36
   molecular structure, 36–37
   side effects, 37
Procan (*see* procainamide)
Procanbid (*see* procainamide)
Procarbazine, 452
   drug interactions with, 452
      alcohol, 453
      chloramphenicol, 453
      CYP isozymes, 453
      digoxin, 453
      levamisole, 453
      live vaccines, 453
      methotrexate, 453
      phenothiazine antipsychotic drugs, 453
   mechanism of action, 451
   molecular structure, 452
   side effects, 452
Prochlorperazine, 104
   drug interactions, 105
   mechanism of action, 104
   molecular structure, 104
   side effects, 105
Progestogens, 380
   drug interactions, 383, 387
   mechanism of action, 383, 386
   molecular structure of, 386
   side effects, 383, 387
Promethazine, 110, 139, 391
   drug interactions with, 113, 142,
      300, 339, 393
      CYP isozymes, 142
      MAO inhibitors, 142

Promethazine (*Cont;d.*)
    mechanism of action, 112, 141, 300,
        339, 393
    molecular structure of, 392
    side effects, 113, 142, 300, 339, 393
Pronestyl (*see* procainamide)
Propantheline, 166
    drug interactions with
        beta blockers, 167
        cefprozil, 167
        tricyclic antidepressants, 167
    mechanism of action, 166
    side effects, 167
Propranolol, 1, 369
    drug interactions, 3, 43, 47, 371
    mechanism of action, 2, 42, 47, 371
    molecular structure, 42
    side effects, 2–3, 43, 47, 371
Propylthiouracil, 369
    drug interactions, 370
    mechanism of action, 369
    molecular structure of, 369
    side effects, 369–370
Proscar (*see* finasteride)
ProSom (*see* estazolam)
Prostaglandin E-1, molecular structure, 150
Prostate cancer
    medications for
        estramustine, 499–501
        flutamide, 499–500
        goserelin, 499–500
        leuprolide, 499–500
Prostigmin (*see* neostigmine)
Protease inhibitors
    drug interactions, 523–524
    mechanism of action, 521
    molecular structures of, 522
    side effects, 523
Protein-bound drugs, 411
Proton-pump inhibitors, 535
    drug interactions, 148
    mechanism of action, 147
    molecular structures of, 148
    side effects, 148
Protonix (*see* pantoprazole)
Protopic (*see* tacrolimus)
Protriptyline, 263, 267
    drug interactions, 268, 288

    mechanism of action, 268, 288
    members, 287
    molecular structures, 287
    side effects, 268, 288
Provera (*see* medroxyprogesterone)
Prozac (*see* fluoxetine)
Pseudoephedrine, 89, 277, 406
    drug interactions, 93
    mechanism of action, 92
    molecular structure, 27
    side effects, 93
Psoriasis, medications,
        immunosuppressants,
        251–252
Psychosis
    medications for
        antipsychotic drugs, 298–300
        aripiprazole, 298
        clozapine, 298
        olanzapine, 298
        phenothiazine antipsychotic drugs,
            299–300
        quetiapine, 298
        risperidone, 298
        sertindole, 298
Psyllium, 168, 295
    drug interactions, 169
    mechanism of action, 169
    side effects, 169
Pulmicort Respules (*see* budesonide)
Pycnogenol, 181, 279
    drug interactions with
        antihypertensive drugs, 183
        NSAIDs, 183
        oral hypoglycemic agents, 183
    mechanism of action, 182
    side effects, 182
Pyrantel pamoate, 560
    drug interactions, piperazine, 564
    mechanism of action, 563–564
    molecular structure, 563
    side effects, 564
Pyrexia
    treatments for
        acetaminophen, 408–409
        aspirin, 408–412
        ibuprofen, 408, 412
Pyridium (*see* phenazopyridine)

Pyridostigmine, 41, 228
  drug interactions with
    anticholinesterase agents, 229–230
    beta blockers, 229–230
    glucocorticoids, 230
    lithium, 230
  mechanism of action, 228–229
  molecular structure, 228
  side effects, 229
Pyrilamine, 89, 426, 431
  drug interactions, first- and second-
    generation, 93–94
  mechanism of action, 93
  side effects first- and second-
    generation, 93
Pyrimethamine, molecular structures, 67

Q
Qropi (see piracetam)
Quetiapine
  drug interactions, 299
  mechanism of action, 299
  molecular structure, 298
  side effects, 299
Quinaglute (see quinidine)
Quinapril, 1
  drug interactions, 9
  mechanism of action, 6, 9
  molecular structure of, 8
  side effects, 9
Quinidex (see quinidine)
Quinidine, 156, 158, 162, 229
  drug interactions with
    chlorpromazine, 39
    CYP isozymes, 39
    digoxin, 39
    loperamide, 39
  mechanism of action, 36
  side effects, 37
Quinine, 554
  drug interactions with
    amantadine, 553
    baking soda, 554
    CYP isozymes, 554
    digoxin, 554
    diuretics, 554
    molecular structure, 553
    succinylcholine, 554

  mechanism of action, 552
  side effects, 552–553
Quinolone antibiotics, 199
  drug interactions, 175, 200
  mechanism of action, 175, 200
  members of, 175, 199
  side effects, 175, 200
Quinora (see quinidine)

R
Raloxifene
  drug interactions with
    cholestyramine, 212
    levothyroxine, 212
  mechanism of action, 211
  molecular structure, 211
  side effects, 212
Ramace (see ramipril)
Ramipril, 1
  drug interactions, 9, 20
  mechanism of action, 6, 9, 20
  molecular structure of, 8
  side effects, 9, 20
Ranitidine, 146, 166
  drug interactions, 147
  mechanism of action, 147
  side effects, 147
Raptiva (see efalizumab)
Rasagiline
  drug interactions with
    CYP isozymes, 332–333
    pseudoephedrine, 333
    selegiline, 333
    SSRIs, 332
  mechanism of action, 332
  side effects, 332
Refludan (see lepirudin)
Reglan (see metoclopramide)
Relafen (see nabumetone)
Remicade (see infliximab)
Repronex. see Human menopausal
    gonadotropin
Requip (see ropinirole)
Reteplase
  drug interactions, 60
  mechanism of action, 60
  side effects, 60
Retinoids (see acitretin)

Rhinitis, 89
  antihistamines, 93–94
  cromolyn sodium, 90–91
  cyproheptadine, 91–92
  glucocorticoids, 90
  seasonal, medications for
    antihistaminic agents, 89–90
    antihistaminic antiserotonin
      agent, 89
    glucocorticoid nasal sprays, 89
    mast-cell stabilizer, 89
    sympathomimetic agent, 89
  pseudoephedrine, 92–93
Rhinocort (*see* budesonide)
Rhinocort Aqua (*see* budesonide)
Rhinorrhea, 89
Rifampin, 525, 535, 541
  drug interactions with
    caspofungin, 535
    CYP isozymes, 535–536
    halothane, 536
    isoniazid, 536
    ondansetron, 536
  mechanism of action, 533
  side effects, 534
Rifaximin, 143
  drug interactions, 144
  mechanism of action, 144
  molecular structure of, 144
  side effects, 144
Rimantadine, 507
  drug interactions, 507
  mechanism of action, 507
  molecular structure of, 507
  side effects, 507
Risedronate, 411
  drug interactions with
    aminoglycosides, 210
    antacids, 210
    aspirin, 210
    CYP enzymes, 210–211
    estrogens, 211
    NSAIDs, 211
  molecular structures, 210
Risperdal (*see* risperidone)
Risperidone
  drug interactions, 299
  mechanism of action, 299

  molecular structure, 299
  side effects, 299
Ritalin (*see* methylphenidate)
Ritonavir, 162, 319
  mechanism of action, 521
  molecular structures of, 522
  side effects, 523
Rivastigmine
  drug interactions, 302–304
  mechanism of action, 302
  molecular structure, 302
  side effects, 302
Rizatriptan, 395–396
  drug interactions, 404
  mechanism of action, 403–404
  molecular structure of, 398
  side effects, 404
Robaxin (*see* methocarbamol)
Robinul (*see* glycopyrrolate)
Romazicon (*see* flumazenil)
Ropinirole, 326
  drug interactions, 330
  mechanism of action, 330
  molecular structure, 331
  side effects, 330
Rosacea
  medications for
    aluminum acetate, 244–245
    azelaic acid, 244
    metronidazole, 243–244
Rosiglitazone, molecular structure, 350
Rosuvastatin
  drug interactions, 80
  mechanism of action, 79–80
  molecular structures, 79
  side effects, 80
RU-486, see mifepristone

S
St. John's Wort, 281, 403
Salagen (*see* pilocarpine)
Salicylates, 202, 226, 353, 465
Saquinavir
  mechanism of action, 521
  molecular structures of, 522
  side effects, 523
Sarin, molecular structure, 569
Scopolamine, 156

drug interactions, 337, 339
mechanism of action, 336, 338
molecular structure, 163, 337
side effects, 336, 339
Seasonal affective disorder (SAD)
medications for
bupropion, 268
MAO inhibitors, 264–267
SSRIs, 263–264
tricyclic antidepressants, 267–268
Seasonal rhinitis, 89
Second-generation antihistamines
drug interactions, 431
mechanism of action, 431
members of, 431
side effects, 431
Sectral (*see* acebutolol)
Selective estrogen receptor modulators
(SERMs)
CYP enzymes and, 485
drug interactions, 484
mechanism of action, 484
members of, 483
side effects, 484
Selective serotonin reuptake inhibitors
(SSRIs), 309, 332, 402, 405–406, 436
drug interactions, 264, 283
mechanism of action, 263–264, 282
members of, 263, 282
side effects, 264, 282
Selegiline
drug interactions with, 277
CYP isozymes, 276
dextromethorphan, 276
MAO inhibitors, 276
mepcridine, 276
mechanism of action, 276, 332
molecular structure, 261
side effects, 276, 332
Senna-Lax, see sennosides
Sennosides, 34, 168, 170
drug interactions
vitamin K, 171
mechanism of action, 171
side effects, 171
Senokot (*see* sennosides)
Septrim (*see* sulfamethoxazole
trimethoprim)

SERMs. *see* Selective estrogen receptor
modulators
Seroquel (*see* quetiapine)
Serotonin
drug interactions, 92
mechanism of action, 91–92
molecular structure, 92
side effects, 92
Serotonin (5-HT) agonists, 405
Seroxat (*see* paroxetine)
Serotonin agonists (*see* buspirone)
Sertindole
drug interactions, 299
mechanism of action, 299
molecular structure, 299
side effects, 299
Sertraline, 263
drug interactions, 264, 283
mechanism of action, 263–264, 282
members, 282
molecular structure, 282
side effects, 264, 282
Sibutramine, 281, 309, 405
drug interactions with, 437
CYP isozymes, 438
MAO inhibitors, 438
mechanism of action, 436
side effects, 436
Sildenafil, 179, 580
Sildenafil,
drug interactions with, 180
alcohol, 181
CYP isozymes, 181
narcotic analgesics, 181
mechanism of action, 179–180
side effects, 180
Simethicone
drug interactions, 144
mechanism of action, 143
molecular structure of, 143
side effects, 143
Simvastatin
drug interactions, 80
verapamil with, 82
mechanism of action, 78, 80
molecular structures, 79
side effects, 80
Sinequan (*see* doxepin)

Singulair (*see* montelukast)
Sinusitis, 89
  antihistamines, 93–94
  cromolyn sodium, 90–91
  cyproheptadine, 91–92
  glucocorticoids, 90
  medications for
    antihistaminic agents, 89–90
    antihistaminic antiserotonin
      agent, 89
    glucocorticoid nasal sprays, 89
    mast-cell stabilizer, 89
    sympathomimetic agent, 89
  pseudoephedrine, 92–93
Skelaxin (*see* metaxalone)
Skeletal muscle relaxants, 229
Skin cancer
  basal cell carcinoma, 471
  medications for
    fluorouracil, 469–471
    imiquimod, 469, 471–472
SMR. *see* Centrally-acting skeletal muscle
  relaxants
Sodium bicarbonate, 273, 305
Sodium channel blockers, 315
  drug interactions, 37, 316–319
  mechanism of action, 36, 316
  members of, 36
  side effects, 37, 316
Sodium iodine, 369
  drug interactions, 371
  mechanism of action, 371
  side effects, 371
Sodium morrhuate
  drug interactions, 77
  mechanism of action, 77
  side effects, 77
Sodium nitrite, 180, 569, 580
  drug interactions, 579–580
  mechanism of action, 579
  side effects, 579
Sodium nitroprusside, 180
  drug interactions, 19–20
  mechanism of actions, 17
  molecular structure, 17
  side effects, 18
Sodium polystyrene sulfonate, 569
  drug interactions with
    digoxin, 575

  magnesium hydroxide, 575
  sorbitol, 575
  mechanism of action, 574
  side effects, 574
Solodyn (*see* minocycline)
Soma (*see* carisoprodol)
Soman, molecular structure, 580
Sonata, see zaleplon
Sorafenib tosylate
  CYP enzymes, 467–468
  mechanism of action, 467–468
  side effects, 468
Sorbitol, 123
  drug interactions, 126
  mechanism of action, 126
  side effects, 126
Sotalol, 552–553
  drug interactions, 43
  mechanism of action, 42
  molecular structure, 42
  side effects, 43
Spiriva (*see* tiotropium)
Spironolactone, 184
  mechanism of action, 23
  molecular structure, 24
  side effects, 24
Sprintec ethinyl estradiol +
  norgestimate
SSRIs. *see* Selective serotonin reuptake
  inhibitors
Statins
  CYP enzymes and, 82
  drug interactions, 80–82
    gotu kola with, 81
  mechanism of action, 78, 80
  molecular structures, 79
  side effects, 80–81
Stavudine, 535
  drug interaction with
    hydroxyurea, 515
    ribavirin, 515
  mechanism of action, 509
  molecular structure of, 516
  side effects, 509
Strattera (*see* atomoxetine)
Streptokinase
  drug interactions, 60
  mechanism of action, 60
  side effects, 60

Stress and anxiety
  medications for
    benzodiazepines, 257–259
    buspirone (BSP), 259–261
    hydroxyzine, 261–262
Succinic semialdehyde, molecular
    structure, 292
Succinylcholine, 102
  molecular structure, 583
Sucralfate, 146
  drug interactions, 150
  mechanism of action, 150
  side effects, 150
Sucrets (see dyclonine)
Sudafed (pseudoephedrine)
Sulfamethoxazole (SMZ), 465, 478
  drug interactions, 531
    cyclosporine, 201
    CYP isozymes, 201–202
    digoxin, 201
    pyrimethamine, 202
  mechanism of action, 530–531
  molecular structure, 200
  side effects, 201
  sulfamethoxazole + trimethoprim, 525
  drug interactions, 531
  mechanism of action, 530
  side effects, 531
Sulfasalazine, 465
  molecular structure, 31
Sulfinpyrazone, 149
  drug interactions with
    CYP isozymes, 226
    hydroxyurea, 226–227
    nitrofurantoin, 227
    tolbutamide, 227
    warfarin, 227
  mechanism of action, 223
  molecular structure, 224
  side effects, 223
Sulfonamide chemotherapeutics, 353, 510
Sulfonated phenol topical solution, 127
  drug interactions, 128
  mechanism of action, 128
  side effects, 128
Sulfonylureas
  drug interactions with, 353
    acitretin, 353
    alcohol, 354

    clarithromycin, 353–354
    CYP isozymes, 354
    disopyramide, 354
    MAO inhibitors, 354
    medroxyprogesterone, 354
    tetracycline antibiotics, 354
  mechanism of action, 352
  members of, 352
  molecular structure, 227
  side effects, 352
Sumatriptan, 309, 396
  drug interactions, 404
  mechanism of action, 403–404
  molecular structure of, 398
  side effects, 404
Sumycin, see tetracycline
Sunitinib malate
  CYP enzymes, 469
  drug interactions, 469
  mechanism of action, 468
  side effects, 469
Surfak (see docusate sodium)
Surmontil (see trimipramine)
Sutent (see sunitinib malate)
Symmetrel (see amantadine)
Sympathomimetic drugs, 353, 356, 427
Synarel nafarelin, 378
Synthroid (see levothyroxine)

T
Tabun, molecular structure, 580
Tacrine, 156
  drug interactions, 302–304
  mechanism of action, 302
  molecular structure, 302
  side effects, 302
Tacrolimus, 246
  drug interactions with, 248
    alcohol, 249
    azole antifungal drugs, 249
    clotrimazole, 249
    CYP isozymes, 249
    danazol, 249
    live vaccines, 249
    NSAIDs, 249–250
  mechanism of action, 246–247
  molecular structure, 247
  and picrolimus vs CYP enzymes, 248
  side effects, 248

Tadalafil, 179, 580
  drug interactions with, 181
    alcohol, 181
    CYP isozymes, 181
    narcotic analgesics, 181
Tamiflu (*see* oseltamivir)
Tamoxifen, 483–484
  drug interactions with
    black cohosh, 485
    CYP isozymes, 485
    mitomycin, 485
  mechanism of action, 484
  molecular structure, 484
  side effects, 484
Tamsulosin, 180
  drug interactions, 188, 206
  mechanism of action, 188, 206
  side effects, 188, 206
Tapazole (*see* methimazole)
Taxol (*see* paclitaxel)
Taxotere (*see* docetaxel)
Tegaserod, 159
  drug interactions, 165
  mechanism of actions, 165
  side effects, 165
Tegretol (*see* carbamazepine)
Telithromycin, 95, 525, 527
  drug interactions, 101, 528
  mechanism of action, 98,
      100, 528
  molecular structures, 100
  side effects, 100–101, 528
Telmisartan, 1
Temazepam, 413
  drug interactions, 416
  mechanism of action, 416
  side effects, 416
Temodal (*see* temozolomide)
Temodar (*see* temozolomide)
Temozolomide
  drug interactions, 454
  mechanism of action, 453–454
  molecular structure, 454
  side effects, 454
Teniposide
  drug interactions, 478
    live vaccines with, 477
  mechanism of action, 477

  molecular structures, 441
  side effects, 477
Tenofovir
  drug interaction with
    CYP isozymes, 516–517
    didanosine, 516
    indinavir, 516
  mechanism of action, 509
  molecular structure of, 509, 514
  side effects, 509
Tenoxicam, 219
  drug interactions, 219
  mechanism of action, 219
  side effects, 219
Terazosin, 1, 180
  drug interactions, 4, 188
  mechanism of action, 3, 188
  members of, 3
  molecular structure of, 3
  side effects, 3–4, 188
Terbinafine, 537, 541
  drug interactions with
    cimetidine, 543
    CYP isozymes, 542–543
    tricyclic antidepressants, 543
  mechanism of action, 541–542
  molecular structure of, 542
  side effects, 542
Testicular cancer
  medications for
    cisplatin, 498
    etoposide, 498–499
    ifosfamide, 498–499
Testosterone
  drug interactions with, CYP
      isozymes, 214
  mechanism of action, 213
  molecular structure, 189, 213
  side effects, 213
Tetracap (*see* tetracycline)
Tetracycline, 127, 525
  antibiotics, 107, 419
  drug interactions, 129, 527
  mechanism of action,
      128–129, 526
  members, 526
  molecular structures of, 138
  side effects, 129, 527

Tetrahydrofolic acid, molecular
  structures, 66
Tetraiodothyronine, molecular
  structure, 374
Teveten (*see* eprosartan)
TFV (*see* tenofovir)
Theophylline, 197, 364
  molecular structure of, 120
Therapeutic classifications of drugs, 589–595
Thiabendazole, 560
  drug interactions, 563, 565
  mechanism of action, 564
  molecular structure, 564
  side effects, 564
Thiamazole (*see* methimazole)
Thiazide diuretics, 34, 38, 171, 202, 225,
    352–353, 356, 364, 545
Thioamides
  drug interactions, 370
  mechanism of action, 369
  side effects, 369–370
Thioguanine, 588
Thorazine (*see* chlorpromazine)
Thrombolytic agents, 149, 410
  drug interactions, 60
  mechanism of action, 60
  side effects, 60
Thrombosis
  medications for
    enoxaparin, 48
    heparin, 48
    lepirudin, 48, 51–52
    low-molecular-weight heparin
      (LMWH), 48
    oral anticoagulants, 48, 52–57
  medications
  oral anticoagulants
    warfarin, 48
  site of action, 50
Thromboxane, molecular structure, 56
Thyrogen (*see* thyrotropin alfa)
Thyroid cancer
  medications for
    cisplatin, 469
    doxorubicin, 469
Thyrolar (liotrix), 372
Thyrotropin alfa, 372
  drug interactions, 375

  mechanism of action, 375
  side effects, 375
Tiazac (*see* diltiazem)
Timolol, 1
  drug interactions, 3
  mechanism of action, 2
  side effects, 2–3
Tiotropium, 110
  drug interactions, 112, 115
  mechanism of action, 114–115
  molecular structure, 115
  side effects, 115
Tipranavir
  mechanism of action, 521
  molecular structures of, 522
  side effects, 523
Tirofiban, 411
Tizanidine, 234, 236
  drug interactions with
    alcohol, 237
    CYP isozymes, 237–238
  mechanism of action, 237
  molecular structure of, 237
  side effects, 237
Tobramycin, 95
  drug interactions, 101–102
  mechanism of action, 101
  side effects, 101
Tocainide
  drug interactions with
    acetazolamide, 37
    antiarrhythmic drugs, 37
    CYP isozymes, 37
  mechanism of action, 36
  molecular structure, 37
  side effects, 37
Tofranil (*see* imipramine)
Tolazoline, molecular structure, 125
Tolbutamide, 201, 319, 478
  molecular structure, 225
Tolterodine
  drug interactions, 192
    CYP isozymes with, 194
  mechanism of action, 191–192
  side effects, 192
Tonocard (*see* tocainide)
Topamax (*see* phenobarbital;
    topiramate)

Topiramate, 396
    drug interactions with, 407
        alcohol, 322
        CYP isozymes, 322
        diuretics, 322
    mechanism of action, 320, 407
    molecular structure, 320
    side effects, 320, 407
Topotecan (TCN), 463
    drug interactions with, 443, 494
        aminoglycoside antibiotics, 444
        CYP isozymes, 444
        live vaccines, 444
    mechanism of action, 442, 493
    molecular structures, 443
    side effects, 443, 493
Toprol-XL (*see* metoprolol)
Toremifene
    CYP enzymes and, 485
    drug interactions with
        CYP isozymes, 486
        thiazide D, 486
    mechanism of action, 484
    molecular structure, 484
    side effects, 484
Totacillin (*see* ampicillin)
Tramadol, 281, 395, 405, 437
    drug interactions with
        benzodiazepine antianxiety
            drugs, 402
        CYP isozymes, 402
        MAO inhibitors, 403
        St. John's Wort, 403
        sibutramine, 403
        warfarin, 403
    mechanism of action, 401
        molecular structure of, 399
    side effects, 402
Tandate (*see* labetalol)
Transderm-Nitro (*see* nitroglycerin)
Transderm-Scop (*see* scopolamine)
Tranylcypromine, 263
    drug interactions with, 264–265
        alcohol, 266
        antihistamine, 267
        atomoxetine, 267
        buspirone, 267
        chlorpropamide, 267

        CYP isozymes, 267
        ginseng, 267
        mechanism of action, 264
        molecular structure, 106
        side effects, 264
Trastuzumab
    drug interactions with, 487
        paclitaxel, 486
        warfarin, 486
    mechanism of action, 486
    side effects, 486
Trazodone, 309, 405
    drug interactions with
        alcohol, 283
        CYP isozymes, 283
        digoxin, 284
        MAO inhibitor, 284
        St. John's Wort, 284
        triptans, 284–285
    mechanism of action, 283
    mirtazapine vs CYP enzymes, 284
    side effects, 283
Triamcinolone, 89, 116, 127, 426, 430
    drug interactions, 90, 121, 130, 250
    mechanism of action, 90, 120–121, 129–
        130, 250
    molecular structure, 129
    side effects, 90, 121, 130, 250
Triamterene, 15, 184
Triazolam, 319, 413
    drug interactions, 416
    mechanism of action, 416
    side effects, 416
Trichlormethiazide,
    drug interactions, 195
    members of, 195
    side effects, 195
Tricor (*see* fenofibrate)
Tricyclic antidepressants, 106, 124, 164, 169,
        193, 277, 309, 402, 427, 436
    drug interactions, 268, 288
    mechanism of action, 268, 288
    members, 267, 287
    molecular structures, 287
    side effects, 268, 288
Trihexane (*see* trihexyphenidyl)
Trihexyphenidyl
    drug interactions, 328

mechanism of action, 327
side effects, 327
Triiodothyronine, molecular structure
    of, 374
Trileptal (*see* oxcarbazepine)
Trimethoprim, 465
    drug interactions with, 531
        antacids, 202
        dapsone, 203
        phenylbutazone, 203
        phenytoin, 203
        pyrimethamine, 203
        zidovudine, 203
    mechanism of action, 200, 530–531
    molecular structure, 200
    side effects, 201, 531
Trimipramine, 263, 267
    drug interactions, 268, 288
    mechanism of action, 268, 288
    members, 287
    molecular structure, 287–288
    side effects, 268, 288
Trimox (*see* amoxicillin)
Trinessa ethinyl estradiol + norgestimate, 417
Triprolidine, 90, 426, 431
    drug interactions, first- and second-
        generation, 93–94
    mechanism of action, 93
    side effects, first- and second-
        generation, 93
Triptans, 281, 402, 406, 437
    drug interactions, MAO inhibitors with, 404
    mechanism of action, 403–404
    members of, 403
    side effects, 404
Tri-Sprintec (ethinyl estradiol +
    norgestimate)
Tritace (*see* ramipril)
Trivastal (*see* piribedil)
Trivora-28, ethinyl estradiol +
    levonorgestrel, 417
Tussionex (*see* chlorpheniramine +
    hydrocodone)
Tussis
    medications for
        benzonatate, 110, 115
        codeine, 110–113
        dextromethorphan, 110, 113–114

hydrocodone, 110–111
        tiotropium, 110, 114–115
Tylenol (*see* acetaminophen)
Tyramine-rich foods, 452
Tyrosine, molecular structure, 326

U

Ultracet (*see* acetaminophen + tramadol)
Ultram (*see* tramadol)
Unisom (*see* doxylamine)
Urecholine (*see* bethanechol)
Uric acid, molecular structure, 222
Uricosuric agents
    mechanism of action, 223
    members of, 223
    side effects, 223
Uridine and thymidine, molecular
    structures, 470
Urinary incontinence. *see* Bed-wetting
Urinary retention
    medications for
        alfuzosin, 206
        alpha blockers, 206
        5-alpha reductase inhibitors, 206–207
        bethanechol, 206
        doxazosin, 206
        finasteride, 206
        tamsulosin, 206
Urinary tract infections (UTIs), 199
Urokinase
    drug interactions, 60
    mechanism of action, 60
    side effects, 60
Uromitexan (*see* mesna)
UroXatral (*see* alfuzosin)
Uterine cancer
    medications, for
        carboplatin, 489–490
        cisplatin, 489–490
        doxorubicin, 489–490
        paclitaxel, 489–490
UTIs (*see* urinary tract infections), 199

V

Valacyclovir
    drug interactions with
        aminoglycoside antibiotics, 503
        CYP isozymes, 503–504

Valacyclovir (*Cont'd.*)
   mycophenolate mofetil, 503
   probenecid, 504
  mechanism of action, 502
  molecular structure, 503
  side eff ects, 503
Valium (*see* diazepam)
Valproic acid
  CYP isozymes and, 294
  drug interactions with
   alcohol, 292
   aspirin, 292
   carbamazepine, 292–293
   cholestyramine, 293
   didanosine, 293
   divalproex, 293
   lamotrigine, 293–294
  mechanism of action, 292
  molecular structure, 291
  side effects, 292
Valsartan, 1
  drug interactions, 22
  mechanism of action, 22
  side effects, 22
Valtrex (*see* valacyclovir)
Vancenase (*see* beclomethasone)
Vancomycin, 102
Vantin (*see* cefpodoxime)
Vardenafil, 179, 580
  drug interactions with, 180-181
   alcohol, 181
   CYP isozymes, 181
   narcotic analgesics, 181
  mechanism of action, 179–180
  side effects, 180
Varicose vein
  medications for
   ethanolamine oleate, 76
   polidocanol, 76
   sodium morrhuate, 76
Vasodilators
  drug interactions, 18–20, 45
  mechanism of action, 17, 45
  medications for
   acebutolol, 45
   beta blockers, 45, 47
   bisoprolol, 45
   calcium-channel blockers, 45

   diltiazem, 45
   isosorbide mononitrate, 45
   metoprolol, 45
   nadolol, 45
   nitroglycerin sublingual, 45
   pindolol, 45
   propranolol, 45
   vasodilators, 45
   verapamil, 45
  members of, 17, 45
  nitroglycerin, 17
  side effects, 17–18, 45
  sodium nitroprusside, 17
Vasopressin
  drug interactions, 63, 360
  mechanism of action, 62, 360
  molecular structure, 62
  side effects, 62, 360
Vasotec (*see* enalapril)
Vectrin (*see* minocycline)
Vecuronium, 558
Veetids (*see* penicillin-V)
Velban (*see* vinblastine)
Venlafaxine, 402, 405
  drug interactions with
   alcohol, 281
   CYP isozymes, 281
   MAO inhibitors, 281–282
  mechanism of action, 280
  molecular structure, 280
  side effects, 281
Vepesid (*see* etoposide)
Verapamil (1, 319, 497)
  drug interactions, 10, 42
  mechanism of action, 10, 42
  molecular structure, 42
  side effects, 10, 42
Verelan (*see* verapamil)
Vermox (*see* mebendazole)
Versed (*see* midazolam)
Vertigo
  medications for
   anticholinergic agents, 334
   antihistaminic antiemetics, 334–336
   betahistine, 334–336
   dimenhydrinate, 334
   meclizine, 334
   piracetam, 334, 336

promethazine, 334
scopolamine, 334, 336–337
vinpocetine, 334, 337
Viagra (*see* sildenafil)
Vibramycin (*see* doxycycline)
Vicodin (*see* hydrocodone)
Vinblastine, 454
  drug interactions with
    asparaginase, 458
    CYP isozymes, 458
    dactinomycin, 458
    mitomycin, 458
    phenytoin, 458
    zidovudine, 459
  mechanism of action, 455
  side effects, 456
Vinca alkaloids, molecular structures, 511
Vincristine
  drug interactions with, 461
    L-asparaginase, 496–497
    CYP isozymes, 497
    digoxin, 497
    mitomycin, 498
  mechanism of action, 460, 496
  side effects, 461, 496
Vinorelbine
  drug interactions with
    cisplatin, 449
    CYP isozymes, 449
    didanosine, 449
    live vaccines, 449–450
  mechanism of action, 449
  side effects, 449
Vinpocetine
  drug interactions, 312, 337
  mechanism of action, 311, 337
  molecular structure, 311
  side effects, 311, 337
Viread (*see* tenofovir)
Visine-A (*see* naphazoline)
Visken (*see* pindolol)
Vistaril (*see* hydroxyzine)
Vitamin A-1, molecular structure, 253
Vitamin D
  drug interactions with
    antacids, 216
    calcium-channel blockers, 216
    cholestyramine, 216

digoxin, 216
glucocorticoids, 216
orlistat, 216
thiazide diuretics, 216
mechanism of action, 215
side effects, 215–216
Vivactil, see protriptyline
Voltaren, see diclofenac
Vomiting
  dimenhydrinate, 141–142
  meclizine, 141–142
    antihistamines, 139
    metoclopramide, 139–141
    ondansetron, 139–140
    promethazine, 141–142
Voriconazole, 537
  drug interactions, 538–539
  mechanism of action, 537
  molecular structure of, 538
  side effects, 538
Vumon (*see* teniposide)
Vytorin (*see* ezetimibe)

W

Warfarin, 102, 201, 213, 215, 364,
    370, 553
  drug interactions with, 53
    anabolic steroids, 54
    bismuth subsalicylate, 54
    cholestyramine, 54
    clofibrate, 54–55
    coumarin-like herbs, 55
    cyclophosphamide, 55
    CYP isozymes, 55
    gemfibrozil, 55
    glucagon, 56
    grape juice, 56
    herbal, 55–56
    leflunomide, 56
    metabolic clearance, 56
    omega-3 fatty acids, 57
    piracetam, 57
    tramadol, 57
    valproic acid, 57
  mechanism of action, 52
  side effects, 53
Wellbutrin XL, see bupropion
Wymox (*see* amoxicillin)

X

Xanax (*see* alprazolam)
Xanthine oxidase site of action, 513
Xeluda, see capecitabine
Xenical, see orlistat
Xerostomia
   medications
      cevimeline, 123–125
      pilocarpine, 123, 125
      sorbitol, 123, 126
Xifaxan (*see* rifaximin)
Xopenex (*see* levalbuterol)
Xylocaine (*see* lidocaine)

Y

Yasmin 28 ethinyl estradiol +
   drospirenone.

Z

Zafirlukast, 411, 426
   drug interactions, 429–430
   mechanism of action, 428–429
   molecular structure of, 429
   relation with CYP enzymes, 430
   side effects, 429
Zalcitabine, 497, 510–511, 535
Zaleplon, 413, 578
   drug interactions, 414
   mechanism of action, 413–414
   molecular structure of, 413
   side effects, 414
Zanaflex (*see* tizanidine)
ZDV (*see* zidovudine)
Zebeta (*see* bisoprolol)
Zelnorm (*see* tegaserod)
Zestril (*see* lisinopril)
Zetia (*see* ezetimibe)

Zidovudine, 442–443, 446, 478
   drug interaction with
      acetaminophen, 517
      atovaquone, 518
      azathioprine, 518
      methadone, 518
      probenecid, 518
      stavudine, 518
   mechanism of action, 510
   molecular structure of, 509
   side effects, 510
Zileuton, 426
   drug interactions, 429–430
   mechanism of action, 429
   molecular structure of, 429
   relation with CYP enzymes, 430
   side effects, 429
Zithromax (*see* azithromycin)
Zofran (*see* ondansetron)
Zoladex (*see* goserelin)
Zolmitriptan, 396
   drug interactions, 404
   mechanism of action, 403–404
   molecular structure of, 404
   side effects, 404
Zolof (*see* sertraline)
Zolpidem, 413, 578
   drug interactions, 414
   mechanism of action, 413–414
   molecular structure of, 414
   side effects, 414
Zomig (*see* zolmitriptan)
Zopiclone, 578
Zyflo, see zileuton
Zyloprim, see allopurinol
Zyprexa, see olanzapine
Zyrtec, see cetirizine